D0900414

LAW
&
MENTAL
HEALTH
PROFESSIONALS

PENNSYLVANIA

Law & Mental Health Professionals Series

Bruce D. Sales and Michael Owen Miller, Series Editors

ARIZONA: Miller and Sales
CALIFORNIA: Caudill and Pope
FLORIDA: Petrila and Otto
GEORGIA: Remar and Hubert
MASSACHUSETTS, 2ND ED.: Brant
MINNESOTA: Janus, Mickelsen, and Sanders
NEVADA: Johns and Dillehay
NEW JERSEY, 2ND ED.: Wulach
NEW YORK: Wulach
PENNSYLVANIA: Bersoff, Field, Anderer, and Zaplac
TEXAS, 2ND ED.: Shuman
WASHINGTON: Benjamin, Rosenwald, Overcast, and Feldman
WISCONSIN: Kaplan and Miller
WYOMING: Blau

LAW & MENTAL HEALTH PROFESSIONALS

PENNSYLVANIA

Donald N. Bersoff
Robert I. Field
Stephen J. Anderer
Trudi Zaplac

American Psychological Association
Washington, DC

First Printing October 1998
Second Printing March 2002

Published by
American Psychological Association
750 First Street, NE
Washington, DC 20002

Copies may be ordered from
APA Order Department
P.O. Box 92984
Washington, DC 20090-2984

Typeset in Palatino by GGS Information Services, York, PA
Cover Designer: Rubin Krassner, Silver Spring, MD
Printer: Edwards Brothers, Inc., Ann Arbor, MI
Project Manager: Debbie K. Hardin, Reston, VA

Library of Congress Cataloging-in-Publication Data
Law and mental health professionals. Pennsylvania / by Donald
    Bersoff . . . [et al.].
        p.   cm.
    Includes bibliographic references and index.
    ISBN 1-55798-555-3
    1. Mental health personnel—Legal status, laws, etc.—
Pennsylvania.   2. Mental health laws—Pennsylvania.   I. Bersoff,
Donald N.
KFP326.P73L39   1999
344.748'044—dc21   98-25722
                                                               CIP

Printed in the United States of America

Contents

Editors' Preface

The Need to Know the Law

For years, providers of mental health services (hereinafter mental health professionals or MHPs) have been directly affected by the law. At one end of the continuum, their practice has been controlled by laws covering such matters as licensure and certification, third-party reimbursement, and professional incorporation. At the other end, they have been courted by the legal system to aid in its administration, providing such services as evaluating the mental status of litigants, providing expert testimony in court, and engaging in therapy with court-referred juveniles and adults. Even when not directly affected, MHPs find themselves indirectly affected by the law because their clients sometimes become enmeshed in legal entanglements that involve mental status issues (e.g., divorce proceedings or termination of parental rights hearings).

Despite this pervasive influence, most professionals do not know about, much less understand, most of the laws that affect their practice, the services they render, and the clients they serve. This state of affairs is particularly troubling for several reasons. First, not knowing about the laws that affect one's practice typically results in the MHPs not gaining the benefits that the law may provide. Consider the law relating to the incorporation of professionals. It confers significant benefit, but only if it is known about and applied. The fact that it has been enacted by the state legislature does not help the MHP, any more than an MHP will be of help to a distressed person who refuses to contact the MHP.

Second, not knowing about the laws that affect the services they render may result in incompetent performance of, and liability for, the MHP either through the civil law (e.g., malpractice law) or through criminal sanctions. A brief example may help underscore this point. When an MHP is asked to evaluate a party to a lawsuit and testify in court, the court (the law's term for the judge) is asking the professional to assess and testify about whether that litigant meets some legal standard. The court is often not concerned with the defendant's mental health per se, although this may be relevant to the MHP's evaluation of the person. Rather, the court wants to know whether the person meets the legal standard as it is set down by the law. Not knowing the legal standard means that the MHP is most likely evaluating the person for the wrong goal and providing the court with irrelevant information, at least from the court's point of view. Regretfully, there are too many cases in which this has occurred.

Third, not knowing the law that affects the clients that MHPs serve may significantly diminish their capability for handling their clients' distress. For example, a client who is undergoing a divorce and a child custody dispute may have distorted beliefs about what may happen during the legal proceedings. A basic understanding of the controlling law in this area will allow the therapist to be more sensitive in rendering therapy.

The Problem in Accessing Legal Information

Given the need for this information, why have MHPs not systematically sought it out? Part of the reason lies in the concern over their ability to understand legal doctrines. Indeed, this is a legitimate worry, especially if they had to read original legal materials that were not collected, organized, and described with an MHP audience in mind. This is of particular concern because laws are written in terms and phrases of "art" that do not always share the common law definition or usage, whereas some terms and phrases are left ambiguous and undefined or are used differently for different legal topics. Another part of the reason is that the law affecting MHPs and their clients is not readily available—even to lawyers. There are no compendiums that identify the topics that these laws cover or present an analysis of each topic for easy reference.

To compound the difficulty, the law does not treat the different mental health professional disciplines uniformly or always specify the particular disciplines as being covered by it. Nor does the law emanate from a single legal forum. Each state enacts its own rules and regulations, often resulting in wide variations in the way a topic is handled across the United States. Multiply this confusion by the one hundred or so topics that relate to mental health practice. In addition, the law within a state does not come from one legal source. Rather, there are five primary ones: the state constitution; state legislative enactments (statutes); state agency administrative rules and regulations; rules of court promulgated by the state supreme court; and state and federal court cases that apply, interpret, and construe this existing state law. To know about one of these sources without knowing how its pronouncements on a given topic have been modified by these other sources may result in one's making erroneous conclusions about the operation of the law. Finally, mental health practice also comes under the purview of federal law (constitutional and statutory law, administrative rules and regulations, and case law).

Federal law authorizes direct payments to MHPs for their services to some clients, sets standards for delivery of services in federal facilities (e.g., Veterans Administration hospitals), and articulates the law that guides cases that are tried in federal courts under federal law.

Purposes of This Series

What is needed, therefore, is a book for each state, the District of Columbia, and the federal jurisdictions that comprehensively and accurately reviews and integrates all of the law that affects MHPs in that jurisdiction (hereinafter state). To ensure currency, regular supplements to these books will also need to be drafted. These materials should be written so that they are completely understandable to MHPs, as well as to lawyers. To accomplish these goals, the editors have tried to identify every legal topic that affects mental health practice, making each one the subject of a chapter. Each chapter, in turn, describes the legal standards that the MHP will be operating under and the relevant legal process that the MHP will be operating within. If a state does not have relevant law on an issue, then a brief explanation of how this law works in other states will be presented while noting the lack of regulation in this area within the state under consideration.

This type of coverage facilitates other purposes of the series. Although each chapter is written in order to state exactly what is the present state of the law and not argue for or against any particular approach, it is hoped that the comprehensiveness of the coverage will encourage MHPs to question the desirability of their states' approach to each topic. Such information and concern should provide the impetus for initiating legislation and litigation on the part of state mental health associations to ensure that the law reflects the scientific knowledge and professional values to the greatest extent possible.

In some measure, states will initially be hampered in this proactivity because they will not know what legal alternatives are available and how desirable each alternative actually is. When a significant number of books in this series is available, however, it will allow for nationally oriented policy studies to identify the variety of legal approaches that are currently in use and to assess the validity of the behavioral assumptions underlying each variant and, ultimately, lead to a conclusion as to the relative desirability of alternate approaches.[1] Thus, two other purposes of this

---

1. Sales, B. D. (1983). The legal regulation of psychology: Professional and scientific interactions. In C. J. Scheirer & B. L. Hammonds (Eds.), *The master lecture series: Vol. 2. Psychology and law* (pp. 5–36). Washington, DC: American Psychological Association.

book are to foster comprehensive analyses of the laws affecting MHPs across all states and of the validity of the behavioral assumptions underlying these laws, and to promote political, legislative, and legal action to change laws that are inappropriate and impede the effective delivery of services. Legal change may be required because of gaps in legal regulation, overregulation, and regulation based on invalid behavioral and social assumptions. We hope that this process will increase the rationality of future laws in this area and improve the effectiveness and quality of mental health service delivery nationally.

There are three remaining purposes for this series. First, although it will not replace the need for legal counsel, this series will make the MHP an intelligent consumer of legal services. This ability is gaining importance in an era of increasing professionalization and litigiousness. Second, it will ensure that MHPs are aware of the law's mandates when providing expert services (e.g., evaluation and testimony) within the legal system. Although chapters will not address how to assess clinically for the legal standard, provider competency will increase because providers now will be sure of the goals of their service (e.g., the legal standard that they are to assess for) as well as their roles and responsibilities within the legal system as to the particular topic in issue. Third and finally, each book will make clear that the legal standards that MHPs are asked to assess for by the law have typically not been translated into behavioral correlates. Nor are there discussions of tests, scales, and procedures for MHPs to use in assessing for the behavioral correlates of the legal standards in most cases. This series will provide the impetus for such research and writing.

Content and Organization of Volumes

Each book in this series is organized into eight sections. Section 1 addresses the legal credentialing of MHPs. Section 2 deals with the different business forms for conducting one's practice, insurance reimbursement, and tax deductions that clients may receive for using mental health services. With the business matters covered, the book then turns to the law directly affecting service delivery. Section 3 covers the law that affects the maintenance and privacy of professional information and discusses the law that limits service delivery and sets liability for unethical and illegal behavior as a service provider. Sections 4 through 8 consider each area of law that may require the services of MHPs: adults, minors, and families; other civil matters; topics that apply similarly in both civil and criminal cases; criminal matters; and voluntary and involuntary receipt of state services by the clients of mental health services.

Collectively, the chapters in these sections represent all topics pertaining to the law as it affects MHPs in their practices. Two caveats are in order, however. First, the law changes slowly over time. Thus, a supplement service will update all chapters on a regular basis. Second, as MHPs become more involved in the legal system, new opportunities for involvement are likely to arise. To be responsive to these developments, the supplements will also contain additional chapters reflecting these new roles and responsibilities.

Some final points about the content of this book are in order. The exact terms that the law chooses are used in the book even if they are a poor choice from an MHP's point of view. Where terms are defined by the law, that information is presented. The reader will often be frustrated, however, because, as has already been noted, the law does not always define terms or provide detailed guidance. This does not mean that legal words and phrases can be taken lightly. The law sets the rules by which MHPs and their clients must operate; thus, the chapters must be read carefully. This should not be too arduous a task because chapters are relatively short. On the other hand, such brevity will leave some readers frustrated because chapters may appear not to go far enough in answering their questions. Note that all of the law is covered. If there is no law, however, there is no coverage. If a question is not answered in the text, it is because Pennsylvania law has not addressed the issue. Relatedly, if an obligation or benefit is created by a professional regulation (i.e., a rule of a professional organization) but is not directly recognized by the law, it is not covered. Thus, for example, professional credentials are not addressed in these volumes.

Finally, we want to point out that, in some instances, the pronoun "he" is used generically to refer to both genders. Most notably, the pronoun is used when quoting directly from the law. Legal language is generally consistent in its preference for using the masculine form of the pronoun; it is not always feasible to attempt a rewording.

Bruce D. Sales
Michael Owen Miller
Series Editors

Authors' Preface

This book is principally a treatment of state law applicable to mental health professionals (MHPs). A comprehensive treatment of federal law, which is also relevant to the actions of MHPs, is beyond the scope of this work as it would expand it by volumes or require a more limited treatment of the subject. A separate volume dedicated to federal law is planned for this series. The sources of state law treated in this work include the state constitutions, state statutes, state administrative rules, state judicial decisions, and state judicial rules.

The Pennsylvania Constitution establishes the framework for state government and describes various individual rights that occupy a high degree of importance in the commonwealth. Citations to the Pennsylvania Constitution appear in the following form: PA. CONST. art. I, § 1. This reference indicates that the citation is to the first section of the first article in the Pennsylvania Constitution.

Citations to state statutes, which result from legislation passed by the Pennsylvania General Assembly made up of the Senate and House of Representatives, appear in the following two forms: PA. STAT. ANN. tit. 50, § 7401 and 18 PA. CONS. STAT. ANN. § 315. These particular citations are references to the green-bound volumes of statutes called *Purdon's Pennsylvania Statutes Annotated* and *Purdon's Pennsylvania Consolidated Statutes Annotated*, respectively, published by West. The laws are first described by title and then enumerated by section. In addition, the Commonwealth of Pennsylvania Legislative Resource Bureau issues a series of blue-bound volumes of statutes, titled *Pennsylvania Consolidated Statutes*.

Purdon's compilation of statutes and the Pennsylvania Constitution contain additional useful material. The compilers attempt to include a citation and a one-sentence summary of any reported cases that have discussed the statute or constitutional provision in question. A researcher may use these case annotations to begin research on how the statute or constitutional provision has been interpreted by the courts. The compilations also contain references to prior statutes that have been repealed. A review of these repealed statutes may be necessary to understand an earlier judicial opinion interpreting them or to resolve an ambiguity in the intent of the legislature in changing the statute.

State administrative rules are created by the state agencies operating under the authority delegated to them by the legislature to carry out specific agency functions. For example, the legislation creating the State Board of Psychology does not list all types of professional misconduct, but rather gives the Board the authority to make administrative rules delineating specific types of misconduct that can result in the suspension or revocation of a license. These rules do not appear in the blue or green volumes of statutes but instead are kept in a three-ring notebook series titled *Pennsylvania Code,* published by Fry Communications, Inc. References to the administrative code appear in the following form: 49 PA. CODE § 41.41. The administrative rule referred to by this citation can be found in the volume containing Section 41.41 of Title 49.

State judicial decisions are the product of judge-made law. Reported decisions are typically those of appellate courts. They consist of decisions of the Pennsylvania Supreme Court, which is the highest state court, and of the lower appellate divisions. Citations to state supreme court decisions appear in the following format: Commonwealth v. Proctor, 585 A.2d 454 (Pa. 1991). A reference to an intermediate appellate court decision would appear in the following manner: Commonwealth v. Stewart, 448 A.2d 598 (Pa. Super. Ct. 1981). Pennsylvania also has the Commonwealth Court of Pennsylvania that has, with certain exceptions, original jurisdiction of all civil actions or proceedings by or against the commonwealth government.[1] A reference to a case decided by this court would appear in this manner: Konhaus v. Lutton, 344 A.2d 763 (Pa. Commw. Ct. 1975).

Pennsylvania appellate and supreme court decisions are reported in the *Atlantic Reporter,* one of a series of bound volumes designated by geographic region. The state supreme court decision cited previously is located in the second series of that compilation. The number 585 represents the volume in which the case appears, and 454 is the page of the volume on which the case begins. The parties to the case are the commonwealth and Stewart.

State judicial rules, as contrasted with judicial decisions, are the product of judges acting in a legislative rather than a judicial capacity. In this role, judges make rules of general application in the courts, not usually in the context of deciding cases. The Pennsylvania supreme court promulgates court rules that relate to civil procedure, criminal procedure, civil appellate procedure, and practice in the other courts. They are cited in the following form: PA. CT. Rule 3.1.

---

1. 42 PA. CONS. STAT. ANN. § 761.

Although the focus of this work is on state rather than federal law applicable to MHPs in Pennsylvania, occasional reference is of necessity made to federal decisions interpreting or limiting state law. The citations to these decisions are from the U.S. District Court (F. Supp.), the U.S. Court of Appeals (F., F.2d, or F.3d), and the U.S. Supreme Court (U.S.). As is the case with the reports of state decisions, the number preceding the reporter is the volume number and number following is the page. References to federal legislation appear in the form 26 U.S.C. § 213(a) (1997). This particular citation to the U.S. Code, the repository of federal legislation, is from title 26, section 213(a), current as of 1997. In addition, there are citations to treatises and law review articles. These references may provide a fuller background of an issue of interest to MHPs.

Finally, although some chapters were updated until the manuscript went to press, the reader should consider the entire volume current as of March 1997.

Donald N. Bersoff

Acknowledgments

This volume could not have been written without the aid of students in the Law and Psychology Program jointly sponsored by Villanova Law School and the Department of Clinical and Health Psychology of the Allegheny University of the Health Sciences. We are particularly indebted to Lawrence Dodds, Jennifer Evans, and the late Charles Fisher (who tragically died during his work on the book), all of whom did the research vital to the development and completion of this book.

Financial support was provided to the senior author by former dean Steven Frankino of Villanova Law School in the form of summer research grants. We are also indebted to the law school's library staff for their help in locating hard-to-find materials, and to our secretaries Grayce Smith and Robin Lewis. Our work was much improved by the critiques provided by Sam Knapp, EdD, of the Pennsylvania Psychological Association, and Alex Siegel, JD, PhD, a lawyer and psychologist in private practice in Philadelphia.

This book is dedicated to the memory of the senior author's father, Irving Bersoff, who would have been proud of this work.

Legal Credentialing

1.1

Licensure and Regulation of Mental Health Professionals

Pennsylvania law provides for the general licensing procedures and the regulation of professionals. The licensing and regulation of all professionals, including MHPs, is supervised by individual licensing boards, which are administered by the Bureau of Professional and Occupational Affairs in the Department of State (hereinafter Bureau).[1] Unlike some other states, there is no general licensing law in Pennsylvania. Specific licensing laws for each mental health profession and the regulations established by the corresponding boards are covered in the remainder of this section of the book.

---

1. 63 Pa. Cons. Stat. § 2201.

Licensure and Regulation of Psychiatrists

The licensure and regulation of psychiatrists is governed by statutory law that establishes a State Board of Medicine and a State Board of Osteopathic Medicine, delineates qualifications and procedures for the licensure of physicians, defines the practice of medicine, regulates the conduct of physicians, establishes exceptions to licensure, and recommends sanctions for violations of the statute. (Physicians are also regulated by the general licensing law that governs all boards and professions; see chapter 1.1.) Although psychiatrists in Pennsylvania must be licensed as physicians there are no specialized licensing provisions for the practice of psychiatry; the law is a generic one that regulates the practice of medicine without regard to specialty. Specialized certification is obtained through the National Board of Psychiatry and Neurology.

(A) State Boards of Medicine and Osteopathic Medicine

The commonwealth has two regulatory boards that govern the licensure and regulation of psychiatrists and all other physicians. The State Board of Medicine, established by the Medical Practice Act of 1985, regulates physicians with MD degrees.[1] The State Board of Osteopathic Medicine, established by the Osteopathic Medical Practice Act, regulates physicians with DO degrees.[2]

---

1. PA. STAT. ANN. tit. 63, §§ 422.1–.45; 49 PA. CODE §§ 16.1–.97, 17.1–.8.
2. PA. STAT. ANN. tit. 63, §§ 271.1–.18; 49 PA. CODE §§ 25.1–.291.

Each Board consists of the Commissioner of Professional and Occupational Affairs, the Secretary of Health, and a specified number of physicians, other medical professionals, and persons who are not involved with the medical profession, representing the public at large. The State Board of Medicine includes six physicians who have held unrestricted licenses for at least 5 years immediately preceding appointment, one nurse midwife or physician assistant or certified registered nurse practitioner, and two persons who are not members of the medical profession.[3] The State Board of Osteopathic Medicine includes five doctors of osteopathy who have been licensed and practicing for at least 5 years and two persons who are not members of the medical profession.[4] The professional and public members of the Boards are appointed by the governor, with the advice and consent of the state Senate. All members serve 4-year terms.[5]

(B) License

The legislature and the Boards of Medicine and Osteopathic Medicine have established general and specific requirements for licensure. The legislature's general requirements for physician licensure are that an applicant must

1. be of good moral character,
2. not be addicted to drugs or alcohol, and
3. have graduated from a medical school or an osteopathic medical college.[6]

An applicant who has been convicted of a felony under The Controlled Substance, Drug, Device and Cosmetic Act is not eligible for licensure unless 10 years have passed since the conviction and the applicant can demonstrate through personal rehabilitation that the applicant will not present substantial risk to the health and safety of patients or the public, or of further criminal violations.[7]

In addition, the State Board of Medicine and Board of Osteopathic Medicine require applicants to

---

3. Pa. Stat. Ann. tit. 63, § 422.3.
4. Pa. Stat. Ann. tit. 63, § 271.2(a).
5. Pa. Stat. Ann. tit. 63, §§ 271.2(a), 422.3.
6. Pa. Stat. Ann. tit. 63, §§ 271.6, 422.22.
7. Pa. Stat. Ann. tit. 63, §§ 271.6, 422.22.

1. be of legal age,
2. pass a licensing examination, and
3. complete 2 to 3 years of graduate medical training.[8]

Whereas the State Board of Medicine makes accommodations for graduates of unaccredited medical colleges, the State Board of Osteopathic Medicine requires applicants to have graduated from Board-approved osteopathic medical colleges.[9]

Both Boards may also grant licenses to applicants who do not satisfy all licensure requirements, provided the applicant's education and experience are endorsed by the Board as equivalent to the standard requirements.[10] Once licensed, physicians must renew their licenses every 2 years.[11] Doctors of Medicine and Doctors of Osteopathy must complete specified continuing education requirements during each 2-year period to qualify for license renewal.[12] All physicians must carry adequate medical malpractice insurance to be licensed and to receive license renewal.[13]

Reciprocity
The State Boards of Medicine and Osteopathic Medicine have discretionary authority to issue a reciprocal license to a physician who is licensed in another state.[14]

Restricted Licenses
Both State Boards grant limited licenses that allow for training and consultation but not full-time private practice. Graduates of medical school or osteopathic programs are granted 1-year limited licenses that permit them to practice only within their assigned teaching hospitals.[15] Medical school graduates may also be granted a limited license permitting practice outside of their assigned teaching hospitals.[16]

Physicians holding unrestricted licenses in other states may be granted limited licenses to teach and to practice in Pennsylvania. Fully licensed physicians in adjoining states who practice near the boundary of the commonwealth may be granted a limited license that permits them to treat patients who reside in

---

8. 49 PA. CODE § 17.1; 49 PA. CODE. § 25.241.
9. 49 PA. CODE §§ 17.1, 25.241.
10. 49 PA. CODE §§ 17.2, 25.242.
11. 49 PA. CODE §§ 16.15, 25.271.
12. 49 PA. CODE § 25.271.
13. 49 PA. CODE §§ 16.32, 25.281.
14. PA. STAT. ANN. tit. 63, §§ 271.8(c), 422.27.
15. 49 PA. CODE §§ 17.5, 25.244.
16. 49 PA. CODE § 17.7.

Pennsylvania.[17] Short-term or temporary licenses may be granted to any physician who holds an unrestricted license in any other state.[18] Furthermore, an MD who holds an unrestricted license in another state may be granted a limited institutional license that permits teaching and medical practice within one specific institution.[19] Any physician's license may be restricted for disciplinary reasons.[20]

Medical Students
Medical and osteopathy students, as "clinical clerks," may make notes on a patient's chart, conduct physical examinations, and perform medical procedures or laboratory tests under the supervision of attending and resident physicians at the hospital in which the service is performed.[21] Notes made on a patient's chart by a clinical clerk must be countersigned by an attending or resident physician, and clinical clerks may not prescribe or dispense drugs.[22]

(B)(1) Exceptions to Licensing

The licensing laws of Pennsylvania do not apply to physicians who are employed by the federal government or who are licensed in another state and acting as a consultant to a licensed physician in Pennsylvania.[23]

(C) Regulation

(C)(1) Disciplinary Actions

The State Boards of Medicine and Osteopathic Medicine may discipline physicians who violate Board regulations or state laws. When a complaint is received, the Boards act as investigatory bodies. If the investigation reveals that a physician has violated an applicable regulation or statute, the Boards may enforce criminal penalties by seeking fines and imprisonment in court.[24] If a physician is practicing without a license, the Board may petition the courts to issue an injunction against further practice.[25] In

---

17. 49 PA. CODE §§ 17.4, 25.243.
18. 49 PA. CODE §§ 17.6, 25.246.
19. 49 PA. CODE § 17.3.
20. PA. STAT. ANN. tit. 63, §§ 271.15, 422.42.
21. PA. STAT. ANN. tit. 63, §§ 271.2, 271.10, 422.11.
22. PA. STAT. ANN. tit. 63, § 422.11(d).
23. PA. STAT. ANN. tit. 63, §§ 271.10, 422.16, 422.18.
24. PA. STAT. ANN. tit. 63, §§ 271.11(a), 422.39(a).
25. PA. STAT. ANN. tit. 63, §§ 271.16(b), 422.38.

addition to criminal penalties, the Boards may impose civil penalties through fines and license restriction or revocation.[26]

Furthermore, the Boards may automatically suspend a physician's license if the physician is committed to an institution because of mental incompetency, convicted of a felony under the Pennsylvania Controlled Substance, Drug, Device and Cosmetic Act,[27] or convicted of an offense under the laws of another jurisdiction that would be an offense under the Controlled Substance, Drug, Device and Cosmetic Act if it were committed within the jurisdiction of Pennsylvania.[28]

Other grounds for disciplinary action include

1. failing to meet qualifications for licensure;
2. making misleading, deceptive, untrue, or fraudulent representations in the practice of medicine or osteopathy, or fraudulently procuring a license or admission to medical school;
3. being convicted of a felony or misdemeanor relating to a health profession or involving moral turpitude;
4. having a license or authorization to practice revoked or suspended in another state;
5. being unable to practice the profession with reasonable skill or safety by reason of illness, addiction to drugs or alcohol, mental incompetence, or conviction of a felony related to controlled substances (see chapter 5.1);
6. violating a Board regulation;
7. knowingly maintaining a professional connection or association with any person who is in violation of either the Medical Practice Act or the Osteopathic Medical Practice Act or assisting another person in violating Board regulations;
8. being guilty of immoral, unprofessional, or unethical conduct even when actual injury to a patient cannot be established;
9. acting in such a manner as to present an immediate and clear danger to public health or safety;
10. acting outside the scope of a license or certificate; and
11. making a false or deceptive biennial registration with the Board.[29]

(C)(2) Disciplinary Boards

In this capacity as investigatory agents, the Boards have the power to issue subpoenas; to compel the production of books,

---

26. PA. STAT. ANN. tit. 63, §§ 271.11(c), 422.39(b).
27. PA. STAT. ANN. tit. 35, §§ 780-101–780-144 (West 1996 & Suppl. 1998).
28. PA. STAT. ANN. tit. 63, §§ 271.14(b), 422.40(b).
29. PA. STAT. ANN. tit. 63, §§ 271.15, 422.41.

records, documents, and papers; to call and cross-examine witnesses; and to administer oaths.[30]

Before instituting disciplinary action, the Boards provide the physician with notice of the allegations, a hearing, an adjudication, and a right of appeal.[31] If a physician poses an immediate and clear danger to public health and safety, however, the Boards may temporarily suspend the physician's license without a hearing.[32] To do so, the Boards must provide the physician with immediate notice of the suspension, as well as enumerations of the allegations that prompted the suspension.[33] A hearing must follow within 30 days of the suspension.[34] If the suspension is upheld, it may remain in effect for a maximum of 180 days, including the time that preceded the hearing.[35]

(C)(3) Penalties for Violations

Penalties for violations may include

1. denial of licensure;

2. public reprimand with or without probation;

3. revocation, suspension, limitation, or restriction of a license;

4. mandatory psychological counseling or medical treatment (see chapter 5.1);

5. mandatory refresher educational courses;

6. probation; and

7. monetary penalties.[36]

Impaired Physicians
Each Board administers a program for the identification, treatment, and rehabilitation of impaired physicians (see chapter 5.1). If an impaired physician is making satisfactory progress in treatment, the Board may defer and ultimately dismiss any corrective actions taken against the physician.[37] When any hospital, health care facility, peer, or colleague has substantial evidence that a physician has an active addictive disease and is not seeking treatment or is diverting controlled substances, or is mentally or physically incompetent to carry out the duties of the license, that facility or individual must report the physician's impairment to either the Board of Medicine or the Board of Osteopathic Medi-

---

30. PA. STAT. ANN. tit. 63, § 271.16(a); 49 PA. CODE § 16.53.
31. PA. STAT. ANN. tit. 63, §§ 271.15(d), 422.39(b).
32. PA. STAT. ANN. tit. 63, §§ 271.14(a), 422.40(a).
33. *Id.*
34. *Id.*
35. *Id.*
36. PA. STAT. ANN. tit. 63, §§ 271.15(c), 422.42.
37. PA. STAT. ANN. tit. 63, §§ 271.15(c), 422.4(b).

cine, whichever governs the impaired physician.[38] Failure to make a required report will subject the facility or individual to a fine, not to exceed $1000.[39] When a facility or individual makes a report in good faith, there can be no civil or criminal liability arising from that report.[40] If the facility or individual is providing treatment for the impaired physician, reporting is not required.[41]

---

38. PA. STAT. ANN. tit. 63, §§ 271.16c(f), 422.4(f).
39. Id.
40. Id.
41. Id.

Licensure and Regulation of Psychiatric Nurses

The licensure and regulation of psychiatric nurses is governed by the Professional Nursing Law,[1] which establishes a State Board for Nursing, defines the practice of nursing, establishes qualifications and procedures for the licensure of registered professional nurses and nurse practitioners, establishes exceptions to licensure, and regulates the conduct of licensed nurses. In addition, the Board promulgates rules and regulations to carry out the provisions of the law. Nurses are also regulated by the general licensing law that governs all boards and professions (see chapter 1.1). There is no separate licensure pertaining to the practice of psychiatric nursing: The law is a generic one that regulates the practice of nursing without regard to specialty. Certification in psychiatric and mental health nursing is obtained through the American Nurses Association.

(A) State Board of Nursing

The State Board of Nursing is the primary administrative agency that licenses and regulates nurses. The Board consists of the Commissioner of Professional and Occupational Affairs and ten members who are appointed by the governor and approved by the state Senate. Seven members of the Board are nurses who have been engaged in nursing for the 5 years immediately preceding appointment. Of the seven nurses, five must be registered nurses and two must be licensed practical nurses. At least three of the registered nurses must have master's degrees. The three re-

---

1. PA. STAT. ANN. tit. 63, §§ 211–226.

maining members are not nurses and serve as representatives of the public at large.[2] All members serve 6-year terms.[3]

(B) Licensure

Applicants are licensed as professional nurses if they have furnished evidence to the Board that they

1. are of good moral character,
2. have completed work equal to a standard high school course as evaluated by the Board,
3. have satisfactorily completed an approved program of professional nursing, and
4. have passed a written examination administered by the Board.[4]

The Board will not issue a nursing license to any applicant who has been convicted of a felony under the Pennsylvania Controlled Substance, Drug, Device and Cosmetic Act or any other drug-related felony.[5] An applicant who has been convicted of such an act may be licensed, however, if 10 years have passed since the conviction and the applicant can show through personal rehabilitation that he or she is not expected to create a substantial risk of harm to patients or the public or to commit further criminal violations.[6]

Licenses must be renewed every 2 years.[7] A nurse may elect to be placed on inactive status rather than to renew the license.[8] A nurse who is on inactive status may request active status at any time. However, after 5 years of inactive status, the nurse will be required to satisfy the Board's regulations for ensuring continued competence.[9]

(B)(1) Exceptions

Temporary Practice Permit
The licensure examination is offered only once a year. As a result, new nursing school graduates and transfer applicants who are licensed in other states may have to wait as long as 12 months

---

2. PA. STAT. ANN. tit. 63, § 212.1(a).
3. PA. STAT. ANN. tit. 63, § 212.1(b).
4. PA. STAT. ANN. tit. 63, § 216.
5. *Id.*
6. PA. STAT. ANN. tit. 63, § 216(1)–(2).
7. PA. STAT. ANN. tit. 63, § 221(a).
8. PA. STAT. ANN. tit. 63, § 221(b).
9. *Id.*

before taking the exam and becoming licensed. To permit new applicants to practice professional nursing during this time, the Board may issue a temporary practice permit.[10] A temporary practice permit is valid for 1 year. If an applicant fails to pass the licensing examination within 1 year, the temporary practice permit will expire.[11]

Nurses Employed by the Federal Government
Individuals who are employed as nurses by the federal government are not required to comply with the nursing licensure requirements.[12]

Providing Home Care for Friends, Relatives, or Employers
The Professional Nursing Law does not require licensure for the home care of friends, relatives, or employers, as long as care givers do not represent themselves as licensed nurses.[13] Churches and their adherents are not required to be licensed to care for the sick when no compensation or personal profit is received and when the care is given solely in connection with practice of the religion.[14]

(C) Regulation

(C)(1) Disciplinary Actions

The State Board of Nursing may discipline nurses who violate Board regulations or state laws. When a complaint is received, the Board acts as an investigatory body. If the investigation reveals that a nurse has violated an applicable regulation or statute, the Board may enforce criminal penalties by seeking in court the imposition of fines and imprisonment.[15] If a nurse is practicing without a license, the Board may petition a court to issue an injunction against further practice.[16] In addition to criminal penalties, the Board may impose civil penalties through fines and restriction or revocation of the license.[17]

Furthermore, the Board may automatically suspend a nurse's license if the nurse is committed to an institution because of mental incompetency, convicted of a felony under the Pennsylva-

---

10. Pa. Stat. Ann. tit. 63, § 214.1.
11. *Id.*
12. Pa. Stat. Ann. tit. 63, § 214(6).
13. Pa. Stat. Ann. tit. 63, § 214(1)–(2).
14. Pa. Stat. Ann. tit. 63, § 214(2).
15. Pa. Stat. Ann. tit. 63, § 223(a).
16. Pa. Stat. Ann. tit. 63, § 225.4.
17. Pa. Stat. Ann. tit. 63, § 223(b).

nia Controlled Substance, Drug, Device and Cosmetic Act,[18] or convicted of an offense under the laws of another jurisdiction that would be an offense under the Controlled Substance, Drug, Device and Cosmetic Act if it were committed within Pennsylvania's jurisdiction.[19]

The Board may take disciplinary action against a nurse for any of the following reasons:

1. repeated occasions of negligent or incompetent nursing;

2. mental or physical illness or dependence on drugs or alcohol that impairs the nurse's ability to exercise reasonable nursing skill (see chapter 5.1);

3. willful or repeated violations of the Professional Nursing Law or Board regulations;

4. fraud or deceit in the practice of nursing or in gaining admission to either the practice of nursing or nursing school;

5. conviction of a crime of moral turpitude;

6. suspension or revocation of license or other profession-related disciplinary action in another state;

7. presenting an immediate and clear danger to public health or safety; or

8. possession, use, acquisition, or distribution of a controlled substance for other than an acceptable medical purpose.[20]

(C)(2) Investigations by the Board

When conducting an investigation, the Board has the power to issue subpoenas, to compel the production of books, records, documents, and papers, to call and cross-examine witnesses, and to administer oaths.[21] Before instituting disciplinary action, the Board must provide the nurse with notice of the allegations, a hearing, an adjudication, and a right of appeal.[22] If a nurse poses an immediate and clear danger to public health and safety, the Board may temporarily suspend the nurse's license without a hearing.[23] However, the Board must provide the nurse with immediate notice of the suspension as well as of the allegations that prompted the suspension.[24] A hearing must follow within 30 days of the suspension.[25] If the suspension is upheld, it may

---

18. PA. STAT. ANN. tit. 35, §§ 780-101–780-144.
19. PA. STAT. ANN. tit. 63, § 225.1(b).
20. PA. STAT. ANN. tit. 63, § 224(a).
21. PA. STAT. ANN. tit. 63, § 225.5(a).
22. PA. STAT. ANN. tit. 63, § 225.
23. PA. STAT. ANN. tit. 63, § 225.1(a).
24. *Id.*
25. *Id.*

remain in effect for a maximum of 180 days, including the time that preceded the hearing.[26]

(C)(3) Penalties for Violations

Penalties for violations may include

1. denial of application for a license;
2. public reprimand;
3. revocation, suspension, limitation, or restriction of the license;
4. required treatment with a physician or psychologist (see chapter 5.1); and
5. placement on probation.[27]

A nurse who violates the Professional Nursing Law or Board regulations may also face criminal prosecution and civil penalties.[28] If a nurse is practicing without a license, the Board may petition the court to issue an injunction against further practice without a license.[29]

Impaired Nurses

The Board administers a program for the identification, treatment, and rehabilitation of impaired nurses (see chapter 5.1). If an impaired nurse is making satisfactory progress in treatment, the Board may defer and ultimately dismiss any corrective actions taken.[30] When a hospital, health care facility, peer, or colleague has substantial evidence that a nurse has an active addictive disease and is not seeking treatment or is diverting controlled substances, or is mentally or physically incompetent to carry out the duties of the license, that facility or individual must report the nurse's impairment to the Board of Nursing.[31] Failure to make a required report will subject the facility or individual to a fine, not to exceed $1000.[32] When a facility or individual makes a report in good faith, there can be no civil or criminal liability arising from that report.[33] If the facility or individual is providing treatment for the impaired nurse, reporting is not required.[34]

---

26. *Id.*
27. Pa. Stat. Ann. tit. 63, § 224(b).
28. Pa. Stat. Ann. tit. 63, § 223(b).
29. Pa. Stat. Ann. tit. 63, § 225.4.
30. Pa. Stat. Ann. tit. 63, § 224.1(b).
31. Pa. Stat. Ann. tit. 63, § 224.1(f).
32. *Id.*
33. Pa. Stat. Ann. tit. 63, § 224.1(e).
34. Pa. Stat. Ann. tit. 63, § 224.1(f).

1.4

Licensure and Regulation of Psychologists

The licensure and regulation of psychologists is governed by the Professional Psychologists Practice Act,[1] which establishes a State Board of Psychology, defines the practice of psychology, establishes qualifications and procedures for the licensure of psychologists, establishes exceptions to licensure, regulates the conduct of licensed psychologists, and provides for administrative hearings. In addition, the Board promulgates rules and regulations to carry out the provisions of the statute. Psychologists are also regulated by the general licensing law that governs all boards and professions (see chapter 1.1).

(A) State Board of Psychology

The State Board of Psychology is responsible for licensing and regulating psychologists. The Board consists of the Commissioner of Professional and Occupational Affairs as well as eight members who are appointed by the governor and approved by the state Senate.[2] Of the eight appointees, six must be currently licensed to practice psychology, and the other two must be nonpsychologists who represent the public at large. The six psychologists are to be broadly representative of the practice areas of psychology. All of the Board members must be citizens of the United States and Pennsylvania residents for at least 3 years.

---

1. PA. STAT. ANN. tit. 63, §§ 1201–1218.
2. PA. STAT. ANN. tit. 63, § 1203.1.

(B) Licensure

Individuals are eligible for licensure if they

1. are of acceptable moral character;
2. have received a doctoral degree from an approved school of psychology or a doctoral degree in a field related to psychology;
3. have 2 years of acceptable supervised experience, one of which must be postdoctoral;
4. have passed an examination adopted by the Board;[3] and
5. have paid all appropriate fees.[4]

An applicant who has been convicted of a felony under the Pennsylvania Controlled Substance, Drug, Device and Cosmetic Act[5] is not eligible for licensure unless at least 10 years have passed since the conviction and the applicant demonstrates that, because of personal rehabilitation, licensure will create neither a substantial risk of harm to public health and safety nor a substantial risk of further violations on the part of the applicant.[6]

All licenses are valid for 2 years, beginning on December 1 of each odd-numbered year.[7] Psychologists must complete a minimum of 30 hours of continuing professional education during every 2-year renewal period.[8]

A psychologist licensed for independent practice in another state or province of Canada may practice psychology on temporary assignment for no longer than 6 months if the psychologist

1. holds a current license to practice,
2. is in good standing with the issuing Board of Psychology,
3. provides written notice to the Pennsylvania Board of Psychology, and
4. receives in writing from the Board temporary permission to practice.[9]

The Board may grant one extension, not to exceed 6 months. Requests for extensions must be submitted in writing. If the temporary assignment in the commonwealth does not exceed 14

---

3. 49 PA. CODE § 41.41.
4. PA. STAT. ANN. tit. 63, § 1206.
5. PA. STAT. ANN. tit. 35, §§ 780-101–780-144.
6. PA. STAT. ANN. tit. 63, § 1206(a)(5).
7. 49 PA. CODE § 41.11(d).
8. 49 PA. CODE § 41.59.
9. PA. STAT. ANN. tit. 63, § 1203(7); 49 PA. CODE § 41.52.

days, a psychologist does not have to notify the Board of the temporary practice.

Licensure of Nondoctoral Applicants

A doctoral degree has not always been required for licensure.[10] Prior to 1988, the Board granted licenses to applicants who had completed master's degrees in psychology. After the requirements were changed and a doctoral degree became mandatory for licensure, the Board adopted a window of opportunity to permit licensure of certain applicants with master's who, as of September 1986, were either enrolled in or had completed a master's degree in psychology or behavioral science.[11] To benefit from the window, applicants had to complete both the educational and supervision requirements for licensure as well as the application for licensure by December 31, 1994.[12]

Reciprocity

The Board may waive the licensing examination requirement for persons who are licensed to practice psychology in another state if the Board finds the other state's licensure requirements are equivalent to the requirements in Pennsylvania.[13] The Board may waive the examination in cases that are exceptional by virtue of the applicant's international or national reputation for making an extraordinary contribution to the science or practice of psychology if the Board finds the applicant competent to practice.[14]

(B)(1) Exceptions to Licensing

The Professional Psychologists Practice Act does not require licensure of all persons who do work of a psychological nature. The following classes are exempt from the licensure requirements:

1. persons licensed to practice any of the healing arts in Pennsylvania;[15]

2. qualified members of other professions, including, but not limited to clergy, drug and alcohol abuse counselors, mental health counselors, social workers, marriage counselors, family counselors, crisis intervention counselors, pastoral counselors, rehabilitation counselors, psychoanalysts, and volunteers who provide crisis or emergency services;

---

10. *See* chapter 1.5.
11. 49 PA. CODE § 41.54.
12. 49 PA. CODE § 41.54(a).
13. 49 PA. CODE § 41.52(a).
14. 49 PA. CODE § 41.43.
15. The commonwealth has defined the healing arts as "the science and skill of diagnosis and treatment in any manner whatsoever of disease or any ailment of the human body." PA. STAT. ANN. tit. 63, § 422.2.

3. persons employed as psychologists by the federal, state, or county government;

4. persons certified and employed as school psychologists in a public or private school;

5. social psychologists meeting applicable qualifications;

6. a faculty or staff member of an accredited institution of higher education, hospital, or state-approved nonpublic school;

7. students in psychology pursuing an official course of graduate study at an approved educational institution, provided the students are designated by titles such as *psychology intern* or *psychology trainee;*

8. employees of businesses or industrial organizations who use principles of psychology for placement, evaluation, selection, promotion, or job adjustment of their own employees;

9. school psychologists certified by the Department of Education who perform in private practice acts that they are permitted to perform in the school system.[16]

(C) Regulation

(C)(1) Disciplinary Actions

The State Board of Psychology may discipline psychologists who violate Board regulations or state laws. When a complaint is received, the Board acts as an investigatory body. If the investigation reveals that a psychologist has violated an applicable regulation or statute, the Board may enforce criminal penalties by seeking the imposition of fines and imprisonment in court.[17] If a psychologist is practicing without a license, the Board may petition a court to issue an injunction against further practice.[18] In addition to criminal penalties, the Board may impose civil penalties through fines and restriction or revocation of the license.[19]

Furthermore, the Board may automatically suspend a psychologist's license if the psychologist is committed to an institution because of mental incompetency, convicted of a felony under the Pennsylvania Controlled Substance, Drug, Device and Cosmetic Act,[20] or convicted of an offense under the laws of another jurisdiction that would be an offense under the Controlled Sub-

---

16. Pa. Stat. Ann. tit. 63, § 1203.
17. Pa. Stat. Ann. tit. 63, § 1211(a).
18. Pa. Stat. Ann. tit. 63, § 1211(c).
19. Pa. Stat. Ann. tit. 63, § 1211(b).
20. Pa. Stat. Ann. tit. 35, §§ 780-101–780-144.

stance, Drug, Device and Cosmetic Act if it were committed within Pennsylvania's jurisdiction.[21]

Other grounds for disciplinary action include

1. failing to demonstrate the qualifications or standards for a license;
2. making misleading, deceptive, untrue, or fraudulent representations in the practice of psychology;
3. practicing fraud or deceit in obtaining a license to practice psychology;
4. displaying gross incompetence, negligence, or misconduct in carrying on the practice of psychology;
5. submitting a false or deceptive biennial registration to the Board;
6. being convicted of a felony or being convicted of a misdemeanor in the practice of psychology;
7. having a license to practice suspended, revoked, or refused or receiving any other disciplinary action by another state's licensing authority;
8. being unable to practice psychology with reasonable skill and safety by reason of illness, drunkenness, excessive use of drugs, narcotics, chemicals, or any other type of material, or as a result of any mental or physical condition (see chapter 5.1);
9. violating a board regulation;
10. knowingly aiding, assisting, procuring, or advising any unlicensed person to practice psychology;
11. committing immoral or unprofessional conduct;
12. soliciting any engagement to perform professional services by any direct, in-person, or uninvited solicitation through the use of coercion, duress, compulsion, intimidation, threats, overreaching, or harassing conduct;
13. failing to perform any statutory obligation placed on a licensed psychologist;
14. intentionally submitting to any third-party payor a claim for a service or treatment that was not actually provided to a client;
15. failing to maintain professional records in accordance with regulations prescribed by the Board.[22]

---

21. PA. STAT. ANN. tit. 63, § 1208(e).
22. PA. STAT. ANN. tit. 63, § 1208(a).

(C)(2) Investigations by the Board

When conducting an investigation, the Board has the power to issue subpoenas, to compel the production of books, records, documents, and papers, to call and cross-examine witnesses, and to administer oaths.[23] Before instituting disciplinary action, the Board must provide the psychologist with notice of the allegations, a hearing, an adjudication, and a right of appeal.[24] If a psychologist poses an immediate and clear danger to public health and safety, the Board may temporarily suspend the psychologist's license without a hearing.[25] However, the Board must provide the psychologist with immediate notice of the suspension and of the allegations that prompted it.[26] A hearing must follow within 30 days of the suspension.[27] If the suspension is upheld, it may remain in effect for a maximum of 180 days, including the time that preceded the hearing.[28]

(C)(3) Penalties for Violations

After the Board finds a violation has been made, it may

1. deny a licensure application;
2. administer a public reprimand;
3. revoke, suspend, limit, or otherwise restrict a license;
4. require a licensee to submit to the care, counseling, or treatment of a physician or psychologist designated by the Board (see chapter 5.1);
5. place a licensee on probation;
6. restore a suspended license while imposing any disciplinary or corrective measure.[29]

Impaired Psychologists
The Board administers a program for the identification, treatment, and rehabilitation of impaired psychologists (see chapter 5.1). If an impaired psychologist is making satisfactory progress in treatment, the Board may defer and ultimately dismiss any corrective actions taken against him or her.[30] When any hospital, health care facility, peer, or colleague has substantial evidence that a psychologist has an active addictive disease and is not seeking treatment or is diverting controlled substances, or is men-

---

23. Pa. Stat. Ann. tit. 63, § 1211.1.
24. Pa. Stat. Ann. tit. 63, § 1208(c).
25. Pa. Stat. Ann. tit. 63, § 1208(d).
26. *Id.*
27. *Id.*
28. *Id.*
29. Pa. Stat. Ann. tit. 63, § 1208(b).
30. Pa. Stat. Ann. tit. 63, § 1218(b).

tally or physically incompetent to carry out the duties of the license, that facility or individual must report the psychologist's impairment to the Board.[31] Failure to make a required report will subject the facility or individual to a fine, not to exceed $1000.[32] When a facility or individual makes a report in good faith, there can be no civil or criminal liability arising from that report.[33] If the facility or individual is providing treatment for the impaired psychologist, reporting is not required.[34]

---

31. PA. STAT. ANN. tit. 63, § 1218(f).
32. Id.
33. Id.
34. Id.

1.5

Subdoctoral and Unlicensed Psychologists

The status of subdoctoral-level psychologists is an important issue, because it pertains both to the law and to the practice of psychology. For example, in a very few states master's-level psychologists have the right to practice independently, whereas in the vast majority of states the laws recognize that these professionals can be a valuable aid to doctoral-level mental health professionals but cannot practice independently.

(A) Psychologists Exempted From Doctoral Degree

Prior to 1995, a person who had a master's degree in psychology or another behavioral science could become licensed as a psychologist in Pennsylvania (see chapter 1.4). In 1988, the Professional Psychologists Practice Act was revised, and licensure now requires a doctoral degree. The revised law, however, includes a grandparent clause intended to accommodate persons who had begun or finished their master's degrees in anticipation of licensure under the old law.[1] Persons who completed the application for licensure by December 31, 1995 (including all educational and supervision requirements), are eligible for licensure as psychologists.[2] After December 31, 1995, only applicants holding doctoral degrees can be licensed as psychologists.

---

1. 49 PA. CODE § 41.54.
2. 49 PA. CODE § 41.54(a).

(B) Rights and Responsibilities of Subdoctoral and Unlicensed Psychologists

A licensed psychologist may employ an unlicensed professional who has graduate training in psychology. In this type of arrangement, the unlicensed professional must perform all duties under the full direction, control, and supervision of the licensed psychologist.[3] The licensed psychologist must ensure that the professional has met the education requirements (15 graduate semester hours of psychology course work) and the licensed psychologist bears full professional responsibility for the welfare of every client of the employee.[4] Billing and public announcements of the fees for the unlicensed employees' services must indicate the supervised status of the employee.[5]

The supervisory responsibilities of the licensed psychologist include

1. ensuring that the employee possesses skills commensurate with the work assigned;

2. consulting with the employee for the purpose of planning service delivery, including acquiring sufficient knowledge of clients or patients;

3. maintaining a level of supervisory contact consistent with professional standards, including regular face-to-face consultation with the employee and acquainting the employee with the pertinent professional code of ethics (the licensed psychologist is accountable for ethical violations by the employee);

4. being available for emergency consultation and intervention;

5. maintaining an ongoing record of the employee's work, competence, and the outcome of all procedures;

6. ensuring that the employee signs all intraoffice documentation and countersigns all documentation the employee prepares for distribution outside the office;

7. ensuring that the employee's supervised status is made known to all clients and providing clients with specific information regarding the employee's qualifications and functions;

---

3. PA. STAT. ANN. tit. 63, § 1203(12).
4. 49 PA. CODE § 41.58(b).
5. 49 PA. CODE § 41.58(d).

8. informing clients that they may meet with the supervisor, at their own requests or at the request of the supervisor;

9. supervising no more than three full-time employees (or equivalent if some are part-time) at any one time.[6]

---

6. 49 PA. CODE § 41.58(c).

1.6

Licensure and Regulation of Social Workers

The licensure and regulation of social workers is governed by the Social Worker's Practice Act,[1] which establishes a State Board for Social Work, defines terms contained within the Act, and establishes qualifications and procedures for licensure. In addition, the Board is authorized to promulgate rules and regulations to carry out the provisions of the statute. Social workers are also regulated by the general licensing law that governs all boards and professions (see chapter 1.1).

(A) State Board of Social Work Examiners

The State Board of Social Work Examiners is the state agency responsible for licensing and regulating social workers. The Board includes the Commissioner of Professional and Occupational Affairs as well as six members who are appointed by the governor and approved by the state Senate.[2] All Board members must be citizens of the United States and residents of the commonwealth for at least 2 years. Of the six appointees, four must satisfy the educational requirements for licensure. The remaining two members are not social workers and represent the public at large. All members serve 4-year terms.

---

1. PA. STAT. ANN. tit. 63, §§ 1901–1922.
2. PA. STAT. ANN. tit. 63, § 1905(a)(b).

(B) Licensure

Individuals are eligible for licensure if they

1. are of good moral character,
2. have received either a master's or a doctoral degree from an accredited school of social work or social welfare,
3. have passed the licensure examination, and
4. have paid the application fee.[3]

Applicants who have received bachelor's degrees in social work from an accredited school of social work or social welfare are eligible for provisional licenses if they meet the requirements listed previously and

1. are currently enrolled in a master's degree program at an accredited school of social work or social welfare; and
2. have 3 years experience under the supervision of a social worker with a master's or doctoral degree.[4]

An applicant who has been convicted of a felony under the Pennsylvania Controlled Substance, Drug, Device and Cosmetic Act[5] is not eligible for licensure unless at least 10 years have passed since the conviction and the applicant demonstrates significant personal rehabilitation such that licensure will create neither a substantial risk of harm to public health and safety nor a substantial risk of further violations by the applicant.[6]

Licenses to practice social work must be renewed every 2 years. The Board may require continuing education as a condition of renewal.[7]

Reciprocity
The Board may grant a reciprocal license to a social worker who is licensed in another state. The licensing requirements of the other state must equal or exceed those of Pennsylvania and the licensing state must also offer reciprocity to social workers licensed by Pennsylvania.[8]

---

3. PA. STAT. ANN. tit. 63, § 1907(a).
4. *Id.*
5. PA. STAT. ANN. tit. 35, §§ 780-101–780-144.
6. PA. STAT. ANN. tit. 63, § 1907(a)(5).
7. PA. STAT. ANN. tit. 63, § 1918.
8. PA. STAT. ANN. tit. 63, § 1910.

(C) Regulation

(C)(1) Disciplinary Actions

The State Board of Social Work Examiners may discipline social workers who violate Board regulations or state laws. When a complaint is received, the Board acts as an investigatory body. If the investigation reveals that a social worker has violated an applicable regulation or statute, the Board may enforce criminal penalties by seeking the imposition of fines and imprisonment in court.[9] If a social worker is practicing without a license, the Board may petition the courts to issue an injunction against further practice.[10] In addition to criminal penalties, the Board may impose civil penalties through fines and restriction or revocation of the license.[11]

Furthermore, the Board may automatically suspend a social worker's license if the social worker is committed to an institution because of mental incompetency, convicted of a felony under the Pennsylvania Controlled Substance, Drug, Device and Cosmetic Act,[12] or convicted of an offense under the laws of another jurisdiction that would be an offense under the Controlled Substance, Drug, Device and Cosmetic Act if it were committed within Pennsylvania's jurisdiction.[13]

Other grounds for disciplinary action may include

1. being convicted of a felony or a crime of moral turpitude;

2. being found guilty of immoral or unprofessional conduct;

3. violating standards of professional practice or conduct;

4. presenting false credentials or documents or making a false statement in support of an application for a license;

5. submitting a false or deceptive biennial renewal to the Board;

6. having a license to practice social work suspended, revoked, or refused, or receiving any other disciplinary action by the social work licensing authority of any other state, territory, possession, or country;

7. violating a board regulation or an order of the Board previously entered in a disciplinary proceeding;

8. being unable to practice social work with reasonable skill and safety by reason of illness, drunkenness, excessive use of

---

9. PA. STAT. ANN. tit. 63, § 1917(a).
10. PA. STAT. ANN. tit. 63, § 1920.
11. PA. STAT. ANN. tit. 63. § 1917(b).
12. PA. STAT. ANN. tit. 35, §§ 780-101–780-144.
13. PA. STAT. ANN. tit. 63, § 1911(e).

drugs, narcotics, chemicals, or any other type of material or as a result of any mental or physical condition (see chapter 5.1).[14]

(C)(2) Investigations by the Board

In its investigatory role, the Board has the power to issue subpoenas; to compel the production of books, records, documents, and papers; to call and cross-examine witnesses; and to administer oaths.[15] Before instituting disciplinary action, the Board must provide the social worker with notice of the allegations, a hearing, an adjudication, and a right of appeal.[16]

However, if a social worker poses an immediate and clear danger to public health and safety, the Board may temporarily suspend the social worker's license, without a hearing.[17] The Board, however, must provide the social worker with immediate notice of the suspension as well as the allegations that prompted the suspension.[18] A hearing must follow within 30 days of the suspension.[19] If the suspension is upheld, it may remain in effect for a maximum of 180 days, including the time that preceded the hearing.[20]

(C)(3) Penalties for Violations

After the board determines that a violation has occurred, it may

1. deny the application for a license;
2. administer a public reprimand;
3. revoke, suspend, limit, or otherwise restrict a license;
4. require the social worker to undergo counseling or other treatment (see chapter 5.1); and
5. place the social worker on probationary status.[21]

Impaired Social Workers
The Board administers a program for the identification, treatment, and rehabilitation of impaired social workers (see chapter 5.1). If an impaired social worker is making satisfactory progress in treatment, the Board may defer and ultimately dismiss any corrective actions taken against the social worker.[22] When a hospital, health care facility, peer, or colleague has substantial evi-

---

14. PA. STAT. ANN. tit. 63, § 1911(a).
15. PA. STAT. ANN. tit. 63, § 1919.
16. PA. STAT. ANN. tit. 63, § 1911(c).
17. PA. STAT. ANN. tit. 63, § 1911(d).
18. *Id.*
19. *Id.*
20. *Id.*
21. PA. STAT. ANN. tit. 63, § 1911(b).
22. PA. STAT. ANN. tit. 63, § 1915(b).

dence that a social worker has an active addictive disease and is not seeking treatment or is diverting controlled substances, or is mentally or physically incompetent to carry out the duties of the license, that facility or individual must report the social worker's impairment to the Board.[23] Failure to make a required report will subject the facility or individual to a fine not to exceed $1000.[24] When a facility or individual makes a report in good faith, there can be no civil or criminal liability arising from that report.[25] If the facility or individual is providing treatment for the impaired social worker, no report is required.[26]

---

23. Pa. Stat. Ann. tit. 63, § 1915(f).
24. Id.
25. Id.
26. Id.

1.7

Certification and Regulation of School Psychologists

In Pennsylvania, school psychologists who are employed in primary and secondary educational settings are certified by the State Board of Education. The Public School Code of 1949[1] contains the laws that govern certification of school psychologists. The certification is entirely independent of the Board of Psychologist Examiners, with school psychologists being specifically exempted from the regular certification procedures.[2] Nevertheless, persons who have completed graduate work in school psychology may also be eligible for licensure as psychologists.[3]

(A) Certification

School psychologists are certified as educational specialists.[4] Applicants are eligible for certification if they

1. are of good moral character;
2. are neither mentally nor physically unable to perform their professional duties;
3. are at least 18 years old;
4. have graduated and received recommendation for certification from a Board-approved university program in school psychology,[5] or graduated and received recommendation for certifica-

---

1. PA. STAT. ANN. tit. 24, §§ 12-1201–12-1214.
2. *See* chapter 1.4.
3. *Id.*
4. PA. STAT. ANN. tit. 24, § 2070.1(4); 22 PA. CODE § 49.72(a)(5).
5. 22 PA. CODE § 49.71.

tion from a non-Board approved university program in school psychology (e.g., an out-of-state program) whose educational requirements are equivalent to those of Board-approved programs in school psychology;[6] and

5. have successfully completed the certification examination.[7]

Continuing professional education is required for maintenance of the certificate.[8]

Applicants who have been convicted of certain offenses within the 5 years immediately preceding application for certification will not be certified.[9] This disqualification provision does not apply to employees who are under 21 years of age, who are hired for 90 days or less, or who are part of a job development or training program.[10]

(A)(1) Reciprocity

The Superintendent of Public Instruction may endorse a certificate that was granted by another state if it finds that the requirements for certification in the issuing state are equivalent to the certification requirements of Pennsylvania.[11]

State Board of Education
The State Board of Education is responsible for setting and enforcing the requirements for certification of all school personnel.[12] The Board consists of 21 members who serve 6-year terms. All are appointed by the governor and approved by the state Senate. Ten are members of the Council of Basic Education, and ten are members of the Council of Higher Education. The remaining member, designated by the governor as chair of the board, serves on both councils.[13] Other than the chair, no more than two members of each council may be employed by a school system (excluding colleges and universities) or the Department of Education.[14] The Council of Higher Education includes three members who are actively employed by a college or university, one of whom must hold an administrative position and one of whom must hold a faculty position.[15] At least two members of each Council must

---

6. 22 Pa. Code § 49.65.
7. 22 Pa. Code §§ 49.12, 49.18.
8. 22 Pa. Code § 49.17.
9. Pa. Stat. Ann. tit. 24, § 1-111.
10. 24 Pa. Code § 1-111(f).
11. Pa. Stat. Ann. tit. 24, § 12-1206.
12. Pa. Stat. Ann. tit. 24, § 12-1201.
13. Pa. Stat. Ann. tit. 24, § 26-2602-B(a).
14. Pa. Stat. Ann. tit. 24, § 26-2602-B(f).
15. *Id.*

have previous experience with vocational–technical education or training.[16]

Professional Standards and Practices Commission
The Professional Standards and Practices Commission is an arm of the State Board of Education. The Commission makes recommendations to the Board on issues such as standards for teacher certification and teacher training programs in colleges and universities, and takes disciplinary action against teachers and other professional educators in the event of wrongdoing.[17] The Commission consists of 13 members who are appointed by the governor and approved by the state Senate. Members serve 3-year terms of office. Seven members are classroom teachers, including one educational specialist.[18] Three members are administrators, including one commissioned officer and one principal. One member is an administrator from a college or university, and two members, who represent the public at large, are not professional educators. All educator members must have been working as teachers or educational administrators for 5 of the 8 years immediately preceding appointment to the Commission. The chair of the Board of Education serves as an ex officio member without voting privileges.[19]

Disciplinary Actions
The Professional Standards and Practices Commission may discipline school psychologists who are found guilty (after a hearing) of immorality, incompetency, intemperance, habitual use of drugs or narcotics, cruelty or negligence, or who are convicted of a crime involving moral turpitude.[20] After a complaint is received, the Department of Education determines whether there is probable cause to believe the allegations are true.[21] If probable cause is established, the matter is given to the local school board for investigation and recommendations for discipline, if any.[22] After the local school board has completed its investigation, the Department then determines whether sufficient punishment has been imposed or if a hearing should be initiated.[23]

---

16. *Id.*
17. PA. STAT. ANN. tit. 24, § 2070.5.
18. An *educational specialist* is a person employed by a public school as a certified guidance counselor, nurse, home and school visitor, psychologist, dental hygienist, instructional media specialist, or nutrition specialist. PA. STAT. ANN. tit. 24, § 2070.1(4).
19. PA. STAT. ANN. tit. 24, § 2070.4.
20. PA. STAT. ANN. tit. 24, § 2070.5(11).
21. PA. STAT. ANN. tit. 24, § 2070.9(8).
22. PA. STAT. ANN. tit. 24, § 2070.11.
23. PA. STAT. ANN. tit. 24, § 2070.12.

If the Department decides to initiate a hearing, it must provide the school psychologist with notice of the allegations.[24] The school psychologist may request the hearing be held within 30 days of notification.[25] If the Department determines that immediate discipline is necessary to protect the health, safety, and welfare of school students or personnel, this process may be expedited.[26] The hearing is closed unless the school psychologist in the proceeding requests that it be open.[27] The decision of the hearing officer is final unless either the school psychologist or the Department of Education files an exception to the decision.[28] If the school psychologist prevails on appeal, the employment record will be expunged of all charges pertaining to the matter.[29]

Private Practice by Certified School Psychologists
Certified school psychologists may perform in private practice those acts that they are permitted to perform in public schools and private schools.[30] In addition to being certified, a person engaged in the private practice of school psychology must be employed in a school as a school psychologist in good standing.[31]

---

24. PA. STAT. ANN. tit. 24, § 2070.13(a).
25. *Id.*
26. PA. STAT. ANN. tit. 24, § 2070.13(b).
27. PA. STAT. ANN. tit. 24, § 2070.13(5).
28. PA. STAT. ANN. tit. 24, § 2070.14.
29. PA. STAT. ANN. tit. 24, § 2070.15.
30. PA. STAT. ANN. tit. 63, § 1203(10); 49 PA. CODE § 41.56.
31. PA. STAT. ANN. tit. 24, § 41.56.

1.8

Certification of School Counselors and School Social Workers

In Pennsylvania, school counselors and school social workers are certified by the State Board of Education. The Public School Code of 1949[1] contains the laws that govern certification of all nonteacher school professionals *(educational specialists)*.

The certification process for school counselors and school social workers is the same as for school psychologists (see chapter 1.7). School counselors, however, are not eligible for state licensure or practice outside the school setting.

---

1. 24 PA. CONS. STAT. §§ 12-1201–12-1231.

Licensure and Regulation of Marriage and Family Counselors

Pennsylvania does not provide for licensure of marriage and family therapists. Legislation is under development that would lead to licensure, based on guidelines developed by the American Association of Marriage and Family Therapists.[1]

---

1. American Association for Marriage and Family Therapy (AAMFT): Code of Professional Ethics (Claremont, CA: AAMFT).

1.10

Licensure of Other Types of Mental Health Professionals

In some states, MHPs other than psychiatrists, psychologists, social workers, and substance abuse counselors are eligible for licensure. However, Pennsylvania law does not provide for this type of licensure.

Substance abuse counselors may participate in a voluntary certification program administered by the Pennsylvania Chemical Abuse Certification Board located in Harrisburg, Pennsylvania.

1.11

Licensure and Regulation of Hypnotists

In some states, the law regulates hypnosis and the professional title *hypnotist* by prescribing education, experience, and skills. Pennsylvania, however, does not provide for the licensure or regulation of hypnotists, although private training and certification programs are available.

The use of hypnotically induced testimony in the courtroom is regulated separately (see chapter 6.8).

1.12

Licensure and Regulation of Polygraph Examiners

In some states, the law regulates polygraph examinations and the professional title *polygraph examiner* by prescribing education, experience, and skills. Pennsylvania, however, does not provide for the licensure or regulation of polygraph examiners. The use of polygraph evidence in court is strictly limited by case law (see chapter 6.3).

1.13

Regulation of Unlicensed Mental Health Professionals

Each professional board (e.g., the State Board of Psychology, the State Board of Medicine) has the authority to regulate the unlicensed practice of its profession. (See chapter 1.2 for psychiatry, 1.3 for nursing, 1.4 for psychology, and 1.6 for social work.)

1.14
Sunset of Credentialing Agencies

Some states have sunset laws, which are the means by which legislatures review and revise most facets of state government from entire departments to small commissions. Such laws work by automatically terminating the authority of an agency unless the legislature, after a mandatory review of the entity's past work, extends the termination date. However, Pennsylvania does not have such laws pertaining to MHPs.

1.15

Open Meeting Laws

In Pennsylvania, the Sunshine Act[1] requires state agencies to hold their meetings and hearings in public. The State Boards of Medicine, Osteopathic Medicine, Nursing, Psychology, and Social Work are all subject to the requirements of the Act.

The purpose of the Sunshine Act is to enhance the democratic process by ensuring citizens the right to have notice of and the opportunity to attend any agency meeting during which agency business is discussed or acted on.[2] Agencies must give 3 days public notice of the first meeting of the calendar or fiscal year and public notice of all scheduled meetings for the remainder of the year.[3] The public must also receive notice of any rescheduled or not previously scheduled meetings, unless they are emergency meetings.[4] The public is permitted to participate in agency meetings[5] and minutes must be recorded.[6] The results of a meeting held in violation of the Act may be invalidated by a court[7] and each participant fined $100.

The Act does permit agencies to meet secretly in "executive sessions" in certain instances.[8] For example, an agency may meet in executive session if it is engaging in quasi-judicial deliberations

---

1. Pa. Stat. Ann. tit. 65, §§ 271–286.
2. Pa. Stat. Ann. tit. 65, § 272.
3. Pa. Stat. Ann. tit. 65, § 279(a).
4. Id.
5. Pa. Stat. Ann. tit. 65, § 280.1(a)
6. Pa. Stat. Ann. tit. 65, § 276.
7. Pa. Stat. Ann. tit. 65, § 283.
8. 65 Pa. Cons. Stat. § 284.

or is investigating possible violations of law.[9] Also, any deliberations that if held in public would violate a lawful privilege or would lead to public disclosure of information made confidential by law are exempt from the requirements of the Act.[10]

---

9. 65 PA. CONS. STAT. § 277.
10. 65 PA. CONS. STAT. § 278(5).

Business Matters

2.1

Sole Proprietorships

An MHP who does not work for an employer as a salaried employee typically organizes his or her business into one of three forms: sole proprietorships (this chapter), professional corporations (PCs; see chapter 2.2), or partnerships (see chapter 2.3).

Structure of Sole Proprietorships
MHPs who practice alone and without any formal corporate structure operate as *sole proprietors*. Unlike professional corporations and partnerships, there is no state law directly regulating this type of business entity. Instead, general business law, including contract, agency, employment, tax, and state and local licensing laws govern sole proprietorships. The assets of the proprietorship are the assets of the owner; the liabilities and obligations of the proprietorship are the direct liabilities and obligations of the owner. The owner and all of his or her personal and other assets are subject to these proprietary liabilities. There is no limited liability as there is in some partnerships or in corporations.

2.2

Professional Corporations

A professional corporation (PC) is a second kind of business structure for MHPs. It offers many of the tax and practice benefits of regular incorporation. There are, however, certain rules of incorporation with which MHPs should be familiar.

(A) Benefits of Incorporation

MHPs accrue several benefits from incorporating their practices. First, certain tax deductions are available to professional corporations that are not available to MHPs through other business forms. For example, the purchase of health insurance, death benefits, and retirement plans are all tax-free benefits for the employees of a PC, and they are all tax deductible expenses for the PC itself. Second, incorporation generally limits liability for shareholders to the assets of the corporation, with protection for their personal assets. Third, the requirements that PCs have shareholder meetings, issue reports, and keep business records may lead members to become more sensitive to the business ramifications of practice.

(B) Incorporation and Operation Procedures

A professional corporation is formed by filing articles of incorporation with the Pennsylvania Department of State.[1] The heading of the articles must indicate that the corporation is a professional (rather than a general business) corporation.[2] The incorporators of the PC are generally the owners of the stock of the corporation. All shareholders must be professionals, licensed in Pennsylvania to provide the professional services offered by the PC.[3] There is no requirement that the corporate name contain the words *professional corporation, corporation, incorporated,* or the abbreviation for one of these.[4] Furthermore, the corporate name need not reflect the names of the incorporators.[5]

Although the general rule is that a professional corporation generally may be organized only for the purpose of providing the services of one profession, MHPs of differing disciplines may join together to form a PC that provides mental health services of more than one discipline.[6] For example, a psychologist and a social worker may join together to form a professional corporation.

Nevertheless, a PC may not engage in any business other than the business of providing the professional services for which it was incorporated.[7] The PC may employ support staff and other persons to perform some duties under the direct supervision and control of a licensed person,[8] but some professional services may only be provided by the professionally licensed officers, employees, or agents of the PC.[9]

(C) Liability and Accountability

When MHPs form a professional corporation, each shareholder remains personally and fully liable for his or her professional wrongdoing. The corporation, however, remains liable for negligent or wrongful acts or misconduct committed by any of the

---

1. 15 Pa. Cons. Stat. § 1309.
2. 15 Pa. Cons. Stat. § 2903.
3. 15 Pa. Cons. Stat. § 2923(a).
4. 15 Pa. Cons. Stat. § 2921.
5. *Id.*
6. 15 Pa. Cons. Stat. § 2903(d).
7. 15 Pa. Cons. Stat. Ann. § 2922.
8. 15 Pa. Cons. Stat. Ann. § 2924.
9. *Id.*

other shareholders;[10] its total liability is limited to the value of its assets.[11]

The PC is subject to the applicable rules and regulations of the licensing agency that regulates the profession.[12] If one of the shareholders becomes ineligible to practice or dies, the PC must acquire all of that shareholder's shares,[13] unless other arrangements have been made for their disposition. This process must be completed within 90 days of the shareholder becoming ineligible to practice or within 13 months of the shareholder's death.[14]

(D) Termination of the Professional Corporation

A PC may terminate its status as a PC but maintain status as a general business corporation by amending its articles of incorporation so they no longer indicate that the corporation is a professional corporation.[15] A PC may terminate its status as a corporation by filing a statement of termination with the Pennsylvania Department of State.[16]

(E) Limited Liability Companies and Limited Liability Partnerships

Limited Liability Companies
Limited Liability Companies (LLC) are entities authorized by statute to provide to owners the protection from personal liability afforded by corporate entities but with taxation solely at the level of the individual receiving proceeds, as in partnerships.[17] LLCs are subject to federal tax as partnerships if they have no more than two of the four essential attributes of corporations: (a) indefinite duration of existence, (b) centralized management, (c) transferability of interests, and (d) limitation of personal liability of owners. LLCs may form the legal structure for professional practices, including those of MHPs, in which case they are known as

---

10. 15 PA. CONS. STAT. ANN. § 2925.
11. 15 PA. CONS. STAT. ANN. § 2925(d).
12. 15 PA. CONS. STAT. ANN. § 2925(e).
13. 15 PA. CONS. STAT. ANN. § 2907(b).
14. *Id.*
15. 15 PA. CONS. STAT. ANN. § 2096.
16. 15 PA. CONS. STAT. ANN. § 1902(a).
17. 15 PA. CONS. STAT. ANN. §§ 8901–8908.

Restricted Professional Companies (RPC).[18] Although members of an RPC are protected from liability for actions of other members, they are still responsible for their own professional negligence. LLCs are taxed as corporations for state tax purposes, but RPCs are taxed as limited partnerships.

An LLC is formed by filing a Certificate of Organization with the Department of State. The operating structure is set forth in an Operating Agreement, which addresses such issues as management, restrictions on transfers of ownership interests, and withdrawal of members. RPCs must submit an annual registration statement to the Department of State along with a fee of $300 for each member.[19]

Limited Liability Partnerships
Limited Liability Partnerships (LLP) may conduct professional practices, including those of MHPs, as long as all partners are licensed and the entity registers as an LLP with the Department of State. General partners are shielded from liability for the professional actions of other partners. Owners remain responsible for their own professional negligence and that of others under their direct supervision and control. They also remain personally liable for debts and obligations of the LLP arising from any other cause. General partners who withdraw from LLPs may be able to limit their liability for debts and obligations of the LLPs, if they continue in operation, by filing a Statement of Withdrawal with the Department of State.

LLPs must maintain minimum amounts of liability insurance to retain their status, which are set at $100,000 per partner up to a maximum of $1 million. They must submit an annual registration statement to the Department of State along with a fee of $200 for each general partner residing in or organized in Pennsylvania.[20] LLPs are subject to taxation as partnerships at both the federal and state levels. Thus, profits are taxed solely at the level of the partner receiving proceeds.

Although use of LLCs and LLPs for professional practices has become increasingly common in other states, they are still seldomly used in Pennsylvania.

---

18. 15 PA. CONS. STAT. ANN. § 8995.
19. 15 PA. CONS. STAT. ANN. § 8998.
20. 15 PA. CONS. STAT. ANN. § 8221.

Partnerships

A partnership is an association of two or more persons who agree to carry on a business.[1] Each partner is a co-owner of the business. The partnership is a legal entity in whose name the business is conducted. Partnerships have the advantage of allowing partners to carry on a more complex business than one individual could manage. However, each partner is liable for the actions of the other partners. Thus, a partnership can create greater liability than an individual alone would face. Even if a group of professionals does not expressly agree to create a partnership, the law may determine that a partnership exists if the partners share control, profits, and losses of a business.[2] Therefore, MHPs should be familiar with the laws governing partnerships even if they are not express members of a partnership.

(A) Formation of a Partnership

In general, a partnership is formed when two or more persons agree to carry on a for-profit business as co-owners. The intent to share profits and losses is the most important factor in determining whether a partnership exists.[3] Partners typically enter into a formal partnership agreement, but this is not a prerequisite to the formation of a partnership. The terms of a partnership agreement may establish a method of dividing profits and losses. For example, if one partner contributed $100,000 to the start up of a busi-

---

1. 15 Pa. Cons. Stat. Ann. § 8311(a).
2. 15 Pa. Cons. Stat. Ann. § 8321.
3. 15 Pa. Cons. Stat. Ann. § 8312(4).

ness and another partner contributed $50,000, the partners may agree formally to allocate the profits and losses in a manner proportional to each individual partner's contribution. In the absence of a formal partnership agreement, the law requires the partners to share profits equally.[4]

(B) Rights and Duties Between Partners

A partnership involves more than merely sharing profits and losses of a business. Unless there is a formal agreement to the contrary, partners share equally in the management and conduct of partnership business.[5] Each partner has access to the partnership books at all times.[6] On any partner's demand, the other partners must render true and full information of all things affecting the partnership.[7] Finally, each partner is a fiduciary of the other partners. This means that no partner may retain any profits made from the business if they were derived without the consent of the other partners.[8]

Every partner is considered an agent of the partnership. That is, the actions of any one partner bind the entire partnership.[9] If one partner makes an admission concerning the partnership affairs, this can serve as evidence against the entire partnership.[10] Also, notice to one partner of any matter concerning the partnership business serves as notice to all of the partners.[11] Perhaps most important, the wrongful act of one partner renders the partnership liable to the same extent as the individual partner.[12] In other words, all the partners are held jointly and severally liable.[13] This means that each partner can be made to satisfy a judgment against any other partner and an individual partner may seek contributions from all other partners to satisfy a judgment entered against him or her as an individual. This type of liability is limited to actions taken as part of the partnership business.

---

4. 15 Pa. Cons. Stat. Ann. § 8331(1).
5. 15 Pa. Cons. Stat. Ann. § 8331(5).
6. 15 Pa. Cons. Stat. Ann. § 8332.
7. 15 Pa. Cons. Stat. Ann. § 8333.
8. 15 Pa. Cons. Stat. Ann. § 8334.
9. 15 Pa. Cons. Stat. Ann. § 8321(a).
10. 15 Pa. Cons. Stat. Ann. § 8323.
11. 15 Pa. Cons. Stat. Ann. § 8324.
12. 15 Pa. Cons. Stat. Ann. § 8325.
13. 15 Pa. Cons. Stat. Ann. § 8327(a).

There are certain limitations to the general rule that the acts of one partner are binding on the entire partnership. For example, one or more—but less than all—the partners cannot assign partnership property in trust for creditors, dispose of the goodwill of the business, commit any act that would make it impossible to carry on the business of the partnership, confess a judgment, submit a partnership claim or liability to arbitration, or accept a new partner into the partnership.[14]

(C) Dissolution of a Partnership

A partnership may be dissolved by

1. the terms of the partnership agreement;
2. the express will of any partner to dissolve when no definite term or particular undertaking is specified;
3. the expulsion of any partner according to the terms of the partnership agreement;
4. breach of the partnership agreement by any partner;
5. any event that makes it unlawful to continue to conduct the business of the partnership;
6. the death of any partner;
7. the bankruptcy of any partner or the partnership; or
8. a court decree when:[15]
   a. a partner is shown to be mentally incompetent;
   b. a partner is shown to be incapable of performing the acts required by the partnership agreement;
   c. a partner's conduct negatively affects carrying on of business;
   d. a partner willfully or persistently breaches the partnership agreement or conducts himself or herself in business matters in such a way that it is not reasonably practicable to continue to do business in partnership with him or her;
   e. the partnership business can only be conducted at a loss; or
   f. other circumstances render the dissolution of the partnership a fair resolution for the business.[16]

---

14. 15 Pa. Cons. Stat. Ann. §§ 8321(c), 8331(7).
15. 15 Pa. Cons. Stat. Ann. § 8354.
16. 15 Pa. Cons. Stat. Ann. § 8353.

The dissolution terminates the authority of all partners to conduct any partnership business other than that required to wind up the partnership's affairs.[17] The dissolution does not discharge the existing liabilities of any partner.[18]

---

17. 15 Pa. Cons. Stat. Ann. § 8355.
18. 15 Pa. Cons. Stat. Ann. § 8358(a).

2.4

Health Maintenance Organizations

A health maintenance organization (HMO) is an organization that provides health services to subscribers for a fixed prepaid fee.[1] HMOs in Pennsylvania are regulated jointly by the Department of Health and the Insurance Department.[2] HMO subscribers must first see a designated primary care physician for all covered services. These physicians are either employees of the HMO or have contracted with the HMO to see patients for an aggregate fixed sum or for a prearranged per capita fee, referred to as a *capitation payment.* The primary care physician determines whether or not specialty services, including those of MHPs, are appropriate, and HMO reimbursement for such services is provided only on a referral from a primary care physician. MHPs and other specialist health care providers are generally paid by the HMO based on a discounted fee schedule. The nature and extent of most specialty services are also subject to utilization review by the HMO, and reimbursement can be denied for services that are determined to be medically inappropriate.

(A) Benefits for Mental Health Services

The Health Maintenance Organization Act[3] requires HMOs to offer "basic health services"[4] defined "as a minimum, but not

---

1. PA. STAT. ANN. tit. 40, § 1553.
2. PA. STAT. ANN. tit. 40, § 1564.
3. PA. STAT. ANN. tit. 40, §§ 1551–1568.
4. PA. STAT. ANN. tit. 40, § 1554.

limited to, emergency care, inpatient hospital and physician care, ambulatory physician care, and outpatient and preventive medical services."[5] Thus, HMOs are under no express legal obligation to offer mental health services. However, HMOs are allowed to include mental health services in their benefit packages, and most HMOs provide some coverage for mental health services. In general, such coverage is subject to limits on the maximum number of outpatient visits or of inpatient days per year and to utilization review.

(B) Point-of-Service Plans

A point of service (POS) permits the patient to obtain services from providers outside the HMOs network subject to copayments and deductibles. Such plans may be offered in Pennsylvania under regulations of the Pennsylvania Insurance Department.[6] The regulations require minimum deductibles of $250 per individual and $500 per family per calendar year and minimum coinsurance of 20% for out-of-network utilization. The plan must also contain annual and lifetime limits on out-of-pocket expenses within specified ranges. Under a POS plan, patients may receive reimbursement for the services of a mental health professional without meeting the usual HMO requirement of obtaining a referral from the primary care physician.

---

5. Pa. Stat. Ann. tit. 40, § 1553.
6. 31 Pa. Code §§ 301.201–301.204.

2.5

Preferred Provider Organizations

A Preferred Provider Organization (PPO) is a group of health professionals or hospitals that offer health care services to subscribers at reduced premiums. PPOs typically contract with employers, unions, and third-party payors (such as Blue Cross/Blue Shield). In return for reduced premiums, subscribers must use the selected professionals, referred to as *preferred providers*, exclusively. Preferred providers must discount fees for their services but enjoy the likelihood of increased patient volume. PPO providers typically see patients in their private offices. PPOs are regulated jointly by the Department of Health and the Insurance Department.[1]

(A) Benefits for Mental Health Services

PPOs are under no express legal obligation to offer mental health services as a benefit to subscribers. However, PPOs are free to include mental health services in their benefit packages, and most PPOs provide some coverage for mental health services.

---

1. Pa. Stat. Ann. tit. 40, § 764a.

2.6

Individual Practice Associations

An individual practice association (IPA) is a group of health care providers, including MHPs, that contracts to provide services for an organization that provides a prepaid health plan, frequently an HMO. The members of the IPA practice in their own offices and may, if they choose, provide additional services to private clients. Although the IPA works for the provider organization, members are compensated by the organization on a fee-for-service or fee-per-patient basis. Pennsylvania law does not expressly address IPAs. In the absence of express law, therefore, traditional contract law should apply.

2.7

Hospital, Administrative, and Staff Privileges

Licensed psychologists, although able to practice independently, must apply for privileges if they wish to practice in a regulated institution such as a hospital. The application process varies by institution.

(A) Agency and Administrative Positions

Many states have laws determining which classes of MHPs are eligible for hospital staff privileges and membership on the hospital's medical staff. Pennsylvania traditionally has regulated physician staff privileges at hospitals.[1] Clinical privileges and duties may also be granted to other professionals.[2] Whether nonphysician mental health professionals are included in this classification is not clearly delineated in Pennsylvania's regulations. Pennsylvania case law, however, indicates that nonphysician health care professionals must be granted clinical privileges within the scope of their licenses to the same extent as physicians.[3]

---

1. 28 PA. CODE § 107.
2. 28 PA. CODE § 107.12(5), (14).
3. Weiss v. York Hospital, 745 F.2d 786 (3d Cir. 1984).

(B) Hospital Staff Privileges

Each hospital is required by law to have an organized medical staff accountable to the hospital's governing body and responsible for the quality of care provided to the hospital's patients.[4] To become a member of a medical staff, an MHP must make an application in accordance with the bylaws, rules, and regulations of the hospital and the hospital's medical staff.[5] The medical staff reviews applications and makes recommendations to the hospital's governing body, which in turn makes final determinations for the granting of privileges. Only licensed professionals[6] who "always act in a manner consistent with the highest ethical standards and levels of professional competence" will be granted privileges.[7] Privileges that are granted must be commensurate with the applicant's qualifications, experience, and present capabilities.[8] Privileges may not be denied on the basis of gender, race, creed, color, national origin, or any other reason that lacks professional or ethical justification, "including association with a prepaid group practice."[9]

Any time that staff privileges are terminated or voluntarily withdrawn for the purpose of avoiding disciplinary measures, if there is reasonable cause to believe that malpractice or misconduct has occurred, the hospital must notify the State Board of Medical Education and Licensure or the State Board of Osteopathic Examiners, whichever governs the physician whose privileges were terminated (see chapter 1.2).[10]

---

4. 28 PA. CODE § 107.1.
5. 28 PA. CODE § 107.2.
6. Id.
7. 28 PA. CODE § 107.3(a).
8. 28 PA. CODE § 107.3(b).
9. 28 PA. CODE § 107.3(c).
10. 28 PA. CODE § 448.806a(a).

Zoning for Community Homes

Zoning regulations are used by state and local governments to guide the rate and type of growth of communities, including their residential and commercial buildings. Although local governments are permitted to enact zoning laws that restrict the ways landowners may use their property, some municipalities have used zoning laws to prohibit certain groups of people from living together, including those with mental disabilities.[1] Any zoning of this type, however, must be rationally related to a legitimate governmental interest.[2] For example, such zoning laws are unconstitutional if they are based on prejudice, because prejudice is not a legitimate governmental interest.[3] Although some states have statutes that render group homes for mentally ill or mentally retarded individuals exempt from zoning laws, Pennsylvania does not. However, the Pennsylvania Supreme Court has considered this issue and has upheld the right of private landowners who live in residential areas zoned solely for single-family dwellings to use their homes as community living arrangements. The home may not be run for a profit, and the home may not be established primarily for therapeutic or corrective purposes.[4] To determine whether a home will be permitted, the courts use a functional analysis and consider whether the home resembles a traditional family setting.[5] For example, the residents should live

---

1. *See* Cleburne v. Cleburne Living Center, 473 U.S. 432 (1985) (city's zoning restriction on group home for persons with mental retardation finding unconstitutional because not rationally related to any legitimate government interest).
2. *Id.* at 459–460, 465–468.
3. *Id.*
4. *In re* Miller, 515 A.2d 904, 908 (Pa. 1986).
5. *Id.*

and cook together as a single housekeeping unit.[6] Courts also look to the quality of the relationships between residents rather than at the duration of the relationships.[7] Some zoning boards have prohibited community homes for people with mental disorders from locating in single-family residential neighborhoods even though such a placement would be in the best interests of the community home residents in terms of quality of relationships and the opportunity to live in a family-style setting.

---

6. *Id.*
7. *Id.* at 909.

2.9

Insurance Reimbursement for Services

Health insurance carriers (insurers) typically have provisions providing reimbursement for mental health services. The policies frequently limit reimbursement to certain classes of health care providers, usually physicians, and to particular types of services.

(A) Required Coverage of Psychiatric Services

The ability of insurance providers to discriminate among different types of licensed providers when reimbursing for mental health services is limited. The Reimbursement for Psychological Services Act[1] states that an insured person or any other person covered by the policy, contract, or certificate, is entitled to reimbursement for "psychologically necessary" services within those areas for which psychologists are licensed, whether the service is performed by a licensed physician (e.g., psychiatrist) or by a psychologist.[2] There is no such requirement, however, for HMOs, federal or state (Medicare/Medicaid) governments, and ERISA-exempt businesses, or out-of-state insurers. Furthermore, the Insurance Payment to Registered Nurse Law[3] dictates that an in-

---

1. PA. STAT. ANN. tit. 40, §§ 767–774.
2. PA. STAT. ANN. tit. 40, § 768.
3. PA. STAT. ANN. tit. 40, §§ 3021–3026 (1992).

sured person or any other person covered is entitled to reimbursement for services provided by a licensed certified mental health nurse or licensed certified clinical nurse specialist under the Professional Nursing Law.[4]

---

4. PA. STAT. ANN. tit. 40, § 3024.

2.10

Mental Health Benefits in State Insurance Plans

In some states, the law mandates that any health insurance plan provided for state government employees must include certain mental health benefits. Pennsylvania does not mandate benefits for mental health services (see chapter 2.9). Nevertheless, any insurance or HMO plan is required to provide benefits for drug and alcohol detoxification or treatment.[1] Many insurance plans offer mental health services, however, because of competitive pressures. In contrast, some health maintenance organizations are governed by federal statutes that mandate a minimum mental health treatment benefit of 30 inpatient days.[2]

---

1. PA. STAT. ANN. tit. 40, § 908-2.
2. 42 U.S.C. §§ 300e–300c-17.

2.11

Tax Deductions for Services

Payments for mental health services may be deductible from federal income taxes as either an individual medical deduction or a business expense, depending on the nature of the service and the use by the recipient taxpayer.

(A) Mental Health Services as a Medical Deduction

A taxpayer may deduct expenses for medical care not reimbursed by insurance or otherwise to the extent the expenses exceed 7.5% of the taxpayer's adjusted gross income.[1] The federal Internal Revenue Code defines medical care expenses as "amounts paid for the diagnosis, cure, mitigation, treatment, or prevention of disease, or for the purpose of affecting any structure or function of the body."[2] Taxpayers may deduct expenses for psychologists, psychiatrists, other kinds of psychotherapists, and "others rendering similar type services" related to medical care.[3] Medical expenses of spouses and dependents also may be included.

The federal Internal Revenue Service has interpreted the taxpayer's obligation with regard to deducting medical expenses:

> The Code and the regulations do not require a taxpayer to ascertain whether a practitioner is qualified, is authorized under state law, or is licensed to practice, before obtaining his services

---

1. 26 U.S.C. § 213(a).
2. 26 U.S.C. § 231(d)(1)(A). Medical care expenses also include transportation that is "primarily for and essential to medical care." 26 U.S.C. § 213(d)(1)(B).
3. Rev. Rul. 53-143, 1953-2 C.B. 129; Rev. Rul. 63-91, 1963-1 C.B. 54.

or claiming a medical expense deduction. . . . Accordingly, it is held that amounts paid for medical expenses rendered by practitioners, such as chiropractors, psychotherapists, and others rendering similar services, constitute expenses for "medical care" within the provisions of section 213 of the Code, "even though the practitioners who perform the services are not required by law to be, or are not licensed, certified, or otherwise qualified to perform such services."[4]

(B) Mental Health Services as a Business Deduction

Expenses for some mental health services provided to employees can be deductible to businesses as trade or business expenses. If a business provides an employee assistance program, for example, it may deduct the cost of the program from its corporate income taxes as an ordinary business deduction.[5]

(C) Mental Health Educational Services Received by MHPs

MHPs may not deduct the cost of their basic professional education as a business expense. They may, however, deduct courses if they are employed or self-employed, if they are required to meet the minimum requirements of the job or profession, and if they maintain or improve professional skills, or the MHPs are required by the employer or by law to take the courses to keep their present salary or position.[6]

Educational expenses are not deductible if they are part of a program of study that will lead to a new trade or business.[7] Under this rule, a licensed psychiatrist is permitted to deduct expenses associated with training at a psychoanalytic institute, including a personal psychoanalysis.[8] A tax court permitted a clinical social worker to deduct her own psychoanalysis.[9] Similarly, a psychiatrist was able to deduct the cost of his own psychotherapy.[10]

---

4. Rev. Rul. 63-91, 1963-1, C.B. 54.
5. Welch v. Helvering, 290 U.S. 111 (1933).
6. I.R.C. § 1.162-5(a).
7. I.R.C. § 1.162-5(b)(3).
8. *Id.*
9. Voigt v. Commissioner, 74 T.C. 82 (1980), nonacq., 1981-2, C.B.1.
10. Porter v. Commissioner, 51 T.C.M. (CCH) 477 (1986).

2.12

Integrated Delivery Systems

An integrated delivery system (IDS) is a collection of health care providers under common ownership or control that offers a full range of health services and that is capable of entering into third-party payor contracts to provide all levels of care to patients. An IDS may include MHPs.

An IDS may be structured as a single corporation or as a partnership, association, or other legal entity, including health care professionals in different disciplines and institutions. An IDS may enter into contracts with HMOs under which the IDS providers accept financial risk for the care of patients through capitation or similar arrangements and under which an HMO delegates to the IDS responsibility for provider credentialing, quality assurance, utilization management, and other essential HMO functions under a Statement of Policy of the Department of Health.[1] Such contracts must be approved by the Department of Health and must include, among other requirements, financial protections for HMO members, continued HMO authority to monitor and review functions delegated to the IDS, and compliance with quality assurance standards.

---

1. 28 Pa. Code § 9.402.

Limitations on and Liability for Practice

3.1

Informed Consent for Services

Informed consent should be obtained before administering services, disclosing information concerning the client to a third party, or taking any other action that may be considered professional misconduct by a licensing board (see chapter 3.11) and that renders MHPs liable to a malpractice suit (see chapter 3.10).

(A) Legal Definition of Informed Consent

Informed consent is only required if a treatment involves physically touching the patient or client.[1] Informed consent is not required for the administration of medications.[2] Although the courts have not yet addressed the precise question of informed consent for psychological services, it seems that the law does not require it as long as the services do not involve touching of any kind.

When treatment does involve physical touching, informed consent is satisfied if the MHP discusses with the patient all the facts, risks, and alternatives that a reasonable patient in the same or similar circumstances would deem significant in deciding whether or not to accept the treatment.[3] Because the law of in-

---

1. *See* Gray v. Grunnagle, 223 A.2d 663 (Pa. 1966).
2. Boyer v. Smith, 497 A.2d 646, 649 (Pa. Super. Ct. 1985).
3. PA. STAT. ANN. tit. 40, § 1301.103; Defulvio v. Holst, 414 A.2d 1087 (Pa. Super. Ct. 1979).

formed consent does not apply to most mental health services, MHPs should take guidance from professional codes of ethics.[4]

In the case of voluntary hospitalization, the Pennsylvania legislature requires verbal and written informed consent so that:

> the person understands his treatment will involve inpatient status; that he is willing to be admitted to a designated facility for the purpose of such examination and treatment; and that he consents to such admission voluntarily, without coercion or duress; and, if applicable, that he has voluntarily agreed to remain in treatment for a specified period of no longer than 72 hours after having given written notice of his intent to withdraw from treatment.[5]

Assent to Voluntary Treatment

Any person who is 14 years of age or older may assent to voluntary mental health treatment, but children under 14 may not enter treatment without the cooperation of their parents or guardians.[6] The U.S. Supreme Court has ruled that because there is a risk of error when parents place their children into psychiatric hospitals for treatment, the admission decision must be reviewed by a neutral fact finder who has the authority to refuse admission.[7]

When an MHP treats a child between the ages of 14 and 17, the minor's parents must be promptly notified.[8] If the parents object to the treatment, they may file an objection with the court.[9] Within 72 hours of the notice, a judge or a mental health review officer will hold a hearing to determine whether or not the voluntary treatment is in the minor's best interests.[10] Anyone who is 14 years old or older may seek voluntary treatment as long as that person is able to provide informed consent; if the minor child is under 14, then the parent or guardian may seek treatment for the child.[11]

---

4. *See, e.g.,* American Psychological Association. (1992). Ethical principles and code of conduct. *American Psychologist, 47,* 1597 (Standard 4.02, Informed Consent to Therapy).
5. PA. STAT. ANN. tit. 50, § 7203. *See also* Zinermon v. Burch, 494 U.S. 113 (1990) (treatment facilities must determine patients competence to understand nature and consequences of admitting themselves for voluntary treatment).
6. PA. STAT. ANN. tit. 50, § 7201.
7. Parham v. J. R., 442 U.S. 584, 606–607 (1979). The "neutral fact finder" may be another MHP employed by the admitting institution.
8. PA. STAT. ANN. tit. 50, § 7204.
9. *Id.*
10. *Id.*
11. PA. STAT. ANN. tit. 50, § 7201.

3.2

Extensiveness, Ownership, Maintenance, and Access to Records

An MHP's records are an important, required part of a practice. MHPs should maintain a record of each client's evaluation, treatment, and progress. For most MHPs and in most mental health treatment settings, record-keeping is required by law. Even when not expressly required by law, MHPs should maintain careful records to ensure quality mental health care service delivery. The law in Pennsylvania does not speak to ownership of mental health records. However, hospitals are the owners of medical records created in the course of treatment at the hospital.[1] By analogy, MHPs in other settings should consider themselves to be the owners of records created in the course of treatment.

(A) Psychologists

Extensiveness of Records
The State Board of Psychological Examiners requires all licensed psychologists to "record accurately [the client's] progress through the evaluation and intervention process."[2] Failure to comply with record-keeping requirements can subject a psychologist to disciplinary action.[3] At a minimum, these records must include the following information:

1. the client's name and address, or, if the client is a minor, the client's parents' names and address(es) and any custody arrangements;

---

1. 28 PA. CODE § 115.28.
2. 49 PA. CODE § 41.57(a).
3. 49 PA. CODE § 41.57(e).

2. presenting problem or diagnosis;

3. fee arrangements;

4. date and substance of each service contact;

5. test results, other evaluative results, and basic test data from which they were derived;

6. notation and results of formal consultation with other providers;

7. a copy of test or evaluative reports prepared as part of the professional relationship; and

8. any authorizations for releases of information.[4]

The Board has not published any guidelines for determining how thorough or detailed a psychologist should be in recording the "substance" of service contacts.

Maintenance of Records
Psychologists must maintain records for 5 years after the last date that service was rendered to a client or patient.[5] Although the law does not specify that records of minors should be retained for longer periods of time, it may be prudent for psychologists to maintain the records of minor clients for 5 years after the minor has attained the age of majority or for at least as long as psychiatrists are required to maintain such records, as discussed later. Other laws or regulations may require psychologists to keep records for more than 5 years.[6]

Client Access
Regulations of the State Board of Psychology do not address the issue of client access to a psychologist's records. There are rules of access, however, for MHPs who practice in settings governed by the Department of Public Welfare. These rules are described in section C in this chapter that deals with mental health treatment centers and hospitals.[7]

(B) Psychiatrists

Extensiveness of Records
The State Board of Medicine and the State Board of Osteopathic Medicine require physicians to keep records of the evaluation and

---

4. 49 Pa. Code § 41.57(b)(1–8).
5. 49 Pa. Code § 41.57(d).
6. *Id.*
7. For an extensive discussion of client access to MHP records, see Burkhardt, S. L. (1992). The effect on the content of mental health records when psychiatric patients are permitted access pursuant to "patient access" laws. *Dissertation Abstracts International, 53,* B3149.

treatment of all patients.[8] Medical records must identify the patient and contain information on evaluation, diagnosis, and treatment procedures that are performed by the physician or by any of the physician's agents.[9] Each entry must be signed and dated by the person making the entry.[10]

Maintenance of Records
The State Board of Medicine requires MDs to maintain records for 7 years after the last date of service. For patients who were minors during their treatment, records must be maintained for 1 year after the patient reaches the age of majority.[11] The State Board of Osteopathic Medicine requires DOs to maintain records for 7 years after the last date of service. For patients who were minors during treatment, records must be maintained for 2 years after the patient's 18th birthday or for 7 years, whichever is later.[12]

Client Access
The State Board of Medicine does not speak to patient or client access to the records created by MDs. In contrast, the State Board of Osteopathic Medicine requires DOs to provide patients with a "complete copy" of their medical records.[13] All physicians who practice in a setting governed by the State Department of Public Welfare are subject to the access rules, described in the next section. In addition, the criminal code requires that patients shall have access to all of their medical records and may photocopy them for their own use.[14]

(C) Mental Health Treatment Centers and Hospitals

Extensiveness of Records
The State Department of Health requires hospitals to maintain medical records on all patients.[15] These records must include "sufficient information to identify the patient clearly, to justify the diagnosis and treatment, and to document the results accurately."[16] The State Department of Public Welfare requires all psychiatric outpatient clinics that are governed by its regulations

---

8. 49 PA. CODE §§ 16.95(a), 25.213(a).
9. 49 PA. CODE §§ 16.95(b–d), 25.213(a).
10. 49 PA. CODE §§ 16.95(b), 25.213(a).
11. 49 PA. CODE § 16.95(c).
12. 49 PA. CODE § 25.213(b).
13. 49 PA. CODE § 25.213(d).
14. PA. STAT. ANN. tit. 42, § 6155(b).
15. 28 PA. CODE § 115.31(a).
16. 28 PA. CODE § 115.32(a).

to maintain a record on each patient or client.[17] These records must be legible, permanent,[18] signed by the person who made them,[19] and must include

1. patient identifying information;
2. referral source;
3. presenting problems;
4. appropriately signed consent forms;
5. medical, social, and developmental history;
6. diagnosis and evaluation;
7. treatment plan;
8. treatment progress notes for each contact;
9. medication orders;
10. discharge summary; and
11. referrals to other agencies, when indicated.[20]

Client Access

Regulations of the Department of Public Welfare state that persons who are receiving or have received mental health care, who are 14 years old or older, and who understand the nature of the mental health records[21] must be given access to (meaning an opportunity to view rather than to possess) their mental health care records, unless:

1. the provider or treatment team leader documents that access to the records would have an adverse effect on the client's treatment; or
2. access to the records would disclose information that would reveal the identity of, or breach the confidentiality of, another person who offered information on condition of confidentiality.[22]

This rule only applies to MHPs and facilities operating under the Department of Public Welfare, although it may serve as a guide to other MHPs and facilities.

Regulations of the Pennsylvania Department of Health require hospitals to provide patients with copies of their medical

---

17. 55 PA. CODE § 5200.41(a).
18. 55 PA. CODE § 5200.41(b)(1).
19. 55 PA. CODE § 5200.41(b)(4).
20. 55 PA. CODE § 5300.41(a)(1-8).
21. Parents or guardians control the medical records of persons under 14 years of age. 55 PA. CODE § 5100.33(a) & (e).
22. 55 PA. CODE § 5100.33(c)(1-2).

records.[23] No exceptions are provided for minor patients or for mental health treatments. However, the Mental Health Procedures Act states that records must be kept confidential and may not be released without the patient's consent to anyone other than those treating the patient, the county administrator, a court in the course of legal proceedings, or others as specified under applicable federal rules when treatment is by a federal agency.[24]

Department of Health regulations also provide that relevant portions of mental health records may be released without patient consent to the following or in the following situations:

1. those actively engaged in treating the individual, or those persons at other facilities, including professional staff of state correctional institutions and county prisons, when the person is being discharged to that facility and the information is necessary to provide for continuity of proper care and treatment;

2. third-party payors operated and financed in whole or part by any governmental agency and their agents or intermediaries, who require information to verify that services were provided or when necessary to obtain certification as an eligible provider of services;

3. reviewers and inspectors, including the Joint Commission on the Accreditation of Health Care Organizations (JCAHCO), and commonwealth licensing and certification boards, when necessary to obtain certification as an eligible provider of services;

4. those participating in Professional Standards Review Organization (PSRO) or utilization reviews;

5. the administrator of the Department of Health under applicable statutes and regulations;

6. a court or mental health review officer, in the course of legal proceedings authorized by the Mental Health Procedures Act;

7. appropriate personnel pursuant to § 5100.38 (relating to child or patient abuse);

8. parents or guardians and others when necessary to obtain consent to medical treatment;

9. attorneys assigned to represent the subject of a commitment hearing;

---

23. 28 PA. CODE § 115.29.
24. PA. STAT. ANN. tit. 50, § 7111.

10. in response to a court order requiring the production of documents under § 5100.35 (relating to release to courts); or

11. in response to an emergency medical situation when release of information is necessary to prevent serious risk of bodily harm or death, with release limited to specific information pertinent to the relief of the emergency.[25]

The regulations also require that current patients or the parents of patients younger than 14 be notified of the specific conditions under which information may be released without their consent. Information that is released without consent must be limited to that information relevant and necessary to the purpose for which it is sought and cannot be released to any other third party without consent or for any additional purposes. The fact that information has been requested and the action taken in response to that request must be recorded in the patient's chart.[26]

The Mental Health Procedures Act is controlling in treatment settings that are governed by the Pennsylvania Department of Public Welfare. In the absence of explicit regulations governing them, MHPs in other settings may also take guidance and direction from the Act.

(D) Access by Regulatory Departments and Boards

Access by Hospital Medical Review Boards
Hospitals are required to establish utilization review committees for the purposes of reducing morbidity and mortality and for the improvement of the care of their patients. These utilization review boards have access to patient medical records, including information relating to mental health evaluation, diagnosis, and treatment. Medical records are also periodically reviewed in hospitals for compliance with the hospital's medical staff bylaws.[27]

Access by State Credentialing Agencies
The boards of Psychology, Medicine, and Osteopathic Medicine may have access to patient records if the records are reasonably necessary to complete an investigation into the practice of a licensee (see chapters 1.2 and 1.5). All possible steps, however, must be taken to protect the confidentiality of patients involved.

---

25. 55 Pa. Code § 5100.32.
26. *Id.*
27. 28 Pa. Code § 115.34(a).

Liability for Violation

MHPs who fail to comply with applicable record-keeping rules may be subject to disciplinary action, including suspension, revocation, or failure to renew their licenses (see chapter 1.5). Furthermore, as these rules establish standards for practice, an MHP who fails to comply with them may be exposed to civil liability for any resulting harm (see chapters 3.10 and 3.11).

3.3

Confidential Relations and Communications

A confidential communication is information conveyed by a client to an MHP, either in oral or written form, in the course of a professional relationship. Professional codes of ethics[1] protect the confidentiality of information based on the premise that effective treatment and assessment of a patient requires a guarantee from the therapist that no information obtained will be given to others without the patient's consent.[2] Confidentiality and the duty to protect information obtained from patients are not absolute under the law. In the courtroom, for example, the duty to maintain confidentiality is not a legally recognized justification to disobey a court order to disclose information that is relevant to a case. That issue is addressed under the law of privilege (see chapter 3.4). In addition, the duty to maintain confidentiality is not necessarily a sufficient justification for failing to take actions that may be necessary to protect the patient or others from harm.

Legal confidentiality requirements are based on statutes, on common law, and on professional codes of ethics. In particular, the Mental Health Procedures Act prohibits nonconsensual disclosure of any documents concerning a patient or client, regardless of the contents of the documents, except:

1. to those involved in treating the patient or client;
2. to the county mental health administrator according to provisions set forth in the Act;
3. to a court in the course of commitment proceedings; or

---

1. *See, e.g.,* American Psychological Association. (1992). Ethical principles of psychologists and code of conduct. *American Psychologist, 47,* 1597–1611.
2. *See* Jaffee v. Redmond, 518 U.S. 1 (1996).

4. pursuant to federal rules, statutes, or regulations when treatment is undertaken by a federal agency.[3]

Regulations of the Department of Public Welfare prohibit the disclosure of mental health records, except to those treating the patient, to third-party payors, or to attorneys representing the patient in a commitment hearing unless there is a court order—not merely a subpoena—requiring release of the records.[4] MHPs may be subject to civil liability for improper release of confidential information (see sections 10 and 11 of this chapter).

Under the Pennsylvania Drug and Alcohol Abuse Act of 1972, records of drug and alcohol treatment may only be disclosed with the patient's consent and only to medical personnel involved in treatment or to government or other officials to obtain benefits for the patient.[5] Disclosure may be made without the patient's consent only in an emergency.[6] The Act has no provisions for release of information pursuant to a subpoena or court order.[7] Under the federal Comprehensive Alcohol Abuse and Alcoholism Prevention Act, information concerning the identity, diagnosis, prognosis, or treatment of patients in federally funded drug and alcohol programs may only be released pursuant to a court order in addition to a subpoena without the patient's written consent.[8]

(A) Psychiatrists and Psychologists

All communications between psychiatrists or licensed psychologists and their clients or patients are confidential. However, the extent of confidentiality has limits that must be revealed to clients at the initiation of services. The legal rules governing the confidentiality of the relationship between a psychologist or psychiatrist and a client or patient are the same as those governing the relationship between an attorney and a client.[9]

---

3. PA. STAT. ANN. tit. 50, § 7111 (Supp. 1994). In Hahnemann University Hospital v. Edgar, 74 F.3d 456 (3d Cir. 1996), these exceptions were interpreted extremely narrowly, recognizing the purpose of keeping all records relating to treatment confidential is to ensure adequate treatment. This right to privacy of psychiatric records has been given constitutional status. *Id.* at 463.
4. 55 PA. CODE § 5100.35 (1993).
5. PA. STAT. ANN. tit. 71, § 1690.108.
6. *Id.* An emergency exists when there is an acute need for medical services—for example, when short-term services are needed to deal with the acute effects of abuse and dependence.
7. *Id.*
8. 42 U.S.C. § 290 dd-2. *See also* 42 U.S.C. § 60-III(c).
9. 42 PA. CONS. STAT. ANN. §§ 5944, 5916, & 5928.

Limitations on the Duty

The circumstances under which confidential information may be revealed are limited by law in order to

1. prevent the client from committing a criminal act that the professional believes is likely to result in death or substantial bodily harm or substantial injury to the financial interests or property of another;

2. prevent or rectify the consequences of a client's criminal or fraudulent act in the commission of which the professional's services are being or had been used; or

3. establish a claim or defense on behalf of the professional in a controversy between the lawyer and the client, establish a defense to a criminal charge or civil claim or disciplinary proceeding against the lawyer based on conduct in which the client was involved, or respond to allegations in any proceeding concerning the lawyer's representation of the client.[10]

The duty not to reveal information relating to a client continues after the client–professional relationship has terminated or after the death of the client.

In addition to these limitations on confidentiality, MHPs are bound by law to report incidents of child abuse (see chapter 4.8) and may report incidents of elder abuse (see chapter 4.7). Courts have also found MHPs to have an obligation to warn an identified victim and the police of a specific threat of harm made by a patient or client (see chapter 3.11).[11]

Liability for Violation

Several types of penalties may be imposed for violations of confidentiality restrictions. The State Boards of Medicine, Osteopathic Medicine, and Psychology may suspend or revoke the license of a psychiatrist or psychologist for breaches of ethical standards including duties of confidentiality.[12] Clients harmed by a breach of confidentiality may also bring a civil suit for recovery of damages (see chapter 3.11).

---

10. 42 PA. CONS. STAT. ANN. § 5928.
11. *See* Ms. B. v. Montgomery County Emergency Serv., 799 F. Supp. 534 (E.D. Pa. 1992).
12. PA. STAT. ANN. tit. 63, § 422.41(8)(i) (MD psychiatrists); PA. STAT. ANN. tit. 63, § 271.15(a)(8) (DO psychiatrists); PA. STAT. ANN. tit. 63, § 1208(a)(11) (psychologists).

(B) Social Workers

Communications between social workers and their clients may be subject to legal confidentiality protections within limits. As with psychologists and psychiatrists, confidentiality may be breached by requirements to report child abuse (see chapter 4.8) and by discretion to report elder abuse (see chapter 4.7). The State Board of Social Work Examiners may suspend or revoke the license of a social worker for breaches of standards of professional practice, including breaches of confidentiality.[13] It is not clear whether clients harmed by a breach of confidentiality may also bring a civil suit for recovery of damages (see chapter 3.11).

(C) Marriage and Family Counselors, Educational Psychologists, Guidance Counselors, Mental Health Nurses/School Nurses, Rehabilitation Counselors, and Mental Health Counselors

MHPs working in educational settings are required to not reveal confidential communications with students unless the student or parent or guardian consents to a release of information concerning them.[14] In addition, MHPs working in the field of substance abuse and chemical dependency are required to maintain communications with patients as confidential unless the patient consents to release. In emergency medical situations, in which the patient's life is in immediate jeopardy, patient records may be released without the patient's consent to proper medical authorities for the sole purpose of providing medical treatment to the patient.[15] In addition, as is true with regard to psychologists and psychiatrists, confidentiality may be breached by requirements to report child (see chapter 4.8) and by discretion to report elder abuse (see chapter 4.7).

---

13. PA. STAT. ANN. tit. 63, § 1911(a)(3).
14. 42 PA. CONS. STAT. ANN. § 5945.
15. PA. STAT. ANN. tit. 71, § 1690.108(b)–(c).

(D) Confidentiality of HIV-Related Information

In 1990, the legislature passed the Confidentiality of HIV-Related Information Act[16] that imposed strict confidentiality protections regarding information concerning tests for the presence of Human Immunodeficiency Virus (HIV), the virus that causes Acquired Immune Deficiency Syndrome (AIDS). The Act provides that no person who obtains information concerning whether or not an individual has been tested for HIV status or the results of such a test may disclose such information without the individual's consent.[17] The Act also limits the circumstances in which a court may order release of such information. Those circumstances are the following: (a) the person seeking the information has demonstrated a compelling need for it that cannot be accommodated by other means or (b) the person seeking to disclose the information has a compelling need to do so.[18] In addition, under the Act, written consent is required before an HIV-related test may be conducted. The Act also grants immunity from civil liability to licensed physicians for notifying contacts of the individual receiving an HIV-related test if the physician reasonably believes that disclosure is medically appropriate and there is a significant risk of future infection to the contact, the physician has counseled the individual receiving the test and reasonably believes that he or she will *not* inform the contact or abstain from behavior that could transmit the virus, has notified the individual receiving the test of the intent to make the disclosure, the physician does not reveal the identity of the individual taking the test, and the disclosure to the contact is made in person, unless circumstances reasonably prevent doing so.[19] The Act also created a civil cause of action for persons aggrieved by violations of wrongful disclosure of confidential HIV-related information.[20]

---

16. PA. STAT. ANN. tit. 35, §§ 7601–7612.
17. PA. STAT. ANN. tit. 35, § 7607.
18. *Id.*
19. PA. STAT. ANN. tit. 35, § 7609.
20. PA. STAT. ANN. tit. 35, §§ 7610, 7611.

3.4

Privileged Communications

Two primary areas of law exist that attempt to protect the client's communications from disclosure. The most well-known is confidentiality law, whose principles originated in professional ethics codes and have now been incorporated in legislation and court rulings (see chapter 3.3). It is designed to encourage frank discussion and the exchange of reliable information and protects the client from improper disclosure of information by the MHP in most situations. It does not necessarily, however, protect the client from court orders requiring the MHP to disclose information.

For protection in the courtroom, the communications must be covered under a privileged communication statute. Privilege refers to the right of a client or patient to prohibit disclosure in a legal proceeding of confidential communications made to a professional. Pennsylvania has recognized this fundamental concept in its common law, in statutes, and in professional rules of conduct,[1] and has several privilege statutes.[2] All MHPs should be knowledgeable about the applicability of the privileged communications law relevant to their professions so that they can advise their clients of the limits of confidential information. There are no privileged communication laws for MHPs other than those specifically provided for by the legislature; therefore, their client's disclosures can be revealed in a court hearing if the MHP is required to testify.

---

1. Packel, L., & A. B. Poulin. (1987). *Pennsylvania evidence*. St. Paul, MN: West.
2. 42 PA. CONS. STAT. ANN. § 5943 (clergy); § 5944 (psychiatrists and licensed psychologists); § 5945 (school personnel); § 5945.1 (sexual assault counselors); § 5948 (qualified professionals).

(A) Psychologists and Psychiatrists

Those Covered Under the Statutes

Communications between patients or clients and psychiatrists and licensed psychologists are privileged in Pennsylvania. The patient or client may prevent the psychiatrist or licensed psychologist from being examined in a civil or criminal matter "as to any information acquired in the course of his professional services in behalf of such client."[3] The law furthers states that "the confidential relations and communications between a psychologist or psychiatrist and his or her patient or client shall be on the same basis as those provided or prescribed by law between an attorney and client."[4] The privilege also applies to information communicated by clients to persons employed by licensed psychologists, where the information is given for the purposes of assisting the psychologist in treating the client.[5]

Exceptions to the Privilege

There are several exceptions permitting judges to order that testimony be given despite the privilege. The privilege does not apply in child or elder abuse proceedings,[6] nor when the client brings charges or a malpractice action against the psychologist or psychiatrist. In contrast, psychiatric records of a witness are absolutely privileged and shielded from discovery, absent the consent of the witness.[7]

(B) Social Workers

There is no law in Pennsylvania creating an explicit privilege for communications between a social worker and a client. However, other statutes may apply in cases in which a social worker is acting in the role of a "sexual assault counselor, domestic violence counselor, or advocate,"[8] a divorce and custody counselor,[9] or as a school counselor.[10]

---

3. *Id.*
4. 42 PA. CONS. STAT. ANN. § 5944.
5. Kalenevitch v. Finger, 595 A.2d 1224 (Pa. Super. Ct. 1991).
6. Matter of Adoption of Embick, 506 A.2d 455 (Pa. Super. Ct. 1986), *appeal denied*, 520 A.2d 1385 (Pa. 1987).
7. Commonwealth v. Smith, 606 A.2d 939 (Pa. Super. Ct. 1992).
8. 42 PA. CONS. STAT. ANN. § 5945.1.
9. 42 PA. CONS. STAT. ANN. § 5948.
10. 42 PA. CONS. STAT. ANN. § 5945.

(C) Sexual Assault Counselors, Domestic Violence Counselors, and Advocates

Without written consent, no sexual assault counselor (nor any coparticipant present during the counseling session) may disclose a victim's oral or written communications or consent to be examined concerning them in any civil or criminal proceeding.[11] Where a victim's statements to a counselor are in the possession of the commonwealth (that is, the prosecuting attorney), the statutory privilege does not apply.[12] The privilege terminates on the death of a victim.[13]

(D) School Personnel

With the exception of compliance with child abuse reporting requirements, the student communications privilege covers a broad range of information and people. The general rule is that school employees, including counselors, nurses, psychologists, teachers, and clerical workers, may not be compelled or allowed to reveal confidential information about a student:

1. without the consent of the student, if the student is 18 years of age or over; or
2. without the consent of a parent or guardian, if the student is under the age of 18 years.[14]

(E) Confidential Communications to Clergy, Priests, Rabbis, and Ministers

The Pennsylvania clergy–penitent privilege statute provides that no member of the clergy, priest, rabbi, or minister of any regularly established church or religious organization may be compelled or allowed to reveal confidential communications with a penitent unless the penitent consents to the disclosure.[15]

---

11. 42 PA. CONS. STAT. ANN. § 5945.1(b)(1)(2).
12. Commonwealth v. Cacek, 517 A.2d 992 (Pa. Super. Ct. 1986).
13. 23 PA. CONS. STAT. ANN. § 6116.
14. 42 PA. CONS. STAT. ANN. § 5945.
15. 42 PA. CONS. STAT. ANN. § 5943.

Search, Seizure, and Subpoena of Records

Search of an MHP's office and seizure of any records may occur within the context of a criminal investigation of the MHP or the client. This chapter is limited to the latter situation. In certain circumstances, a court may issue a search warrant authorizing the search of an MHP's office. A court may also issue a subpoena requesting that the MHP bring certain records to court in a civil or criminal proceeding. Both types of request, search and subpoena, are important to MHPs because they provide major exceptions to confidentiality (see chapter 3.3) and privileged communication law (see chapter 3.4). Note, however, that the seizure of records does not necessarily mean that they will ultimately be admissible in court. That determination will be made at trial.

(A) Search and Seizure

In general, before searching a private office a government official must have a warrant. Although warrantless searches are sometimes permissible, they are generally restricted to exigent circumstances such as immediate danger to a police officer. The search warrant is a court order authorizing the search and seizure of specifically identified persons or places. A search warrant may be issued to search for or seize

1. anything illegally possessed or the fruits of a crime,
2. property that is or was used to commit a crime, or
3. property that is evidence of a crime.[1]

---

1. Pa. R. Crim. P. 2002.

A court may not grant a search warrant unless there is probable cause to believe that the persons or property to be searched or seized will be found.[2] Normally, search warrants are executed between the hours of 6:00 A.M. and 10:00 P.M. A stronger showing of cause must be made if a search warrant is to be executed outside those hours.[3] The probable cause for the search must be established through sworn affidavits.[4] The affidavits must contain detailed and specific descriptions of the person or places to be searched or seized, must specify the crime that has been committed, and must set forth the specific facts and circumstances that form the affiant's conclusion that there is probable cause to believe that the items or property are proper for a search and will be found at the location specified in the warrant.[5]

Before entering property, the law enforcement officer executing the search warrant must give, or make reasonable effort to give, notice of his or her identity, authority, and purpose to any person occupying the premises.[6] After announcing his or her identity, authority, and purpose, the officer must wait a reasonable period of time before entering the premises.[7] If the officer is not admitted after waiting a reasonable period of time, he or she may forcibly enter the premises and is permitted to use as much physical force as is necessary to effect the search.[8] In the case of exigent circumstances, a law enforcement officer may forcibly enter the premises without giving notice of identity, authority, or purpose and without waiting a reasonable time to be admitted into the premises.[9]

Whenever a search is executed, the law enforcement officer must leave a copy of the warrant, the supporting affidavits, and a receipt for any property that was seized.[10] This requirement stands whether or not any person was occupying the premises and whether or not any property was seized.[11]

---

2. PA. R. CRIM. P. 2003(a).
3. PA. R. CRIM. P. 2003(c), 2006(g).
4. PA. R. CRIM. P. 2003(a).
5. PA. R. CRIM. P. 2006(a–f).
6. PA. R. CRIM. P. 2007(a).
7. PA. R. CRIM. P. 2007(b).
8. PA. R. CRIM. P. 2007(c).
9. PA. R. CRIM. P. 2007(a–c).
10. PA. R. CRIM. P. 2008.
11. *Id.*

(B) Subpoena

A subpoena is a written order of the court compelling a witness to appear and to give testimony or to provide documents.[12] Subpoenas may be used to compel appearance, testimony, or production of documents at a civil or criminal hearing or trial or a deposition in a civil case.[13] They must contain the name of the court, the title of the action, and the time and place where the appearance or production is to be made.[14]

A subpoena may be served by hand delivery or by mailing a copy directly to the person whose testimony or records are being subpoenaed.[15] Failure to appear at the time and place specified in a subpoena may result in contempt of court proceedings, which can lead to punishment by jail.[16] If appearing or producing the subpoenaed documents would be unreasonable and oppressive, however, a witness may make a timely motion to quash or modify the subpoena or to condition compliance on payment of the reasonable cost of producing such evidence. Further, mere issuance of a subpoena, which is done by a court clerk, does not mean that any applicable privilege is overcome. Rather, the MHP must assert the privilege until the client expressly waives it or the court orders the privilege waived as a matter of law, which may occur when the person holding the privilege has disclosed the information in such a way as to extinguish its confidential nature (see chapter 3.4). Failure by a psychologist or psychiatrist to assert the privilege may result in civil liability (see chapters 1.1, 1.3, 3.10, 3.11) and in criminal liability for psychologists (see chapter 3.12). A hospital must produce a patient's records in response to a subpoena.[17]

---

12. Pa. R. Civ. P. 234.1(a).
13. Pa. R. Civ. P. 234.1(b); Pa. R. Crim. P. 9016.
14. Pa. R. Civ. P. 234.6; Pa. R. Crim. P. 9016.
15. Pa. R. Civ. P. 234.2.
16. Pa. R. Civ. P. 234.5
17. 42 Pa. Cons. Stat. Ann. § 6152.

3.6

State Freedom of Information Act

Pennsylvania's Right to Know Act[1] allows any citizen to examine, inspect, and photocopy any public record of a state agency. Certain information is excluded from the Right to Know Act, however, including information concerning an agency investigation.[2] In addition, any information that may not be published normally because of court order or statute is exempted, as is any information that, if published, would lead to prejudice or impairment of a person's reputation or personal security.[3] Thus, although state mental health agencies are subject to the Right to Know Act, patient records are exempted because of confidentiality protections (see chapter 3.3), privilege (see chapter 3.4), and potential for prejudice or impairment of a person's reputation.

If citizens are denied the right to examine or make copies of public records, they may appeal to the Court of Common Pleas.[4]

---

1. 65 PA. CONS. STAT. ANN. §§ 66.1–66.4.
2. 65 PA. CONS. STAT. ANN. § 66.1(2).
3. *Id.*
4. 65 PA. CONS. STAT. ANN. § 66.4.

3.7

Right to Refuse Treatment

MHPs may be involved in evaluating an individual who has refused or requested discontinuation of life-sustaining treatment. The right to refuse medical treatment is established by the common-law right to self-determination as well as the right to privacy guaranteed by the Fourteenth Amendment to the U.S. Constitution.[1] An individual's right to refuse such treatment, however, will be weighed against the state's interests in preserving life, protecting innocent third parties, preventing suicide, and maintaining the integrity of the medical profession.[2]

People who have the capacity to seek voluntary treatment have, by definition, the capacity to refuse such treatment. The right of involuntarily committed patients to refuse treatment, however, has not always been recognized. The extent to which civilly committed, mentally ill, and developmentally disabled individuals have the right to refuse treatment is discussed in chapters 8.3 and 8.7.

When a person is being treated on a voluntary basis, services may be refused at any time. A person who is receiving voluntary inpatient treatment may withdraw from treatment by giving written notice.[3] Nevertheless, very often, voluntary inpatients have signed an agreement to delay release for up to 72 hours after signing the written notice.[4]

When a person under the age of 14 is being treated on a voluntary basis, the parents or guardian may withdraw the child

---

1. *In re* Doe, 45 Pa. D. & C. 371 (Pa. Commw. Ct. 1987).
2. *Id.*
3. PA. STAT. ANN. tit. 50, § 7206.
4. *Id.*; PA. STAT. ANN. tit. 50, § 7203.

from treatment.[5] In addition, any responsible party who believes the best interests of the child demand removal from voluntary treatment may petition the Juvenile Division of the Court of Common Pleas to release the child or move the child to a less restrictive treatment.[6] Within 10 days of receiving the petition, the court will appoint an attorney for the minor and will hold a hearing to determine what treatment, if any, is in the minor's best interests.[7]

A person who is being treated as an involuntarily committed inpatient may not leave treatment unless the reasons that justified involuntary treatment no longer exist. A person may be treated on an involuntary basis if the person is found to be severely mentally disabled and in need of immediate treatment.[8] A person is *severely mentally disabled* if, as a result of mental illness, the person's "capacity to exercise self-control, judgment and discretion in the conduct of his affairs and social relations or to care for his own personal needs is so lessened that he poses a clear and present danger of harm to others or to himself."[9]

Whether a person is being treated on a voluntary or involuntary basis, the treatment should be in the "least restrictive alternative consistent with affording the person adequate treatment for his condition."[10] Furthermore, "to the extent possible," the patient should participate in and consent to the treatment plan.[11] The courts have not yet decided whether an involuntary patient who refuses psychotropic medications can be medicated absent the patient's consent.[12]

The criteria for testing competency to refuse life-sustaining treatment mandate that the patient

1. understands his current condition;
2. is able to make independent decisions about his welfare and medical treatment;

---

5. PA. STAT. ANN. tit. 50, § 7206(b).
6. *Id.*
7. *Id.*
8. PA. STAT. ANN. tit. 50, § 7301.
9. *Id.*
10. PA. STAT. ANN. tit. 50, § 7107.
11. PA. STAT. ANN. tit. 50, § 7101; *see In re* Gross, 382 A.2d 116 (Pa. 1978); *see also* Washington v. Harper, 494 U.S. 210 (1990) (mentally ill prisoner can be medicated without consent if dangerous to self or others and if decision to medicate is reviewed by administrative panel); Rennie v. Klein, 750 F.2d 266, 269 (3d Cir. 1983) (involuntary patient has constitutional right to refuse medication, but can be medicated absent consent if patient is dangerous to self or others and if in exercise of professional judgment, medications are necessary to prevent the patient from endangering self or others).
12. *In re Gross,* 382 A.2d at 122, n. 12.

3. understands what would happen if the current condition went untreated;

4. understands what the proposed treatment consists of;

5. understands the complications, benefits, and risks of the proposed treatment; and

6. has the ability to perceive the world realistically, think clearly, and make a judgment of the preceding considerations with an accurate understanding of the consequences of such conduct both physically and emotionally to himself, his family, and his loved ones.[13]

---

13. *Id.*

3.8

Regulation of Aversive and Avoidance Conditioning

Behavioral therapies using aversive stimuli are carefully regulated or prohibited in some states when they are intended for use with developmentally disabled or mentally ill individuals. MHPs employing such methods should be aware of these legal and institutional limits. Neither the Pennsylvania courts nor the legislature has spoken on this issue (but see chapters 8.4 and 8.7). Professional codes of ethics may provide guidance on the use of these techniques.

3.9

Quality Assurance for Hospital Care

The law requires that the governing body of every licensed hospital organize the health care providers with privileges to practice in the hospital into committees to review the professional practices within the hospital for the purposes of reducing morbidity and mortality and for the improvement of care of patients in the hospital.

(A) Peer Review

Health care providers, including hospitals, physicians, nurses, and psychologists, are encouraged to create peer review committees.[1] A peer review committee is a group of health care professionals who meet and evaluate the professional skills and abilities of other members of their profession.

(B) Privilege and Immunity

Persons who in good faith provide information to review committees are immune from civil and criminal liability.[2] Likewise, as long as they are exercising due care and are motivated by concerns for improving patient care, the individuals who serve on review committees are immune from liability as well.[3] Further-

---

1. The Peer Review Protection Act, PA. STAT. ANN. tit. 63, §§ 425.1–425.3; Cooper v. Delaware Valley Medical Ctr., 630 A.2d 1 (Pa. Super. Ct. 1993)
2. PA. STAT. ANN. tit. 63, § 425.3.
3. *Id.*

more, the proceedings and records of a review committee are not subject to discovery and may not be introduced into evidence in a civil action against a health care provider.[4] Otherwise admissible material will not be privileged, however, simply because it was evaluated by a review committee.[5]

---

4. 63 Pa. Cons. Stat. § 425.4.
5. *Id.*

3.10

Malpractice Liability

A malpractice suit is a civil action in which the plaintiff alleges that he or she suffered damages as the consequence of an act or omission by a professional who did not exercise the level of ordinary and reasonable care possessed by the average member of that discipline. In an action for malpractice against MHPs a plaintiff must establish three things. First, the plaintiff must show that the MHP owed the plaintiff a duty of care. Second, the plaintiff must show that the MHP breached that duty. Third, the plaintiff must show that the MHP's breach of the duty of care was the proximate cause of the plaintiff's injury.[1] In this way, plaintiffs prove that the MHP did not exercise the professional skills and knowledge ordinarily exercised by a hypothetical reasonable MHP and that this action caused injury to the plaintiff.

(A) Limitations on Liability

The Pennsylvania legislature has established some limitations on liability for MHPs. The Mental Health and Mental Retardation Act of 1966 provides immunity from civil and criminal liability to persons and government agencies for diagnosis, opinion, reports, or any other treatment covered by the Act.[2] As long as the MHP was acting in good faith—not falsely, corruptly, maliciously, or without reasonable cause—there will be no liability unless the

---

1. Collins v. Hand, 246 A.2d 398 (Pa. 1968); Crivellaro v. Pennsylvania Power & Light Co., 491 A.2d 207 (Pa. Super. Ct. 1985).
2. PA. STAT. ANN. tit. 50, § 4603; *see also* Freach v. Commonwealth, 370 A.2d 1163 (Pa. 1977) (§ 4603 applied to officials of the commonwealth, its governmental components, as well as private persons).

MHP was grossly negligent or incompetent.[3] Under this statute, MHPs are not immune from liability for negligent day-to-day care or treatment of patients, but they are immune from liability for admission and discharge decisions.[4]

In a similar fashion, the Mental Health Procedures Act grants immunity from civil and criminal liability to MHPs who work with mentally ill persons.[5] Absent gross negligence[6] or willful misconduct, an MHP's treatment and decisions about treatment, discharge, and reduction of restraint will be immune from civil and criminal liability.[7] This immunity provision does not apply to cases of voluntary outpatient treatment.[8]

(B) Malpractice Arbitration Panels

Malpractice actions against hospitals, physicians, and their employees and administrators are governed by the Health Care Services Act.[9] All claims covered by this Act must first be presented to an arbitration panel rather than a state or federal court of law.[10] The arbitration panels must consist of three members—one attorney, who will serve as chair and determine the questions of law, one health care provider, and one lay person.[11] The parties are free to appeal the decision of the arbitration panel to the court of common pleas.[12] The court of common pleas conducts appeals from arbitration as if the case had never been presented to any decision-making body.[13]

(C) Statute of Limitations

A plaintiff must bring a malpractice lawsuit within 2 years of the date of the malpractice.[14] This time period may be extended if the

---

3. *Id.*
4. Venesky v. Community Medical Ctr., 30 D. & C.3d 96 (1984).
5. Pa. Stat. Ann. tit. 50, § 7114.
6. *Gross negligence* is "substantially more than ordinary carelessness, inadvertence, laxity, or indifference. . . . Behavior of the defendant must be flagrant, grossly deviating from the ordinary standard of care." Bloom v. Dubois Regional Medical Ctr., 597 A.2d 671, 679 (Pa. Super. Ct. 1991).
7. Pa. Stat. Ann. tit. 50, § 7114; Farago v. Sacred Heart Gen. Hosp., 562 A.2d 300, 304 (Pa. 1989).
8. McKenna v. Mooney, 565 A.2d 495, 496 (Pa. Super. Ct. 1989).
9. Pa. Stat. Ann. tit. 40, §§ 1301.101–1301.1006.
10. Pa. Stat. Ann. tit. 40, § 1301.309.
11. Pa. Stat. Ann. tit. 40, § 1301.308.
12. Pa. Stat. Ann. tit. 40, § 1301.509.
13. *Id.*
14. 42 Pa. Cons. Stat. Ann. § 5524.

plaintiff did not discover the wrongful act until more than 2 years after the event.[15] The time period will not be extended for longer than a reasonable person would have taken to discover the wrongful act.[16] The time period will not be extended because the plaintiff was experiencing mental illness that prevented recognition of the malpractice.[17] The time period will only be extended if an ordinary reasonable person (i.e., not mentally disabled) using reasonable diligence would not have discovered the malpractice.[18]

---

15. *See* A. McD. v. Rosen, 621 A.2d 128, 130 (Pa. Super. Ct. 1993).
16. *Id.* at 131.
17. *A. McD.*, 621 A.2d at 131.
18. *Id.* at 131–132.

Other Forms of
Professional Liability

Because malpractice claims are limited to a narrow class of situations (see chapter 3.10), MHPs may also be faced with lawsuits premised on other theories of civil liability.

(A) Intentional Torts

A *tort* is any action that causes injury to another person. Torts can be a result of negligent or intentional behavior. A tort as a result of negligence occurs when a person fails to use the ordinary care that would be exercised by a "reasonable person" in the same or similar circumstances. Malpractice cases are based on negligent behavior. In lawsuits based on intentional torts, the plaintiff does not have to prove that the defendant intended harmful consequences. The plaintiff must simply prove that the defendant intended to perform the act and knew or should have known the act would produce the consequences.

(A)(1) Defamation of Character

Defamation occurs when one person says or publishes something that damages the reputation and good name of another. Written defamation is called *libel* and spoken defamation is called *slander*. The plaintiff must show that the defendant was negligent (i.e., did not use the ordinary care that would have been exercised by a reasonable person in the same or similar circumstances) or that the defendant acted with reckless disregard in ascertaining the truth or falsity of the defamatory message.[1] There is no defamation if the defendant can show that what was communicated was true or that the defendant was otherwise privileged (legally entitled) to make the communication.[2] A privilege may exist when the communication serves a valuable social purpose. For example, when an MHP, in good faith, conducts and publishes research on the efficacy of a publicly funded mental health treatment program, there is no defamation, even when the publication results in damage to the reputation of the program's director.[3]

(A)(2) Invasion of Privacy

The tort of invasion of privacy exists when one person unreasonably and seriously interferes with another's privacy, causing an impairment of the latter person's ability to lead a secluded and private life, "away from the prying eyes, ears and publications of others."[4] MHPs are bound both legally and ethically to maintain the confidentiality of their patients and clients (see chapters 3.3 and 3.4). If an MHP violated a client's confidentiality, the client would likely have a cause of action for invasion of privacy.

(A)(3) Malicious Prosecution, False Imprisonment, and Abuse of Process

When civil or criminal proceedings are instituted without probable cause, with malice, and the proceedings are terminated in favor of the plaintiff, the plaintiff has a cause of action for malicious prosecution.[5] When one person intentionally confines another person to a limited area and the confined person is aware of the confinement, the person who was confined has a cause of action for false imprisonment.[6] When one person makes "use of legal process against another 'primarily to accomplish a purpose for which it is not designed,' " there is a cause of action for abuse of process.[7] MHPs are afforded some protection from liability in these areas by the Mental Health and Mental Retardation Act of 1966 and the Mental Health Procedures Act (see chapter 3.10).[8]

---

1. *See* Rutt v. Bethlehems' Globe Publishing Co., 484 A.2d 72 (Pa. Super. Ct. 1984); *see also* RESTATEMENT (SECOND) OF TORTS § 580B.
2. *Id.*
3. Doman v. Rosner, 371 A.2d 1002 (Pa. Super. Ct. 1977).
4. Moses v. McWilliams, 549 A.2d 950, 955 (Pa. Super. Ct. 1987) (quoting RESTATEMENT (SECOND) OF TORTS § 652A cmt. b (1977)).
5. Kelley v. General Teamsters, Chauffeurs, and Helpers, Local Union 249, 544 A.2d 940 (Pa. 1988).
6. Gagliardi v. Lynn, 285 A.2d 109, 111 (Pa. 1971).
7. Rosen v. American Bank of Rolla, 627 A.2d 190, 192 (Pa. Super. Ct. 1993) (quoting RESTATEMENT (SECOND) OF TORTS § 682).
8. PA. STAT. ANN. tit. 50, §§ 4603, 7114.

(A)(4) Criminal-Related Acts

An MHP who commits a crime (see chapter 3.12) may also face civil liability for the injury that resulted from the criminal behavior. Criminal charges are brought and prosecuted by the district attorney, whereas a civil complaint is brought and prosecuted by the individual who was injured by the defendant's act.

(B) Other Types of Civil Liability

(B)(1) Breach of Contract

Where two parties agree to exchange things of value, they have formed a contract. If one of the parties fails to meet the terms agreed to, the other party has a cause of action for breach of contract. The remedy for a breach of contract usually will be to put each of the parties in the positions they would have been in if the terms of the contract had been met. MHPs must be careful in defining their contractual relationships with clients. If an MHP communicates to a client that therapy will lead to a cure and the client agrees to pay the MHP for therapy, there is a contract and the MHP will be liable for damages if the client pays for therapy but does not receive a cure.

In some states, physicians and MHPs have a duty to avoid abandoning their patients and clients. In those states, MHPs must discuss termination early enough that the client has adequate opportunity to secure the services of another MHP. Sometimes MHPs are required to assist clients in making these transitions. The tort of abandonment is not recognized in Pennsylvania.[9]

Pennsylvania does, however, recognize the torts of negligent and intentional infliction of emotional distress.[10] *Negligent infliction of emotional distress* occurs when the defendant creates an unreasonable risk of causing bodily harm or emotional disturbance, the plaintiff suffers emotional disturbance, and the emotional disturbance is so severe that it produces bodily harm (e.g., headaches, high blood pressure, etc.).[11] *Intentional infliction of emotional distress* occurs when the defendant's behavior is extreme or outrageous and intentionally or recklessly causes severe emotional distress with physical symptoms.[12]

---

9. Abadie v. Riddle Memorial Hosp., 589 A.2d 1143, 1144 (Pa. Super. Ct. 1991).
10. *Id.*
11. *Id.* at 1145.
12. *Id.* at 1146.

(B)(2) Duty to Warn Third Parties

Some jurisdictions require MHPs to warn or protect third parties when patients or clients threaten to harm someone.[13] Pennsylvania has not yet adopted this rule of law. When the lower courts have had the opportunity to discuss this issue, the opinions have stressed the importance of maintaining therapist–patient confidentiality.[14] Although the courts have not adopted this so-called Tarasoff Rule, it is possible the rule would be adopted if the courts were presented with a case in which an MHP's client made threats to harm a specific individual.[15]

---

13. *See, e.g.,* Tarasoff v. Regents of Univ. of CA, 551 P.2d 334 (Cal. 1976). This was the first case in the United States to develop such a standard of care.
14. Dunkle v. Food Serv. East, Inc., 582 A.2d 1342, 1347 (Pa. Super. Ct. 1990); *see also* Leonard v. LaTrobe Area Hosp., 625 A.2d 1228 (Pa. Super. Ct. 1993).
15. *Dunkle,* 582 A.2d at 1347; *Leonard,* 625 A.2d at 1232.

3.12

Criminal Liability

MHPs who practice in accordance with the ethical principles of their professions will rarely run into conflict with the criminal law. When an MHP breaches professional ethics, it is usually not a crime. There are certain ethical breaches, however, that are also crimes.

(A) Improper Treatment of Mentally Retarded Persons

The legislature has criminalized certain acts that would be harmful to persons residing in facilities providing treatment for mentally retarded persons. Any person who helps a residential client to obtain drugs or alcohol, elope from the facility, be detained or committed to a facility when it is unwarranted, or who discloses confidential information about a residential client or any physician who knowingly makes false representations that lead to the unwarranted detention or commitment of a mentally retarded person will be subject to a fine of up to $1,000 and imprisonment of up to 1 year.[1]

---

1. *See supra* chapter 1.

(B) Sexual Offenses

In Pennsylvania, a person commits the crime of rape if the person engages in "sexual intercourse with another person not his spouse: (1) by forcible compulsion; (2) by threat of forcible compulsion that would prevent resistance by a person of reasonable resolution; (3) who is unconscious; (4) who is so mentally deranged or deficient that such a person is incapable of consent."[2] If an MHP engages in sexual intercourse with a client, the MHP could be found to have committed rape as defined by this criminal statute. Even if the conduct is not rape as defined by this statute, however, the legislature has proposed to criminalize all sexual contact between MHPs and their clients for the duration of treatment and 1 year beyond termination of treatment.[3]

(C) Assault

A person is guilty of assault if the person attempts to cause bodily injury; intentionally, knowingly, or recklessly causes bodily injury; negligently causes bodily injury with a deadly weapon; or "attempts by physical menace to put another in fear of imminent serious bodily injury."[4] A person may use force to resist an assault as long as the force used if not excessive.[5] The resistor does not have any duty to attempt a retreat first.[6] This provision has particular relevance for MHPs who must occasionally deal with violent patients.

(D) Involuntary Manslaughter

If a person causes the death of another by doing a lawful or an unlawful act in a reckless or grossly negligent manner, the person is guilty of involuntary manslaughter, a misdemeanor.[7] The negligence required is greater than ordinary negligence and the fatal consequences of the act must have been foreseeable at the time of the act.[8]

---

2. 18 PA. CONS. STAT. ANN. § 3121.
3. *See in general,* Bisbing, S. B., L. M. Jorgenson, & P. K. Sutherland. (1995). *Sexual abuse by professionals: A legal guide.* Charlottesville, VA: Michie.
4. 18 PA. CONS. STAT. ANN. § 2701.
5. Commonwealth v. Presogna, 292 A.2d 476 (Pa. Super. Ct. 1972).
6. Commonwealth v. Banks, 268 A.2d 230 (Pa. Super. Ct. 1970).
7. 18 PA. CONS. STAT. ANN. § 2504.
8. Commonwealth v. Aurick, 19 A.2d 920 (1941).

3.13

Liability of Credentialing Boards

Credentialing boards, like the State Board of Psychology or the State Board of Social Work Examiners, are arms of the commonwealth and therefore enjoy sovereign immunity. The doctrine of sovereign immunity precludes citizens from bringing lawsuits against the government. The doctrine exists so that the government may govern without having to justify through a lawsuit each action it takes. There are some exceptions to sovereign immunity. The legislature has made an exception for occasions on which a local agency acts negligently and ultimately causes injury to a person as a result of this action and if the agency would be have been liable had it been private rather than governmental.[1]

In the case of credentialing boards, sovereign immunity prevents MHPs who were rejected for licensure or who have been sanctioned from suing the members of the board or the board as an entity. The remedy for an MHP unhappy with the decisions or actions of a credentialing board is to appeal the board's decision to the Commonwealth Court. The court will review the credentialing board's decision for violations of constitutional rights, errors of law, and to determine whether the findings of fact are supported by substantial evidence.[2]

---

1. 42 PA. CONS. STAT. ANN. § 8542.
2. *See, e.g.,* Makris v. Bureau of Professional and Occupational Affairs, 599 A.2d 279, 282 (Pa. Commw. Ct. 1991).

3.14

Antitrust Limitations to Practice

Antitrust laws were enacted to prevent the formation of monopolies and prevent the abuses of economic power. In recent years, health care providers and their organizations have increasingly become defendants in antitrust litigation.

(A) Prohibited Activities

Scrutinized activities include price fixing (an agreement among competitors to establish a common price or a system for setting prices), the division of markets (an agreement among competitors to allocate certain markets to certain participants), a group boycott (an agreement among competitors to patronize only certain businesses), and tying arrangements (an arrangement whereby a party agrees to sell a certain product or service only on the condition that the buyer also purchases a different product). All of these fall under the general prohibition of restraint of trade.

(B) Enforcement of the Law

Enforcement is through federal law in federal court. Pennsylvania is the only jurisdiction that does not have a corresponding state antitrust law.

Families and Juveniles

Competency to Marry

The law provides that a marriage license may not be issued "if either of the applicants for [the] license is weak minded, insane, of unsound mind or is under guardianship as a person of unsound mind unless the court decides that it is for the best interest of the applicant and the general public to issue the license."[1] Thus, some minimum level of mental status is required to get a marriage license. Unfortunately, because of the archaic language, it is unclear what the minimum mental status is. As a practical matter, there is no formal screening for mental status prior to the issuance of a marriage license. Nevertheless, in cases of obvious mental impairment or if a person acknowledges mental impairment on questioning, a license might be denied.

Such a restriction on the issuance of marriage licenses seems to run counter to the current guardianship law (see chapter 4.2), although it may not directly conflict. The guardianship law states that unless there is a specific order after specific findings of fact, a guardian shall not have the power to prohibit the marriage of an incapacitated person.[2]

If a marriage license is issued and a marriage takes place, that marriage may still be invalidated on competency grounds. A marriage is deemed void "where either party to such marriage was incapable of consenting by reason of insanity or serious mental disorder or otherwise lacked capacity to consent or did not intend to consent to the marriage."[3] Capacity to consent requires an ability to understand the nature of the marriage

---

1. 23 PA. CONS. STAT. ANN. § 1304. This statutory provision retains archaic language that has been eliminated elsewhere (see chapter 4.2).
2. 20 PA. CONS. STAT. ANN. § 5521(d).
3. 23 PA. CONS. STAT. ANN. § 3304(a)(3).

contract and its consequent effect.[4] One of the parties to the marriage—or someone on his or her behalf—may have the marriage declared void by a judge through an annulment proceeding (see chapter 4.4). Pennsylvania is one of the few states that still recognizes common-law marriages.[5] Presumably, the same level of capacity would be required for a valid consent to a common-law marriage.

Persons under 18 years of age cannot be married without the consent of a custodial parent or guardian.[6] A person under the age of 16 also must have the approval of a judge.[7]

(A) Standard for Voiding a Marriage

The law distinguishes between void and voidable marriages. If a marriage is deemed void, it never existed from a legal standpoint, no matter what the parties say. If a marriage is deemed voidable, a party has an option of invalidating the marriage. In cases of marriages that are voidable, until a decree of annulment is obtained from a court, the marriage is valid.[8]

A marriage is void in the following cases:

1. where either party at the time of the marriage was still married to a third person, except where that party had obtained a decree of presumed death of the third person;

2. where the parties are too closely related;[9]

3. where either party was incapable of consenting by reason of insanity or serious mental disorder or otherwise lacked capacity to consent or did not intend to consent to the marriage (see chapter 4.1); or

4. where either party to a common-law marriage was under 18 years of age.[10]

Marriages that are void under these rules may be confirmed by cohabitation following the removal of the impediment. For example, if a party who was unable to consent at the time of the

---

4. DeMedio v. DeMedio, 257 A.2d 290 (Pa. Super. Ct. 1969).
5. *See* 23 PA. CONS. STAT. ANN. § 1103.
6. 23 PA. CONS. STAT. ANN. §§ 1304(b), 3304(a), 3305(a).
7. 23 PA. CONS. STAT. ANN. § 1304(b).
8. 23 PA. CONS. STAT. ANN. § 3305(b).
9. A person may not marry his or her parent, aunt, uncle, sibling, child, grandchild, or first cousin. 23 PA. CONS. STAT. ANN. § 1304. Although Section 3304 states that marriages between people who are too closely related are void, Section 1703 states that such marriages are voidable. 23 PA. CONS. STAT. ANN. § 1703.
10. 23 PA. CONS. STAT. ANN. § 3304.

marriage cohabits with the other party after becoming capable of consenting, the marriage may be confirmed and will no longer be void.

4.2

Guardianship for Adults

There are two classes of persons for whom guardianship is generally obtained: minors and incapacitated persons. This chapter is limited to a discussion of guardianship for incapacitated adults. Guardianship for minors is discussed in chapter 4.11.

Guardians may be appointed to assist adult individuals who have significant difficulty making or communicating decisions regarding their personal or financial affairs because of an emotional or cognitive disability. Guardianship is not intended to protect a person from normal daily risks, and should not be used simply because the person makes a poor decision or because the person refuses proffered medical or mental health treatment.

Before a guardian is appointed, the impaired individual must be declared *incapacitated* (prior to 1992, the term used was *incompetent*). An MHP may become involved in this process to certify that attendance at a hearing is detrimental to the alleged incapacitated person.[1] In addition, an MHP may be asked to conduct an evaluation to help determine whether the individual should be declared incapacitated[2] and may be asked to testify at a deposition or in court.[3] An MHP may have a role in advising and implementing interventions as alternatives to guardianship.[4] Furthermore, an MHP may assist the guardian in developing plans of supportive services for wards; in obtaining participation of wards in decisions that affect them; in enabling wards to act on their

---

1. 20 PA. CONS. STAT. ANN. § 5511 (alleged incapacitated person must be present at hearing unless licensed psychologist or physician states person would be harmed by attending hearing).
2. 20 PA. CONS. STAT. ANN. §§ 5511, 5518.
3. 20 PA. CONS. STAT. ANN. § 5518.
4. 20 PA. CONS. STAT. ANN. §§ 5512.1, 5518.

own behalf whenever they are able to do so; and in helping wards to develop or regain the capacity to manage their personal affairs.[5]

(A) Application for Guardianship

"Any person interested in the alleged incapacitated person's welfare" may petition to have that person declared incapacitated and to have a guardian appointed.[6] Written notice of the petition and hearing—"in large type and simple language"—must be given to the alleged incapacitated person.[7] Also, the contents and terms of the petition should be explained in language and terms the individual is most likely to understand.[8]

Right to Counsel
The alleged incapacitated person may have an attorney appointed "if the court deems it appropriate."[9] If appointment of an attorney is appropriate and if the alleged incapacitated person is unable to pay for an attorney, the county must pay for one.[10]

Evaluation
To establish incapacity, the petitioner must present testimony from "individuals qualified by training and experience in evaluating individuals with incapacities of the type alleged by the petitioner."[11] Although at one time evidence of incapacity could only be presented by a physician, this statutory provision, enacted in 1992, suggests that the evaluator's training and experience is more important than the evaluator's title. For example, a speech or hearing specialist may be the appropriate person to evaluate someone with a communication disorder. Courts have accepted expert testimony in guardianship proceedings from psychologists and social workers, among others.[12]

The court may order an independent evaluation. If the alleged incapacitated person requests an independent evaluation and demonstrates a reason for such an evaluation, the court is required to order one.[13] If the alleged incapacitated person is

---

5. 20 Pa. Cons. Stat. Ann. § 5521(a).
6. 20 Pa. Cons. Stat. Ann. § 5511.
7. *Id.*
8. *Id.*
9. *Id.*
10. *Id.*
11. 20 Pa. Cons. Stat. Ann. § 5518.
12. 20 Pa. Cons. Stat. Ann. § 5518.
13. 20 Pa. Cons. Stat. Ann. § 5511(d).

unable to pay for the cost of an evaluation, the court can obligate the county to pay this cost.[14]

(B) Guardianship Hearing

The hearing may be closed to the public and may be held at the residence of the alleged incapacitated person.[15] The alleged incapacitated person may choose to have the hearing with or without a jury.[16] If the alleged incapacitated person is in Pennsylvania, he or she must be present at the hearing unless "the court is satisfied, upon the deposition or testimony of or sworn statement by a physician or licensed psychologist, that his physical or mental condition would be harmed by his presence."[17] The burden of proof is the "clear and convincing evidence" standard.[18]

A person who is institutionalized—for example, a person who has been committed to a mental hospital—is not presumed to be incapacitated.[19]

An emergency guardian may be appointed in appropriate circumstances without a full guardianship hearing, but a full hearing must be held shortly thereafter.[20]

Determining Incapacity

An *incapacitated person* is defined as "an adult whose ability to receive and evaluate information effectively and communicate decisions in any way is impaired to such a significant extent that he is partially or totally unable to manage his financial resources or to meet essential requirements for his physical health and safety."[21] The evaluator's testimony must establish "the nature and extent of the alleged incapacities and disabilities and the person's mental, emotional and physical condition, adaptive behavior and social skills."[22] The petitioner also must present evidence

1. regarding the services being used to meet essential requirements for the alleged incapacitated person's physical health

---

14. 20 PA. CONS. STAT. ANN. § 5511(c).
15. 20 PA. CONS. STAT. ANN. § 5518.
16. *Id.* Juries are rarely requested for guardianship proceedings in Pennsylvania.
17. *Id.*
18. 20 PA. CONS. STAT. ANN. § 5511(a).
19. 20 PA. CONS. STAT. ANN. § 5512.1(f).
20. 20 PA. CONS. STAT. ANN. § 5513.
21. 20 PA. CONS. STAT. ANN. § 5501.
22. 20 PA. CONS. STAT. ANN. § 5518.

and safety, to manage the person's financial resources or to develop or regain the person's abilities;

2. regarding the types of assistance required by the person;

3. concerning why no less restrictive alternatives would be appropriate; and

4. regarding the probability that the person's incapacities will significantly change (i.e., the probability that the person's condition will deteriorate or improve).[23]

Testimony about the capacity of the alleged incapacitated person is subject to cross-examination by counsel for the alleged incapacitated person.[24]

After receiving the evidence outlined previously, the court must make the following specific findings of fact:

1. the nature of any condition or disability that impairs the individual's capacity to make and communicate decisions;

2. the extent of the individual's capacity to make and communicate decisions;

3. the need for guardianship services, if any, in light of such factors as the availability of family, friends, and other supports to assist the individual in making decisions and in light of the existence, if any, of advance directives such as durable powers of attorney or trusts;

4. the type of guardian, limited or plenary, of the person or estate; and

5. the duration of the guardianship.[25]

The statute states that the court shall prefer limited guardianships.[26] If the court finds that a person is partially incapacitated and in need of guardianship services, the court must enter an order appointing a limited guardian with powers consistent with the person's incapacity.[27] The court may appoint a plenary (global) guardian of the person or estate only on a finding that the person is totally incapacitated and in need of plenary guardianship services.[28]

---

23. *Id.*, and § 5518.1.
24. 20 PA. CONS. STAT. ANN. § 5518.1.
25. 20 PA. CONS. STAT. ANN. § 5512.1
26. *Id.*
27. *Id.*
28. 20 PA. CONS. STAT. ANN. §§ 5512.1(c), 5512(e).

(C) Appointment and Authority of the Guardian

The court may appoint as guardian any qualified individual, a corporate fiduciary, a nonprofit corporation, a guardianship support agency, a county agency, or the guardian office at a state facility.[29] If appropriate, the court shall give preference to a person named by the incapacitated person.[30]

The powers granted to a guardian must be consistent with the court's findings of limitations.[31] The powers granted to a guardian of the person may include

1. caring, maintaining, and holding custody of the incapacitated person;

2. designating the place for the incapacitated person to live;

3. ensuring that the incapacitated person receives such training, education, medical, and psychological services and social and vocational opportunities as appropriate, as well as assisting the incapacitated person in developing maximum self-reliance and independence; and

4. providing required consents or approvals on behalf of the incapacitated person.[32]

For a guardian of the estate, the court must specify the portion of the assets or income over which the guardian of the estate is assigned powers and duties.[33] Except in those areas over which the limited guardian has power as designated by court order, a partially incapacitated person retains all legal rights.[34]

The court may not grant the guardian powers controlled by other statutes, such as the power to admit an incapacitated person to an inpatient psychiatric facility or the power to consent on behalf of the incapacitated person to relinquishment of the person's parental rights.[35] Also, without prior court approval, a guardian may *not*, on behalf of the incapacitated person,

1. consent to an abortion, sterilization, psychosurgery, electro-convulsive therapy, or removal of a healthy body organ;

2. prohibit marriage or consent to divorce (see chapters 4.1 and 4.5); or

---

29. 20 PA. CONS. STAT. ANN. § 5511(f).
30. *Id.*
31. 20 PA. CONS. STAT. ANN. §§ 5512.1(b), 5512.1(d).
32. 20 PA. CONS. STAT. ANN. § 5512.1(b).
33. 20 PA. CONS. STAT. ANN. § 5512.1(d).
34. 20 PA. CONS. STAT. ANN. § 5512.1.
35. 20 PA. CONS. STAT. ANN. § 5521.

3. consent to participation in experiments or receipt of experimental treatment.[36]

It is the duty of the guardian of the person to assert the rights and best interests of the incapacitated person. Expressed wishes and preferences of the incapacitated person must be respected to the greatest possible extent. Where appropriate, the guardian must participate in the development of a plan of supportive services to meet the person's needs that explains how services will be obtained. The guardian must also encourage the incapacitated person to participate in all decisions that affect him or her, to act on his or her own behalf whenever he or she is able to do so, and to develop or regain the capacity to manage his or her personal affairs.[37]

(D) Review of Guardianship and Annual Reports

The court may set a date for a review hearing in its order establishing the guardianship or hold a review hearing at any time it shall direct. The court must conduct a review hearing on petition if there is a significant change in the person's capacity or the need for guardianship services, or if the guardian fails to perform his or her duties or fails to act in the best interests of the incapacitated person.[38] The guardian must file an annual report and a final report as specified in the statute.[39]

---

36. *Id.*
37. 20 PA. CONS. STAT. ANN. § 5521(a).
38. 20 PA. CONS. STAT. ANN. § 5512.2(a).
39. 20 PA. CONS. STAT. ANN. § 5521(c).

4.3

Conservatorship for Adults

Many states use the term *guardianship* in proceedings relating to care of the person and the term *conservatorship* for proceedings relating to care of property. Some states use the term *conservatorship* to refer to both types of proceedings. Pennsylvania law uses the term *guardianship* when referring to proceedings relating to care of persons or property.

Annulment

Annulment is the process whereby a marriage is declared void and is legally held never to have existed. This distinction between annulment and divorce—which dissolves what was once a valid, functioning marriage—has legal significance. For instance, a widowed spouse of a worker receives compensation benefits until the widow remarries, and if the second marriage ceases by virtue of an annulment rather than divorce, the person regains the benefits. MHPs may contribute to annulment proceedings when annulments are sought on certain grounds, directly through evaluation and testimony or indirectly when they are working with persons who are contemplating the dissolution of their marriage.

(A) Grounds for Annulment

A marriage is voidable and subject to annulment in the following cases:

1. where either party to the marriage was under 16 years of age and the marriage was not authorized by a court;

2. where either party was 16 or 17 years of age, did not have the consent of a parent or guardian, and has not subsequently ratified the marriage on reaching 18 years of age;

3. where either party to the marriage was under the influence of alcohol or drugs;

4. where either party to the marriage was at the time of the marriage and still is incurably impotent unless the condition was known to the other party prior to the marriage; or

5. where one party was induced to enter the marriage because of fraud, duress, coercion, or force attributable to the other party and there has been no subsequent voluntary cohabitation after knowledge of the fraud or release from the effects of fraud, duress, coercion, or force.[1]

In some cases, the action for annulment must begin within 60 days after the marriage ceremony.[2] The validity of a voidable marriage may be confirmed subsequently by the parties to the marriage.[3]

In all cases in which an alleged marriage has been contracted that is void or voidable, either party may bring an action in annulment to have the marriage declared void.[4] Where the validity of a marriage is denied or doubted, either or both of the parties may seek a declaration of the validity or invalidity of the marriage. On proof of the validity or invalidity of the marriage, the marriage shall be declared valid or invalid by decree of the court.[5] In the case of a purported common-law marriage in which a party was under 18 years of age, a parent or guardian of the minor may bring a declaratory judgment proceeding during the party's minority to have the marriage declared void.[6]

MHPs may be consulted where the validity of a marriage is contested on the ground that a party lacked the capacity to consent to the marriage (see chapter 4.1). They also may be consulted where it is alleged that a party was induced to enter the marriage by duress or coercion.

---

1. 23 PA. CONS. STAT. ANN. § 3305.
2. Id.
3. Id.
4. 23 PA. CONS. STAT. ANN. § 3303(a).
5. 23 PA. CONS. STAT. ANN. § 3306.
6. 23 PA. CONS. STAT. ANN. § 3303(b).

Divorce

Prior to 1980, divorce law in Pennsylvania, as in many states, required the petitioning party to allege fault by the other spouse. In 1980, Pennsylvania added "no-fault" grounds to the traditional fault grounds for obtaining divorces. Because the fault grounds are used less often, litigation generally centers around property division, child and spousal support, alimony, and child custody (see chapter 4.6). MHPs may come into contact with this process through clients who are divorced, divorcing, or contemplating divorce. MHPs may provide counseling that is mandated through Pennsylvania's divorce law. An MHP may perform an evaluation of a party's functioning because that party's earning capacity is in question, or the MHP may perform a child custody evaluation. Some MHPs are now becoming involved as mediators to resolve economic and child custody disputes between parties.

(A) Divorce Procedure

An action for divorce begins with the filing of a complaint with the Court of Common Pleas. After appropriate proceedings, the court may either dismiss the complaint or enter a decree of divorce or annulment.[1] Although procedures vary somewhat from county to county, they may include hearings before conference officers (who may or may not be lawyers) and masters (who are lawyers), as well as hearings before judges. If either party desires any matter of fact that is affirmed by one and denied by

---

1. 23 Pa. Cons. Stat. Ann. § 3323(a).

the other to be tried by a jury, that party may petition to have that matter of fact tried by a jury.[2]

Where the matters are raised, a decree granting a divorce or annulment must include an order determining property rights between the parties, custody and visitation rights, child support, alimony, reasonable attorney fees, costs and expenses, and any other related matters, including the enforcement of agreements between the parties.[3] In some cases, the court may enter a decree granting a divorce before resolving the other issues.[4]

In certain cases, the court may order a party to provide health care coverage for a spouse or children or to pay uncovered health care expenses.[5] Health care expenses may include expenses for psychological or psychiatric services if those services are specified in the order.[6]

Grounds for Divorce

A "fault" divorce may be granted to the "innocent and injured spouse" on grounds of desertion, adultery, cruel and barbarous treatment, bigamy, imprisonment for 2 or more years for a criminal conviction, and indignities.[7] The court also may grant a divorce on the ground that insanity or serious mental disorder has resulted in confinement in a mental institution for 18 months before the commencement of the action in the case in which there is no reasonable prospect that the spouse will be discharged from inpatient care during the 18 months subsequent to the commencement of the action.[8]

A no-fault divorce may be granted where both parties consent, it is alleged that the marriage is irretrievably broken, and 90 days have elapsed from the date of commencement of the divorce action.[9] *Irretrievable breakdown* is defined as "estrangement due to marital difficulties with no reasonable prospect of reconciliation."[10]

The court also may grant a no-fault divorce in cases in which it determines that the parties have lived separate and apart for a period of at least 2 years and that the marriage is irretrievably broken, or in which the defendant spouse does not deny the plaintiff spouse's allegations that the parties have lived separate and apart for a period of at least 2 years and that the marriage is

---

2. 23 PA. CONS. STAT. ANN. § 3322. Juries are rarely used in divorce matters.
3. 23 PA. CONS. STAT. ANN. § 3323(b).
4. 23 PA. CONS. STAT. ANN. § 3323(c).
5. 23 PA. CONS. STAT. ANN. §§ 4324, 4326; PA. R. CIV. P. 1910.16-5.
6. 23 PA. CONS. STAT. ANN. § 4326; PA. R. CIV. P. 1910.16-5.
7. 23 PA. CONS. STAT. ANN. § 3301(a).
8. 23 PA. CONS. STAT. ANN. § 3301(b).
9. 23 PA. CONS. STAT. ANN. § 3301(c).
10. 23 PA. CONS. STAT. ANN. § 3103.

irretrievably broken.[11] If a party denies one or more of the allegations in a divorce complaint on the ground of irretrievable breakdown and the court determines that there is a reasonable prospect
of reconciliation, the court must continue the matter for at least 90
days and not more than 120 days unless the parties agree to a
period in excess of 120 days. If the parties have not reconciled at
the expiration of the time period and one party states under oath
that the marriage is irretrievably broken, the court must determine whether the marriage is irretrievably broken. If the court
determines that this is the case, the court must grant the divorce.
Otherwise, the court must deny the divorce.[12]

Competency to Divorce
Much as there is a minimum mental capacity required to get
married (see chapter 4.1), there is a minimum mental capacity
necessary to get divorced. The Superior Court has stated that to
institute a divorce proceeding, a spouse at least must have the
capacity to exercise reasonable judgment as to personal decisions,
understand the nature of the action, and express unequivocally a
desire to dissolve the marriage.[13] Even if a guardian (see chapter
4.2) or guardian *ad litem* (see chapter 4.11) is appointed for the
spouse, the spouse must still meet these criteria.[14]

Counseling
Pennsylvania's divorce law provides that the court may mandate
counseling in certain circumstances. Whenever indignities is the
ground for divorce, the court must require counseling where a
party requests it.[15] Whenever mutual consent is the ground for
divorce, the court must require counseling within the 90 days
following the commencement of the action where a party requests
it.[16] As noted previously, if a party denies allegations in a divorce
complaint on the ground of irretrievable breakdown and the
court determines that there is a reasonable prospect of reconciliation, the court must continue the matter for at least 90 days.
During this period, the court must require counseling where a
party requests it.[17] Also, in a divorce on the ground of irretrievable breakdown, the court may require counseling where the

---

11. 23 PA. CONS. STAT. ANN. § 3301(d).
12. 23 PA. CONS. STAT. ANN. § 3301(d).
13. Syno v. Syno, 594 A.2d 307 (Pa. Super. Ct. 1991).
14. *Id.*
15. 23 PA. CONS. STAT. ANN. § 3302(a).
16. 23 PA. CONS. STAT. ANN. § 3302(b).
17. 23 PA. CONS. STAT. ANN. §§ 3301(d), 3302(c).

parties have at least one child under 16 years of age.[18] The court may require a maximum of three counseling sessions.[19]

The choice of a qualified professional is at the option of the parties, and the professional need not be selected from a list provided by the court.[20] The term *qualified professionals* is defined to include "marriage counselors, psychologists, psychiatrists, social workers, ministers, priests, rabbis or other persons who by virtue of their training and experience, [who] are able to provide counseling."[21] There is a specific statutory provision stating that confidential communications made to such qualified professionals shall be privileged and inadmissible as evidence in divorce and custody proceedings.[22]

Evaluations of Earning Capacity
When a party files for child support, spousal support, alimony *pendente lite*[23] or alimony, the actual earnings of the parties and their earning capacities become relevant.[24] Specifically with regard to alimony, where a divorce decree has been entered, the court may award alimony to either party only if it finds that alimony is necessary.[25] In determining whether alimony is necessary and in determining the nature, amount, duration, and manner of payment of alimony, the court must consider all relevant factors.[26] The factors that the court is to consider include the physical, mental, and emotional conditions of the parties; the relative earnings and earning capacities of the parties; the relative education of the parties and the time necessary to acquire sufficient education or training to enable the party seeking alimony to find appropriate employment; the relative needs of the parties; and whether the party seeking alimony is incapable of self-support through appropriate employment.[27]

MHPs may become involved in alimony or support proceedings to determine whether a party's mental or emotional functioning will interfere with his or her ability to obtain and maintain employment. MHPs may be asked to conduct formal vocational evaluations to assist the court in determining an appropriate earning capacity for a party.

---

18. 23 PA. CONS. STAT. ANN. § 3302(c).
19. 23 PA. CONS. STAT. ANN. § 3302.
20. 23 PA. CONS. STAT. ANN. § 3302(e).
21. 23 PA. CONS. STAT. ANN. § 3103.
22. 42 PA. CONS. STAT. ANN. § 5948.
23. Spousal support and alimony *pendente lite* are two different types of financial support that may be paid to a spouse prior to the entry of a divorce decree.
24. *See, e.g.*, 23 PA. CONS. STAT. ANN. § 4322(a); PA. R. CIV. P. 1910.16-5(c).
25. 23 PA. CONS. STAT. ANN. § 3701(a).
26. 23 PA. CONS. STAT. ANN. § 3701(b).
27. *Id.*

4.6

Child Custody After Marital Dissolution

Child custody determinations can result from changes in the legal status of a marriage—such as separation, annulment, or divorce—or a parent who was never married to the other parent may bring a custody action. In certain circumstances, custody actions may be brought by grandparents, nonrelatives, or the state. Parents or other parties may at any time bring an action to modify an existing custody agreement or order.

MHPs may become involved in child custody determinations in several ways. First, one or more parties or the court may request an evaluation of one or more parties or children to assist in determining the most appropriate custody or visitation arrangement.[1] This evaluation may culminate in a court appearance as an expert witness. Second, an MHP who has provided services to one or more parties or children, whether diagnostic or therapeutic, may be subpoenaed by either party to present evidence as a witness. Third, an MHP may become involved as a mediator to help the parties reach an agreement on the most appropriate custody or visitation arrangement. Fourth, an MHP may be asked to counsel the parties or assist them in addressing parenting issues that arise before or after a custody or visitation arrangement has been determined.

---

1. Ethical issues may arise if an MHP renders an opinion without fully evaluating all parties to a custody dispute. See American Psychological Association. (1992). Ethical principles of psychologists and code of conduct. *American Psychologist, 47,* 1597; American Psychological Association. (1991). Guidelines for child custody evaluations in divorce proceedings. *American Psychologist, 49,* 677; Committee on Ethical Guidelines for Forensic Psychologists. (1991). Specialty guidelines for forensic psychologists. *Law and Human Behavior, 15,* 655.

(A) Categories and Degrees of Custody

There are a number of different types and degrees of child custody. *Legal custody* refers to the legal right to make major decisions affecting the child, including, but not limited to, medical, religious, and educational decisions.[2] Ordinarily, day-to-day decisions are made by the party with physical custody.

Physical custody is the actual physical possession and control of a child.[3] *Partial physical custody* refers to the right to take possession of a child away from the custodial parent for a certain period of time.[4]

Visitation is the right to visit a child; the term does not include the right to remove a child from the custodial parent's control.[5] It merely means that the party may spend time with the child while the child is in the control of another person. This term is sometimes used inappropriately by courts and practitioners to mean partial physical custody.

Shared custody is an order awarding shared legal or shared physical custody, or both, of a child in such a way as to ensure the child frequent and continuing contact with and physical access to both parents.[6] Shared physical custody does not necessarily provide the parties with equal physical possession. For example, one party with shared physical custody may have physical custody throughout the week and the other may exercise custody on designated weekends. In this instance, one party has primary physical custody and the other partial physical custody. Shared legal custody means that the parties have equal rights to make major decisions affecting the child.

Sole custody is the award of legal or physical custody to one party to the exclusion of the other party.[7]

---

2. 23 PA. CONS. STAT. ANN. § 5302.
3. *Id.*
4. *Id.*
5. *Id.*
6. *Id.*
7. 23 PA. CONS. STAT. ANN. § 5303.

(B) Standard in Custody Determinations: Best Interests of the Child

The paramount consideration in custody determinations is the best interests of the child.[8] To ascertain the child's best interests, the court is required to "consider all factors which legitimately impact upon the child's physical, intellectual, moral and spiritual well-being on a case by case basis in deciding how to allocate post-divorce parental authority via legal and physical custody."[9] These factors can include, among other things, the respective parties' parenting skills, past conduct, new relationships, relative stability, work schedules, and ages of the parent; the needs of the child, the child's preference, and the custody arrangements of siblings; the geographic proximity of the parties, relocation of a party, and, to some extent, religion. The court is required to consider each parent and adult household member's violent and abusive conduct.[10] The court also is mandated to consider which parent is more likely to encourage, permit, and allow frequent and continuing contact and physical access between the noncustodial parent and the child.[11] If both parents are equally fit and the child is young, positive consideration is to be given to the party who has been the primary caregiver of the child in the past.[12] Courts no longer rely on the "tender years" presumption that awarded custody of young children to their mothers.[13]

The legislature has declared that it is the public policy of Pennsylvania, when in the best interests of the child, to ensure a reasonable and continuing contact of the child with both parents after a separation or dissolution of the marriage and the sharing of the rights and responsibilities of child rearing by both parents.[14] Nonetheless, the court must award sole custody when it is in the best interest of the child.[15]

An order for shared custody may be awarded when it is in the best interest of the child:

1. on application of one or both parents;

---

8. McMillen v. McMillen, 602 A.2d 845 (Pa. 1992).
9. Zummo v. Zummo, 574 A.2d 1130 (Pa. Super. Ct. 1990).
10. 23 PA. CONS. STAT. ANN. § 5303.
11. *Id.*
12. Mumma v. Mumma, 550 A.2d 1341 (Pa. Super. Ct. 1988); *Com. ex rel.* Jordan, 448 A.2d 1113 (Pa. Super. Ct. 1982); *Com. ex rel.* Williams v. Miller, 385 A.2d 992 (Pa. Super. Ct. 1978).
13. Haag v. Haag, 485 A.2d 1189 (Pa. Super. Ct. 1984).
14. 23 PA. CONS. STAT. ANN. § 5301.
15. 23 PA. CONS. STAT. ANN. § 5303(d).

2. when the parties have agreed to an award of shared custody; or

3. in the discretion of the court.[16]

The Superior Court has announced four factors for courts to consider in deciding whether to order shared custody:

1. the fitness of the parents;

2. the expressed desire of both parents to seek continuing active involvement in the child's life;

3. a relationship between the child and both parents; and

4. the capacity of the parents of a minimum of cooperation with each other.[17]

There is no presumption for or against shared custody.[18] In most circumstances, however, Pennsylvania courts will award two fit parents shared legal custody and shared—though not necessarily equal—physical custody.

To obtain visitation rights—as opposed to partial custody rights—a party must show merely that it is in the child's best interest to have some time with that party.[19] Natural parents, even when they have lost custody of their children, will be awarded visitation "except in extreme circumstances."[20] It will be denied in cases in which the party's "mental or moral deficiencies pose a threat to the child."[21]

Grandparents, Other Relatives, and Nonrelatives

Parents begin custody actions on an even footing.[22] There are different rules for grandparents. The legislature has provided for grandparent partial physical custody or visitation in three instances:

1. when one parent has died;

2. when the parents are divorced or are separated for 6 months or more; or

3. when the child has lived with the grandparents for 1 year or more.[23]

---

16. 23 PA. CONS. STAT. ANN. § 5304.
17. *In re* Wesley, J.K., 445 A.2d 1243 (Pa. Super. Ct. 1982).
18. Zummo v. Zummo, 574 A.2d 1130, 1137 (Pa. Super. Ct. 1990).
19. *Com. ex rel.* Williams v. Miller, 385 A.2d 992 (Pa. Super. Ct. 1978).
20. *In re* Mary Kathryn T., 629 A.2d 988 (Pa. Super. Ct. 1993); *In re* Long, 459 A.2d 403, 405 (Pa. Super. Ct. 1983).
21. Vanaman v. Cowgill, 526 A.2d 1226, 1227 (Pa. Super. Ct. 1987).
22. Sawko v. Sawko, 625 A.2d 692 (Pa. Super. Ct. 1993).
23. 23 PA. CONS. STAT. ANN. §§ 5311–5313.

These statutes do not provide a basis for a grandparent to petition for legal custody or for sole, equally shared, or primary physical custody, although there may be circumstances in which a court would award such custody to a grandparent (e.g., if the parents agreed or if the parents were unfit).

If a parent of a child is deceased, the parents or grandparents of the deceased parent may be granted reasonable partial custody or visitation rights on a finding that such rights would be in the best interest of the child and would not interfere with the parent–child relationship.[24] In the context of proceedings for divorce or annulment, or when parents have been separated for 6 months or more, the court may, on application of the parent or grandparent of a party, grant reasonable partial custody or visitation rights if it finds that such rights would be in the best interests of the child and would not interfere with the parent–child relationship.[25] In both of these types of cases, the court must consider the amount of personal contact between the parents or grandparents of the deceased parent or party and the child prior to the application.[26] If a child has resided with his or her grandparents or great-grandparents for a period of 12 months or more and is subsequently removed from the home by the parents, the grandparents or great-grandparents may petition the court for an order granting them reasonable partial custody or visitation rights to the child. The court must grant the petition if it finds that such rights would be in the best interest of the child and would not interfere with the parent–child relationship.[27] The provisions relating to grandparent custody and visitation do not apply if the child has been adopted by a person other than a stepparent or grandparent.

Relatives other than grandparents and nonrelatives historically have had a heavy burden to overcome before they would be awarded custody of a child when a parent was seeking custody of that child. At the very least, third parties had to prove with convincing reasons that it would be in the child's best interests to have custody lie with them.[28] More recently, however, the Pennsylvania Supreme Court has suggested that the burden for third parties may not be as great, although parenthood is a "factor of significant weight."[29] The state may obtain custody over a child in three ways:

1. by consent of the parent or guardian;

---

24. 23 Pa. Cons. Stat. Ann. § 5311.
25. 23 Pa. Cons. Stat. Ann. § 5312.
26. 23 Pa. Cons. Stat. Ann. §§ 5311, 5312.
27. 23 Pa. Cons. Stat. Ann. § 5313.
28. Ellerbe v. Hooks, 416 A.2d 512 (Pa. 1980).
29. Rowles v. Rowles, 668 A.2d 126 (Pa. 1995).

2. through a dependency action; or

3. by a delinquency adjudication (see chapter 4.15).[30]

(C) Custody Evaluations

The court may order children or parties to submit to evaluations by appropriate experts.[31] Experts are required to deliver detailed written reports setting out findings, results of all tests made, diagnoses, and conclusions within time limits provided in the rules of civil procedure.[32]

In conducting child custody evaluations, MHPs should be aware of statutory provisions and case law governing child custody determinations.[33]

Counseling

The court may require the parents to attend counseling sessions and may consider the recommendations of the counselors prior to entering a custody order. These counseling sessions may include, but shall not be limited to, discussions of the responsibilities and decision-making arrangements involved in different custody arrangements and the suitability of each arrangement to the capabilities of each parent or both parents.[34] The court may require the counselor to submit a report if the court desires and within such reasonable time as the court determines.[35] Even after the court has entered a custody order, the court may require the parties to participate in counseling designed to address ongoing parenting issues.

If a parent has been convicted of or has pleaded guilty or no contest to certain criminal offenses, in making a determination to award custody, partial custody, or visitation to that parent, the court is required to appoint a qualified professional to provide counseling to the parent. The court must take testimony from the professional regarding the provision of such counseling prior to issuing any order of custody, partial custody, or visitation. If the court awards custody, partial custody, or visitation to an offending parent, the court may require subsequent periodic counseling and reports on the rehabilitation of the offending parent and the well-being of the child. If, after hearing these reports, the

---

30. 23 PA. CONS. STAT. ANN. § 2511.
31. PA. R. CIV. P. 1915.8(a).
32. PA. R. CIV. P. 1915.8.
33. *See also* American Psychological Association. (1994). Guidelines for child custody evaluations. *American Psychologist, 49,* 677.
34. 23 PA. CONS. STAT. ANN. § 5305(a).
35. 23 PA. CONS. STAT. ANN. § 5303(c).

court determines that the offending parent poses a threat of harm to the child, the court may schedule a hearing and modify the order of custody or visitation to protect the well-being of the child.[36]

Courts in some Pennsylvania counties are now mandating educational programs for parties engaged in custody litigation. Some courts are encouraging parties to participate in mediation to attempt to resolve custody disputes.

---

36. *Id.*

4.7

Reporting of Adult Abuse

The law requires certain individuals who have reasonable cause to believe that a person is being abused, mistreated, or neglected in a nursing home or residential health care facility to make a report. However, there is no legal duty on any person to report probable abuse in domestic settings, although such abuse or neglect is a crime.

(A) Who Must Report

Some states have laws that require certain professionals to report known or suspected abuse, neglect, or exploitation of adults; Pennsylvania does not. However, any person having reasonable cause to believe that an older adult (60 years of age or older) is in need of protective services may report such information to the agency that is the local provider of protective services.[1] Pennsylvania's Older Adults Protective Services Act is designed to provide protective services to older adults who lack the capacity to protect themselves and are at imminent risk of abuse, neglect, exploitation, or abandonment.[2]

In addition, the Protection From Abuse Act states that any person having reasonable cause to believe that a person is being abused may report the information to the local police department.[3] Under the Protection From Abuse Act, a court may direct a defendant to refrain from abusing a person, may order the defendant to temporarily relinquish weapons, may grant possession of

---

1. 35 PA. CONS. STAT. ANN. § 10215.
2. 35 PA. CONS. STAT. ANN. § 10212.
3. 23 PA. CONS. STAT. ANN. § 6115.

a residence to a person to the exclusion of the defendant, may award temporary custody or visitation rights, may prohibit the defendant from having contact with a person, and may direct the defendant to refrain from stalking or harassing a person.[4] The court may also order the defendant to pay support or pay for losses suffered as a result of abuse.[5]

Older Adults Protective Services Act
The Older Adults Protective Services Act[6] defines certain key terms as follows:

1. An *older adult in need of protective services* is defined as an incapacitated person who cannot perform or obtain services necessary to maintain physical or mental health, who lacks a responsible caregiver, and whose person or property is at imminent risk of danger. A legal finding of incapacity is not necessary (see chapter 4.2).

2. *Abandonment* is defined as the desertion of an older adult by a caretaker.

3. *Abuse* is defined as the infliction of injury, unreasonable confinement, intimidation, or punishment with resulting physical harm, pain, or mental anguish. In addition, the willful deprivation by a caretaker of goods or services that are necessary to maintain physical or mental health is considered abuse. Furthermore, sexual harassment and rape are specifically defined as abuse.

4. *Exploitation* is defined as an act or course of conduct, without the informed consent of the older adult or with consent obtained through misrepresentation, coercion, or threats of force, that results in gain for the perpetrator and loss to the older adult.

5. *Neglect* is defined as the failure to provide for oneself or the failure of a caretaker to provide goods or services essential to avoid a clear and serious threat to physical or mental health.

6. *Protective services* are those activities, resources, and supports provided to older adults to detect, prevent, reduce, or eliminate abuse, neglect, exploitation, and abandonment.[7]

Protection From Abuse Act
Under the Protection From Abuse Act, abuse is defined as the occurrence of certain acts between family or household members,

---

4. 23 PA. CONS. STAT. ANN. § 6108(a).
5. *Id.*
6. 35 PA. CONS. STAT. ANN. § 10213.
7. *Id.*

sexual or intimate partners, or persons who share biological parenthood. These acts include attempting to cause or causing bodily injury, rape, spousal sexual assault, or involuntary deviate sexual intercourse; placing a person in fear of imminent serious bodily injury by physical menace; falsely imprisoning a person; and physically or sexually abusing minor children.[8]

(B) Immunity From Liability

Any person who makes a report under the Older Adults Protective Services Act or the Protection From Abuse Act is immune from civil and criminal liability for the report unless the person acted in bad faith or with malicious purpose.[9] If the reporter of the abuse, however, is also the perpetrator of the abuse, immunity does not apply.[10]

(C) Confidentiality and Privilege

Confidentiality and privilege grant broad immunity from legal liability for making a report. These grants of immunity suggest that MHPs can make reports without fear of liability for breaching the legal and ethical duty of confidentiality. The Protection From Abuse Act provides, however, that unless a victim consents in writing, a domestic violence counselor–advocate[11] shall not disclose confidential communications made to or by the counselor–advocate by or to a victim of domestic violence (see chapters 3.3, 3.4).

The Protection From Abuse Act and Older Adults Protective Services Act do not require the MHP to breach client confidentiality.

The Older Adults Protective Services Act provides some specific rules for preserving the confidentiality of protective service agency records. The release of information that would identify the person who made a report under the Act or cooperated in a subsequent investigation is prohibited, unless the Secretary of Aging of the Commonwealth can determine that such a release will not be detrimental to the safety of such person.

---

8. 23 Pa. Cons. Stat. Ann. § 6102(a).
9. 35 Pa. Cons. Stat. Ann. § 10215(d); 23 Pa. Cons. Stat. Ann. § 6115(c).
10. 35 Pa. Cons. Stat. Ann. § 10215(d).
11. A *domestic violence counselor–advocate* is defined in the statute as an individual who is engaged in a domestic violence program, who provides services to victims of domestic violence, who has undergone 40 hours of training, and who is under the control of a direct services supervisor of a domestic violence program. 23 Pa. Cons. Stat. Ann. § 6102(a).

Reporting of Child Abuse

The law requires that persons who, in the course of their employment, occupation, or practice of their profession, come into contact with a child whom they have reason to believe is being abused, are required to report the suspected abuse to the county child protective service.[1] The definition of *child abuse* in the Child Protective Services Law is set forth in chapter 4.9 of this volume.

(A) Who Must and May Report

Those required to report include, among others, mental health professionals, physicians, interns, nurses, social services workers, school teachers, school administrators, day care center workers, other child-care or foster-care workers, police officers, law enforcement officials, and anyone who comes into contact with children in the course of his or her employment, occupation, or practice of a profession.[2] An MHP does not need to be licensed or certified to be bound by the reporting requirement.

In addition to those persons who are required to report suspected child abuse, any person is permitted to make such a

---

1. 23 PA. CONS. STAT. ANN. § 6311(a). It is essential to emphasize that in Pennsylvania, a report is only required when the relevant professional actually sees the child, as opposed to hearing about it from a parent.
2. 23 PA. CONS. STAT. ANN. §§ 6311(a)–(b). Whenever a staff member of an institution is required to report, that person must immediately notify the person in charge of the institution or the designated agent of the person in charge. The person in charge or the designated agent must then assume the legal obligation to report or cause a report to be made. 23 PA. CONS. STAT. ANN. § 6311(c).

report if that person has reasonable cause to suspect that a child is abused.[3]

(B) When a Report Must Be Made

The requirement to report is triggered when the professional comes into contact with the child in the course of his or her professional duties or employment. The child must come before the MHP in his or her "professional or official capacity."[4] Second-hand reports of abuse, even if they are admissions made by the abuser, do not trigger the requirement to report.

The law pertains only to past events, not to abuse or neglect that may occur in the future. There is no requirement that the abuse be continuing and there is no statute of limitations on reporting. Thus, even if the abuse occurred some time ago and is no longer occurring, the MHP is still required to report.

The fact that the abuser is seeking treatment for the child does not absolve the mandated reporter of the duty to report.

(C) How a Report Must Be Made

An oral report must be made immediately by telephone to the appropriate child protective service.[5] A written report must follow the oral report within 48 hours.[6] The written report must be made to the appropriate child protective service in a manner and on forms prescribed by regulation.[7] The written forms must include the following information if available:

1. the names and addresses of the child and the parents or other person responsible for the care of the child;
2. where the suspected abuse occurred;
3. the age and gender of the child;
4. the nature and extent of the suspected abuse, including any evidence of prior abuse to the child or siblings of the child;
5. the name of the person or persons responsible for causing the suspected abuse;
6. family composition;

---

3. 23 PA. CONS. STAT. ANN. § 6312.
4. 23 PA. CONS. STAT. ANN. § 6311(a).
5. 23 PA. CONS. STAT. ANN. § 6313(a).
6. *Id.*
7. 23 PA. CONS. STAT. ANN. § 6313(c).

7. the relationship of the suspected perpetrator to the child;

8. the name of the person making the report;

9. the person making the report and where that person can be reached;

10. the actions taken by the reporting source, including the taking of photographs and x-rays, removal or keeping of the child, or notifying the medical examiner or coroner; and

11. any other information that may be required by regulation.[8]

(D) Immunity From Liability

Any person or institution participating in good faith in the making of a report, cooperating with an investigation, or testifying in a proceeding arising out of an instance of suspected child abuse is immune from civil and criminal liability for those actions.[9] Mandated reporters are presumed to act in good faith in reporting suspected abuse.[10]

(E) Confidentiality and Privilege

A claim of privileged communication between a professional required to report and the patient or client of that professional is not a basis for failure to report.[11] A claim of privileged communication, except between lawyer and client or minister and penitent, will not be grounds for excluding evidence in a child abuse proceeding.[12]

(F) Failure to Report

A mandated reporter who willfully fails to report a case of suspected child abuse commits a summary offense for the first violation. A second or subsequent violation is a third-degree misdemeanor.[13]

---

8. *Id.*
9. 23 PA. CONS. STAT. ANN. § 6318(a).
10. 23 PA. CONS. STAT. ANN. § 6318(b).
11. 23 PA. CONS. STAT. ANN. § 6311(a).
12. 23 PA. CONS. STAT. ANN. § 6381(c).
13. 23 PA. CONS. STAT. ANN. § 6319.

4.9

Abused and Neglected Children

Procedures for handling child abuse and neglect cases typically involve three stages: taking the child into protective custody, holding a fact-finding hearing, and holding a dispositional hearing. It is generally a hierarchical process that may stop at any point if the allegations are unfounded or on a showing that the parents are currently capable of raising their children in a responsible manner.

Three Pennsylvania civil statutes permit state intervention to protect children from abuse and neglect: the Juvenile Act, the Child Protective Services Law, and the Protection From Abuse Act. These statutes may be employed singularly or in concert. MHPs may be called on to evaluate the abused or neglected child and the alleged abuser(s). In addition, MHPs may be asked to report to a child protective services worker or to testify at an abuse or dependency proceeding.

Neglect: Juvenile Act

The primary authority for intervention in cases of neglect is the Pennsylvania Juvenile Act.[1] A judicial determination of "dependency" is required before the state may exercise jurisdiction and enter an order of court providing for the disposition of a child. One definition of a *dependent child* is a child who "is without proper parental care or control, subsistence, education as required by law, or other care or control necessary for his physical, mental, or emotional health, or morals."[2] The statutory definition of *dependent child* also includes children who have been placed for

---

1. 42 PA. CONS. STAT. ANN. §§ 6301–6365.
2. 42 PA. CONS. STAT. ANN. § 6302.

adoption in violation of state law; have been abandoned; are without a parent; are habitually truant; are habitually disobedient, are ungovernable, and are found to be in need of care, treatment, or supervision; and are younger than 10 years old and have committed a delinquent act.[3] Chapter 4.15 describes the procedures under the Juvenile Act.

Abuse: Child Protective Services Law
The Child Protective Services Law (CPSL)[4] and its implementing regulations[5] define *child abuse* as, "Serious physical or mental injury which is not explained by the available medical history as being accidental, sexual abuse, sexual exploitation or serious physical neglect of a child under 18 years of age."[6] To be considered child abuse, the injury, abuse, or neglect must have "been caused by the acts or omissions of the child's parents or by a person responsible for the child's welfare, or any individual residing in the same home as the child, or a paramour of the child's parent."[7] *Sexual abuse* is defined as, "The obscene or pornographic photographing, filming or depiction of children for commercial purposes or the rape, molestation, incest, prostitution or other forms of sexual exploitation of children under circumstances which indicate the child's health or welfare is harmed or threatened thereby."[8]

(A) Protective Custody

The CPSL provides that the child may be taken into protective custody as provided in the Juvenile Act (see chapter 4.15).[9] In addition, the CPSL provides that a child may be taken into protective custody by a treating or examining physician or a director of a hospital or medical institution where the child is being treated if such custody is immediately necessary to protect the child from further serious physical injury, sexual abuse, or serious physical neglect.[10] The child may not be kept for longer than 24 hours unless child protective services is immediately notified of the custody and they obtain a proper court order allowing the child to

---

3. *Id.*
4. 23 PA. CONS. STAT. ANN. §§ 6301–6384.
5. 55 PA. CODE §§ 3490.1–3490.210.
6. 23 PA. CONS. STAT. ANN. § 6303.
7. *Id.*
8. *Id.*
9. 23 PA. CONS. STAT. ANN. § 6315(a)(1).
10. 23 PA. CONS. STAT. ANN. § 6315(a)(2). The parents, guardian, or other custodian of the child must be notified of the custody in writing within 24 hours.

be held longer.[11] Custody may not exceed 72 hours unless a detention hearing is held before the court.[12]

Reporting Abuse
See chapter 4.8 for a description of requirements and procedures for reporting child abuse.

(B) Investigation and Report

The CPSL requires the local child protective service to commence an investigation within 24 hours of receiving a report of suspected child abuse.[13] The investigation must include a determination of the risk to the child or children if they continue in the existing home environment as well as a determination of the nature, extent, and cause of any condition enumerated in the report.[14] MHPs may be questioned as part of an investigation. The investigation must be completed within 30 days of the initial report.[15] The report must be characterized as *indicated,* meaning that there was a finding by the child protective service of substantial evidence of abuse; *founded,* meaning that there was a judicial adjudication that the child was abused; or *unfounded,* which encompasses all other reports.[16] Alleged perpetrators of indicated and founded reports are listed in the Statewide Central Child Abuse Register.[17]

Evidentiary Requirements
In court proceedings concerning abuse brought under the CPSL, the rules of evidence are somewhat relaxed. If a required reporter such as an MHP (see chapter 4.8) is unavailable because the MHP has been removed from the jurisdiction of the court (i.e., has moved out of town or has died), the MHP's written report is admissible in civil proceedings arising out of child abuse even if hearsay.[18] The court may give "appropriate" weight to any hearsay statements, but cannot base an abuse adjudication solely on hearsay.[19] Privileged communications, such as those between psychotherapist and patient, are admissible at any proceeding regarding child abuse or its cause. However, privileged commu-

---

11. 23 Pa. Cons. Stat. Ann. § 6315(b).
12. 23 Pa. Cons. Stat. Ann. § 6315(d).
13. 23 Pa. Cons. Stat. Ann. § 6368(a).
14. 23 Pa. Cons. Stat. Ann. § 6368.
15. 23 Pa. Cons. Stat. Ann. § 6368(c).
16. 23 Pa. Cons. Stat. Ann. §§ 6303, 6368.
17. 23 Pa. Cons. Stat. Ann. § 6331.
18. 23 Pa. Cons. Stat. Ann. § 6381.
19. *Id.*

nications between lawyer–client and minister–penitent are not admissible at child abuse proceedings.[20]

(C) Disposition

Based on the investigation and evaluation conducted, the child protective service must provide or contract with agencies to provide for the protection of the child. The services are to be provided at home whenever possible, but the child protective service must provide for services necessary for adequate care of the child when the child is placed in protective custody.[21] The child protective service can provide or arrange for and monitor rehabilitative services for children and their families on a voluntary basis or under a final or intermediate order of the court.[22] If the child protective service finds that the placement for temporary or permanent custody, care, or treatment is for any reason inappropriate or harmful to the physical or mental well-being of the child, it must take immediate steps to remedy these conditions, including petitioning the court.[23]

Abuse: Protection From Abuse Act
In the Protection From Abuse Act (PFAA),[24] *abuse* is defined as the occurrence of certain acts between family or household members, sexual or intimate partners, or persons who share biological parenthood (see chapter 4.7). These acts include physically or sexually abusing minor children as defined in the CPSL.[25]

Petition and Proceedings
Any parent, adult household member, or guardian *ad litem* may petition for an order of protection on behalf of the child.[26] If a plaintiff petitions for a temporary order for protection from abuse and alleges immediate and present danger of abuse to the plaintiff or minor children, the court must conduct an *ex parte* proceeding. The court may enter a temporary order to protect the plaintiff or minor children when it finds they are in immediate and present

---

20. *Id.*
21. 23 PA. CONS. STAT. ANN. § 6370.
22. 23 PA. CONS. STAT. ANN. § 6371.
23. 23 PA. CONS. STAT. ANN. § 6372.
24. 23 PA. CONS. STAT. ANN. §§ 6101–6117.
25. 23 PA. CONS. STAT. ANN. § 6102(a).
26. 23 PA. CONS. STAT. ANN. § 6106. PA. DIST. JUST. RULE 1205 provides that emergency relief from abuse may be sought by the abused child, a parent, or any adult household member.

danger of abuse.[27] Within 10 days of the filing of a petition, a hearing must be held before the court, at which the allegation of abuse must be shown to be more likely to be true than not.[28] The court may then enter such order as is necessary to protect the child, including awarding temporary custody or visitation rights or restraining the accused abuser from having any contact with the child.[29] An advantage to proceeding under the PFAA is that a court may order the abusing party to vacate the home. A domestic violence counselor–advocate may accompany a party to a PFAA hearing.[30]

Confidentiality of Victim's Communication

Unless written permission is given by the victim, a domestic violence counselor–advocate is not permitted to testify or to otherwise disclose confidential communications made between the counselor–advocate and a victim.[31]

---

27. 23 PA. CONS. STAT. ANN. § 6107(b). In some counties, after business hours, emergency relief may be obtained by filing petitions with the minor judiciary. 23 PA. CONS. STAT. ANN. § 6110. In an emergency, it may be advisable to first contact the local police.
28. 23 PA. CONS. STAT. ANN. § 6107(a).
29. 23 PA. CONS. STAT. ANN. § 6108(a).
30. 23 PA. CONS. STAT. ANN. § 6111.
31. 23 PA. CONS. STAT. ANN. § 6116.

4.10

Termination of Parental Rights

After child abuse, neglect, or maltreatment has been reported and a finding is made (see chapters 4.8 and 4.9), the question will sometimes arise as to whether parental rights should be terminated. Parental rights may be relinquished voluntarily[1] or terminated involuntarily.[2] The laws favor keeping the family intact, and involuntary termination is a drastic measure that is reserved for extreme situations—for example, situations in which there is a pattern of repeated abuse or neglect of the child that the parent is unable to correct. If a determination is made to petition for involuntary termination of parental rights, the parent is afforded a range of procedural due process rights. MHPs may be asked to assess the child, the parent(s), parent–child relationships, and the familial living situation to assist the court in its decision.

(A) Voluntary Relinquishment

The parent or parents of a child may petition the court for permission to relinquish forever all parental rights and duties with respect to their child. The child may be relinquished to an agency that is caring for the child or to an adult intending to adopt the child (see chapter 4.14).[3] A hearing must be held on the petition.[4]

The court must compile and make available a list of qualified counselors and counseling services available to counsel natural

---

1. 23 PA. CONS. STAT. ANN. §§ 2501–2504.
2. 23 PA. CONS. STAT. ANN. §§ 2511–2513.
3. 23 PA. CONS. STAT. ANN. §§ 2501–2502.
4. 23 PA. CONS. STAT. ANN. § 2503.

parents contemplating relinquishment or termination of parental rights.[5] The court also may refer the parent for counseling.[6]

Filing the Involuntary Termination Petition
The petition can be filed by one parent against the other, by an agency, or by an individual having custody or standing *in loco parentis* to the child and who has filed a report of intention to adopt the child.[7] The petition must specifically set forth the grounds and facts that are the basis of the request for termination.[8]

Prehearing Requirements
The court must schedule a hearing to take place not less than 10 days after the filing of the petition.[9] The parents whose rights are at issue must be given proper notice of the hearing.[10] The court may terminate the rights of the parent at the close of this hearing.

(B) Grounds for Termination

The rights of a parent may be terminated on any of the following grounds:

1. For a period of 6 months, the parent either has evidenced a settled purpose of relinquishing parental claim to a child or has refused or failed to perform parental duties.

2. Repeated and continued incapacity, abuse, neglect, or refusal of the parent has caused the child to be without essential parental care, control, or subsistence necessary for his or her physical or mental well-being, and the parent cannot or will not remediate the problem.

3. The parent is the presumptive but not the natural father of the child.[11]

4. The child is in the custody of an agency, having been found under such circumstances that the identity or whereabouts of the parent is unknown and cannot be ascertained by diligent

---

5. 23 PA. CONS. STAT. ANN. § 2510.
6. *Id.*
7. 23 PA. CONS. STAT. ANN. § 2512(a). *See* chapter 4.14 for a description of adoption procedures.
8. 23 PA. CONS. STAT. ANN. § 2512(b).
9. 23 PA. CONS. STAT. ANN. § 2513(a).
10. The parent(s) whose rights are to be terminated must be given a minimum of 10 days notice. 23 PA. CONS. STAT. ANN. § 2513(b).
11. A child born during wedlock will be presumed to be the child of the married couple, even where a woman's husband is not the natural (biological) father of the child.

search and the parent does not claim the child within 3 months after the child is found.

5. The child has been removed from the care of the parent by the court or under a voluntary agreement with an agency for a period of at least 6 months; the conditions that led to the removal or placement of the chid continue to exist; the parent cannot or will not remedy those conditions within a reasonable period of time; the services or assistance reasonably available to the parent are not likely to remedy the conditions that led to the removal or placement of the child within a reasonable period of time; and termination of the parental rights would best serve the needs and welfare of the child.

6. In the case of a newborn child, the parent knows or has reason to know of the child's birth; does not reside with the child; has not married the child's other parent; has failed for a period of 4 months immediately preceding the filing of the petition to make reasonable efforts to maintain substantial and continuing contact with the child; and has failed during the same 4-month period to provide substantial financial support for the child.

7. The parent is the father of a child who was conceived as a result of rape.[12]

The court in terminating the rights of a parent must give primary consideration to the needs and welfare of the child.[13] The conditions needed to justify termination of parental rights must be established by clear and convincing evidence.[14]

Effect of Termination

After hearing, the court must make a finding regarding the grounds for involuntary termination and on such finding may enter a decree of termination of parental rights.[15] A termination decree shall award custody to an agency or person.[16] That agency or person shall stand *in loco parentis* to the child and shall have the same the authority concerning the child as does a natural parent.[17] A termination decree shall extinguish the power or right of the parent to object to, or receive notice of, adoption proceedings.[18]

---

12. 23 Pa. Cons. Stat. Ann. § 2511(a).
13. 23 Pa. Cons. Stat. Ann. § 2511(b).
14. *In re* T.R., 465 A.2d 642 (Pa. 1983).
15. 23 Pa. Cons. Stat. Ann. § 2513(d).
16. 23 Pa. Cons. Stat. Ann. § 2521(b).
17. 23 Pa. Cons. Stat. Ann. § 2521(c).
18. 23 Pa. Cons. Stat. Ann. § 2521(a).

4.11

Guardianship for Minors

The law permits the appointment of guardians for children. Such a guardian may be appointed in situations in which the custodial parent(s) is unable to care for the child because of death, legal termination of parental rights, or other circumstances. It is the guardian's responsibility to protect the person and assets of the child. MHPs may become involved in the guardian selection process or provide follow-up services.

(A) Appointing a Guardian

A guardian may be appointed by the parent(s) of a minor or by the court. Parents can indicate who they wish to care for their child or their child's property in the event of their deaths by placing provisions in their wills designating testamentary guardians.[1] The court also may appoint a guardian of the person or estate of a minor.[2]

A *guardian of the person* is responsible for the physical well-being of the child. A *guardian of the estate* is entrusted with the control of the child's property, including money, real estate, and business enterprises. The same person may be appointed both as guardian of the minor's estate and guardian of the minor's person.

---

1. 20 PA. CONS. STAT. ANN. § 2519.
2. 20 PA. CONS. STAT. ANN. § 5111.

Court Appointment of a Guardian

A petition for the appointment of a guardian for the estate or person of a minor must be filed by the minor, if the minor is over 14 years of age.[3] If minors are under 14 years of age, petitions for the appointment of guardians for their estates or persons must be filed by their parents, persons with whom they reside or by whom they are maintained, or by any persons as next friends of the minors.[4] The petition must set forth, among other things:

1. that the minor's parents consent to the petition, if it is not filed by them, or the reason why they do not consent;

2. the necessity of the appointment of a guardian and that the minor has no guardian or that a guardian already appointed has died, been discharged, or removed by the court;

3. the name of the proposed guardian and his relationship to the minor, if any;

4. the nature of any interest of the proposed guardian adverse to that of the minor;

5. if the petition is for the appointment of a guardian of the person, the religion of the parents of the minor and of the proposed guardian;

6. if the petition is for a guardianship of the estate, an itemization of the assets of such estate; and

7. if the minor is entitled to receive any money as a party to any action or proceeding in any court, a reference to the court record and the amount to which the minor is entitled.[5]

The proposed guardian's written consent must be attached to the petition.[6]

Custodianship for the Transfer of Property to a Minor

Under the Pennsylvania Uniform Gifts to Minors Act, property may be transferred to a minor, but held on his or her behalf by a custodian.[7] A *custodian* is similar to a guardian of the estate except that the custodian's area of control is limited to the specific property named in the appointment.

---

3. Pa. Orphans' Ct. R. 12.5(a).
4. *Id.*
5. Pa. Orphans' Ct. R. 12.5(b).
6. Pa. Orphans' Ct. R. 12.5(c).
7. 20 Pa. Cons. Stat. Ann. §§ 5301–5320.

(B) Guardianship Hearing

The court may appoint a guardian *ad litem* during the course of certain legal proceedings (e.g., child abuse proceedings or parental rights termination proceedings).[8] The guardian *ad litem* may be charged with representing the best interests of the child in those proceedings.[9]

The primary consideration of the court in appointing a guardian for a minor's estate is whether the appointment of such a guardian will be in the best interests of the minor's estate. There are few cases discussing the standard for appointment of a guardian of the person, presumably because disputes over the child's physical well-being are more likely to be resolved through child custody proceedings (see chapter 4.6).

The court next determines who should be appointed guardian. The court will prefer a specific person nominated by the child if the minor is over the age of 14.[10] Preference is also given to a guardian who is of the same religion as the child.[11] The ability to serve the best interests of the minor in all respects, however, is the paramount consideration of the court in choosing a guardian.

(C) Duties of the Guardian

The powers and responsibilities of a guardian of the estate of a minor are specified in the statutes.[12] The powers and responsibilities of a guardian of the person of a minor are not so specified.

(D) Termination of Guardianship

The guardianship remains in effect until the child reaches the age of 18 or dies, unless the guardian is discharged or removed for cause. Grounds for removal of the guardian include wasting or mismanaging the estate, failing to discharge duties as a result of physical or mental incapacitation, failing to remain in Pennsylva-

---

8. 23 Pa. Cons. Stat. Ann. §§ 2313, 6382; Pa. Orphans' Ct. R. 12.4.
9. 23 Pa. Cons. Stat. Ann. § 6382.
10. 20 Pa. Cons. Stat. Ann. § 5113.
11. *Id.*
12. *See* 23 Pa. Cons. Stat. Ann. §§ 5141–5167.

nia, or generally jeopardizing the estate by continued service.[13] The guardian may be ordered to refute the charges or the court may summarily dismiss the guardian to protect the rights of those with an interest in the estate.[14]

---

13. 20 PA. CONS. STAT. ANN. § 3182. Although the law does not specifically address the issue, presumably a guardian of the person could be removed if he or she were not properly attending to the needs of the child. *See, e.g.,* Scientific Living, Inc. v. Hohensee, 270 A.2d 216, 223 (Pa. 1970) (explaining fiduciary guardian may be removed if his continued service is harmful to the estate).

14. 20 PA. CONS. STAT. ANN. § 5131, referring to 20 PA. CONS. STAT. ANN. § 3183.

Conservatorship for Minors

Many states distinguish between proceedings relating to care of the person (using the term *guardianship*) and those related to care of property (using the term *conservatorship*). Some states use the term *conservatorship* to refer to both types of proceedings. Pennsylvania only uses the term *guardianship* (see chapters 4.2, 4.3, and 4.11).

4.13

Foster Care

Foster care is a service designed to provide substitute care for a child until a parent is able to receive help and develop the skills necessary to provide adequate care to his or her children or until someone adopts the child (see chapter 4.14). It usually involves providing residential housing and support for children who are not able to live in their own homes. Although foster care is ideally a temporary arrangement (and may last as short as one night), children frequently live in foster care settings for years. MHPs may assist in determining whether foster care or some other alternative is appropriate for a child or may provide treatment to a family as an alternative to, or in conjunction with, foster care.

There is a strong presumption in favor of keeping the child in the care of the biological parents (see chapter 4.15).[1] Pennsylvania's policy is that

1. the unique bond that exists between parent and child must be recognized as fundamental to the growth and development of children; and

2. the treatment of neglected and abused children must include a commitment to strengthening the families of these children through the intensive application of social services and family therapy.[2]

Through establishment of Family Preservation Programs, Pennsylvania has attempted to reduce the "expensive and poten-

---

1. 62 Pa. Cons. Stat. Ann. § 2172.
2. *Id.*

tially damaging incidence of out-of-home placement in foster care or group homes."[3]

Those families in which one or more children are at imminent risk of separation from their families through placement in foster care, a group home, or other appropriate facility are eligible to receive family preservation services.[4] Pennsylvania regulations state that provision of services to children and their families without placement is the primary objective of children and youth services.[5] Returning the child home is the major objective for any placement into care. Only when return home is unlikely after a reasonable period of time and after services have been offered to a family should the remaining options be considered.

Regulations require the county agency to prepare, within 30 days of accepting a family for services, a written Family Service Plan. The plan must include a description of the circumstances under which the case was accepted, the service objectives, the services to be provided, each party's responsibilities, and the dates by which the various actions must be completed.[6]

(A) Placement of Children Into Foster Homes

If a child is found to be a "dependent child" (see chapter 4.15), the child may be removed from the familial home and placed in foster care.[7] Prior to placement of the child outside of the familial home, the court must make certain findings (see chapter 4.15).

Foster care may take place in a foster family home, a group home, or an institution. A wide variety of specialized programs, including therapeutic foster care, is available according to a child's individual needs. Dependency Court has broad authority to require the provision of any and all services "best suited" to a child's needs.[8]

---

3. 62 PA. CONS. STAT. ANN. § 2174.
4. *Id.* Families in which children are at imminent risk of sexual abuse or physical endangerment perpetrated by a member of their immediate household are not eligible to receive family preservation services. *Id.*
5. 55 PA. CODE §§ 3130.13(b)(4), 3130.67. Case law has also approved court orders directing agencies to provide in-home services before removing children from their families. *See* Interest of Pernishek, 408 A.2d 872 (Pa. Super. Ct. 1979); Interest of Whittle, 397 A.2d 1225 (Pa. Super. Ct. 1979); Matter of DeSavage, 360 A.2d 237 (Pa. Super. Ct. 1976).
6. 55 PA. CODE § 3130.61.
7. 42 PA. CONS. STAT. ANN. § 6351(a).
8. *See* 42 PA. CONS. STAT. ANN. § 6351(a); *In re* Tameka M., 580 A.2d 750 (Pa. 1990); *In re* Lowry, 484 A.2d 383 (Pa. 1984).

(B) Prospective Foster Parents

Extended family caregivers are playing an increasingly important and pervasive role as placement resources for children who cannot live with their parents. Many family caretaking situations are informal and temporary. Grandparents, aunts and uncles, and others may assume legal or physical custody (see chapter 4.6). Custody may be transferred by agreement between two parties and then ratified by the court, or may be transferred after a dependency or custody hearing.

Persons who wish to become foster parents must be investigated to determine their suitability. Prospective foster parents must submit information concerning any criminal history in the form of a report from the state police or a statement from the state police that no criminal history information exists.[9] They also must obtain certification from child protective services that they have not been identified in the central register as the perpetrator of child abuse.[10]

(C) Placement Review

Under the Juvenile Act, the court must review each placement every 6 months to determine whether placement continues to be best suited for the protection and physical, mental, and moral welfare of the child.[11]

---

9. 23 PA. CONS. STAT. ANN. §§ 6344(b) & (d).
10. Id.
11. 42 PA. CONS. STAT. ANN. §§ 6351(e)–(h). After the third review hearing, subsequent disposition review hearings must be held at least every 12 months. The Pennsylvania Foster Care Regulations require the County Children and Youth Agency to request a court or administrative review of all children in placement at least once every 6 months. 55 PA. CODE § 3130.71.

4.14

Adoption

The laws of Pennsylvania provide that any individual, regardless of age or residence, may be adopted.[1] Although the law also provides that anyone may become an adoptive parent, certain requirements must be met by the prospective adoptive parent(s) and the adoptive home. An adopted child and his or her natural parents also have certain rights and responsibilities that must be fulfilled for the adoption to be valid. MHPs may be called on to evaluate the child, the prospective adoptive parents, and the prospective adoptive home environment. In some cases, they may be called on to provide counseling to the natural parents, the adoptive parents, or the adoptive child.

(A) Adoption Requirements

The parental rights of a natural parent must be terminated before an adoption may occur (see chapter 4.10).[2] A decree terminating parental rights extinguishes the power or the right of the parent to object to adoption proceedings.[3]

A child may not be placed into the care or custody of a prospective adoptive parent unless a home study containing a favorable recommendation has been completed within the preceding 3 years and has been supplemented within the prior year.[4]

---

1. 23 PA. CONS. STAT. ANN. § 2311.
2. 23 PA. CONS. STAT. ANN. § 2901.
3. 23 PA. CONS. STAT. ANN. § 2521(a).
4. 23 PA. CONS. STAT. ANN. § 2530. In some cases, a child may be placed in the physical care or custody of a prospective adoptive parent while a home study is in the process of being completed.

The home study must be conducted by a local public child care agency, an adoption agency, or a licensed social worker designated by the court. A preplacement report must be prepared by the agency or person conducting the home study. Among other things, this report must

1. set forth all pertinent information relating to the fitness of the adopting parents as parents;

2. be based on a study that includes an investigation of the home environment; family life; parenting skills; age; physical and mental health; social, cultural, and religious background; facilities and resources of the adoptive parents; and their ability to manage their resources; and

3. include a determination regarding the fitness of the adopting parents as parents.[5]

Prospective adoptive parents must submit information concerning any criminal history in the form of a report or statement from the state police that no criminal history information exists.[6] They also must obtain certification from child protective services that they have not been identified in the central register as the perpetrator of child abuse.[7]

Prospective adoptive parents must file a report of intention to adopt.[8] Within 6 months after filing this report, the intermediary arranging the adoption placement must make a written report to the court containing information about the adoption.[9]

(B) Petition for Adoption and Hearing

A petition for adoption must be filed, and in some cases, the consents of certain parties must be attached to the petition.[10] The consents must evidence an intent to permanently relinquish all rights to the child.[11]

---

5. 23 Pa. Cons. Stat. Ann. § 2530(c).
6. 23 Pa. Cons. Stat. Ann. § 2530; *see also* 23 Pa. Cons. Stat. Ann. § 2535 (requiring the court to ensure that an investigation is conducted).
7. 23 Pa. Cons. Stat. Ann. §§ 6344(b) & (d).
8. *Id.*
9. 23 Pa. Cons. Stat. Ann. § 2531. When the prospective adoptive parent is a relative, a report of intention to adopt may not be required. *Id.*
10. 23 Pa. Cons. Stat. Ann. § 2533.
11. 23 Pa. Cons. Stat. Ann. §§ 2701–2714. The consent of the parents is not required if a decree of termination of parental rights has been entered. 23 Pa. Cons. Stat. Ann. § 2714.

The court must hold a hearing on the petition, giving proper notice to all parties whose consent is required.[12] The adoptive parent(s) and the adoptee must appear at the hearing, unless the court determines their presence is unnecessary.[13] The court may require testimony and further investigation in support of the petition.[14] The court must decide the desirability of the proposed adoption on the basis of the physical, mental, and emotional needs and welfare of the child.[15] The court may request the services of an MHP to assist in making this determination.

(C) Adoption Decree

If the court is satisfied that the statements made in the petition are true, that the needs and welfare of the person proposed to be adopted will be promoted by the adoption, and that all legal requirements have been met, a decree of adoption may be entered.[16] The person proposed to be adopted shall have all the rights of a child and heir of the adopting parent or parents and shall be subject to the duties of a child.[17]

---

12. 23 PA. CONS. STAT. ANN. §§ 2711, 2714.
13. 23 PA. CONS. STAT. ANN. § 2721.
14. 23 PA. CONS. STAT. ANN. § 2723.
15. 23 PA. CONS. STAT. ANN. § 2724.
16. Id.
17. 23 PA. CONS. STAT. ANN. §§ 2901–2902.

4.15

Delinquency and Persons in Need of Supervision

The Court of Common Pleas is charged with making provisions for the care and supervision of dependent or delinquent minors. The court may request information from MHPs to assist in determining the child's need for services.

(A) Juvenile Delinquency

(A)(1) Terms and Definitions

The Pennsylvania Juvenile Act provides the authority for state intervention on behalf of dependent (see chapter 4.9) and delinquent minors.[1] The Juvenile Act defines the following terms:

1. *Delinquent act* is one designated as a crime by federal or state law or local ordinances. The term does not apply to murder, nor does it apply to summary offenses unless the child fails to comply with the sentence imposed. The term does not include any of the following prohibited conduct if the child was 15 years of age or older at the time of the conduct and a deadly weapon was used during the commission of the offense: rape; involuntary deviate sexual intercourse; aggravated assault; robbery; robbery of motor vehicle; aggravated indecent assault; kidnapping; voluntary manslaughter; or an attempt, conspiracy, or solicitation to commit murder or any of these crimes. The term does not include any of the following prohibited conduct when the child was 15 years of age or older at the time of the offense and has been previously adjudicated delin-

---

1. 42 Pa. Cons. Stat. Ann. §§ 6301–6365.

quent of any of the following prohibited conduct: rape; involuntary deviate sexual intercourse; robbery; robbery of motor vehicle; aggravated indecent assault; kidnapping; voluntary manslaughter; or an attempt, conspiracy, or solicitation to commit murder or any of these crimes. The term does not include a crime committed by a child who has been found guilty in a criminal proceeding for other than a summary offense.

2. *Delinquent child* is a child 10 years of age or older whom the court has found to have committed a delinquent act and is in need of treatment, supervision, or rehabilitation.

3. *Dependent child* is a child who "is without proper parental care or control, subsistence, education as required by law, or other care or control necessary for his physical, mental, or emotional health, or morals." The statutory definition of *dependent child* also includes children who have been placed for adoption in violation of state law; have been abandoned; are without a parent; are habitually truant; are habitually disobedient, are ungovernable, and are found to be in need of care, treatment, or supervision; or are under 10 years old and have committed a delinquent act.[2]

(A)(2) Initiation of Proceedings

Proceedings under the Juvenile Act may begin with the child being taken into custody, transferred from criminal proceedings, or on the filing of a petition.[3] A child may be taken into custody:

1. pursuant to a court order,

2. pursuant to the laws of arrest,

3. by a law enforcement officer or officer of the court if there are reasonable grounds to believe that the child is suffering from illness or injury or is in imminent danger from his or her surroundings, and that the child's removal is necessary,

4. by a law enforcement officer or officer of the court if there are reasonable grounds to believe that the child has run away from his or her parents, guardian, or other custodian, or

5. by a law enforcement officer or court order if there are reasonable grounds to believe that the child has violated conditions of his or her probation.[4]

The child taken into custody cannot be detained or placed into shelter care prior to a hearing unless:

---

2. 42 PA. CONS. STAT. ANN. § 6302.
3. 42 PA. CONS. STAT. ANN. § 6321.
4. 42 PA. CONS. STAT. ANN. § 6324.

1. the child's detention or care is required to protect the person or property of others or of the child;
2. the child may leave the jurisdiction of the court;
3. the child has no one who is able to provide supervision and care for him or her and return him or her to the court when required; or
4. an order for his or her detention or shelter care has been made by the court.[5]

If the child is taken into custody, his or her parent, guardian, or other custodian must be notified with all reasonable speed.[6] The child may only be detained in certain designated detention or shelter care facilities or homes, and the child may not be detained in a facility with adults.[7]

A petition may be filed under the Juvenile Act by any person alleging that it is in the best interests of the child and the public that the proceeding be brought, and if delinquency is alleged, that the child is in need of treatment, supervision, or rehabilitation.[8]

In some cases of delinquency or dependency, there may be an informal resolution of the matter—for example, by referral to a public or private social agency. Such agencies and the probation officer or other officer of the court may give counsel and advice to the parties with a view toward resolution without formal judicial proceedings.[9] In these cases, the services of an MHP could be requested. Cases also may be resolved by agreement (consent decree).[10]

(A)(3) Detention or Shelter Care Hearing

Once a child is taken into custody, there must be prompt hearings and disposition. When a child is placed into detention or shelter care, a petition must be filed within 24 hours, and an informal hearing must be held within 72 hours.[11] The child has rights to notice, to counsel, to be heard, to introduce evidence, and to cross-examine witnesses, and the right to remain silent with respect to allegations of delinquency.[12]

---

5. 42 PA. CONS. STAT. ANN. § 6325.
6. 42 PA. CONS. STAT. ANN. § 6326(a).
7. 42 PA. CONS. STAT. ANN. § 6327.
8. 42 PA. CONS. STAT. ANN. § 6334.
9. 42 PA. CONS. STAT. ANN. § 6323.
10. 42 PA. CONS. STAT. ANN. § 6340.
11. 42 PA. CONS. STAT. ANN. §§ 6331–6332.
12. 42 PA. CONS. STAT. ANN. §§ 6332, 6337–6338.

(A)(4) Adjudication Hearing

If the court orders protective custody at the 72-hour shelter-care hearing, an adjudication hearing must be held on the petition within 10 days of its filing.[13] If protective custody is not taken, there is no time limit for holding the adjudication hearing. At the hearing, the court must decide if the evidence supports finding the child to be dependent or delinquent. In the case of delinquency, the court must find "beyond a reasonable doubt" that the child committed the delinquent acts alleged.[14] The court must find "clear and convincing" evidence that the child is dependent.[15]

Rules of Evidence

Strict rules of evidence apply in an adjudication. Hearsay statements are not admissible at the adjudication stage. Furthermore, privileged communications, such as doctor–patient, husband–wife, and psychotherapist–patient communications are not admissible at the adjudication stage.

Expert testimony may be used to prove dependency. For example, an expert may testify about observations of the parent–child visits, the parent's emotional problems, and the parent's ambivalence about the child's return.[16] An MHP's subjective impressions alone are insufficient.[17]

Mental Health Evaluations

During the pendency of proceedings, the court may order the child to be evaluated by a physician or psychologist.[18] If the allegations of the petition are admitted, if the child has been given notice of a hearing on transfer to criminal proceedings (see chapter 4.18), or if the court has found that the child committed a delinquent act or is a dependent child, the court may direct that a social study and written report to the court be made.[19]

---

13. 42 PA. CONS. STAT. ANN. § 6335. There are some exceptions to this rule. *Id.* If the child causes the delay by being unavailable for the hearing or asking for a continuance, then this rule is not applicable. § 6335(f).
14. 42 PA. CONS. STAT. ANN. § 6341(b).
15. 42 PA. CONS. STAT. ANN. § 6341(c).
16. *In re* Clouse, 368 A.2d 780, 782 (Pa. Super. Ct. 1976).
17. Commonwealth *ex rel.* Bankert v. Children's Services, 307 A.2d 411, 415 (Pa. Super. Ct. 1973).
18. 42 PA. CONS. STAT. ANN. § 6339(b).
19. 42 PA. CONS. STAT. ANN. § 6339(a). The social study concerns the child, the child's family, the child's environment, and other matters relevant to the disposition of the case. *Id.*

(A)(5) Disposition Phase

Rules of Evidence

At the disposition stage, as distinguished from the adjudication stage, a court may consider all relevant oral and written evidence even if it contains hearsay so long as parties or their counsel can examine and controvert written reports as well as cross-examine individuals making the reports. Confidential sources of information need not be disclosed.[20]

Dependent Child

If the court finds that the child is dependent at the 10-day adjudication hearing, the court may immediately make a disposition of the case, but in no event can this occur later than 20 days after adjudication if the child has been removed from home.[21] The court has wide discretion in determining the disposition that is best suited to the protection and physical, mental, and moral welfare of the child. Court orders may require children to remain with their parents in their homes, conditioned on supervision or on parental or child participation in needed treatment programs.[22] The court also may transfer custody temporarily to an individual or a private or public agency.[23] If, at a hearing, evidence indicates that the child may be subject to commitment or detention under the provisions of the Mental Health and Retardation Act of 1966 or the Mental Health Procedures Act (see chapter 4.19), the court must proceed under the provisions of the appropriate statute.[24]

Before a court may order removal of a child from home, the court must find that continuation of the child in the home would be contrary to the welfare of the child and determine

1. whether reasonable efforts were made prior to the placement of the child to prevent or eliminate the need for removal of the child from home, if the child has remained home pending such disposition; or

2. if preventive services were not offered because of the need for an emergency placement, whether such lack of services was reasonable under the circumstances; or

3. if the court has previously determined that reasonable efforts were not made to prevent the initial removal of the child from

---

20. 42 Pa. Cons. Stat. Ann. § 6341(d).
21. 42 Pa. Cons. Stat. Ann. § 6341(c).
22. 42 Pa. Cons. Stat. Ann. § 6351.
23. Id.
24. 42 Pa. Cons. Stat. Ann. § 6356; see also Pa. Stat. Ann. tit. 50, § 7401(c) (Mental Health Procedures Act applies to children committed under Juvenile Act); In re McMullins, 462 A.2d 718 (Pa. Super. Ct. 1983).

home, whether reasonable efforts are under way to make it possible for the child to return home.[25]

Case law suggests that before placement outside the home, the court must make a finding of clear necessity for the removal, make a determination regarding the feasibility of ordering the commonwealth to instruct parents in needed skills, and provide follow-up supervision in the home. In *Clouse*,[26] the Superior Court stated that many factors must be considered to determine whether "clear necessity" requires separation of the biological parent and child:

1. the age and mental development of the child;
2. the nature of the child's relationship with his or her natural parents (e.g., is it healthy or destructive); and
3. the nature of the relationship between the child and the foster parents and to what degree is that relationship like that of a natural family.[27]

Pennsylvania administrative regulations require the least restrictive setting, with services to children in their homes as the preferred alternative.[28]

Delinquent Child

If the court finds that the child is delinquent at the 10-day adjudication hearing, the court may immediately hear evidence as to whether the child is in need of treatment, supervision, or rehabilitation, but in no event must this occur later than 20 days after adjudication if the child is in detention.[29] Testimony of MHPs may be helpful at this stage. The court must determine which disposition is best suited to the treatment, supervision, rehabilitation, and welfare of the child. The court may

1. order any of the options available for disposition of the dependent child;
2. place the child on probation under supervision of a probation officer;

---

25. 42 Pa. Cons. Stat. Ann. § 6351.
26. 369 A.2d at 784.
27. *Id.*
28. 55 Pa. Code §§ 3130.13(b)(4), 3130.67; *see also* 42 Pa. Cons. Stat. Ann. § 6351. Emergency shelter may be ordered for 30 days to develop necessary service plans. Temporary removal occurs only when (a) removal is required for the immediate protection of the child; (b) the child presents a danger to himself or to others; or (c) the child would abscond if he or she were living at home. 55 Pa. Code § 3130.37.
29. 42 Pa. Cons. Stat. Ann. § 6341(b).

3. commit the child to an institution, youth development center, camp, or other facility for delinquent children;

4. order payment of fines, costs, or restitution; or

5. order the child to participate in a program of service or education that may include payment of restitution.[30]

When confinement is necessary, the court must impose the minimum amount of confinement that is consistent with the protection of the public and the rehabilitation needs of the child.[31]

Review
Under the Juvenile Act the court must review each placement or commitment every 6 to 12 months.[32] The court must hold a disposition review hearing at least every 9 months.[33]

---

30. 42 PA. CONS. STAT. ANN. § 6352.
31. *Id.*
32. 42 PA. CONS. STAT. ANN. §§ 6351, 6353; *see* 55 PA. CODE § 3130.71 (foster care regulations require county Children and Youth Agency to request review of all children in placement at least once every 6 months).
33. 42 PA. CONS. STAT. ANN. § 6353.

4.16

Competency of Juveniles to Stand Trial

The law has not addressed whether juveniles who face delinquency proceedings under the Juvenile Act (see chapter 4.15) have the same rights regarding competency to stand trial as do adults in criminal proceedings (see chapter 7.5). If the juvenile is being tried as an adult in criminal proceedings (see chapter 4.18), the court would be obligated to follow the procedures outlined for adult prosecutions.

Children who appear before the juvenile court have many of the procedural protections available to adult criminal defendants (see chapter 4.15). In addition, the legislature intended that all rights granted to adults by the Mental Health Procedures Act[1] be granted to juveniles who are 14 years of age or older, and that if juveniles are younger than 14, their parents, guardians, or other person *in loco parentis* act for them.[2] Therefore, it would appear that the procedural safeguards concerning competency to stand trial that are contained in the Mental Health Procedures Act would be available to juveniles 14 years of age or older to the same extent they are available to adults (see chapter 7.5). This issue, however, has not been settled.[3]

---

1. 50 PA. CONS. STAT. ANN. §§ 7101–7116.
2. *In re* McMullins, 462 A.2d 718 (Pa. Super. Ct. 1983).
3. A provision of the Juvenile Act states that children in delinquency proceedings may be committed or detained under the provisions of the Mental Health Procedures Act. *See* 42 PA. CONS. STAT. ANN. § 6356. This may be read to include the provision of the Mental Health Procedures Act pertaining to competency to stand trial. That provision of the Mental Health Procedures Act, however, only refers to criminal charges, not delinquency charges. *See* PA. STAT. ANN. tit. 50, § 7402; *see also* PA. STAT. ANN. tit. 50, § 7401(c) (civil provisions of act apply to proceedings for examination and treatment of juvenile). *But see In re* McMullins, 462 A.2d 718 (Pa. Super. Ct. 1983) (stating that §§ 7405 and 7406 of Mental Health Procedures Act apply to juveniles).

4.17

Nonresponsibility Defense

If a juvenile is being tried as an adult (see chapter 4.18), the court is obligated to follow the procedures outlined for adult prosecutions, and the juvenile could raise the insanity defense in the same manner as an adult defendant (see chapter 4.18). The law has not conclusively addressed the issue of whether a juvenile can raise the insanity defense in a delinquency proceeding. As discussed later, however, the Pennsylvania Superior Court has suggested that the insanity defense is unavailable to a juvenile in a delinquency proceeding.

At one time, children between the ages of 7 and 14 years were presumed to lack the capacity to commit crimes. More recently, the Pennsylvania Superior Court held that this so-called infancy defense was abolished by the Juvenile Act.[1] Therefore, it cannot be claimed that a child is not responsible for acts of delinquency simply because of his or her age. In addition, the Superior Court stated more broadly that the capacity of the juvenile to differentiate right from wrong is irrelevant in delinquency proceedings.[2] Children 10 years of age or older (and therefore covered by the delinquency provisions of the Juvenile Act) are conclusively presumed to have the capacity to commit delinquent acts.[3] This decision suggests that the insanity defense—which is based on a claim that a person does not have sufficient capacity to be held responsible for his or her acts—may be irrelevant in delinquency proceedings.

---

1. In the Interest of G.T., 597 A.2d 638 (Pa. Super. Ct. 1991).
2. *Id.*
3. *Id.*

Transfer of Juveniles to Stand Trial as Adults

In general, when a child under the age of 18 years commits an act that may be considered a crime, the child will be subject to delinquency proceedings under the Juvenile Act (see chapter 4.15). There are circumstances, however, in which a juvenile may be prosecuted as an adult in criminal proceedings. Most notably, this is the case when a child is charged with murder or certain other offenses that are expressly excluded from the definition of delinquent act (see chapter 4.15). Judges may order that juveniles be tried as adults for other crimes as well. The court, the prosecuting attorney, or the defense attorney may request an evaluation by an MHP to provide evidence at a hearing to transfer the matter from delinquency proceedings to criminal proceedings or vice versa. Specifically, MHPs may be asked whether the juvenile is amenable to treatment, supervision, or rehabilitation as a juvenile and whether the juvenile is committable to an institution for mentally retarded or mentally ill individuals.

(A) Transfer Requirements for Charges Other Than Serious Crimes Deemed Nondelinquent

When a child is charged with a crime other than murder or certain other offenses that are expressly excluded from the definition of delinquent act (see chapter 4.15), proceedings will either begin in the juvenile justice system or will be transferred to the juvenile system from the criminal justice system "forthwith."[1]

The judge is not granted unlimited discretion to transfer cases from the juvenile system to the criminal system. First, all of the following conditions must exist:

1. the child must have been 14 years of age or older when the conduct occurred;

2. the court must hold a hearing on whether the transfer should be made;

3. notice of the time, place, and purpose of the hearing must be given at least 3 days before the hearing to the child and his or her parents, guardian, or other custodian; and

4. the court must find that there is a prima facie case that the child likely committed the delinquent act and that the delinquent act would be a felony if committed by an adult.[2]

In addition, the court must find that there are reasonable grounds to believe the following:

1. that the public interest is served by the transfer of the case for criminal prosecution. In determining whether the public interest can be served, the court must consider the following factors:

   a. the impact of the offense on the victim or victims;

   b. the impact of the offense on the community;

   c. the threat to the safety of the public or any individual posed by the child;

   d. the nature and circumstances of the offense allegedly committed by the child;

   e. the degree of the child's culpability;

   f. the adequacy and duration of dispositional alternatives available under the chapter and in the adult criminal justice system; and

   g. whether the child is amenable to treatment, supervision, or rehabilitation as a juvenile taking into account age, mental capacity, maturity, degree of criminal sophistication, previous records, the nature and extent of any prior delinquent history, including the success or failure of previous rehabilitation attempts, whether the child can be rehabilitated prior to the expiration of the juvenile court jurisdic-

---

1. 42 Pa. Cons. Stat. Ann. § 6322.
2. 42 Pa. Cons. Stat. Ann. § 6355.

tion, probation or institutional reports, and any other relevant factors; and

2. that the child is not committable to an institution for mentally retarded or mentally ill individuals.[3]

If all of these conditions are met the court may transfer the case for adult criminal proceedings.

An MHP may be asked whether the juvenile is amenable to treatment, supervision, or rehabilitation as a juvenile. The MHP should attend to the specific statutory factors outlined previously for determining amenability to treatment. The evaluation requires more than an assessment of the juvenile; it also requires knowledge of the facilities available in the juvenile system, because the evaluator must predict the outcome for the juvenile if a disposition is reached through juvenile proceedings. The MHP also may be asked whether the juvenile is committable to an institution for people with mental retardation or with mental illness. Furthermore, the MHP may be asked to evaluate what threat the child poses to the safety of others or may be asked to provide evidence relating to the child's level of culpability.

(B) Transfer Requirements for Murder Charges

When a child is charged with a crime other than murder or certain other offenses that are expressly excluded from the definition of delinquent act (see chapter 4.15), the burden generally is placed on the state to prove that the juvenile should be tried as an adult.[4] However, when a child is charged with murder or these other offenses, the burden is placed on the child to show that the case should be heard in juvenile court.[5] The child must show that retaining the case in juvenile court serves the public interest and that he or she is amenable to rehabilitation, supervision, or treatment as a juvenile, considering the factors enumerated previously.

---

3. *Id.*
4. 42 PA. CONS. STAT. ANN. § 6355(g).
5. 42 PA. CONS. STAT. ANN. §§ 6322, 6355(g).

4.19

Voluntary Admission and Commitment of Minors

Although in certain circumstances minors (persons under 18) come under the same mental health laws as adults, in many instances there are different procedures. The most important factors in determining which procedures will be invoked are the age of the child and the wishes of parents. Also, different laws apply to persons with mental retardation.

(A) Voluntary Admission of Minors

Voluntary Admission of Children Under 14 Years of Age
When a child is younger than 14 years old, a parent, guardian, or person standing *in loco parentis* may subject that child to examination and treatment under the Mental Health Procedures Act, and "in doing so shall be deemed to be acting for the child."[1] Thus, the adult may arrange for a "voluntary" admission of the child into a hospital for mental health care (see chapter 8.3). The admission may be considered voluntary even when the child objects.

The parent, legal guardian, or person standing *in loco parentis* also may effect the child's release from hospitalization. In addition, "If any responsible party believes that it would be in the best interest of a person under 14 years of age in voluntary treatment to be withdrawn therefrom or afforded treatment constituting a less restrictive alternative," that person may file a petition requesting a withdrawal from or modification of treatment.[2] If such a petition is filed, the child is entitled to an attorney and a hearing

---

1. PA. STAT. ANN. tit. 50, § 7201.
2. PA. STAT. ANN. tit. 50, § 7206.

within 10 days to determine what inpatient treatment, if any, is in the minor's best interest.[3]

Voluntary Admission of Minors 14 Years Old or Older
A minor 14 years of age or older "who believes that he is in need of treatment and substantially understands the nature of voluntary treatment" may apply for examination and treatment under the Mental Health Procedures Act, "provided that the decision to do so is made voluntarily."[4] The procedures are the same as for adults (see chapter 8.3).

After accepting an application for examination and treatment by a child 14 years or older but younger than 18 years of age, the director of the facility must promptly notify the minor's parents, guardian, or person standing *in loco parentis* and inform them of the right to file an objection.[5] If an objection is filed, a hearing must be held within 72 hours to determine whether or not the voluntary treatment is in the best interest of the minor.[6]

(B) Involuntary Civil Commitment

If minors 14 years of age or older object to treatment, the procedures used for involuntary commitment of adults must be followed (see chapter 8.4), even if their parents want them to be hospitalized. As noted previously, minors younger than 14 may be admitted "voluntarily" by a parent, guardian, or person standing *in loco parentis* even when the minors object. Minors younger than 14 years of age may be admitted "involuntarily" over the objection of a parent, guardian, or person standing *in loco parentis.* Again, the procedures used for involuntary commitment of adults must be followed.

Developmental Disabilities
The Mental Health Procedures Act, adopted in 1976, does not apply to persons with mental retardation (see chapter 8.7). Rather, the law that applies to such persons is the Mental Health and Mental Retardation Act of 1966.[7] Mental retardation is defined as "subaverage general intellectual functioning which originates during the developmental period and is associated with impairment of one or more of the following: (1) maturation, (2) learning

---

3. *Id.*
4. PA. STAT. ANN. tit. 50, § 7201.
5. PA. STAT. ANN. tit. 50, § 7204.
6. *Id.*
7. PA. STAT. ANN. tit. 50, §§ 4201–4203.

and (3) social adjustment."[8] Under the Mental Health and Mental Retardation Act of 1966, any person 18 years of age or older may apply for voluntary admission or commitment to a facility for examination and treatment.[9] If the person to be admitted or committed is 18 years of age or younger, a parent, guardian, or individual standing *in loco parentis* to that person may apply for admission or commitment to a facility for examination and treatment.[10] Persons 18 years of age or younger with mental retardation may be committed "involuntarily" over the objection of a parent, guardian, or person standing *in loco parentis*.[11] The procedures used for involuntary commitment of adults with mental retardation must be followed (see chapter 8.7).

---

8. PA. STAT. ANN. tit. 50, § 4102.
9. PA. STAT. ANN. tit. 50, §§ 4402–4403.
10. *Id.*
11. PA. STAT. ANN. tit. 50, §§ 4404–4406.

Education for Gifted and Handicapped Children

The law has specific provisions designed to ensure that children who have disabilities or outstanding abilities receive educations that meet their needs. MHPs may evaluate these children, consult with parents and educational personnel, make recommendations for services, provide services, or testify at due process hearings.

(A) Terms and Definitions

To understand the process by which a child may be deemed eligible for special education services, it is necessary to understand how certain terms are defined in Pennsylvania's special education law.

1. *Special education* means specially designed instruction to meet the needs of an exceptional child.

2. *Exceptional children* are children of school age who deviate from the average in physical, mental, emotional, or social characteristics to such an extent that they require special education facilities or services. All children in detention homes are classified as exceptional.

3. *Early intervention* means an appropriate program of educational–developmental services and programs specially designed to meet the needs of eligible young children and address the strengths and needs of the family to enhance the child's development. The need for these services and programs must be in one or more of the following developmental areas: physical, sensory, cognitive, language and speech, social–emotional, and self-help.

4. *Educational placement* means the overall educational environment in which special education and related services or early intervention services and programs are provided to an exceptional student or eligible young child.

5. *Eligible student* means a school-age individual who was receiving services for persons with disabilities prior to July 1, 1990, or a school-age individual who meets the criteria in paragraphs (a) and (b).

   a. the individual has one or more of the following physical or mental disabilities:

      i.   autism–pervasive developmental disorder;
      ii.   serious emotional disturbance;
      iii. neurological impairment;
      iv.   deafness–hearing impairment;
      v.   specific learning disability;
      vi.   mental retardation;
      vii. multihandicap;
      viii. other health impairment;
      ix.   physical disability;
      x.   speech and language impairment; or
      xi.   blindness–visual impairment.

   b. the individual is determined by an Individualized Education Program team (discussed later), based on recommendations in a multidisciplinary evaluation, to need special education.

6. *Eligible young child* means a child who is younger than the age of beginners and at least 3 years of age and who meets the criteria in paragraph (a) or (b):

   a. the child has one or more of the 11 physical or mental disabilities set forth in paragraph 5(a); or

   b. the child has a developmental delay.[1]

Definitions of Disabilities

Specific definitions of the 11 physical and mental disabilities relevant to eligibility are provided in the law:

1. *Autism/pervasive developmental disorder* is a severe neurological disorder characterized by qualitative distortions in the devel-

---

1. PA. STAT. ANN. tit. 24, § 13-1371; 22 PA. CODE §§ 14.1, 342.1. In addition to provisions specifically applicable to this state, Pennsylvania special education law implements and complies with the federal Individuals with Disabilities in Education Act. 20 U.S.C. §§ 1400–1491(o).

opment of cognitive, language, social, or motor skills. Determination of autism–pervasive developmental disorder must include a full assessment and comprehensive report of diagnosis by a physician qualified to render a diagnosis and by a public school psychologist specifying the nature and degree of the disorder. Symptoms are typically manifested before 3 years of age, are not usual for any stage of child development, and shall include two or more of the following:

a. impairment in reciprocal social interaction;

b. impairment in communication and imaginative activity including verbal and nonverbal skills;

c. markedly restricted repertoire of activities and interests, often involving resistance to change and motor or verbal stereotypes; or

d. abnormal or inconsistent responses to sensory stimuli in one or more of the following areas: sight, hearing, touch, pain, balance, smell, taste, posture, and motor behavior.

2. *Serious emotional disturbance* is a condition exhibiting one or more of the following characteristics over a long period of time and to a marked degree adversely affects educational performance—an inability to learn that cannot be explained by intellectual, sensory, or health factors; an inability to build or maintain satisfactory interpersonal relationships with peers and teachers; inappropriate behavior or feelings under normal circumstances; a general pervasive mood of unhappiness or depression; or a tendency to develop physical symptoms or fears associated with personal or school problems. The term does not include students who are socially maladjusted, unless it is determined that they are also seriously emotionally disturbed. A student may not be determined to have a serious emotional disturbance for disciplinary reasons alone. Determination of serious emotional disturbance must include a full assessment and comprehensive report by a certified public school psychologist and may include the diagnosis of a licensed psychiatrist.

3. *Neurological impairment* is an injury to the brain, as identified by a neurological examination, resulting in behavior or learning disorders, or both. Persons whose behavior and learning disorders are primarily the result of visual, hearing, or motor handicaps, mental retardation, emotional factors, or environmental disadvantage are not neurologically impaired. The term does not include minimal brain dysfunction (but see the definition of *specific learning disability* in this section). Determination of neurological impairment must include a neurologi-

cal report from a physician and a psychological report from a certified public school psychologist and must specify the nature and degree of the impairment.

4. *Deafness or hearing impairment* is a hearing loss that interferes with the development of communication skills and results in failure to achieve educational potential. Determination of the hearing impairment must include a report by an audiologist or otologist, or both, specifying the nature and degree of the impairment.

5. *Specific learning disability* is

   a. a chronic condition of presumed neurological origin that selectively interferes with the development, integration, or demonstration of language, spoken or written, or of nonverbal abilities;

   b. the condition manifests itself as a severe discrepancy between achievement and intellectual ability in one or more of the following areas:

      i. oral expression;

      ii. listening comprehension;

      iii. written expression;

      iv. basic reading skill;

      v. reading comprehension;

      vi. mathematics calculation; or

      vii. mathematics reasoning.

   c. The term is not synonymous with underachievement. The term includes specific deficits in receptive and expressive language and deficiencies in initiating or sustaining attention, impulsivity, and other specific conceptual and thinking difficulties, such as nonverbal reasoning, integrating problems, motor coordination, and social perception. Examples of the condition include minimal brain dysfunction, dyslexia, and developmental aphasia, if the evaluation clearly indicates that the person can demonstrate normal or above normal intellectual functioning on an appropriate measure of intelligence. The term does not include learning conditions that are primarily the result of sensory impairment, physical disability, mental retardation, emotional factors, or environmental, cultural, or economic disadvantage. Determination of the learning disability must include a full assessment and comprehensive report by a certified public school psychologist specifying the nature and degree of the disability.

6. *Mental retardation* means impaired mental development that adversely affects the educational performance of a person. The term includes a person who exhibits significantly impaired adaptive behavior in learning, maturation, or social adjustment as a result of subaverage intellectual functioning. The term does not include persons with IQ scores of 80 or higher. Determination of mental retardation must include a full assessment and comprehensive report by a certified public school psychologist specifying the nature of the impairment and the level of functioning.

7. *Multihandicap* (multiple disabilities) are concomitant impairments, such as mental retardation and a physical disability, the combination of which results in needs requiring extraordinary service delivery. The term does not include students who are "deaf–blind."

8. *Other health impairments* are conditions in which a person exhibits limited strength, vitality, or alertness as a result of chronic or acute health problems, including a heart condition, spina bifida, tuberculosis, rheumatic fever, nephritis, asthma, sickle-cell anemia, hemophilia, epilepsy, environmental illness, such as lead poisoning, leukemia, or diabetes, the conditions of which adversely affect a child's educational performance. Determination of other health impairments must include reports from a physician and a certified public school psychologist and must specify the nature and degree of the impairment.

9. *Physical disability* is a functional limitation that affects one or more of the following: physical mobility, speech or other forms of nonvocal communication, writing, arm and hand movement, eye and head movement, or one or more of the precursor developmental steps that lead up to full attainment of these skills necessary for success in education. Determination of physical disability must include reports from a physician and a public school psychologist, must specify the nature and degree of the impairment and, when appropriate, the student's ability to profit from assistive technology.

10. *Speech and language impairment* are impairments of language, voice, fluency, or articulation not resulting from sensory impairment or developmental delay but that are present to such a degree that academic achievement is affected and the condition is significantly disabling to the affected person. Determination of speech and language impairment must include the report of a certified speech clinician specifying the nature and degree of the impairment.

11. *Blindness or visual impairment* is a visual impairment adversely affecting the educational performance of the person. Determination of visual impairment must include a full assessment and comprehensive report by an eye specialist specifying the nature and degree of the impairment.[2]

Developmental Delay

Developmental delay, which is relevant to the eligibility of a young child, also is defined in the law. A child is considered to have a developmental delay when one of the following exists:

1. The child's score, on a developmental assessment device (using an instrument that yields a score in months) indicates that the child is delayed by 25% of the child's chronological age in one or more developmental areas: cognitive, language–speech, physical, social–emotional, and self-help.
2. The child is delayed in one or more of the following developmental areas: cognitive, language–speech, physical, social–emotional, and self-help, as documented by test performance of 1.5 standard deviations below the mean on standardized tests.[3]

In addition, the child must need early intervention services because of the delay.

Determination of developmental delay must specify the nature and degree of the delay and must include a full assessment and comprehensive report by a certified public school psychologist, speech correctionist, pediatrician, or psychiatrist.

Mentally Gifted

Mentally gifted is defined as outstanding intellectual and creative ability, the development of which requires special services and programs not ordinarily provided in the regular education program. This term includes a person who has an IQ of 130 or higher and when multiple criteria as set forth in department guidelines indicate gifted ability. Determination of gifted ability is not based on IQ score alone. A person with an IQ score lower than 130 may be admitted to gifted programs when other educational criteria in the profile of the person strongly indicate gifted ability. Determination that a student is mentally gifted must include a full assessment and comprehensive report by a public school psychologist specifying the nature and degree of the ability.[4]

---

2. 22 PA. CODE § 342.1.
3. 22 PA. CODE § 342.1.
4. *Id.*

(B) Referral and Multidisciplinary Evaluation

Before special education services will be provided, students must be evaluated to determine the need for those services. Parents who suspect that their child is exceptional may make a written request for a "multidisciplinary evaluation" at any time, or the school may initiate such an evaluation under certain circumstances.[5] Such evaluations must be conducted by multidisciplinary teams (MDTs). The MDT must comprise the student's parents, persons familiar with the student's educational experience and performance, persons knowledgeable in each area of suspected exceptionality, persons trained in the appropriate evaluation techniques and, when possible, persons familiar with the student's cultural background. The multidisciplinary evaluation must be sufficient in scope and depth to investigate information relevant to the student's suspected exceptionality, including academic functioning, adaptive behavior, social behavior, learning problems, learning strengths, and educational needs.[6]

Multidisciplinary evaluations also must be conducted by school districts for children who are at least 3 years of age—but not yet of the age of those thought to be eligible for early intervention—and who are referred for evaluation by the child's parents, an attending physician, or an agency that has provided services to the child.[7]

Parents have the right to obtain an independent educational evaluation of the student or young child. If parents obtain an independent educational evaluation at private expense, the results of the evaluation must be considered by the district in educational decisions made for the student, and the results may be presented as evidence at a due process hearing regarding that student (discussed later). Parents of applicable children have the right to an independent evaluation at public expense if the parents disagree with an evaluation obtained by the school. The school may initiate an impartial due process hearing, however, to show that its evaluation was appropriate.[8]

---

5. 22 PA. CODE § 14.25. In the years between kindergarten and the end of sixth grade, public school students may receive "instructional support" prior to the initiation of a multidisciplinary evaluation. 22 PA. CODE § 14.24.
6. 22 PA. CODE § 14.25.
7. 22 PA. CODE § 14.53.
8. 22 PA. CODE § 14.67.

Multidisciplinary Team Report

The MDT must prepare a comprehensive written report that brings together all of the information and findings from the evaluation concerning the student's educational needs and strengths and includes an interpretation of assessment results and information on observations in the classroom and other settings. The report must

1. make recommendations as to whether the student is exceptional;

2. indicate the bases for those recommendations; and

3. provide recommendations for the student's educational program, regardless of whether the student is found to be exceptional.[9]

Each exceptional student must be reevaluated by an MDT at least once every 2 years. In addition, reevaluation must occur before a change in educational placement is recommended for the student, or prior to applying disciplinary action that would change an exceptional student's educational placement.

(C) Individualized Education Program

An Individualized Education Program (IEP) team must be appointed to review the recommendations of the MDT and, if it determines a student is exceptional, to develop an IEP for the student. An IEP is a written plan for the appropriate education of an exceptional student.[10] Each IEP team must include

1. one or both of the student's parents;

2. the student, if 18 years of age or older, or if younger and the parents choose to have the student participate;

3. a representative of the district, other than the student's teacher, who:

   a. is qualified to provide or supervise the provision of special education;

   b. can ensure that the services specified in the student's IEP will be provided; and

   c. will serve as the chair of the IEP team.

---

9. 22 Pa. Code § 14.25.
10. 22 Pa. Code § 14.31.

4. one or more of the student's current teachers;

5. the persons who initiated the screening–identification process of the student;

6. A person who is familiar with the placement options of the district;

7. a member of the instructional support team, if appropriate;

8. one or more members of the MDT that completed the most recent evaluation of the student;

9. a person qualified to conduct a diagnostic examination of students if a student is suspected of having a specific learning disability; and

10. other individuals at the discretion of either the parents or the district.[11]

A single member of the IEP may meet two or more of the qualifications specified.

The IEP of each exceptional student must include

1. a statement of the student's present levels of performance;

2. a statement of annual goals and short-term learning outcomes responsive to the learning needs identified in the evaluation report.

3. a statement of the specific special education services and programs and related services to be provided to the student;

4. projected dates for initiation and anticipated duration of special education services and programs and each related service;

5. appropriate objective criteria, assessment procedures, and timelines for determining, on at least an annual basis, whether the goals and learning outcomes are being achieved;

6. a description of the extent to which the eligible student will participate in programs and activities with noneligible students and of the adaptations, if any, to activities that are necessary to ensure meaningful participation;

7. a plan for the completion of necessary credits for graduation developed at least 3 years prior to the anticipated year of graduation; and

8. signatures and positions of IEP team participants documenting participation in the meeting, and the date of the meeting.[12]

---

11. 22 Pa. Code § 14.32.
12. *Id.*

A copy of the IEP must be provided to the parents, along with a notice of parental rights. The IEP team meetings must be convened at least annually, or more frequently if conditions warrant, following an evaluation. An IEP team meeting must also be convened at the request of a member of the IEP team.

IEPs also must be prepared to outline the plan for provision of appropriate early intervention services to an eligible young child.[13]

(D) Parental Rights

Parents must be given written notice within a reasonable time prior to one or more of the following events if the school district:

1. proposes to conduct a multidisciplinary evaluation or reevaluation of the student or young child;

2. refuses to provide independent evaluation at public expense;

3. proposes to initiate or change the identification, evaluation, or educational placement of the student or young child, or proposes to make any significant changes in the IEP and the provision of an appropriate program to the student or young child; or

4. refuses to initiate or change the identification, evaluation, or educational placement of the student or young child, or refuses to make changes requested by the parents in the IEP and the provision of an appropriate program to the student or young child.[14]

The notice must be detailed and written in language understandable to the general public and, if appropriate, in the native language or other mode of communication used by the parents. If necessary the content of notices must be communicated orally or directly.[15]

Written parental consent must be obtained prior to conducting an initial multidisciplinary evaluation or initially placing an exceptional student or eligible young child in a special education or early intervention program.[16]

Prehearing Conference
If the parents do not approve of the recommended assignment following an IEP conference, the school district superintendent

---

13. 22 Pa. Code § 14.54.
14. 22 Pa. Code § 14.61.
15. *Id.*
16. 22 Pa. Code § 14.62.

must convene a prehearing conference within 10 days of receipt of notice of the disapproval. If the prehearing conference results in agreement as to a recommended assignment, the student's IEP shall be implemented. If the prehearing conference does not result in agreement as to a recommended assignment, the parents may request an impartial due process hearing. The parents or the school district may waive the right to a prehearing conference and immediately request an impartial due process hearing.[17]

Impartial Due Process Hearing

If parents disagree with a school district's identification, evaluation, or placement of, or the provision of a free appropriate public education to, a student or young child, the parents may request an impartial due process hearing. Also, a school district may request a hearing to proceed with an initial evaluation or an initial educational placement when the district has not been able to obtain consent from the parents. The hearing is conducted by a hearing officer and must be held in the local school district at a place reasonably convenient to the parents. Parents may be represented by any person, including legal counsel. A written transcript of the hearing must be made on request and provided to parents at no cost. A party has the right to present evidence and testimony, including expert medical, psychological, or educational testimony, and the right to compel the attendance of and question witnesses.

The decision of the impartial hearing officer may be appealed to a panel of three appellate hearing officers. The panel's decision may be appealed further to a court of competent jurisdiction.[18]

As an alternative, parents and agencies involved in an early intervention or special education dispute may obtain the assistance of an impartial mediator in attempting to reach a mutually agreeable settlement.[19]

---

17. 22 PA. CODE § 14.63.
18. 22 PA. CODE § 14.64.
19. 22 PA. CODE § 14.65.

Consent, Confidentiality, and Services for Minors

Whenever a minor requests or receives services without a parent's knowledge or consent (see chapter 3.1), legal issues arise concerning the minor's capacity to give informed consent and the scope of the confidential relations between the minor and the MHP. Failure to obtain consent from the appropriate person before providing services and failure to maintain confidential information are grounds for loss of licensure, a malpractice suit (see chapter 3.10), or other types of civil (see chapter 3.11) or criminal liability (see chapter 3.12). It is important, therefore, for MHPs to identify who the client is from a legal perspective—the minor or the parent. The law does not broadly address these issues, however.

(A) Consent for Mental Health Treatment for Minors

The Minors' Consent to Medical, Dental and Health Services Act provides that any person who is 18 years of age or older, or has graduated from high school, or has married, or has been pregnant, may give effective consent to medical, dental, and health services for himself or herself.[1] Also, "medical, dental and health services may be rendered to minors of any age without the consent of a parent or legal guardian when, in the physician's judgment, an attempt to secure consent would result in delay of treatment which would increase the risk to the minor's life or

---

1. Pa. Stat. Ann. tit. 35, § 10101.

health."[2] In all other circumstances, the consent of a parent or guardian is necessary before providing services to minors.

Any minor who has been married or has borne a child may give effective consent to medical, dental, and health services for his or her child.[3]

Confidentiality and privileged communication are discussed generally in chapters 3.3 and 3.4. When a minor receives mental health services, however, questions arise regarding whether parents or guardians may be given information about that treatment and whether minors or their parents or guardians control the privilege.

For involuntary inpatient and outpatient treatment and for voluntary inpatient treatment, the implementing regulations of the Mental Health Procedures Act provide the rules. If a patient is 14 years of age or older and "understands the nature of documents to be released and the purpose of releasing them," that patient shall control release of his or her records.[4] If a patient lacks the necessary understanding, any person chosen by the patient may control release of records, if the director of the facility finds that the chosen person is acting in the patient's best interest.[5] If the patient is younger than 14 years of age (or has been adjudicated legally incapacitated), control over release of the patient's records may be exercised by a parent (or guardian).[6]

There is no specific statute or regulation governing control of information when minors receive outpatient mental health services on a voluntary basis. It might be argued that when a parent's consent is required for such services, the parent should have access to the information relating to those services. Therefore, an MHP who believes certain information should remain within the control of the minor may wish to enter into an agreement with the parents of that minor regarding the release of information.

Minors of any age can consent to diagnosis or treatment for alcoholism and other drug abuse, and parents do not need to be informed. Although there is no specific statutory provision, it may be presumed that minors receiving diagnostic or treatment services for substance abuse can control the information relating to such services.

If it is determined that a child's parents should control information about that child's evaluation or treatment, a problem may arise when the child's parents are separated or divorced. The

---

2. PA. STAT. ANN. tit. 35, § 10104.
3. PA. STAT. ANN. tit. 35, § 10102.
4. 55 PA. CODE § 5100.33.
5. Id.
6. Id.

general rule is that both parents are to be provided access to all of their child's records, unless a court specifically determines otherwise.[7]

(B) Treatment for Alcohol and Substance Abuse

Under the Pennsylvania Drug and Alcohol Abuse Control Act,[8] minors of any age can consent to medical care or counseling related to diagnosis or treatment for the abuse of alcohol and other drugs.[9] The minor's consent is as valid and binding as the consent of an adult. Physicians or any agencies or organizations operating drug abuse programs who provide counseling to minors using controlled or harmful substances may inform the parents or legal guardians of such minors about treatments given or needed, but they are not obligated to do so.[10]

Voluntary Admission to Mental Health Centers
Minors 14 years of age or older may seek voluntary admission to hospitals for mental health treatment (see chapter 4.19). For children younger than 14, a parent, guardian, or person standing *in loco parentis* may arrange for the child's "voluntary" admission into a hospital for mental health treatment (see chapter 4.19).

Voluntary Outpatient Mental Health Treatment and Partial Hospitalization
There are no specific statutory provisions relating to minors providing consent to outpatient mental health treatment or partial hospitalization. As noted previously, under the Minors' Consent to Medical, Dental and Health Services Act, persons must be 18 years of age or older, have graduated from high school, have married, or have been pregnant to be able to give effective consent to medical and health services for themselves. (See chapter 4.19 explaining parents providing consent for treatment of their children.) The Act does not list psychological services specifically, but psychological treatment services may be considered "health services." Thus, a strict reading of the statute suggests that in nonemergency situations, parental consent is required for outpa-

---

7. 23 PA. CONS. STAT. ANN. § 5309. The court may not order disclosure of the address of a shelter for battered spouses and their dependent children or of otherwise confidential information of a domestic violence counselor. *Id.*
8. PA. STAT. ANN. tit. 71, §§ 1690.101–1690.115.
9. PA. STAT. ANN. tit. 71, § 1690.112.
10. *Id.*

tient psychological treatment or partial hospitalization of minors younger than 18 years of age (unless they have graduated from high school, married, or been pregnant).

Because the Mental Health Procedures Act provides that minors 14 years of age or older may seek voluntary admission to hospitals for mental health treatment, arguably such minors should be able to consent to outpatient mental health treatment or partial hospitalization. Until the legislature adopts a specific statutory provision, however, the safest course for an MHP is to obtain the consent of a parent or guardian before undertaking to provide mental health treatment to a minor of any age.

4.22

Consent for Abortion

The U.S. Constitution forbids states from imposing regulations giving parents veto power over a minor woman's right to an abortion.[1] Nevertheless, the state may impose parental consent or notification requirements when there is an opportunity to bypass that consent or notification through judicial proceedings. Pennsylvania has adopted a statute requiring either parental consent or judicial bypass of parental consent. MHPs may become involved in this process by evaluating and testifying about whether the minor woman is mature enough to make the decision without parental consent or whether the abortion decision is in the minor's best interests.

(A) Standard for Consent

Parental or Guardian Consent
In general, except in the case of a medical emergency, if a pregnant woman is younger than 18 years old and not emancipated, a physician is prohibited from performing an abortion for her unless the physician first obtains the informed consent both of the pregnant woman and one of her parents.[2] If both parents have died or are otherwise unavailable to the physician within a reasonable time and in a reasonable manner, consent of the pregnant woman's guardian or guardians is sufficient. If the pregnant

---

1. Planned Parenthood of S.E. Pennsylvania v. Casey, 505 U.S. 833 (1992); Planned Parenthood of Central Missouri v. Danforth, 428 U.S. 52 (1976).
2. 18 PA. CONS. STAT. ANN. § 3206(a). Pennsylvania has detailed requirements for the procedures for obtaining informed consent to abortion. 18 PA. CONS. STAT. ANN. § 3205.

woman's parents are divorced, consent of the parent having custody is sufficient (a problem may arise if the divorced parents have "shared" custody; see chapter 4.23). If neither a parent nor a legal guardian is available to the physician within a reasonable time and in a reasonable manner, consent of any adult person standing *in loco parentis* is sufficient.[3]

If a pregnant woman has been adjudged an incapacitated person (see chapter 4.2), a physician is prohibited from performing an abortion on her unless the physician first obtains the informed consent of her guardian.[4]

Judicial Bypass of Parental or Guardian Consent
If both of the parents or guardians of the pregnant woman refuse to consent to the performance of an abortion or if she elects not to seek the consent of either of her parents or of her guardian, the court may authorize a physician to perform the abortion. The pregnant woman must file a petition or motion and the court must hold a hearing. If the court determines that the pregnant woman is mature and capable of giving informed consent to the proposed abortion, and has, in fact, given such consent, the court must authorize the physician to perform the abortion.[5] If the court determines that the pregnant woman is not mature and capable of giving informed consent or if the pregnant woman does not claim to be mature and capable of giving informed consent, the court must determine whether the performance of an abortion would be in her best interests. If the court determines that the performance of an abortion would be in the best interests of the woman, it must authorize a physician to perform the abortion.[6]

(B) Notification Hearing

At the hearing, the court must hear evidence relating to the emotional development, maturity, intellect, and understanding of the pregnant woman; the fact and duration of her pregnancy; the nature, possible consequences, and alternatives to the abortion; and any other evidence that the court may find useful in determining whether the pregnant woman should be granted full capacity for the purpose of consenting to the abortion or whether the abortion is in the best interests of the pregnant woman.[7] Such evidence may be provided by MHPs.

---

3. 18 PA. CONS. STAT. ANN. § 3206(b).
4. 18 PA. CONS. STAT. ANN. § 3206(a).
5. 18 PA. CONS. STAT. ANN. § 3206(c).
6. 18 PA. CONS. STAT. ANN. § 3206(d).
7. 18 PA. CONS. STAT. ANN. § 3206(e).

The pregnant woman may participate in proceedings in the court on her own behalf and the court may appoint a guardian *ad litem* to assist her. The court must provide the pregnant woman with court-appointed counsel unless she wishes to appear with private counsel or has knowingly and intelligently waived representation by counsel.[8] There are provisions in the law for expedited proceedings in these matters and for preservation of confidentiality.[9]

---

8. *Id.*
9. 18 PA. CONS. STAT. ANN. §§ 3206(f) & (h).

4.23

Evaluation and Treatment of Children at the Request of a Noncustodial Parent

MHPs may be asked to provide services to children at the request of noncustodial parents. Some states' laws provide that where one parent has custody, that person exercises exclusive authority over the care and upbringing of the child; the noncustodial parent does not have the authority to give legal consent to evaluation or treatment decisions regarding the child. MHPs who provide services at the request of a noncustodial parent without first obtaining the permission of the custodial parent may be vulnerable to a malpractice claim on the basis that consent to the services was not given (see chapter 3.10).

(A) Noncustodial Parent

In Pennsylvania, the parent with legal custody (as opposed to physical custody) has the right to make major decisions concerning the child (see chapter 4.6). If no legal determination regarding legal custody has been made, either parent may ask an MHP to provide services to his or her child. If only one person has been granted legal custody, only that person may request that an MHP provides services to his or her child. If the MHP provides services to the child at the request of a person who does not have legal custody, the MHP is vulnerable to a malpractice claim on the basis that consent to the services was not given (see chapters 3.1, 3.10).

(B) Joint Custody

Problems may arise in two situations: (a) when no legal determination regarding custody of the child has been made and one parent consents but the other parent objects; and (b) when two people, most likely the parents, have been awarded shared legal custody (see chapter 4.6). There is no specific state statute or case law to guide MHPs in the first situation. In the second situation, current case law suggests that a parent with shared legal custody cannot unilaterally authorize an MHP to provide services; that parent must obtain the consent of the other parent or the authorization of a court.[1] The safest course of action for the MHP in either situation is to refuse to provide services until the issue is resolved, if necessary through a petition by one of the parents to the court. This course of action avoids putting the child and the therapist in the middle of a parental dispute.

---

1. Hill v. Hill, 619 A.2d 1086 (Pa. Super. Ct. 1993); Vender v. Luppold, No. 86-1448-00 (C.C.P. Berks March 26, 1996).

Other Civil Matters

Mental Status of Licensed or Certified Professionals

The law governing the licensure or certification of professionals (see chapter 1.2) often includes a provision concerning the mental status of these professionals. It may pertain to the regulation procedures (i.e., disciplinary action, suspension, and revocation of licensure) or it may be a condition of application. Also, licensure and certification laws often include provisions regarding the identification and treatment of so-called "impaired professionals." MHPs may be asked to evaluate and testify before the credentialing board or a court concerning the professional's mental status and its effect on job performance. MHPs also may be asked to treat the professional.

Almost all licensure laws contain a provision that a license may be revoked if the person is unable to practice in a competent manner. It is obvious that some mental disorders can hinder or prevent competent practice. For example, the architects' licensure law provides that a certificate may be revoked for incompetence in the practice of architecture, and an architect suffering from paranoid schizophrenia might not be able to rationally interact with a building inspector. This chapter, however, is limited to laws that specifically mention mental status or mental examinations.

(A) Laws Affecting Specific Professions

(A)(1) Attorneys

If an attorney is declared incompetent (the proper term is now *incapacitated;* see chapter 4.2) or is involuntarily committed to an institution on the grounds of incompetency or disability (see chapter 8.4), a certificate regarding the incapacity determination or commitment must be filed with the Supreme Court.[1] The Pennsylvania Supreme Court, on proper proof of the incapacity declaration or civil commitment, must immediately transfer the attorney to inactive status for an indefinite period until further order of the court.[2]

(A)(2) Dentists and Dental Hygienists

The State Board of Dentistry may not license dentists or dental hygienists if they are "addicted to the use of intoxicating liquor or narcotic drugs."[3] In addition, the Board may refuse, revoke, or suspend the license of any dentist or dental hygienist for being unable to practice as a dentist or dental hygienist with reasonable skill and safety to patients by reason of illness, drunkenness, excessive use of drugs, or as the result of any physical or mental condition.[4] The Board, on finding of probable cause, has authority to compel a dentist or dental hygienist to submit to a mental or physical examination by physicians designated by the Board.[5] MHPs other than physicians are not expressly designated as qualified to conduct the mental examinations. The Board may require a licensee to submit to the care, counseling, or treatment of a physician or psychologist designated by the Board.[6]

(A)(3) Nurses

The State Board of Nursing may refuse, suspend, or revoke any license if the Board finds that the licensee is unable to practice professional nursing with reasonable skill and safety to patients by reason of mental or physical illness or condition or dependence on alcohol or drugs that tend to impair coordination or

---

1. PA. RULES OF DISCIPLINARY ENFORCEMENT (hereinafter R.D.E.) 301(a)–(c). The clerks of the Pennsylvania courts and Pennsylvania Disciplinary Counsel have responsibility for filing such certificates. *Id.*
2. PA. R.D.E. 301(c).
3. PA. STAT. ANN. tit. 63, §§ 122(c)–(d).
4. PA. STAT. ANN. tit. 63, § 123.1.
5. *Id.*
6. *Id.*

judgment so long as the dependence continues.[7] The Board, on probable cause, has authority to compel a licensee to submit to a mental or physical examination as designated by it.[8] Also, the Board may require a licensee to submit to the care, counseling, or treatment of a physician or a psychologist designated by the Board.

(A)(4) Pharmacists

The State Board of Pharmacy has the power to refuse, revoke, or suspend the license of any pharmacist on proof satisfactory to it that the pharmacist (a) is unfit to practice pharmacy because of intemperance in the use of alcoholic beverages, controlled substances, or any other substance that affects the intellect and judgment to such an extent as to impair the performance of professional duties; or (b) is unfit or unable to practice pharmacy by reason of a physical or mental disease or disability. On finding probable cause, the Board has the authority to compel a pharmacist to submit to a mental or physical examination by physicians or psychologists approved by the Board.[9] Also, the Board may require a licensee to submit to the care, counseling, or treatment of a physician or a psychologist designated by the Board.[10] Furthermore, a pharmacist's license must automatically be suspended on the legal commitment to an institution because of mental incompetency (see chapter 8.4) from any cause on filing with the Board a certified copy of such commitment.[11]

(A)(5) Physicians, Physician Assistants, and Midwives

The State Board of Medicine has authority to impose disciplinary or corrective measures on a Board-regulated practitioner for being unable to practice the profession with reasonable skill and safety to patients by reason of illness, addiction to drugs or alcohol, or if he or she has become mentally incompetent. The Board, on finding probable cause, has authority to compel a practitioner to submit to a mental or physical examination by a physician or a psychologist approved by the Board.[12] Also, the Board may require the Board-regulated practitioner to submit to the care, counseling, or treatment of a physician or a psychologist designated by the Board.[13]

---

7. PA. STAT. ANN. tit. 63, § 224.
8. *Id.*
9. PA. STAT. ANN. tit. 63, § 390-5(a).
10. PA. STAT. ANN. tit. 63, § 390-5(c).
11. PA. STAT. ANN. tit. 63, § 390-7.
12. PA. STAT. ANN. tit. 63, § 422.41.
13. PA. STAT. ANN. tit. 63, § 422.42(a).

(A)(6) Psychologists

The State Board of Psychology may refuse to issue a license or may suspend, revoke, limit, or restrict a license or reprimand a licensee for being unable to practice psychology with reasonable skill and safety by reason of illness, drunkenness, excessive use of drugs, or as a result of any mental or physical condition. The Board, on finding probable cause, has authority to compel a psychologist to submit to a mental or physical examination when directed by the Board.[14] The Board may require a licensee to submit to the care, counseling, or treatment of a physician or a psychologist designated by the Board.[15] A psychologist's license must be suspended automatically on the legal commitment of the licensee to an institution because of mental incompetence from any cause (see chapter 8.4) on filing with the Board a certified copy of the commitment.[16]

(A)(7) Social Workers

The State Board of Social Work may refuse to issue a license or may suspend, revoke, limit, or restrict a license or reprimand a licensee for being unable to practice social work with reasonable skill and safety by reason of illness, drunkenness, excessive use of drugs, or as a result of any mental or physical condition. The Board, on probable cause, has authority to compel a social worker to submit to a mental or physical examination by a physician approved by the Board.[17] The Board may require a licensee to submit to the care, counseling, or treatment of a physician designated by the Board.[18] MHPs other than physicians are not expressly designated as qualified to conduct the mental examinations or treatment. A social worker's license must automatically be suspended on the legal commitment of the licensee to an institution because of mental incompetence from any cause (see chapter 8.4) on filing with the Board a certified copy of the commitment.[19]

---

14. PA. STAT. ANN. tit. 63, § 1208(a).
15. PA. STAT. ANN. tit. 63, § 1208(b).
16. PA. STAT. ANN. tit. 63, § 1208(e).
17. PA. STAT. ANN. tit. 63, § 1911(a).
18. PA. STAT. ANN. tit. 63, § 1911(b).
19. PA. STAT. ANN. tit. 63, § 1911(e).

(B) Laws Common to Multiple Professions

Impaired Professionals

The laws regarding impaired professionals are consistent across many different professions, including dentists and dental hygienists;[20] nurses;[21] pharmacists;[22] physicians, physician assistants, and midwives;[23] physical therapists;[24] podiatrists;[25] psychologists;[26] and social workers.[27] In general, these laws address the identification, treatment, rehabilitation, and discipline of "persons with physical or mental impairments," including professionals with drug and alcohol dependency disorders as well as other mental or emotional disorders. The State Boards may defer and ultimately dismiss corrective action for an impaired professional as long as the professional is progressing satisfactorily in an approved treatment program. The impaired professional who enrolls in an approved treatment program must enter into an agreement with the Board under which the professional's license is suspended or revoked. However, enforcement of that suspension or revocation may be stayed for the length of time the professional remains in the program and makes satisfactory progress, complies with the terms of the agreement, and adheres to any limitations on his or her practice imposed by the Board to protect the public. Failure to enter into such an agreement disqualifies the professional from the impaired professional program and activates an immediate investigation and disciplinary proceeding by the Board. If, after consultation with the treatment provider, the consultant believes that an impaired professional who is enrolled in an approved treatment program has not progressed satisfactorily, the consultant must disclose to the Board all information in the consultant's possession regarding the professional, and the Board must institute proceedings to determine if the impaired professional's license will be suspended or revoked.

Mandatory Reporting of Impaired Professionals

The laws regarding mandatory reporting of impaired professionals are consistent across different professions that have im-

---

20. PA. STAT. ANN. tit. 63, § 130g.
21. PA. STAT. ANN. tit. 63, § 224.1.
22. PA. STAT. ANN. tit. 63, § 390-7.
23. PA. STAT. ANN. tit. 63, § 422.4.
24. PA. STAT. ANN. tit. 63, § 1313.
25. PA. STAT. ANN. tit. 63, § 42.21b.
26. PA. STAT. ANN. tit. 63, § 1218.
27. PA. STAT. ANN. tit. 63, § 1915.

paired professional laws discussed previously. In general, these laws state that a hospital or health care facility, peer, or colleague having substantial evidence that a professional has an active addictive disease for which the professional is not receiving treatment, is diverting a controlled substance, or is mentally or physically incompetent to carry out the duties of his or her license must make or cause to be made a report to the Board. Any person or facility acting in a treatment capacity to an impaired physician in an approved treatment program is exempt from the mandatory reporting requirements. Any person or facility who reports in good faith and without malice is immune from any civil or criminal liability arising from such report. Failure to provide such a report within a reasonable time from receipt of knowledge of such impairment subjects the person or facility to a fine not to exceed $1000 dollars.[28]

28. *See* chapters 1.2–1.6.

5.2

Workers' Compensation

Workers' Compensation law provides employees with protection against the treatment costs and income losses resulting from work-related accidents or disease. The employer purchases compensation insurance (or is self-insured) to provide the benefits for employees. These benefits are awarded regardless of whether anyone—the employee or employer—is at fault. In return, the employee relinquishes the right to sue the employer.

MHPs may become involved in this process in two ways. An employee, employer, or insurance company may request that the MHP conduct an evaluation to determine the nature, extent, and cause of an employee's injury and possibly to testify about the findings at a hearing. Also, an MHP may be asked to treat an injured employee with the cost for these services being paid for by Workers' Compensation insurance.

(A) Scope of the Coverage

There are two statutes governing Workers' Compensation—the Pennsylvania Workers' Compensation Act[1] and the Pennsylvania Occupational Disease Act.[2] Only the Pennsylvania Workers' Compensation Act covers accident claims, whereas benefits for disabilities as a result of occupational diseases may be claimed under either act. In the ordinary course, the differences between the two acts should not be a concern for MHPs. Therefore, this chapter focuses primarily on the Workers' Compensation Act.

---

1. PA. STAT. ANN. tit. 77, §§ 1–28.
2. PA. STAT. ANN. tit. 77, §§ 1201–1209.

Workers' Compensation benefits are payable for personal injuries (including death) that arise in the course of employment.[3] The injury must be causally connected to the course of employment. The term *injury* has been broadly defined to encompass all work-related harm.[4]

(B) Workers' Compensation and Mental Stress–Disorder

Disabilities involving psychological elements may be considered to be injuries under the Workers' Compensation Act and, therefore, compensable if the other elements needed to establish a claim are met. For example, the claimant alleging a compensable mental illness or psychiatric injury must establish that the condition is causally connected to the employment. Disabilities involving psychological elements fall into three discrete areas: (a) psychological stimulus causing physical injury; (b) physical stimulus causing psychological injury; and (c) psychological stimulus causing psychological injury.[5] Courts consider the third category to be the most troublesome.[6]

Psychological Stimulus Causing Physical Injury
Physical injuries that are caused by job-related stress are compensable for Workers' Compensation purposes, particularly in cases in which there is a direct connection between stress and a physical injury leading to death, such as a fatal heart attack caused by work-related stress.[7]

Physical Stimulus Causing Psychological Injury
Psychological disorders resulting from physical injuries are compensable. A disability resulting from a work-related physical injury later supplemented by a psychological component is referred to as a *functional overlay*, and because it is a result of the work-related injury, it is fully compensable.[8] Where the work-

---

3. PA. STAT. ANN. tit. 77, § 431
4. Pawlosky v. Workmen's Compensation Appeal Bd., 525 A.2d 1204 (Pa. 1987).
5. Boeing Vertol Co. v. Workmen's Compensation Appeal Bd. (Coles), 528 A.2d 1020 (Pa. Commw. Ct. 1987).
6. *Id.*
7. 39 STANDARD PENNSYLVANIA PRACTICE 2D § 167, 135 (1993) (citing Krawchuk v. Philadelphia Electric Co., 439 A.2d 627 (Pa. 1981)).
8. 39 STANDARD PENNSYLVANIA PRACTICE 2D § 167, 86 (1993) (citing County of Dauphin v. Workmen's Compensation Appeal Bd. (Davis), 82 A.2d 434 (Pa. Commw. Ct.), *appeal denied*, 596 A.2d 160 (Pa. 1990)).

related psychological disability is associated with physical injury, the claimant essentially needs only to prove the basic requirements of Workers' Compensation disability—that is, that the injury resulted in the course of employment and was related to it.[9]

Psychological Stimulus Causing Psychological Injury

Psychological disorders that are caused by job-related stress are compensable for Workers' Compensation purposes. Although the work-related psychiatric disability alone can be compensable, the practical difficulties in evaluating the merits of such claims has led the courts to adopt additional evidentiary safeguards for these types of claims. These additional requirements of proof arise because of a perception that psychiatric and mental injuries are not susceptible to the same objective standard of proof as are physical injuries and other illnesses. Diagnosis of psychological or mental injuries is believed to be more subjective in nature. The additional evidentiary safeguards are intended to provide a more reliable basis for making factual determinations and to deter frivolous claims.

A claimant seeking to recover for mental illness caused by work-related stress has the burden of establishing that the mental injury is caused by an "objective reaction" to "abnormal work conditions."[10] There must be objective evidence that the claimant has suffered a psychiatric injury and objective evidence of the working conditions that caused the injury—rather than subjective evidence of the employee's reaction or feelings or apprehensions regarding working conditions.[11] Only when the court is satisfied that the actual events could cause the psychological injury is the grant of benefits proper.[12]

A claimant generally cannot rely solely on his or her own account of the working environment to meet the burden of showing that a psychiatric injury was not caused by a subjective reaction to normal working conditions; in most cases, the claimant's testimony of abnormal working conditions must be corroborated by other evidence.[13] In some cases, however, such as sexual harassment, the testimony of the claimant regarding actual events

---

9. *Id.*
10. *See, e.g.,* Berry v. Workmen's Compensation Appeal Bd. (United Minerals & Grain Corp.), 602 A.2d 415 (Pa. Commw. Ct. 1992).
11. *Id.*
12. Calabris v. Workmen's Compensation Appeal Bd. (American General Cos.), 595 A.2d 765 (Pa. Commw. Ct. 1991).
13. Waldo v. Workmen's Compensation Appeal Bd. (Erie Metro Transit Authority), 582 A.2d 1147 (Pa. Commw. Ct. 1990).

may be sufficient evidence to support a finding that abnormal working conditions existed.[14]

Abnormal working conditions does not necessarily refer to a single, specific incident, but can refer to a combination of events or circumstances. The claimant alleging a mental injury absent a physical injury must establish either that there were actual extraordinary events that occurred at work, for which specific events can be pinpointed in time, or that the existence of abnormal working conditions over a longer period of time caused the psychiatric injury.[15] Extremely stressful conditions can be abnormal working conditions. However, exposure to highly stressful conditions, where such exposure is a usual part of that employment, does not support the finding of a work-related and compensable mental injury.[16]

Conduct directed toward an employee by the employer or employer's supervisors (e.g., harassment), may create abnormal working conditions sufficient to support a finding that the resulting mental or psychological disability was work related and compensable.[17]

Although intentionally self-inflicted injuries or deaths generally are not compensable for Workers' Compensation purposes, self-inflicted injuries or deaths arising from mental illness or psychiatric condition that are work-related are compensable on showing of proper proof.[18] A claimant seeking to recover for the suicide of the deceased has the burden of proving that abnormal work conditions caused the employee's severe mental disorder and resultant suicide.[19]

(C) Processing a Claim

A claimant seeking compensation under the Workers' Compensation Act is required to notify the employer that the employee in question received an injury in the course of employment at a specific time and place.[20] Unless the employer has knowledge of the occurrence of the injury, if notice is not given within 21 days, the claimant will not be entitled to compensation until such notice

---

14. Archer v. Workmen's Compensation Appeal Bd. (General Motors), 587 A.2d 901 (Pa. Commw. Ct. 1991).
15. 39 STANDARD PENNSYLVANIA PRACTICE 2D § 167, 189 (citing Calabris, 595 A.2d 765).
16. 39 STANDARD PENNSYLVANIA PRACTICE 2D § 167, 191 (1993).
17. Marsico v. Workmen's Compensation Appeal Bd. (Pennsylvania Dept. of Revenue), 588 A.2d 984 (Pa. Commw. Ct. 1991).
18. Martin v. Ketchum, Inc., 568 A.2d 159 (Pa. 1990).
19. *Id.*
20. PA. STAT. ANN. tit. 77, §§ 631–633.

is given.[21] Furthermore, except in the case of death claims, for compensation to be permitted at all, an employer must receive notice of the employee's injury within 120 days after its occurrence unless the employer has actual knowledge of the injury.[22] The notice period begins on the date the claimant knows, or should know, that the injury is severe enough to be compensable and that the injury was caused by the employment.[23]

In the event that the employer, or the employer's insurer, fails to agree with the employee or the employee's dependent with respect to the facts or compensation that may be due, the employee or the dependents are entitled to present a claim for compensation to the Department of Labor and Industry.[24] After a claim is presented, the Department will assign it to a workers' compensation judge (previously called a *referee*) to be heard.[25] Workers' compensation judges are appointed to conduct hearings by and subject to the general supervision of the secretary of the department. They are civil service employees and need not be attorneys.

A party who is adversely affected by a workers' compensation judge's decision to award or disallow compensation has the right to take an appeal to the Workmen's Compensation Appeal Board.[26] The appeal must be timely. Final orders of the Board may be appealed directly to the Commonwealth Court.[27]

Expert Witnesses

The workers' compensation judge has discretion similar to that of a trial judge in determining whether a medical witness is qualified as an expert.[28] Experts may be qualified by reason of their knowledge or experience. The Commonwealth Court has held that a clinical psychologist is competent to testify to the history, diagnosis, and treatment of a claimant's condition, although psychologists are not physicians.[29] The expert's testimony and conclusions should be supported by proper and relevant findings;

---

21. PA. STAT. ANN. tit. 77, § 631.
22. *Id.* Actual knowledge is defined as "awareness of such information as would cause a reasonable person to inquire further; such awareness considered as a timely and sufficient substitute for actual notice." MERIAM WEBSTER'S DICTIONARY OF LAW 278–279 (1996).
23. *See, e.g.,* Sun Oil Co. v. Workmen's Compensation Appeal Bd. (Davis), 600 A.2d 684 (Pa. Commw. Ct. 1991).
24. PA. STAT. ANN. tit. 77, § 751; 34 PA. CODE § 131.32(a).
25. PA. STAT. ANN. tit. 77, § 775.
26. PA. STAT. ANN. tit. 77, § 853.
27. 42 PA. CONS. STAT. ANN. § 763.
28. Workmen's Compensation Appeal Bd. (Carl A. Lindbom) v. Jones & Laughlin Steel Corp., 349 A.2d 793 (Pa. Commw. Ct. 1975).
29. Serrano v. Workmen's Compensation Appeal Bd. (Chain Bike Corp.), 553 A.2d 1025 (Pa. Commw. Ct. 1989).

testimony that merely recites a legal standard is insufficient.[30] A medical expert may give an opinion about whether the employee is disabled to perform the employee's job when the expert is familiar with the position.[31]

---

30. *Id.*
31. Bethlehem Mines Corp. v. Workmen's Compensation Appeal Bd., 423 A.2d 479 (Pa. Commw. Ct. 1980).

5.3

Vocational Disability Determinations

The State Board of Vocational Rehabilitation administers a program funded jointly by the state and federal governments for persons who have physical or mental disabilities that currently prevent them from obtaining (or maintaining) employment but who might be able to engage (or to continue) in gainful occupations if given vocational rehabilitation services. MHPs may become involved to conduct evaluations or to provide rehabilitation services.

(A) The Vocational Rehabilitation Act

The purpose of the Vocational Rehabilitation Act is to develop and implement programs of vocational rehabilitation to meet the needs of individuals with disabilities to maximize their employability, independence, and integration into the workplace and the community.[1]

Vocational rehabilitation services are any goods or services, as defined by federal law,[2] that are provided directly or indirectly through public or private sources and that are found to be necessary for an individual with a disability to: (a) overcome employment handicaps and engage in a gainful occupation or profession; (b) achieve such ability of independent living as to function more independently within the family and within the community and engage in or continue to engage in employment; or (c) engage in competitive work in integrated settings through the provision of

---

1. PA. STAT. ANN. tit. 43, § 682.2.
2. 29 U.S.C. §§ 706, 723.

training and time-limited postemployment services leading to supported employment.[3]

The Office of Vocational Rehabilitation within the Department of Labor and Industry has the responsibility for providing vocational rehabilitation services to individuals with disabilities who are determined to be eligible for them.[4] Any individual who is applying for or receiving vocational rehabilitation and who is aggrieved by any action or inaction of any officer or agent of the office is entitled to a fair hearing.[5]

(B) Vocational Rehabilitation Recipient Eligibility Requirements

Vocational rehabilitation services must be provided to any individual with a disability whose vocational rehabilitation the office determines can be satisfactorily achieved or who is eligible for such services under the terms of an agreement with another state or the federal government. Except as otherwise provided by law or agreement, vocational rehabilitation services are provided at public cost only to individuals found to require financial assistance. The following services, however, are provided at public cost to individuals with disabilities without any consideration of economic need for financial assistance: (a) evaluation of rehabilitation potential, including diagnostic and related services, incidental to the determination of eligibility for, and the nature and scope of, services to be provided; and (b) counseling, guidance, referral, and placement services, including follow-up and follow-along services.[6]

"The office may make money payments necessary to meet living requirements for disabled or injured individuals and their families during the period of vocational rehabilitation and training and for an additional 60-day trial period of employment if the disabled or injured individual is cooperative and demonstrates satisfactory progress."[7]

The Vocational Rehabilitation Act and the Workers' Compensation Act are to be read together to provide both rehabilitation assistance and compensation to employees who have been

---

3. *Id.*
4. PA. STAT. ANN. tit. 43, § 682.7.
5. PA. STAT. ANN. tit. 43, § 682.13.
6. PA. STAT. ANN. tit. 43, § 682.10.
7. PA. STAT. ANN. tit. 43, § 682.11(b). The focus is on a person's wage-earning capacity, such that anyone able to work should, but those who truly need more time to recover should be allotted the needed time.

injured in the course of their employment. Receipt of benefits under the Workers' Compensation Act does not preclude receipt of rehabilitation assistance under the Vocational Rehabilitation Act.[8]

---

8. PA. STAT. ANN. tit. 43, § 682.11; Burgess v. Workmen's Compensation Appeal Bd. (Plaza Foods), 612 A.2d 542 (Pa. Commw. Ct.), *appeal denied,* 618 A.2d 403 (1992).

Emotional Distress as a Basis for Civil Liability

Emotional distress (also known as *mental suffering*) may be the basis for a civil tort suit (i.e., a lawsuit alleging physical or personal injury) or may be part of a larger claim. The cause of the distress, the nature of the injury, and the motivations of the injuring person determine whether a lawsuit requesting compensation for emotional distress must be part of a larger claim or can stand by itself. MHPs may be asked to evaluate the person who claims to have suffered the distress and to testify about its etiology, severity, and duration, as well as methods of treating it.

(A) Intentional Infliction of Emotional Distress

The lower state courts and federal courts applying the law have held that the law permits a person to sue for intentional infliction of emotional distress. However, the Pennsylvania Supreme Court has expressed some reservation about this type of claim, and the Superior Court has not expressly adopted the standard definition of intentional infliction of emotional distress.[1] Nevertheless, court decisions suggest that such a claim would require that: (a) the defendant's conduct is capable of being characterized as "extreme and outrageous"; (b) the conduct was either intended to cause emotional distress or recklessly disregarded the near certainty

---

1. Strain v. Ferroni, 592 A.2d 698, 703 (Pa. Super. Ct. 1991).

that such distress would result from the conduct; and (c) severe emotional distress occurred as a result of the conduct.[2]

The availability of recovery for intentional infliction of emotional distress is limited.[3] The first requirement will only be met in cases in which the defendant's conduct has been so outrageous and so extreme in degree as to go beyond all possible bounds of decency and to be regarded as atrocious and utterly intolerable in a civilized community.[4] As an example, to conceal the negligent treatment of a patient, a hospital and physicians allegedly prepared a false report that a patient's death resulted from assault by the plaintiff and as a result the plaintiff was prosecuted for assault and homicide. Such behavior by the hospital and physicians was held to be sufficient to state a claim for intentional infliction of emotional distress.[5]

The last element requires proof that the plaintiff actually experienced severe emotional distress. The Pennsylvania Supreme Court has stated that "given the advanced state of medical science, it is unwise and unnecessary to permit recovery to be predicated on an inference based on the defendant's outrageousness' without expert medical confirmation that the plaintiff actually suffered the claimed distress."[6] The court concluded that in an action for intentional infliction of emotional distress "at the very least, existence of the alleged emotional distress must be supported by competent medical evidence."[7]

The Pennsylvania Supreme Court has stated that the reluctance of courts to allow recovery for purely psychological injury can be traced to three principal concerns: medical science's difficulty in proving causation, the danger of fraudulent or exaggerated claims, and the perception that recognition of such a cause of action would precipitate excessive litigation.[8]

---

2. *Id.* (citing § 46 of RESTATEMENT (SECOND) OF TORTS).
3. *Id.*; Ford v. Isdaner, 542 A.2d 137 (Pa. Super. Ct. 1988); Kazatsky v. King David Memorial Park, Inc., 527 A.2d 988 (Pa. 1987).
4. D'Ambrosio v. Pennsylvania Nat. Mut. Casualty Ins. Co., 431 A.2d 966 (Pa. 1981).
5. Banyas v. Lower Bucks Hosp., 437 A.2d 1236 (Pa. Super. Ct. 1981) (disapproved on other grounds by *Kazatsky*, 527 A.2d 988.
6. *Kazatsky*, 527 A.2d at 995.
7. *Id.*
8. *Kazatsky*, 527 A.2d at 993 (citations omitted).

(B) Negligent Infliction of Emotional Distress

The law permits a person to sue for negligent infliction of emotional distress. In a negligence action, the plaintiff must show that the defendant owed a duty to him or her, a breach of that duty, damages, and a causal connection between the damages and breach of the duty owed.[9] The courts have limited liability by holding that defendants only owe a duty to "foreseeable" plaintiffs. The courts also have limited liability by holding that the breach of the duty must be the "proximate" or "legal" cause of the damages—the courts can determine that at some point the chain of causation is so attenuated that the defendant will not be held liable. Thus, to prove negligent infliction of emotional distress, the plaintiff must show that the defendant, through the defendant's breach of a duty, was the proximate cause of the emotional injury to a foreseeable plaintiff.

There are a variety of situations in which plaintiffs may be able to recover for negligent infliction of emotional distress. Where a plaintiff has suffered emotional distress directly traceable to the peril in which the defendant's negligence placed him or her, that distress is a legitimate element of damages, if it was preceded or accompanied by some independent bodily injury or impact, however slight.[10] Traditionally there was no recovery for negligently inflicted emotional distress in the absence of physical impact on the plaintiff. The Pennsylvania Supreme Court, however, has established a cause of action for negligent infliction in the absence of physical impact.[11] It is not necessary to demonstrate a physical impact in a case in which the plaintiff was in personal danger of physical impact because a negligent force was directed against him or her; and the plaintiff actually did fear physical impact.[12] This is known as the *zone of danger rule*.

A more recent line of cases allows plaintiffs who are outside of the zone of danger to recover for negligent infliction based on the emotional distress caused by observing someone else to be injured.[13] The defendant's liability for psychological injury to such a bystander plaintiff depends on meeting three require-

---

9. Morena v. South Hills Health System, 462 A.2d 680 (Pa. 1983). *See generally,* Douglas B. Marlowe. (1988). Comment: Negligent infliction of mental distress: A jurisdictional survey of existing limitation devices and proposal based on an analysis of objective versus subjective indices of distress. *Villanova Law Review,* 33, 781.
10. Stoddard v Davidson, 513 A.2d 419 (Pa. Super. Ct. 1986).
11. Niederman v. Brodsky, 261 A.2d 84 (Pa. 1970).
12. *Id.* at 413, 261 A.2d at 90.
13. Sinn v. Burd, 404 A.2d 672 (Pa. 1979).

ments: (a) The plaintiff must be located near the scene of the accident as contrasted with one who is a distance away; (b) the shock must result from a direct emotional impact on the plaintiff from the "sensory and contemporaneous observance" of the accident; and (c) the plaintiff and the victim must be closely related.[14] With regard to the second element, it is not necessary that the plaintiff see the accident; hearing the impact may be sufficient.[15] With regard to the third element, recovery is dependent on a familial relationship between the plaintiff and the injured victim, although this need not be a blood relationship (e.g., husband and wife relationships and foster parent and foster child relationships have been held to be sufficient).[16]

In many states, to recover for emotional distress in the absence of a physical impact, the emotional distress itself must result in some physical injury. The requirement of resulting physical injury is another synthetic device to guarantee the authenticity of the claim, and the Pennsylvania Supreme Court has suggested that advances in science make it possible to prove psychological injury even without a physical manifestation of that injury.[17] Nevertheless, the Pennsylvania Supreme Court has not directly addressed, and the lower courts are divided over, the issue of whether recovery for negligent infliction of emotional distress is dependent on a physical manifestation of the emotional distress.[18]

---

14. Mazzagatti v. Everingham, 516 A.2d 672 (Pa. 1986); Sinn v. Burd, 404 A.2d 672 (Pa. 1979).
15. Krysmalski v. Tarasovich, 622 A.2d 298 (Pa. Super. Ct. 1993); Neff v. Lasso, 555 A.2d 1304 (Pa. Super. Ct.) *appeal denied,* 565 A.2d 445 (Pa. 1989). At least one court, however, has required that aural observances be accompanied by prior and subsequent visual observances to allow recovery for negligent infliction of emotional distress. *Id.*
16. Strain v. Ferroni, 592 A.2d 698 (Pa. Super. Ct. 1991) (allowing recovery where relationship between victim and plaintiff was husband and wife); Neff v. Lasso, 555 A.2d 1304 (Pa. Super. Ct. 1989) (same); and Kratzer v. Unger, 17 Pa. D. & C.3d 771 (Bucks Co. 1981) (foster parent).
17. Sinn v. Burd, 404 A.2d 672, 679 (Pa. 1979).
18. Banyas, III v. Lower Bucks Hosp., 437 A.2d 1236 (Pa. Super. Ct. 1981) (physical harm needed); Wall v. Fisher, 565 A.2d 498 (Pa. Super. Ct. 1989), *appeal denied,* 584 A.2d 319 (Pa. 1990) (physical harm needed); Strain v. Ferroni, 592 A.2d 698 (Pa. Super. Ct. 1991) (physical harm needed); Krysmalski v. Tarosovich, 622 A.2d 298 (Pa. Super. Ct. 1993) (no bodily harm in addition to emotional distress required for recovery).

(C) Emotional Distress as an Element of Damages

Both of the foregoing claims require the presence of emotional distress. There are other claims, however, in which emotional distress is not an essential element of the claim but in which the plaintiff may be able to recover damages for emotional distress along with other damages. For example, when a person is severely physically injured in a car accident as a result of a defendant's negligence, that person may sue for physical injuries, loss of earnings, and emotional distress damages. The emotional distress damages must be causally connected to the defendant's acts.

The law also recognizes claims for emotional distress as part of a wrongful death action. In this type of action, the decedent's spouse, children, and parents have a claim against the defendant for any damages they may have suffered as a result of the defendant's wrongful conduct against the decedent.

Finally, there are some other claims that invoke, directly or indirectly, some measure of emotional distress, such as false imprisonment, malicious prosecution, slander, or invasion of privacy. These are referred to as dignity torts (i.e., an injury to the person's reputation or personal sense of worth), yet it is clear that the damage is largely to one's emotional well-being. Although these claims do not require evidence of emotional harm to the plaintiff to prove liability, the size of the damage award may hinge on such proof.

Insanity of Wrongdoers and Civil Liability

A person's mental status may affect whether he or she is liable under civil law for injurious behavior he or she caused to another and whether the person can participate in civil litigation. MHPs may be asked to evaluate a defendant's mental status at the time of the alleged wrongdoing for the purpose of determining that defendant's liability. MHPs also may be asked to evaluate a plaintiff's or defendant's mental status during the course of civil litigation to determine his or her capacity to participate in the litigation. In either case, the MHP may be asked to testify.

(A) The Civil Liability of a Mentally Disabled Person

Mentally disordered adults are generally civilly responsible for injuries they cause to others or property.[1] "The law is that 'mental deficiency [short of insanity] does not relieve the actor from liability for conduct which does not conform to the standard of a reasonable man under the circumstances.' "[2] The mentally deficient person is held to the standard of conduct of a reasonable person. There are few recent cases on the issue, but testimony regarding the mental condition of the defendant may be relevant in cases in which wrongful or malicious intent is an essential

---

1. Priese v. Clement, 70 Pa. D. & C.2d 47 (Del. Co. 1974).
2. *Id.* at 63 (quoting RESTATEMENT (SECOND) OF TORTS § 283(B)); *see also* Wolf's Case, 46 A. 72 (Pa. 1900); Lancaster County Nat'l Bank v. Moore, 78 Pa. 407 (1875) ("A person with a mental deficiency is civilly liable for his torts.").

element of the cause of action (e.g., fraud, slander and malicious prosecution).[3]

(B) Insanity and Liability Insurance

Insurance policies almost always contain exclusionary provisions denying coverage for personal injuries or property damage caused by the intentional acts of the insured. The exclusion may also extend to the costs of legal representation. The question arises whether insureds can raise an "insanity" defense (though in a civil context), claiming that they were able to form the specific intent to cause the injury, thereby compelling the insurer to provide coverage. The issue has not been definitively resolved. One appellate court has indicated, however, that the proper test to apply in such cases is the *M'Naughton* insanity rule used in criminal cases (see chapter 7.9).[4]

(C) Capacity to Participate in Civil Litigation

The law provides that a party to a civil lawsuit who is "incapacitated" (formerly *incompetent*) must be represented by a guardian or by a guardian *ad litem* who shall supervise and control the conduct of the action on his or her behalf.[5] The standard for determining incapacity is whether the person's "ability to receive and evaluate information effectively and communicate decisions in any way is impaired to such a significant extent that the person is partially or totally unable to manage financial resources or to meet the essential requirements for physical health and safety."[6] This is the same incapacity standard that is found in guardianship law (see chapter 4.2). If the court finds that a party is incapacitated and that party has not had a guardian appointed (see chapter 4.2), the court may appoint a guardian *ad litem* who has responsibility for the incapacitated person only as it pertains to the suit. The guardian as litem does not take responsibility for any other aspect of the person's life. Frequently the guardian *ad litem* is an attorney, but this is not a requirement.

---

3. Wolf's Case, 46 A. 72 (Pa. 1900) (citing Insurance Co. v. Showalter, 3 Pa. Super. 452 (1896)).
4. Germantown Insurance Co. v. Martin, 595 A.2d 1172 (Pa. Super. Ct. 1991).
5. PA. R. CIV. P. 2053; see also PA. R. CIV. P. 2056.
6. PA. R. CIV. P. 2051.

5.6

Competency to Contract

A person wishing to enter into a contract to buy or sell anything of value (including real estate) must have a minimum mental capacity. In general, people are presumed to have sufficient capacity to enter into their contracts. An issue may arise prior to a contract, however, when the capacity of one of the potential parties to the contract is in doubt. Also, an issue may arise after parties have entered into a contract when one of the parties (or that person's legal representative, such as a guardian) wishes to be excused from the obligation to fulfill his or her part of the agreement. Therefore, either before a contract or after, an MHP may be asked to evaluate the capacity of the person to enter into the contract, and an MHP may be asked to testify about that capacity.

(A) Legal Standard of Competency to Contract

A claim that a person lacked the capacity (or competency) to enter into a contract is distinct from a claim that he or she is generally incapacitated (see chapter 4.2).

In evaluating a person's competency to enter into a contract, the Pennsylvania Supreme Court focused on the party's lucidity, ability to act with deliberation, and capacity to understand or comprehend the contract.[1] Although the standard is not clear, being controlled by common law and not by statute, it appears that the courts will focus on the person's orientation ('lucidity') and cognitive understanding of the contract. Thus, an assessment of competency to contract should focus on whether the party is able to understand the nature and consequences of the transaction.

The Pennsylvania Supreme Court has suggested that "reasonableness" and "rationality" are not necessary for competency to contract.[2] In addition, this case suggests that the courts should be reluctant to overturn contracts on the grounds that a party lacked the capacity to contract. In one of the rare cases in which the court found that a release should be set aside because of an enfeebled physical and mental condition, these facts were coupled with fraud and misrepresentation.[3] Cases involving releases and gifts that were contested on grounds of incompetency are consistent with the competency to contract cases; the courts have not drawn distinctions among the standards for competency to contract, to make a gift, and to execute a release.

A person who has been adjudicated a "partially incapacitated person" (see chapter 4.2) is by law incapable of making any contract or gift or any instrument in writing in those specific areas in which the person has been found to be incapacitated.[4] A person who has been adjudicated as "totally incapacitated" (see chapter 4.2) is by law incapable of making any contract or gift or any instrument in writing.[5]

(B) Determination of Competency

The courts have established the following general evidentiary principles to be followed in competency to contract cases:

1. It is presumed that an adult is competent to enter into an agreement, and thus, a signed document yields the presumption that it accurately expresses the state of mind of the signing party.[6] Therefore, once a signed contract is produced, the party

---

1. Estate of McGovern v. Commonwealth State Employees' Retirement Board, 517 A.2d 523 (Pa. 1986); accord Weir by Gasper v. Estate of Ciao, 556 A.2d 819 (Pa. 1989) (lucidity relevant); Taylor v. Avi, 415 A.2d 894 (Pa. Super. Ct. 1979) (ability to understand nature of business being transacted relevant); Law v. Mackie, 95 A.2d 656 (Pa. 1953) (ability to comprehend facts and circumstances leading to settlement agreement negotiation relevant).
2. McGovern, 517 A.2d 523.
3. Jenkins v. Peoples Cab Co., 220 A.2d 669 (Pa. Super. Ct. 1966).
4. 20 PA. CONS. STAT. ANN. § 5524.
5. Id.
6. McGovern, 517 A.2d 523; Taylor v. Avi, 415 A.2d 894.

claiming that the contracting person was incompetent has the burden of proving incompetence.

2. The burden of proof to set aside a transaction on the basis of mental incompetency is "clear, precise and convincing."[7] This is an intermediate standard of proof designed to make it more difficult to prove that a person was incompetent to contract. Incompetence must be proved by more than a "preponderance of the evidence" (the general civil liability standard), although it need not be proved "beyond a reasonable doubt" (the general criminal liability standard).

3. The determination as to mental capacity depends on the condition of the person at the time he executed the contract.[8]

4. A person's mental capacity is best determined by his spoken words and his conduct, and the testimony of persons who observed such conduct on the date of the contract outranks testimony as to observations made before and after that date.[9]

5. Mere "mental weakness" will not authorize a court to set aside a contract, if it does not amount to inability to comprehend the contract, and is unaccompanied by evidence of imposition or undue influence.[10] (See chapter 5.7 discussing the legal concept of "undue influence" in the context of wills.)

6. A presumption of mental incapacity does not arise merely because of an unreasonable or unnatural disposition of property.[11]

---

7. *McGovern*, 517 A.2d at 526; Elliot v. Clawson, 204 A.2d 272 (Pa. 1964); *Taylor*, 415 A.2d 894; *Jenkins*, 220 A.2d 669.
8. *Weir by Gasper v. Estate of Ciao*, 556 A.2d 819, 824 (Pa. 1989); *McGovern*, 517 A.2d at 526; Sobel v. Sobel, 254 A.2d 649, 651 (Pa. 1969).
9. *Weir*, 556 A.2d at 824; *McGovern*, 517 A.2d at 526; *Sobel*, 254 A.2d at 651.
10. *McGovern*, 517 A.2d at 526; *Law v. Mackie*, 95 A.2d 656 (Pa. 1953).
11. *McGovern*, 517 A.2d at 526; *Lawrence's Estate*, 132 A. 786 (Pa. 1926).

Competency to Sign a Will

Persons who make wills or amend existing ones (referred to as *testators*) must meet minimum mental status requirements. If it is later shown that the person did not have the required minimum mental status, the testator's estate will be distributed according to the terms of a previous valid will, if any, or by the intestacy (i.e., without a will) statutes.

An MHP may be asked to conduct an evaluation of the testator specifically to determine whether the testator has or had the mental capacity necessary to execute a will. An MHP also may be consulted when he or she treated the testator or evaluated the testator for some other purpose (but see chapters 3.3 and 3.4 for limitations on use of such information). In some cases (e.g., after the testator has died), an MHP may be asked to provide an opinion of the testator's mental status based on reports of other witnesses and any other relevant information. In addition, in circumstances similar to the those discussed, MHPs may be consulted regarding issues arising in the context of an allegation that someone has used undue influence in getting a testator to execute a will.

(A) Legal Test of Testamentary Capacity

A statute provides, "Any person 18 or more years of age who is of sound mind may make a will."[1] Over the years, the courts have

---

1. 20 Pa. Cons. Stat. Ann. § 2501.

determined what "sound mind" (or testamentary capacity) means for purposes of executing a will. A testator possesses testamentary capacity if the testator knows (a) those who are the "natural objects of his or her bounty"; (b) of what his or her estate consists; and (c) what he or she desires done with the estate.[2] The *natural objects of one's bounty* are those people who have a natural claim to the estate property (i.e., family members). The courts have not developed specific definitions for each of these three elements.

(B) Proving Testamentary Incapacity

The Pennsylvania Supreme Court has established a few basic rules when a will is contested on the basis that the testator lacked testamentary capacity:

1. The burden of proving testamentary capacity is initially with the proponent of the will.

2. A presumption of testamentary capacity arises on proof of execution by two subscribing witnesses. Thereafter, the burden of proof as to incapacity shifts to the contestants to overcome the presumption by clear, strong, and compelling evidence.

3. The condition of the testator at the very time of execution is crucial; however, evidence of capacity or incapacity for a reasonable time before and after execution is admissible as indicative of capacity.

4. Old age, sickness, distress, or debility of body neither proves nor raises a presumption of incapacity.[3]

Because the inquiry focuses on the time when the will is executed, most decisions have accorded more weight to the testimony of persons actually present at the execution than that of persons who can only give an opinion based on facts as they existed before or after execution (e.g., MHPs).[4] Therefore, if an

---

2. *In re* Estate of Kuzma, 408 A.2d 1369, 1371 (Pa. 1979).
3. Kuzma, 408 A.2d 1369.
4. *See, e.g., In re* Estate of Ziel, 359 A.2d 728 (Pa. 1976) (physician's opinion testimony entitled to little weight in cases in which it is based on observations made more than 1 year before execution of will and codicils; testimony of attorney–scrivener and lay witnesses who had seen testator on relevant dates accorded more weight). *But cf.* Masciantonio Will, 141 A.2d 362 (Pa. 1958) (error for lower court to accord less weight to opinion testimony of two physicians who examined decedent within several hours before and after execution of will than to direct evidence of attorney–scrivener and subscribing witnesses who were interested parties).

MHP is consulted prior to the drafting of a will, the evaluation of testamentary capacity should take place as close in time as possible to the execution of the will.

(C) Undue Influence

The Pennsylvania Supreme Court has defined undue influence as:

> Control acquired over another that virtually destroys his free agency.... To constitute undue influence sufficient to void a will, there must be imprisonment of the body or mind . . . fraud, or threats, or misrepresentations, or circumvention, or inordinate flattery or physical or moral coercion, to such a degree as to prejudice the mind of the testator, to destroy his free agency and to operate as a present restraint upon him in the making of a will.[5] When the proponent of a will has established that the formalities of execution have been followed, a presumption of lack of undue influence arises.[6] The burden then shifts to the contestant to prove, through either direct or circumstantial evidence, that there was undue influence exerted to procure the testamentary provisions being contested.[7]

If the contestant seeks to prove undue influence circumstantially, he or she must establish by clear and convincing evidence "that (1) when the will was executed the testator was of weakened intellect, and (2) that a person in a confidential relationship with the testator (3) receives a substantial benefit under the will."[8] The first element, *weakened intellect,* need not rise to the level of testamentary incapacity.[9] The second element, *confidential relationship,* exists between a testator and another person when circumstances make it certain that the parties do not deal on equal terms.[10] There is either "overmastering influence" on one side or weakness, dependence, or trust, justifiably reposed, on the other.[11] Such a set of circumstances creates the opportunity for the person in the confidential relationship to take unfair advantage of the testator.[12] Once the contestant establishes each of these three elements, a presumption of undue influence arises. The burden then shifts back to the proponent to refute that presumption by clear

---

5. Williams v. McCarroll, 97 A.2d 14, 20 (Pa. 1953) (*quoted with approval* in Estate of Ziel, 359 A.2d 728, 733 (Pa. 1976)).
6. Estate of Clark, 334 A.2d 628 (Pa. 1975).
7. *Id.*
8. Estate of Fickert, 337 A.2d 592, 594 (Pa. 1975).
9. *Ziel,* 359 A.2d at 734 (citing Estate of Clark, 334 A.2d at 633).
10. *Ziel,* 359 A.2d at 734.
11. *Id.*
12. *Id.*

and convincing evidence.[13] To prevail, the proponent must establish that the bequest was the free, voluntary, and clearly understood act of the testator.[14]

When an allegation of undue influence has been made, an MHP may be consulted for an opinion regarding the testator's susceptibility to coercion, the coercive impact of actions by the person exerting influence, the relationship between the testator and the person exerting influence, the "weakened intellect" of the testator, or the understanding of the testator.

---

13. *Id.*
14. Thompson's Estate, 126 A.2d 740 (Pa. 1956).

Competency to Vote

The right to vote can be denied or revoked based on a person's mental status, although such determinations are rare. A person must be qualified to vote and MHPs may be asked to evaluate a person in this regard.

(A) Competency to Vote

The Pennsylvania Constitution and the Pennsylvania Election Code[1] state the qualifications that are necessary to vote.[2] There is no requirement in the Constitution or in the Code that a person have a specific mental status, nor has a definitive standard for competency to vote been developed in court cases. The attorney general of Pennsylvania has stated that a mentally retarded or mentally ill person cannot be disenfranchised solely because he or she is undergoing treatment for a mental disability or is known to reside in an institution for the treatment of the mentally disabled.[3] A court, however, has held that a person who would not understand for whom his or her votes were being cast and would not be aware of the effect of his or her vote may be denied the right to

---

1. PA. STAT. ANN. tit. 25, §§ 2600–3591.
2. *See* PA. CONST. art. VII, § 1; PA. STAT. ANN. tit. 25, § 2811; *see also* PA. STAT. ANN. tit. 25, § 951-22 (who may register).
3. 73 Op. Att'y. Gen. 48. (1973).

vote.[4] This is as close as the courts have come to articulating a standard for competency to vote.

(B) Patients Confined in Mental Institutions

The Pennsylvania Election Code provides that certain persons are entitled to vote by absentee ballots. The Code, however, specifically states that persons confined in mental institutions are not qualified to vote by absentee ballot.[5] Nevertheless, such persons may vote at their places of institutional residence.[6]

---

4. *In re* 233 Absentee Ballot Appeals, 81 York 137 (1967) (where because of cerebral difficulty voter would not have understood for whom votes were being cast and would not have been aware of effect of vote, legislature indicated its intent that such person should not be entitled to vote); *see also* Thompson v. Ewing, 1 Brewst. 92 (1861) (vote of "lunatic" may be rejected though there has been no finding of "lunacy")
5. PA. STAT. ANN. tit. 25, § 3146.1.
6. *See* 73 Op. Att'y. Gen. 48 (1973) (denial of absentee ballot to mentally disabled, institutionalized person does not prohibit that person from voting at his or her place of institutional residence).

Competency to Obtain a Driver's License

The law provides that certain disorders or disabilities may render a person incompetent to drive a motor vehicle. Physicians have an obligation to report to the Department of Transportation when someone has one of these conditions and it interferes with the ability to drive safely. In addition, physicians may be asked to conduct evaluations of these conditions and the ability to drive safely.

Specified Disorders or Disabilities
The law provides that a "Medical Advisory Board shall define disorders characterized by lapses of consciousness or other mental or physical disabilities affecting the ability of a person to drive safely."[1] State regulations provide that a person afflicted by certain specified conditions may not drive if, in the opinion of the examining physician, the conditions are likely to interfere with the ability to control and safely operate a motor vehicle. The following listed conditions are particularly relevant to MHPs:

1. periodic loss of consciousness, attention, or awareness from whatever cause;

2. mental deficiency or marked mental retardation in accordance with the International Classification of Diseases. The regulations specify that for diagnostic categories, terminology and concepts to be used in classification, the physician should refer to the *Diagnostic and Statistical Manual*[2] of the American Psychiatric Association and the *Manual on Terminology and Classifi-*

---

1. 75 PA. CONS. STAT. ANN. § 1518(a).
2. American Psychiatric Association. (1994). *Diagnostic and statistical manual of mental disorders* (4th ed.). Washington, DC: Author.

cation in Mental Retardation[3] of the American Association on Mental Deficiency;

3. mental or emotional disorder, whether organic or functional;

4. use of any drug or substance, including alcohol, known to impair skill or functions, regardless of whether the drug or substance is medically prescribed; or

5. another condition that, in the opinion of the examining licensed physician, could interfere with the ability to control and safely operate a motor vehicle.[4]

Mandatory Reporting

All physicians and other persons authorized to diagnose or treat disorders and disabilities defined by the Medical Advisory Board must report to the Department of Transportation in writing within 10 days the full name, date of birth, and address of every person over 15 years of age diagnosed as having any of the specified disorders or disabilities.[5] Although the phrase "other persons authorized to diagnose or treat disorders or disabilities defined by the [board]" could be construed to include MHPs other than physicians, other portions of the relevant statutes and regulations suggest that only physicians have the duty to file the reports. Presumably, these reports only need be made if in the opinion of the examiner, the conditions are likely to interfere with the ability to control and safely operate a motor vehicle. In addition, the person in charge of every mental hospital, institution, or clinic, or any alcohol or drug treatment facility is responsible for ensuring that these reports are filed.[6] The reports are to be kept confidential and not used for any purpose other than determining the qualifications of any person to drive.[7] No civil or criminal action may be brought against any person or agency for providing the required information.[8]

If the Department of Transportation has cause to believe that a licensed driver or applicant may not be physically or mentally qualified to be licensed, the Department may obtain the advice of a physician to cause an examination to be made or to designate

---

3. American Association on Mental Deficiency. (1977). *Manual on terminology and classification in mental retardation.* Washington, DC: Author. *See also* Luckasson, R., et al. (1992). *Mental retardation: Definition, classification and systems of support.* Washington, DC: American Association of Mental Retardation.

4. 67 PA. CODE § 83.5.

5. 75 PA. CONS. STAT. ANN. § 1518(b).

6. 75 PA. CONS. STAT. ANN. § 1518(c).

7. 75 PA. CONS. STAT. ANN. § 1518(d).

8. 75 PA. CONS. STAT. ANN. § 1518(e). There is no statutory provision or case law on the effects on MHPs in terms of legal liability if the MHP voluntarily files a report when not mandated by law.

any other qualified physician to handle the advising of the Department. The licensed driver or applicant may have a written report sent to the Department by a physician of the driver's or applicant's choice. Then the Department must appoint one or more qualified persons to consider all medical reports and testimony and determine the competency of the driver or the applicant to drive.[9] The examiner may be compelled to testify in proceedings for recall of operating privileges.[10]

The Department must recall the operating privilege of any person whose incompetency has been established as described previously. The recall is for an indefinite period until satisfactory evidence is presented to the Department to establish that the person is competent to drive a motor vehicle.[11]

These laws create an exception to the psychotherapist–patient and physician–patient privileges.

---

9. 75 PA. CONS. STAT. ANN. § 1519(a).
10. 75 PA. CONS. STAT. ANN. § 1519(b).
11. 75 PA. CONS. STAT. ANN. § 1519(c).

5.10

Product Liability

The term *product liability* covers any liability of a manufacturer or other seller of a product where personal injury or damage to some other property is caused by a defect in that product. Although a product liability claim may be based on principles of negligence[1] or warranty,[2] this chapter is limited to a third basis, strict tort liability. The central element of this claim is that the product was unreasonably dangerous to the user. MHPs who have special expertise in human factors[3] may be asked to evaluate the dangerousness of a product and testify in court as to the results.

(A) Elements of a Product Liability Claim

The law on strict liability[4] provides that a seller[5] of a product is subject to liability for physical harm to the user or the user's property caused by the product if the product is in a "defective

---

1. *Negligence* means that the wrongdoer's conduct fell below the standard of what is expected of the reasonably prudent person in the particular circumstances.
2. A *warranty* claim alleges that the product did not work as promised or as represented by the seller or manufacturer.
3. This is an interdisciplinary field that focuses on the interrelationship of people's abilities and the requirements of a product's design within a specified environment.
4. Pennsylvania follows the RESTATEMENT (SECOND) OF TORTS § 402A; *see also* Webb v. Zern, 220 A.2d 853 (Pa. 1966).
5. A *seller* means any person engaged in the business of selling products for use or consumption. It applies to manufacturers, wholesalers, distributors, or retailers. RESTATEMENT (SECOND) OF TORTS § 402A, cmt. f.

condition [and] unreasonably dangerous." *Defective condition* refers to its state at the time it left the seller. A product is defective when a reasonable seller would not sell the product if he or she knew of the risks involved or if the risks are greater than a reasonable buyer would expect.[6] A product is *unreasonably dangerous* if the product is more dangerous than an ordinary consumer would expect when it is used in the intended or reasonably foreseeable manner.[7] It is not enough that the product is potentially unsafe. For example, a sharp knife or chain saw can be very dangerous, but their inherent risks are well-known. But even with these kinds of products, a seller may be strictly liable if he or she fails to provide adequate warnings or instructions concerning the use of the product.[8]

(B) Defenses to a Product Liability Claim

The law provides for certain defenses to a strict liability claim. Negligence of the injured party may be a defense, but it is not a defense when the negligence consists merely of a failure to discover the defect in the product or to guard against the possibility of its existence.[9] Also, assumption of risk[10] by an injured party, if established, completely bars a strict liability action.[11] Misuse of a product (e.g., using it for an abnormal purpose, in a manner that was not reasonably be foreseeable by the seller, or in an manner that was not intended) may bar recovery in a strict liability claim.[12] A substantial alteration to the product that was not reasonably foreseeable by the seller may preclude imposition of liability if the injury is caused by the alteration.[13]

---

6. AMERICAN LAW OF PRODUCTS LIABILITY 3D § 17, 4.
7. AMERICAN LAW OF PRODUCTS LIABILITY 3D § 17, 30.
8. Mackowick v. Westinghouse Elec. Corp., 575 A.2d 100 (Pa. 1990).
9. McCown v. International Harvester Co., 342 A.2d 381 (Pa. 1975).
10. A plaintiff assumes the risk when he or she consents to relieve the defendant of an obligation to exercise care for the plaintiff's protection and agrees to take his or her chances as to injury from a known or possible risk.
11. Ferraro v. Ford Motor Co., 223 A.2d 746 (Pa. 1966).
12. Dorney Park Coaster Co. v. General Electric Co., 669 F. Supp. 712 (E.D. Pa. 1987).
13. Merriweather v. E.W. Bliss Co., 636 F.2d 42 (3d Cir. 1980).

5.11

Unfair Competition

Business competitors may engage in fierce battles to win a share of the market. They cannot, however, use tactics that do not serve the public interest or have been judicially declared to be "unfair," such as defaming competitors or their goods, stealing trade secrets, or starting a business with a former employer's customer lists. A large area of unfair competition of interest to MHPs, particularly psychologists, is a type of marketing that attempts to confuse the consumer into believing that one business's products or services were produced by another. MHPs may be asked to conduct consumer surveys to determine whether the defendant's business practices resulted in such confusion and to testify in court about their findings.

(A) Legal Test of Unfair Competition

One form of false marketing that constitutes unfair competition is referred to as "palming off." This is an attempt to make the purchaser believe that the product of the subsequent entrant is that of a better known competitor.

(B) Trademark Confusion

A trademark is a word, name, symbol, device, or any combination thereof that is used by a person to designate his or her goods. Trademarks are typically registered under federal law. The general purpose of trademark law is to avoid public confusion and unfair competition. An owner of a trademark acquires the right to prevent the goods to which the mark is applied from being confused with those of others and to prevent the owner's trade from being diverted to competitors from their use of misleading marks. A person may manufacture and sell a product indistinguishable in appearance from an original competing product unless the original has become associated in the public mind with its producer, provided one identifies his or her own product and does not infringe a patent, trademark, or copyright.[1] When a name becomes associated with certain products, groups, services, or goodwill in the public's mind, a competitor may not usurp that name and by doing so unjustly acquire the goodwill associated with the original product.[2]

The relevant inquiry generally turns on whether the mark has an established distinctiveness. For example, in one case, the court found that the evidence established that the defendant trying to sell luggage and stationery items had deliberately chosen the logotype ("Miss Seventeen") most closely resembling distinctive script of the plaintiff ("Seventeen"), a publisher of a monthly magazine, to take advantage of the likelihood of confusion of two reproductions of the same word and to permit the defendant to capitalize on the goodwill attached to the plaintiff's trademark.[3]

The Lanham Act[4] was passed to provide national protection of trademarks and thereby secure to the owner of the trademark the goodwill of his or her business and protect the ability of consumers to distinguish among competing producers.[5]

(C) Product Confusion

Product confusion occurs when a business sells a product that is very similar in appearance to a competitor's product. There are two elements in proving product confusion. First, the product must have acquired "special significance" whereby the public identifies it as made by a particular manufacturer. Second, the copier's product must confuse the public (i.e., the public cannot tell who made which product or must be unaware that the product is a copy of the original).

---

1. Gum, Inc. v. Gumakers of America, 136 F.2d 957 (3d Cir. 1943).
2. United States Jaycees v. Philadelphia Jaycees, 490 F. Supp. 688 (E.D. Pa. 1979), *vacated*, 639 F.2d 134 (3d Cir. 1981).
3. Triangle Publications, Inc. v. Standard Plastic Products, Inc., 241 F. Supp. 613 (E.D. Pa. 1965).
4. 15 U.S.C. §§ 1051–1072.
5. Park N Fly, Inc. v. Dollar Park & Fly, Inc., 469 U.S. 189 (1985).

Employment Discrimination

The law prohibits employers from engaging in discriminatory employment practices. This applies to professionals who have employees as well as to management consultants who advise employers concerning personnel selection, discharge, and promotion. MHPs should be aware of this law as it pertains to industrial consulting and test construction.

Relationship to Federal Employment Discrimination Law
The employment discrimination provisions in the Human Relations Act[1] largely parallel Title VII of the Federal Civil Rights Act of 1964[2] in its provisions and the spirit in which the courts interpret them. The provisions of the Human Relations Act are accorded considerable deference by the federal government.

(A) Who Is Affected by Employment Discrimination Law

The Human Relations Act defines employer to include the commonwealth or any political subdivision, administrative agency, or other governmental body, and any "person" (including partnerships, corporations, and other business entities [see chapters 2.1–

---

1. PA. STAT. ANN. tit. 43, §§ 951–962.2
2. 42 U.S.C. §§ 2000e-2(a), 2000e-17. There are several other applicable federal laws, such the Rehabilitation Act of 1973 (29 U.S.C. §§ 701–796), and the Americans With Disabilities Act (42 U.S.C. §§ 12101–12213), with which MHPs should be familiar.

2.3]) employing four or more persons within the state.[3] The antidiscrimination provisions applicable to employers are also extended to employment agencies and labor organizations.[4]

(B) Unlawful Employment Practices

The Act protects against discrimination on the basis of race, color, religion, ancestry, age, national origin, gender, handicap or disability, or use of guide dogs or other guide animals.[5] It protects members of these enumerated groups from discrimination in hiring, tenure, compensation, terms, conditions, or privileges of employment.[6]

MHPs who engage in personnel selection or employment consulting need to be sensitive to possible ways that their selection measures may discriminate, or appear to discriminate, against protected groups.

---

3. PA. STAT. ANN. tit. 43, § 954(b).
4. PA. STAT. ANN. tit. 43, § 955.
5. PA. STAT. ANN. tit. 43, § 952(a).
6. PA. STAT. ANN. tit. 43, § 955(a).

Section 6

Civil and Criminal Trial Matters

6.1

Jury Selection

A jury is composed of six to twelve people who have been selected from a much larger group of potential jurors through a process called *voir dire*. The jurors, in fact, are not *selected*. Jury selection is a process by which potential jurors are excluded. In the end, the jury is composed of the requisite number of persons who were not excluded during the process of jury selection. MHPs may play a role in jury selection by conducting pretrial surveys, evaluating potential jurors, and designing questions for use in the selection process.

(A) Juror Qualifications

Each year, the jury selection commissions for each county prepare master lists of all prospective jurors for their respective counties. These lists contain the names of all persons on the voter registration lists. They may also be supplemented by the names of persons listed in the telephone, city, and municipal directories; persons listed on the taxpayer rolls; persons who participate in state, county, local, or federal programs; persons on school census lists; and any other qualified person who applies to the commission for inclusion on the master list of prospective jurors.[1]

Persons are qualified for jury service if they are of voting age (18 years old) and reside in the county.[2] Persons are not qualified for jury service if they are unable to read, write, speak, and understand English; if they are incapable of rendering efficient

---

1. 42 Pa. Cons. Stat. Ann. §§ 4521(a)(1)–(5).
2. 42 Pa. Cons. Stat. Ann. § 4502.

jury service by reason of mental or physical infirmity; or if they have been convicted of a crime that was punishable by imprisonment of a year or more (unless pardoned.)[3]

Furthermore, a person may be disqualified 'for cause' from jury service if the person has a fixed bias, or a relationship with a party, witness, or counsel.[4] Potential jurors may be exempted from jury service if they are on active military duty; have served on a jury within the previous 3 years (at least 3 days within 1 year); or can demonstrate undue hardship or extreme inconvenience.[5]

(B) Criminal Trials

(B)(1) When a Jury Is Allowed

Almost all criminal defendants have the right to a jury trial. The federal constitution guarantees a jury trial to any criminal defendant charged with a crime that would require a jury trial if tried in a federal court.[6] The Pennsylvania constitution guarantees a jury trial to any criminal defendant charged with a crime that would have required a jury trial at common law.[7] Basically, any criminal defendant, other than a petty offender, is guaranteed a jury trial.[8]

Any criminal defendant may waive the right to a jury trial as long as the waiver is made knowingly and intelligently.[9] The waiver will only be considered knowing and intelligent if the court has discussed the essential elements of a jury trial with the defendant. The court must inform the defendant that the jury will be chosen from the community, the verdict must be unanimous, and the defendant must be allowed to participate in selecting the jurors.[10] This discussion between the court and the defendant

---

3. 42 PA. CONS. STAT. ANN. §§ 4502(1)–(3).
4. *See, e.g.,* Commonwealth v. Delligatti, 538 A.2d 34, 41–42, *appeal denied,* 552 A.2d 250 (1988); Commonwealth v. Johnson, 517 A.2d 1311, 1314–1315 (1986).
5. 42 PA. CONS. STAT. ANN. §§ 4503(a)(1)–(3).
6. U.S. CONST. AMEND. VI. Originally, the Sixth Amendment only applied to the federal government. Later, the U.S. Supreme Court held that the due process clause of the Fourteenth Amendment makes the Sixth Amendment applicable to the states. Duncan v. Louisiana, 391 U.S. 145, 159 (1968).
7. Blum v. Merrell Dow Pharmaceuticals, Inc., 626 A.2d 537 (Pa. 1993). In 1862, Pennsylvania adopted the "Laws Agreed Upon in England." *See id.* at 542. Those laws make up what we now refer to as the common law.
8. Duncan, 391 U.S. at 159–162.
9. PA. R. CRIM. P. 1101.
10. Commonwealth v. Williams, 312 A.2d 597 (Pa. 1973); Commonwealth v. Polston, 616 A.2d 669 (Pa. Super. Ct. 1992).

must be included in the court's record and the actual waiver must be in writing.[11]

(B)(2) Jury Size

A jury normally consists of 12 members.[12] The judge may also direct that a reasonable number of alternates be selected.[13] If one or more jurors become unable to complete the trial, an alternate will fill in. If no alternates are needed, they will be dismissed prior to the beginning of deliberations.[14] If one or more jurors is unable to complete the trial and there are no alternates, the defendant may consent to being tried by a jury of fewer than twelve.[15] This is only after a jury of 12 has been properly selected and sworn and before deliberations have begun. In any event, a jury may not have fewer than six members.[16]

(B)(3) Unanimity Requirement

The Pennsylvania constitution requires that verdicts in criminal trials be unanimous.[17]

(B)(4) Change of Venue

If criminal defendants believe they cannot receive a fair trial in the community in which they are to be tried, they may request changes of venue. A change of venue may be granted only if "substantial prejudice" will result if the change is not made.[18] MHPs may aid courts in assessing community attitudes and possibly presenting research to aid the court in deciding whether to grant a motion for change of venue. The court may appoint an MHP to this role or either party could hire an MHP to present expert witness testimony at a pretrial hearing on this issue.

---

11. PA. R. CRIM. P. 1101.
12. *See* Blum, 626 A.2d at 543-44.
13. PA. R. CRIM. P. 1108.
14. *Id.*
15. PA. R. CRIM. P. 1103; Commonwealth v. Proctor, 585 A.2d 454, 460 (Pa. 1991); Commonwealth v. Stewart, 448 A.2d 598, 601 (Pa. Super. Ct. 1981) (defendant must object to loss of juror or right to 12-member jury waived); *see also* Williams v. Florida, 399 U.S. 78, 102 (1970) (juries in criminal cases of as few as six members are constitutional).
16. PA. R. CRIM. P. 1103; *see also* Ballew v. Georgia, 435 U.S. 223, 239 (1978) (juries of fewer than six members are unconstitutional).
17. PA. CONST. art. I, § 9; Smith v. Times Publishing Co., 36 A. 296 (Pa. 1897); *see also* Commonwealth v. Fugmann, 198 A. 99, 111 (Pa. 1938). The federal constitution permits state courts to acquit and convict on the basis of nonunanimous jury decisions. Johnson v. Louisiana, 406 U.S. 356, 360 (1972). If the state has a jury of only six members, the verdict must be unanimous. Burch v. Louisiana, 441 U.S. 130, 138 (1979).
18. PA. R. CRIM. P. 25.

(B)(5) Voir Dire

Voir dire is the process by which the jury is selected from the larger jury pool. The *voir dire* may be conducted by the judge or by the attorneys in the presence of a judge. Prospective jurors may be questioned as a group or individually. If the jury will hear a capital case, *voir dire* must be conducted individually.[19] Jurors may be excluded by either a "peremptory challenge" or a "challenge for cause."

A juror may be excluded from service on a challenge for cause if, in the discretion of the judge, the juror cannot be impartial, or the juror has such a close relationship, be it familial, financial, or situational with a party, counsel, victim, or witness that the court should presume prejudice.[20] A juror may also be excused on a challenge for cause if a physical disability, such as a severe hearing impairment that prevents the juror from hearing material testimony, will interfere with proper discharge of juror duties.[21]

An attorney uses peremptory challenges to disqualify jurors who cannot be challenged for cause. A peremptory challenge does not require any reason or explanation. No juror, however, may be excused on the basis of race, color, religion, gender, national origin, or economic status.[22] In trials involving only one defendant, each party has five peremptory challenges in a trial involving a misdemeanor; seven peremptory challenges in a trial involving a noncapital felony; and twenty peremptory challenges in a trial involving a capital felony.[23] If the trial involves more than one defendant, the defendants must divide equally the number of peremptory challenges that would be given to the defendant with the highest grade of offense if that defendant had been tried individually. Each defendant must have at least two peremptory challenges and the judge has discretion to increase the number of these peremptory challenges. The commonwealth is given the same number of peremptory challenges as the total for all the defendants combined.[24]

---

19. PA. R. CRIM. P. 1106(a)–(e).
20. Commonwealth v. Stamm, 429 A.2d 4 (Pa. Super. Ct. 1981).
21. Commonwealth v. Golson 456 A.2d 1063 (Pa. Super. Ct. 1983).
22. 42 PA. CONS. STAT. § 4501(3); *see also* J. E. B. v. Alabama, 511 U.S. 127 (1994) (equal protection clause of the federal constitution prohibits exclusion of jurors on the basis of gender in state trials); Batson v. Kentucky, 476 U.S. 79 (1986) (same as to race).
23. PA. R. CRIM. P. 1126(a)(1)–(3).
24. PA. R. CRIM. P. 1126(b)(1)–(3).

(C) Civil Trials

The right to a jury trial in a civil matter exists when a claim is based on a common law cause of action[25] or on a statute that expressly provides for the right to a jury trial.[26] A party must serve a written demand for a jury trial within 20 days of the last permissible pleading. If this written demand is not made, the party has permanently waived the right to a jury trial.[27]

An important exception to this general rule is compulsory arbitration.[28] MHPs may serve as witnesses in these proceedings.[29] In most counties, claims equal to or less than $50,000 may not be brought in the Court of Common Pleas. Instead, these claims must be submitted for arbitration by a panel of three attorneys. In addition to these relatively smaller civil claims, all medical malpractice cases must be submitted for arbitration before being heard by the Court of Common Pleas.[30]

The decision of an arbitration panel has the same power and effect as a decision by the Court of Common Pleas. If any party is displeased with the results of arbitration, the issue may be appealed to the Court of Common Pleas.[31] This court will hear and decide the appeal as if the case had originated in it.

(C)(1) Jury Size

The Pennsylvania Constitution guarantees civil litigants a right to a jury of 12 members.[32]

(C)(2) Unanimity Requirement

There is no requirement of unanimity in civil jury trials. A verdict rendered by five sixths of the jury will have the same effect as the verdict of a unanimous jury.[33]

(C)(3) Change of Venue

If the court finds that a "fair and impartial trial cannot be held" in the county in which the lawsuit is originally brought, the court

---

25. PA. CONST. art. I., § 6.
26. *In re* Friedman, 457 A.2d 983 (Pa. Commw. Ct. 1983).
27. PA. R. CIV. P. 1007.1(a).
28. 42 PA. CONS. STAT. § 7361; PA. R. CIV. P. 1301–1309.
29. 42 PA. CONS. STAT. § 7309.
30. Health Care Services Malpractice Act, PA. STAT. ANN. tit. 40, §§ 1301.101–1301.1006; *see also* PA. R. CIV. P. 1801–1809.
31. 42 PA. CONS. STAT. § 7361(d).
32. PA. CONST. art. I, § 6; Blum, 626 A.2d at 546.
33. PA. R. CIV. P. 5104(b).

may order a change of venue.[34] MHPs may be able to assist the court in making such a determination.[35]

(C)(4) *Voir Dire*

As in the criminal context, *voir dire* in the civil context should be conducted with the purpose of securing a competent, fair, and impartial jury.[36] Questioning should be designed to ascertain any interest a juror might have in the parties or the outcome of the litigation.[37] Challenges for cause in the civil context are analogous to those used in the criminal context. In civil cases, each party is entitled to four peremptory challenges.[38]

---

34. PA. R. CIV. P. 1006(d)(2).
35. *See* section on Criminal Trials, this chapter. *See also* chapter 7 regarding Criminal Matters.
36. Bentivoglio v. Ralston, 288 A.2d 745, 749 (Pa. 1972) (*citing* Commonwealth v. Corbin, 231 A.2d 138 (Pa. 1967)).
37. *Id.* (*citing* Clay v. Western Md. R.R. Co., 70 A. 807 (Pa. 1908)).
38. PA. R. CIV. P. 221.

Expert Witnesses

Expert witnesses are used to assist the judge or jury in understanding scientific or technical evidence. MHPs may be called to serve as expert witnesses when a case involves understanding social science research, clinical mental health issues, or any other issue that is beyond the understanding of the judge or jury but within the realm of the expert's specialized knowledge or training.

(A) Qualifying as an Expert Witness

Before an expert is allowed to testify, the judge must rule that the expert is qualified to give an opinion on the matter and that what the expert wishes to testify about meets general scientific acceptance.[1] The qualification of an expert is "a matter within the sound discretion of the trial court and will be reversed only for clear abuse of discretion."[2] An expert will be qualified if he or she "has any reasonable pretension to specialized knowledge on the subject under investigation"[3] or if the expert has "sufficient skill,

---

1. Packel, L., & A. B. Poulin. (1987). *Pennsylvania evidence.* St. Paul, MN: West (*citing* Walker v. General Motors Corp., 557 A.2d 1 (Pa. Super. Ct.), *appeal granted*, 569 A.2d 1369 (Pa. 1989)). All discussion of evidentiary issues in this text is based on Packel & Poulin's treatise, the leading authority on Pennsylvania Rules of Evidence.

   Although the U.S. Supreme Court has interpreted the federal rules of evidence to require that admissibility be based on scientific validity, Daubert v. Merrell Dow Chemical Co, 509 U.S. 579 (1993), the courts retain the more traditional scientific acceptance test. *See* chapter 6.8, n. 1.
2. Ruzzi v. Butler Petroleum Co., 588 A.2d 1 (Pa. 1991).
3. Kuisis v. Baldwin-Lima-Hamilton Corp., 319 A.2d 914, 924 (Pa. 1974).

knowledge, or experience in that field or calling as to make it appear that his opinion or inference will probably aid the trier in his search for truth."[4]

A witness may be qualified on the basis of education,[5] but formal education and training is not required if the expert has sufficient experience.[6] In a licensed profession, a witness who has the requisite education but is not yet licensed (e.g., medical intern) may qualify as an expert.[7] And a witness who specializes in one area is not usually disqualified from testifying about another specialty area within the same discipline.[8]

(B) When an Expert Witness May Be Called to Testify

Expert witness testimony is only allowed if the subject matter is "distinctly related to a science, skill, or occupation beyond the knowledge or experience of the average layman."[9] If the jury can understand the facts without the assistance of an expert's testimony, the expert testimony will not be allowed because courts do not want the jury to be unduly influenced.[10]

On the other hand, in medical malpractice cases, expert testimony is often required[11] and may also be required to establish negligent practice in other professions.[12] As with medical malpractice cases, expert testimony will not be required in cases in which laypersons could understand the evidence and reasonably come to a conclusion of negligence.[13]

---

4. Dambacher by Dambacher v. Mallis, 485 A.2d 408, 415 (Pa. Super. Ct. 1984).
5. See Kravinsky v. Glover, 396 A.2d 1349 (Pa. Super. Ct. 1979) (clinical psychologist with PhD and experience in psychological research and practice qualified to testify on diagnosis, prognosis, and cause of emotional disturbance).
6. Ruzzi, 588 A.2d 1; Commonwealth v. Gonzalez, 546 A.2d 26 (Pa. 1988); Commonwealth v. Henry, 569 A.2d 929 (Pa. 1990); see also Commonwealth v. Young, 572 A.2d 1217 (Pa. 1989) (master's-level psychologist licensed in clinical psychology and associated with academic program of law and psychology for more than 20 years qualified to testify as expert in psychology).
7. Commonwealth v. Davenport, 295 A.2d 596 (Pa. 1972).
8. Commonwealth v. Berrena, 617 A.2d 1278 (Pa. Super. Ct. 1992) (psychiatrist qualified to testify about effects of ingesting certain substances).
9. Commonwealth v. O'Searo, 352 A.2d 30, 32 (Pa. 1976).
10. Collins v. Zediker, 218 A.2d 776 (Pa. 1966).
11. See Robinson v. Wirts, 127 A.2d 706, 710 (Pa. 1956).
12. Thomas M. Durkin & Sons, Inc. v. Nether Providence Township Sch. Auth., 460 A.2d 800 (Pa. Super. Ct. 1983), rev'd on other grounds, 476 A.2d 904 (Pa. 1984).
13. Rizzo v. Haines, 555 A.2d 58 (Pa. 1989); Jones v. Harrisburg Polyclinic Hosp., 437 A.2d 1134 (Pa. 1984)).

(C) Form and Content of Testimony

The judge has broad discretion to determine whether the expert witness testimony will be allowed.[14] This means that a decision to include or exclude expert witness testimony will rarely be overturned on appeal. Decisions involving expert witness testimony of MHPs have been inconsistent.[15] Sometimes, psychiatric testimony has been allowed to show a criminal defendant's state of mind at the time of the crime. Other times, such testimony has not been allowed.[16]

Expert testimony on rape trauma syndrome (see chapter 6.7) or similar psychological phenomena intended to enhance credibility of witnesses in cases of rape, child sexual abuse, or incest is not allowed in Pennsylvania.[17] In contrast, expert testimony on battered woman's syndrome has been allowed (see chapter 6.6).[18] Expert testimony on the typical profile of an abusive spouse, however, has not been allowed.[19]

Although a lay witness may only give opinions that are reasonably based on personal knowledge, the expert witness may rely on both personal knowledge and facts about which the expert has no personal knowledge.[20] In most cases, however, the facts on which the expert bases an opinion must be supported by evidence in the record.[21] A direct or cross-examination question that asks an expert's opinion on facts that are part of the record, but not

---

14. *See* Walasavage v. Marinelli, 483 A.2d 509 (Pa. Super. Ct. 1984).
15. Packel & Poulin, *supra* note 1, at 508.
16. Commonwealth v. O'Searo, 352 A.2d 496 (Pa. 1981) (psychiatric testimony not allowed to show that murder defendant acted unintentionally or accidentally); Commonwealth v. Jones, 327 A.2d 10 (Pa. 1974) (psychiatric testimony allowed to assist jury in determining weight to be given to defendant's testimony); Commonwealth v. Light, 326 A.2d 288 (Pa. 1974) (psychiatric testimony admitted to show that murder defendant acted in self-defense); Commonwealth v. McCusker, 292 A.2d 286 (Pa. 1972) (psychiatric testimony admitted to show that murder defendant acted in heat of passion); Commonwealth v. Battle, 433 A.2d 496 (Pa. Super. Ct. 1981) (psychiatric testimony not allowed to show that murder defendant acted in self-defense); Commonwealth v. Newman, 555 A.2d 151 (Pa. Super. Ct. 1989) (psychiatric testimony not allowed to show defendant acted under belief he was victim of voodoo).
17. Commonwealth v. Sees, 605 A.2d 307 (Pa. 1992); Commonwealth v. Dunkle, 602 A.2d 830 (Pa. 1992); Commonwealth v. Gallagher, 54 A.2d 355 (Pa. 1988).
18. Commonwealth v. Stonehouse, 555 A.2d 772 (Pa. 1989); Commonwealth v. Kacsmar, 617 A.2d (Pa. Super. Ct. 1992).
19. Commonwealth v. Garcia, 588 A.2d 951 (Pa. Super. Ct. 1991), *appeal denied*, 604 A.2d 248 (Pa. 1992).
20. Packel & Poulin, *supra* note 1, at 515 (citing McCormick on Evidence § 14 (3d ed. 1984)).
21. Commonwealth v. Rounds, 542 A.2d 997 (Pa. 1988) (pediatrician's opinion on child abuse was not allowed because factual basis not in record); Commonwealth v. Paskings, 290 A.2d 82 (Pa. 1972).

part of the expert's first-hand knowledge, is known as a *hypothetical question.* An expert may also base an opinion on facts that are not in the record if those facts are "of a type reasonably relied upon by experts in the particular field in forming opinions or inferences upon the subject."[22] For example, an MHP could base an opinion on medical records or evaluations completed by other professionals because these are types of information that MHPs commonly use to form opinions and inferences.[23]

Whether an expert may give an opinion on the "ultimate issue" in a case is unclear.[24] The *ultimate issue* is "one of the issues which constitutes an element of a party's charge, claim, or defense."[25] With regard to both laypersons' and experts' testimony, the courts have ruled that witnesses may give opinion testimony on the ultimate issue unless that issue is the mental condition of a criminal defendant.[26] This means that an MHP cannot testify about whether a criminal defendant was insane at the time of a crime. Although expert witnesses traditionally have been permitted to give an opinion on ultimate issues (other than the mental condition of a criminal defendant),[27] a decision by the Pennsylvania Supreme Court suggests that experts may not be permitted to testify on the ultimate issue.[28] Although this area of the law is unsettled, what remains clear is that even if an expert is permitted to testify on the ultimate issue, an expert's testimony must not be unduly prejudicial or confusing to the jury.[29]

---

22. FED. R. EVID. 703.
23. Commonwealth v. Thomas, 282 A.2d 693 (Pa. 1971) (psychiatrist could base opinions on evaluation prepared by psychologist).
24. Packel & Poulin, *supra* note 1, § 704.
25. *Id.* at 519.
26. Lewis v. Mellor, 393 A.2d 941 (Pa. Super. Ct. 1978) (court adopted FED. R. EVID. 704, which provides in relevant part that "No expert witness testifying with respect to the mental state or condition of a defendant in a criminal case may state an opinion or inference as to whether the defendant did or did not have the mental state or condition constituting an element of the crime charged or of a defense thereto").
27. Commonwealth v. Daniels, 390 A.2d 172 (Pa. 1978).
28. Kozak v. Struth, 531 A.2d 420 (Pa. 1987).
29. Commonwealth v. Terry, 521 A.2d 398 (Pa.), *cert. denied*, 482 U.S. 920 (1987).

6.3

Polygraph Evidence

Polygraph examinations are governed by laws regulating the licensure of polygraph examiners and the submission of test results at trial. These laws apply to all MHPs.

(A) Polygraph Examinations

The use of polygraph ("lie detector") tests under the law is very limited. The legislature has forbidden the use of polygraph tests as a condition for employment or continuation of employment.[1] It is curious to note that the legislature has carved out an exception allowing law enforcement agencies to use polygraph testing for employment decisions.[2] For all other employers, the use of the polygraph for these purposes is a misdemeanor.[3] It is also a misdemeanor to use any psychological-stress evaluator or audio-stress monitor to judge truth or falsity without the consent of the person who is being tested.[4] This applies to all settings, not just employment.

Pennsylvania has not yet regulated pencil-and-paper honesty or integrity tests being used with increasing frequency in employment settings. Because of problems with test construction, especially construct validity, the use of these tests may present serious ethical problems at this time.[5]

---

1. 18 PA. CONS. STAT. ANN. § 7321.
2. 18 PA. CONS. STAT. ANN. § 7321(b).
3. 18 PA. CONS. STAT. ANN. § 7321.
4. 18 PA. CONS. STAT. ANN. § 7507.
5. *See* Wayne J. Camara & Dianne L. Schneider. (1994). Integrity tests. *American Psychologist, 49,* 112.

(B) Admissibility of Polygraph Examinations

The courts have limited the use of polygraph tests even further.[6] Because of the perceived inherent unreliability of the polygraph examination, the results of a polygraph are not admissible in court, even if the parties knowingly, intelligently, and voluntarily stipulate to their admission.[7] Furthermore, evidence that a party refused or agreed to take a polygraph is not admissible.[8]

---

6. *See* Packel & Poulin, at 531. *See also* United States v. Scheffer, 118 S. Ct. 1261 (1998) (explaining limiting on admissibility of evidence).
7. Commonwealth v. Nelson, 456 A.2d 1383 (Pa. Super. Ct. 1983).
8. *Id.*

6.4

Competency to Testify

A witness in a civil or criminal trial must have the mental capacity to testify accurately and reliably in court; any other rule would open the fairness of the trial to question. Thus, when there is some doubt regarding a witness' ability to give accurate and reliable testimony, the court must determine whether the witness is competent to testify. Although the final decision is made by the judge, an MHP may be asked to evaluate witnesses of questionable competency. The court may question a witness' competency because of youth, emotional condition, or intellectual functioning. Typically, there is no age or diagnostic condition that automatically renders a witness competent or incompetent to testify. Rather, determinations of competency to testify are highly variable and idiosyncratic.

(A) Legal Test of Competency to Testify

Historically, any person with an interest in the outcome of a case, including parties and their spouses, were not permitted to testify.[1] By the middle of the nineteenth century, the prevailing theory was that interested parties should be permitted to testify because more information, by way of more testimony, would lead to more accurate results.[2] In 1869, the legislature abolished the

---

1. Packel & Poulin at 365 (citing 2 JOHN H. WIGMORE, EVIDENCE §§ 575–576 (Chadbourn rev. 1979)).
2. *Id.*

rule that made interested parties incompetent as witnesses. The result is that courts today will usually presume that a witness is competent to testify.[3] There are a few exceptions to the general rule of competency, including persons who have been convicted of perjury, surviving parties in cases of death or mental incapacity (the Dead Man's Rule),[4] some children, some persons with mental disabilities, and persons who have undergone hypnosis to "remember" their testimony.[5] In the case of perjury, a witness will not be found incompetent unless the witness has actually been sentenced for perjury.[6]

(B) Determination of Witness Competency

Children who are 14 years old or older are presumed to be competent witnesses,[7] although a child as old as 15 has been found incompetent to testify.[8] When a witness is under 14 years old, the court must make a searching inquiry into the child's mental capacity.[9] Usually, the judge will conduct the evaluation, but attorneys have done so in some cases.[10] Factors to be considered in the competency evaluation include the ability to communicate, which includes the ability to understand questions and the ability to express intelligent answers; the mental capacity to observe and remember the matter about which the child is to testify; and a "consciousness of the duty to speak the truth."[11] Typically, courts have focused primarily on the child's ability to understand the responsibility to be truthful.[12]

When it is brought to the court's attention that the witness may be incompetent because of mental disability, the court has

---

3. *Id.* The relevant modern statutes are 42 PA. CONS. STAT. ANN. § 5921 (establishing general rule of competency in civil trials) and 42 PA. CONS. STAT. ANN. § 5911 (establishing general rule in criminal trials).
4. 42 PA. CONS. STAT. ANN. § 5930. The Dead Man's Rule prevents a person from testifying when that person's interests are adverse to those of the deceased party's. This does not apply if the witness is also a party to the action. *See* Packel & Poulin, *supra* n. 1, at 377–387.
5. *See* Packel & Poulin, *supra* n. 1, §§ 601.1–601.8.
6. 42 PA. CONS. STAT. ANN. §§ 5912, 5922.
7. Rosche v. McCoy, 156 A.2d 307 (Pa. 1959).
8. Commonwealth v. Mazzaccoli, 380 A.2d 786 (Pa. 1977).
9. Commonwealth v. Stohr, 329 A.2d 589 (Pa. Super. Ct. 1987).
10. Packel & Poulin, *supra* n. 1, at 387–388 (citing Commonwealth v. Short, 420 A.2d 694 (Pa. 1980)).
11. *Rosche,* 156 A.2d at 310.
12. Packel & Poulin, *supra* n. 1, at 389 (citing *Mazzoccoli,* 380 A.2d 786).

the discretion to order a psychiatric examination.[13] When a person has been committed to a mental hospital or found incompetent to stand trial because of mental disability or insanity, the presumption of competency is reversed and the party who called the witness has the burden of proving that the witness is competent to testify.[14]

The test for competency of a mentally retarded person is the same as for a child.[15] The court must presume the mentally retarded person is competent to testify.[16] The courts have not defined the test for competency of a mentally ill person quite so clearly. The test for any mentally disabled person centers on perception, memory, and communication.[17] The witness must have been able to perceive the event when it occurred and must be able to perceive, recollect, and testify accurately about the event at the time of the trial.[18]

A witness whose testimony is based on hypnotically refreshed memories may not be competent. The state may not make a rule that hypnotically refreshed testimony is automatically invalid.[19] Testimony that is remembered before hypnosis will be admissible at trial, but testimony remembered only after hypnosis will not be.[20] The party seeking to admit this kind of testimony must prove by clear and convincing evidence that the testimony was recalled prior to undergoing hypnosis.[21]

(C) Competency of Rape Victims to Testify

Questions of competency to testify can be especially sensitive when a rape victim witness is mentally retarded, mentally ill, or a child. Often the victim is the only witness to the crime. If the

---

13. Packel & Poulin, *supra* n. 1, at 391 (citing Commonwealth v. Garcia, 387 A.2d 46 (Pa. 1978)).
14. *Id.* (citing and discussing Commonwealth v. Mozzillo, 278 A.2d 874 (Pa. 1971) (commitment to a psychiatric facility created presumption of incompetency); *but see* Syno v. Syno, 594 A.2d 307 (Pa. Super. Ct.), *appeal denied*, 600 A.2d 1259 (Pa. 1991) (witness may be competent to testify although adjudicated as incompetent for other purposes)).
15. Commonwealth v. Anderson, 552 A.2d 1064 (Pa. Super. Ct. 1988), *appeal denied*, 571 A.2d 379 (1989).
16. *Id.* at 1069.
17. Commonwealth v. Ware, 329 A.2d 258 (Pa. 1974); Packel & Poulin, *supra* n. 1, at 392.
18. *Ware*, 329 A.2d at 269–270; Packel & Poulin, *supra* note 1, at 392–393.
19. Rock v. Arkansas, 483 U.S. 44 (1987).
20. Commonwealth v. Smoyer, 476 A.2d 1304 (Pa. 1984).
21. Commonwealth v. DiNicola, 502 A.2d 606 (Pa. Super. Ct. 1985).

victim is incompetent to testify, there may be no evidence against the defendant, making a conviction very unlikely.

The Pennsylvania Supreme Court has dramatically limited the testimony that can be given by expert witnesses in child sexual abuse cases.[22] In child sexual abuse cases, expert witnesses may not testify about the general behavior reactions of child sexual abuse victims, why a child would delay reporting an incident, why a child would give incomplete details of an incident, or why a child might not recall the exact date and time of an incident.[23] The court believed that ordinary jurors could understand these issues without the help of an expert.[24]

The legislature has enacted a Rape Shield Law protecting rape victim witnesses from having to give testimony about their past sexual conduct with people other than the defendant.[25] Furthermore, questions about prior sexual contact with the defendant may only be asked if consent is at issue.[26]

---

22. P. A. Korey. (1993). Evidence-rehabilitative expert testimony in child sexual abuse cases: The Supreme Court of Pennsylvania shuts the door on effective prosecutions—Commonwealth v. Dunkle, 602 A.2d 830 (Pa. 1992). *Temple Law Review*, 66, 589.
23. Commonwealth v. Dunkle, 602 A.2d 830 (Pa. 1992).
24. *Id.*
25. 18 PA. CONS. STAT. ANN. § 3104.
26. *Id.*

6.5

Psychological Autopsy

The motivations and mental state of a person prior to death or being reported missing are frequently critical issues in subsequent litigation. MHPs may contribute to the resolution of these issues by providing a retrospective psychological profile called a *psychological autopsy*. A psychological autopsy is an attempt by an MHP to reconstruct the mental state of a deceased or missing person at some earlier time.[1] The results of the psychological autopsy may be helpful in determining whether a death was a suicide, a murder, or an accident.[2] Such information may be of interest to the courts, insurance companies, beneficiaries, and family members. A psychological autopsy includes interviews with significant others as well as evaluation of medical and school records.[3]

(A) Admissibility of Psychological Autopsies

The courts have not yet addressed the question of admissibility of psychological autopsy evidence. The Superior Court did reject a criminal defendant's request to admit evidence derived from an analogous technique, "psychological reconstruction," which is similar to psychological autopsy, but the subject is a living per-

---

1. J. R. Ogloff & Randy K. Otto. (1993). Psychological autopsy: Clinical and legal perspectives. *St. Louis University Law Journal, 37,* 607.
2. *Id.*
3. *Id.*

son.[4] Other courts that have addressed this question have come to differing conclusions. Some have allowed evidence obtained through psychological autopsy, and others have ruled this type of evidence inadmissible.[5]

---

4. Pennsylvania v. Ahearn, 516 A.2d 45, 47 (Pa. Super. Ct. 1986).
5. *See* Ogloff & Otto, *supra* note 1, for a review of cases addressing admissibility of psychological autopsy evidence. *See also* N. Poythress, R. K. Otto, J. Darkes, & L. Starr. (1993). APA's expert panel in the congressional review of the USS Iowa Incident. *American Psychologist, 48,* 8.

6.6

Battered Woman's Syndrome

The Supreme Court of Pennsylvania has acknowledged the presence of the battered woman's syndrome,[1] although it is still debating the role that the syndrome should have in criminal trials. The court has adopted the definition of a *battered woman* as a "woman who is repeatedly subjected to any forceful physical or psychological behavior by a man in order to coerce her to do something he wants her to do without any concern for her rights."[2] The Superior Court has recognized that this syndrome may apply equally to men when a man is the victim of the physical or psychological abuse.[3]

Currently in Pennsylvania, the battered woman's syndrome is not recognized as a defense to a crime or as a legal justification relieving the accused of criminal liability for a killing.[4] Courts do allow psychiatric testimony, however, regarding the battered woman's syndrome when such testimony is related to the accused's state of mind at the time of the offense.[5] This testimony is similar to testimony allowed for provocation (see chapter 7.6) and for diminished capacity (see chapter 7.8).

The use of force against another person is legally justified if the actor "believes that such force is immediately necessary for the purpose of protecting himself against the use of unlawful

---

1. Commonwealth v. Stonehouse, 555 A.2d 772 (Pa. 1989), *rev'g* 517 A.2d 540 (Pa. Super. Ct. 1986).
2. *Id.* (quoting Walker, L. (1979). The battered woman. New York: Harper & Row.)
3. Commonwealth v. Kacsmar, 617 A.2d 725 (Pa. Super. Ct. 1992), *appeal denied*, 639 A.2d 25 (Pa. 1994).
4. Commonwealth v. Ely, 578 A.2d 540 (Pa. Super. Ct. 1990).
5. Commonwealth v. Stonehouse, 555 A.2d 772 (Pa. 1989), *rev'g* 517 A.2d 540 (Pa. Super. Ct. 1986).

force by such other person on the present occasion."[6] The use of deadly force is legally justified when the actor "believes that such force is necessary to protect himself against death, serious bodily injury, kidnapping or sexual intercourse compelled by force or threat."[7] Under this statute, for a self-defense claim to be successful, the accused must establish that he did not provoke or encourage the confrontation that led to the killing, that he "reasonably believed that he was in imminent danger of death or great bodily harm, and that there was a necessity to kill in order to save himself," and that the accused could not have retreated to a safe place.[8] Pennsylvania does not recognize the battered woman's syndrome, by itself, as a legally justified self-defense to a killing.[9]

Expert testimony on the battered woman's syndrome is admissible, however, to establish that because of a long history of physical or psychological abuse, the accused reasonably feared imminent death or serious bodily harm. For the defense to be successful, it must be proven that at the time of the offense, it was reasonable to believe that death or serious bodily harm was imminent.[10]

In one case, a concurring opinion discussed the acceptable use of expert testimony regarding the battered woman's syndrome.[11] This opinion suggested that testimony may demonstrate how the battering relationship alters the accused's perspective on danger, imminent danger, and the need for force. In addition, expert testimony might be used to explain why the accused remained in the abusive relationship, why the abused individual never reported the abuse, or why the individual feared future violence.[12] Another opinion stated that expert testimony might discuss how an abused individual views the attacker, or how the final incident before the killing may be perceived as more severe or life-threatening than other episodes.[13]

---

6. 18 PA. CONS. STAT. ANN. § 505(a).

7. 18 PA. CONS. STAT. ANN. § 505(b)(2).

8. Commonwealth v. Grove, 526 A.2d 369, 372 (Pa. Super. Ct. 1987), *appeal denied*, 539 A.2d 810 (Pa. 1987) (quoting Commonwealth v. Simmons, 475 A.2d 1310, 1312–1313 (Pa. 1984)).

9. Commonwealth v. Ely, 578 A.2d 540 (Pa. Super. Ct. 1990).

10. Commonwealth v. Grove, 526 A.2d 369 (Pa. Super. Ct. 1987), *appeal denied*, 539 A.2d 810 (Pa. 1987) (it is not reasonable to believe that a sleeping person poses a threat of imminent harm).

11. Commonwealth v. Dillon, 598 A.2d 963 (Pa. 1991) (Nix, C.J., concurring).

12. *Id.*

13. Commonwealth v. Stonehouse, 555 A.2d 772 (Pa. 1989).

6.7

Rape Trauma Syndrome

Rape Trauma Syndrome (RTS) is an umbrella term for the broad spectrum of physical, psychological, and emotional reactions of rape victims.[1] Courts throughout the United States have debated the admissibility of RTS at trial. Some jurisdictions allow expert testimony on RTS to prove that the victim did not consent to the perpetrator's act or to corroborate testimony that a rape occurred. Jurisdictions that allow RTS testimony believe that it aids the jury in understanding a subject beyond the knowledge and experience of the average juror. Many jurisdictions, however, do not allow testimony on RTS because it either does not reliably prove that a rape occurred or that there was a lack of consent. Other jurisdictions refuse RTS syndrome testimony on the theory that it only addresses the victim's credibility, and determining credibility is a proper role for the jury, not an expert.[2]

The courts have wavered on accepting testimony on RTS. In 1986, the Superior Court accepted expert testimony on RTS and recognized that experts from many fields could assist the jury in understanding the effects of rape trauma syndrome.[3] In 1988, however, the court reversed the previous decision and ruled that expert testimony on the RTS improperly usurped the function of the jury.[4] This decision did not address whether RTS was sufficiently accepted by the scientific community to allow expert testi-

---

1. For the seminal article on the topic, *see* A. Burgess & L. Holmstrom. (1974). Rape trauma syndrome. *American Journal of Psychiatry, 131,* 981.
2. For a review of the leading rulings on RTS, *see* Commonwealth v. Gallagher, 510 A.2d 735 (Pa. Super. Ct. 1986), *rev'd,* 547 A.2d 355 (Pa. 1988).
3. *Id.*
4. Commonwealth v. Gallagher, 547 A.2d 355 (Pa. 1988), *rev'g,* 510 A.2d 735 (Pa. Super. Ct. 1986).

mony at trial. Instead, the decision stated that expert testimony on RTS was introduced to bolster the credibility of the victim. Determining the victim's credibility is the sole province of the jury, and expert testimony that usurps the jury's function is consistently rejected.[5] Further, the Superior Court has refused to admit expert testimony on RTS when the purpose of the testimony is to prove that the victim did not consent to the activities.[6] Subsequent cases have indicated that RTS testimony may be admitted under certain circumstances. One decision recognized that expert testimony on the syndrome was not admissible, but that layperson testimony about the victim's behaviors after the alleged attack could assist the jury and should be admitted.[7] A second opinion ruled that expert testimony was admissible when the expert testified to the general symptoms of RTS and did not testify to whether the victim was experiencing any of the symptoms.[8]

---

5. *Id.* (citing Kozak v. Struth, 531 A.2d 420 (Pa. 1987)).
6. Commonwealth v. Zamarripa, 549 A.2d 980 (Pa. Super. Ct. 1988).
7. Commonwealth v. Pickford, 536 A.2d 1348 (Pa. Super. Ct. 1987), *appeal dismissed,* 564 A.2d 158 (Pa. 1989).
8. Commonwealth v. Cepull, 568 A.2d 247 (Pa. Super. Ct. 1990), *appeal denied,* 578 A.2d 411 (Pa. 1990).

6.8

Hypnosis of Witnesses

In the course of a criminal investigation or a criminal trial, both the prosecution and the defense sometimes use MHPs trained in hypnosis to interview witnesses. Hypnosis is used in an attempt to stimulate the witnesses' recall of the event, especially when that person's memory has failed because of the trauma associated with the event. The admissibility of hypnotically refreshed testimony into a trial has raised scientific and legal questions.

In 1981, the Supreme Court of Pennsylvania reviewed the relevant literature on hypnosis and the arguments for and against the admissibility of hypnotically refreshed testimony. The court applied the Frye rule for admitting expert scientific evidence and determined that hypnotically refreshed testimony is not admissible.[1] The court reasoned that the scientific community does not have established criteria sufficient to evaluate the accuracy of hypnotically refreshed testimony, especially because the hypnotized person is prone to suggestibility and a desire to satisfy the hypnotist. However, the court did not establish a per-se rule

---

1. Commonwealth v. Nazarovitch, 436 A.2d 170 (Pa. 1981). In Frye, the federal court wrote that "just when a scientific principle or discovery crosses the line between the experimental and demonstrable stages is difficult to define. Somewhere in this twilight zone the evidential force of the principle must be recognized, and while courts will go a long way in admitting expert testimony deduced from a well-recognized scientific principle or discovery, *the thing from which the deduction is made must be sufficiently established to have gained general acceptance in the particular field in which it belongs.*" Id. at 172 (quoting Frye v. United States, 293 F. 1013, 1014 (D.C. Cir. 1923)) (emphasis in original). The U.S. Supreme Court ruled that the Frye general acceptance standard was superseded by the FED. R. OF EVID. 402, which allows all relevant evidence to be admitted. Daubert v. Merrell Dow, Pharmaceuticals, Inc., 509 U.S. 579 (1993). How this decision will affect expert testimony in state courts is unclear and has not yet been addressed in Pennsylvania.

against the admissibility of hypnotically refreshed testimony. If more conclusive proof of the reliability of hypnotically refreshed testimony is presented, the court may consider admitting hypnotically refreshed testimony.[2]

Testimony that is adduced from hypnosis is not admissible; however, testimony that is not adduced from the hypnotic session is admissible.[3] Whenever a person who has been hypnotized is to testify to material not adduced from the hypnotic session, the party wishing to introduce the testimony must establish that certain safeguards were present during the hypnotic session.[4] The party must inform the court that the witness was hypnotized before testifying, must demonstrate that the testimony to be presented was established and existed before the hypnotic session, must establish that the person who conducted the hypnotic session is trained in hypnosis and is not connected to either party in the case.[5] In addition, the trial judge must inform the jury that the witness was previously hypnotized and that the jury should carefully scrutinize the testimony.[6]

Under this standard, testimony of a previously hypnotized witness is admissible when the testimony is based on a recollection of the facts that existed before the hypnotic session.[7] However, before a hypnotically refreshed witness can testify to a prehypnotic recollection, the information must be verified by clear and convincing evidence.[8] The requirement of the hypnotist's neutrality can be demonstrated by a tape recording of the session, exhibiting the hypnotist's impartial nature.[9] In another case, a brief review of the facts presented to the hypnotist prior to the hypnotic session did not violate the hypnotist's impartiality.[10] Although these cases have allowed hypnotically refreshed witnesses to testify to information not adduced by the hypnotic session, a relatively recent court decision reinforced the opinion that there is no adequate scientific evidence to admit hypnotically refreshed testimony.[11]

---

2. Commonwealth v. Nazarovitch, 436 A.2d 170 (Pa. 1981).
3. Commonwealth v. Smoyer, 476 A.2d 1304 (Pa. 1984), *rev'g*, 448 A.2d 1190 (Pa. Super. Ct. 1982).
4. *Id.*
5. *Id.*
6. *Id.*
7. Commonwealth v. Romanelli, 485 A.2d 795 (Pa. Super. Ct. 1984), *aff'd*, 560 A.2d 1384 (Pa. 1989).
8. Commonwealth v. DiNicola, 502 A.2d 606 (Pa. Super. Ct. 1985), *appeal denied*, 531 A.2d 1118 (Pa. 1987), *cert. denied*, 484 U.S. 1028 (1988).
9. Commonwealth v. Romanelli, 485 A.2d 795 (Pa. Super. Ct. 1984), *aff'd*, 560 A.2d 1384 (Pa. 1989).
10. Commonwealth v. Mehmeti, 500 A.2d 832 (Pa. Super. Ct. 1985).
11. Commonwealth v. Reed, 583 A.2d 459 (Pa. Super. Ct. 1990), *appeal denied*, 598 A.2d 282 (Pa. 1991).

Eyewitness Identification

Eyewitnesses play an important role in many criminal trials. There is a growing body of professional literature that addresses the reliability of eyewitness identifications. Some federal courts have ruled that mental health experts may testify to the reliability of eyewitness identifications under limited circumstances.[1] The courts refuse to allow expert testimony on the matter.[2] The courts reason that expert testimony on the reliability of eyewitness identifications would provide information that is common knowledge and would intrude on the jury's function of assessing witness credibility.

---

1. United States v. Downing, 753 F.2d 1224 (3d Cir. 1985). On remand, the specific testimony offered in this case was not admitted. The district court found that the offered expert testimony on eyewitness identifications was unreliable, would mislead the jury, and possessed only a weak connection to the disputed facts of the case. United States v. Downing, 609 F. Supp. 784 (E.D. Pa. 1985), *aff'd*, 780 F.2d 1017 (3d Cir. 1985).
2. Commonwealth v. Spence, 627 A.2d 1176 (Pa. 1993); Commonwealth v. Smith, 434 A.2d 115 (Pa. Super. Ct. 1981).

Criminal Matters

Screening of Police Officers

The Municipal Police Officers' Education and Training Commission, chaired by the commissioner of the state police,[1] establishes the standards for hiring, removing, educating, and training police officers.[2] Of the commission's many duties, those relevant to MHPs include the power to:

1. revoke an officer's certification when the officer fails to comply with required in-service training programs, is convicted of a criminal offense, or is determined to be physically or mentally unfit to perform the duties of a police officer;
2. require all police officers to submit to a background investigation prior to employment, to determine the person's suitability for the position; and
3. require minimum standards for physical fitness, psychological evaluations, and educational levels for employment as a police officer.[3]

(A) Screening State Police Officers

An applicant for the position of state police officer must be a citizen of the United States, between the ages of 21 and 40 years old, and must be "of sound constitution . . . [and] of good moral character."[4] In addition, the applicant must satisfactorily pass the

---

1. PA. STAT. ANN. tit. 53, § 2163(a)(1)(i).
2. PA. STAT. ANN. tit. 53, § 2164.
3. *Id.*
4. PA. STAT. ANN. tit. 71, § 1193(a).

physical and mental examination required of officers in cities of the first class.[5]

(B) Screening for Lethal Weapons Training

All persons who are privately employed to provide guard watch, a protective patrol, detective services, or criminal investigative services and carry a lethal weapon as part of their employment are required to attend a Lethal Weapons Training Program.[6] The program is administered by the Commissioner of the Pennsylvania State Police[7] who has the authority to implement, administer, or approve the physical and psychological testing and screening of all candidates and will bar from the program all candidates "not physically or mentally fit to handle lethal weapons."[8] A person who wishes to be certified under this program must be 18 years old, must properly complete all necessary application forms and fees, and must submit to a physical and mental examination.[9]

---

5. *Id.* Philadelphia is a city of first class, being one of the largest cities in Pennsylvania.
6. PA. STAT. ANN. tit. 22, § 44(b).
7. PA. STAT. ANN. tit. 22, § 44(a).
8. PA. STAT. ANN. tit. 22, § 45(2).
9. There are a few exceptions to the physical and psychological examination requirement. For instance, applicants who have been employed continuously as full-time police officers since June 19, 1974, and submitted to the physical and psychological examination requirement for that position are not required to submit to the physical and psychological examination for lethal weapons training. Further, a retired police officer who did not retire because of a disability and who has worked as a privately employed agent for 3 years is not required to submit to the examinations. 37 PA. CODE § 21.15.

7.2

Competency to Waive the Rights to Silence, Counsel, and a Jury

All persons who are subject to a criminal prosecution have certain rights guaranteed to them by the constitutions of the United States and Pennsylvania. Among others, these rights include the right to remain silent, the right to have an attorney, and the right to trial by jury.[1] The criminal defendant may waive any or all of these rights during the criminal process. There are strict standards for accepting a waiver of these rights, however, and MHPs may be asked to evaluate the defendant to determine whether he or she was competent to waive the rights.

(A) Right to Silence

The U.S. Supreme Court has interpreted the Fifth Amendment to require that whenever a criminal defendant is in police custody, the authorities must follow procedural safeguards before a statement from the defendant can be received.[2] The procedural safeguards are commonly referred to as *Miranda* warnings and include a warning to the defendant that "he has a right to remain silent, that any statement he does make may be used as evidence against him, and that he has a right to the presence of an attorney, either retained or appointed."[3] After the warnings have been given, the defendant may waive these rights and answer any questions asked by the police, including providing a confession.

---

1. U.S. CONST. amends. V, VI; PA. CONST. art. I, § 9.
2. Miranda v. Arizona, 384 U.S. 436 (1966).
3. *Id.* at 444.

In any event, the waiver must be made "voluntarily, knowingly, and intelligently."[4]

The courts recognize a relationship between a defendant's IQ, mental age, and ability to waive the right to silence,[5] although a low IQ alone does not indicate that a defendant is incapable of understanding these rights. For example, in one case, the Superior Court ruled that a defendant with low intelligence adequately understood the warnings to effectuate a valid waiver, because the defendant had been arrested previously, had repeated exposure to the warnings, and the defendant had entered guilty pleas on other occasions.[6]

The courts also have considered whether a mental illness can prevent a defendant from effectuating a valid waiver of the right to silence, although with varying results. In one case, a court ruled that a person suffering from undifferentiated chronic schizophrenia could not waive the right to silence because the mental illness prevented him from understanding the right.[7] In an earlier case, the court decided that a person diagnosed as mentally ill may be capable of waiving the right to silence, as it was not established that the mental illness interfered with the defendant's ability to understand the waived right.[8]

(B) Right to Counsel

A defendant in a criminal investigation has the right to be represented by an attorney at all phases of the criminal process.[9] This right to counsel is fundamental to the notion of a fair trial.[10] As with the right to remain silent, the defendant must be informed of the right to have an attorney. The warning must come as soon as feasible after the criminal process has started. The defendant may make a voluntary, knowing, and intelligent waiver of the right to counsel.[11]

---

4. *Id.*
5. Commonwealth. v. Brown, 583 A.2d 805 (Pa. Super. Ct. 1990), *cert. denied*, 502 U.S. 946 (1991).
6. *Id.*
7. Commonwealth. v. Cephas, 522 A.2d 63 (Pa. Super. Ct. 1987), *appeal denied*, 531 A.2d 1118 (Pa.), *cert. denied*, 484 U.S. 981 (1987).
8. Commonwealth v. Neely, 444 A.2d 1199 (Pa. Super. Ct. 1982), *overruled by* 461 A.2d 1268 (Pa. Super. Ct. 1983) (overruled on separate grounds).
9. U.S. CONST. amend. VI.; PA. CONST. art. I, § 9.
10. Gideon v. Wainwright, 372 U.S. 335 (1963).
11. PA. R. CRIM. P. 318(a).

(C) Right to Waive a Jury Trial

A criminal defendant may waive the right to a jury trial and instead be tried in front of the judge at a bench trial.[12] When a jury trial is waived, the judge must question the defendant to determine whether the waiver is made knowingly and intelligently.[13] The judge's questioning of the defendant must appear in the official record of the court proceedings.[14] The waiver must be in writing and signed by the defendant, the judge, and the defendant's attorney.[15] At anytime before the trial begins, the defendant may withdraw the waiver, or if the trial has started, the judge may order the withdrawal of the waiver.[16]

For the waiver to be considered informed and intelligently made, the judge must determine that the defendant knows the essential protections in a jury trial and the consequences of not proceeding with a jury trial.[17] These protections mandate that a defendant must be informed of the fact that the jury is composed of peers chosen from the defendant's community, that the defendant can participate in selecting the jury, and that every member of the jury must be convinced beyond a reasonable doubt that the defendant is guilty to convict the defendant on the charges.[18]

12. PA. R. CRIM. P. 1101.
13. Id.
14. Id.
15. Id.
16. PA. R. CRIM. P. 1102(b).
17. Id.
18. Id.

7.3

Precharging and Pretrial Evaluations

In some states, the prosecutor may request a precharging mental health evaluation to decide whether a person should be charged with a criminal offense or, as an alternative, be placed into the mental health system. Pennsylvania does not use precharging evaluations. Instead, Pennsylvania employs a postcharging Accelerated Rehabilitative Disposition (ARD) program that diverts certain criminal cases out of the criminal system and may involve pretrial mental health evaluations.[1] MHPs may be involved both in a defendant's evaluation for acceptance into an ARD program and in a defendant's treatment during an ARD program.

Accelerated Rehabilitative Disposition
The ARD program serves two primary purposes. The first goal is to rehabilitate the offender. The second goal is to expedite the criminal court process by eliminating extended and costly criminal trials and proceedings. ARD is intended to offer offenders a fresh start and a chance for a clean record after completing the program.[2]

The rules of criminal procedure do not explicitly establish who is eligible for ARD programs. The committee introduction to the rules indicates that ARD programs should be available to 'first offenders who lend themselves to treatment and rehabilitation rather than punishment [when] the crime charged is relatively minor and does not involve a serious breach of the public trust.'[3]

---

1. PA. R. CRIM. P. 160–186.
2. PA. R. CRIM. P. 160, committee introduction.
3. *Id.*

The commonwealth may initiate proceedings to admit the defendant to an ARD program.[4] If such proceedings are started, there is an open hearing before a judge, attended by the defendant, the defendant's attorney, the attorney for the commonwealth, and any victims of the offense.[5] At the ARD hearing, it must be determined that the defendant understands that if an ARD program is offered by the commonwealth and accepted by the defendant, it offers the chance to have the charges dismissed on successful completion of the program.[6] The defendant must also understand that failure to complete the program may result in full prosection of the charges and that, during any enrollment period in an ARD program, the defendant waives the appropriate statute of limitations for prosecuting the offense and the right to a speedy trial.[7]

If the defendant understands these conditions, the prosecutor will present the facts of the case to the judge. If the judge believes that ARD is appropriate, then the judge will state the conditions of the program.[8] Conditions of an ARD program may include any condition appropriate for a defendant placed on probation (see chapter 7.12).[9] As such, the defendant may be required to (a) receive appropriate medical or psychiatric treatment, either as an inpatient or as an outpatient; (b) participate in a drug or alcohol treatment program;[10] or (c) "satisfy any other conditions reasonably related to the rehabilitation of the defendant and not unduly restrictive of his liberty or incompatible with his freedom of conscience."[11] In all cases, the ARD program may not last longer than 2 years.[12]

If the defendant refuses to accept the conditions of the ARD program, the judge will deny the ARD motion and the case will proceed in court.[13] If the defendant agrees to the terms of the ARD program, successfully completes the program, and subsequently petitions the court, the case will be dismissed and the criminal charges will be removed from the defendant's record.[14]

---

4. PA. R. CRIM. P. 160, 161, 176, 42 PA. CONS. STAT. ANN. (1989 & Supp. 1993).
5. PA. R. CRIM. P. 160–161, 176.
6. PA. R. CRIM P. 178.
7. Id.
8. PA. R. CRIM. P. 179.
9. PA. R. CRIM. P. 182(a).
10. 42 PA. CONS. STAT. ANN. § 9754(c)(3) & (12).
11. 42 PA. CONS. STAT. ANN. § 9754(c)(13).
12. PA. R. CRIM P. 182(b).
13. PA. R. CRIM. P. 183.
14. PA. R. CRIM. P. 185–186.

Other Pretrial Evaluations

MHPs may be asked to conduct pretrial evaluations of defendants in a number of situations discussed in other sections of this volume. For example, MHPs may be asked to evaluate the defendant's competency to stand trial (see chapter 7.5), to determine whether the defendant should be involuntarily committed before trial (see chapter 8.4), or to determine the defendant's capacity to form the required mental state to commit the charged crime (see chapters 7.6–7.9).

Bail Determinations

Almost all persons charged with a crime are eligible for bail to secure their release from jail pending trial.[1] Bail is not available to persons charged with a capital offense.[2] The purpose of bail is to ensure that the person charged with a crime will attend future court proceedings related to the criminal charges. The amount of bail required of the person cannot be excessive.[3] In addition to persons charged with criminal offenses, persons who are material witnesses in criminal cases may be required to post a bail.[4]

The statutes related to bail determinations do not require that an MHP evaluate the accused. The court, however, will consider the person's mental condition and possible addiction to drugs or alcohol when establishing the appropriate bail.[5] In this regard, an MHP may be asked to consult with the court or other professionals in the criminal law system.

(A) Standards for Setting Pre-Verdict Bail

Pre-verdict bail refers to bail set at any stage of the criminal proceedings before the defendant is found guilty.[6] In establishing

---

1. PA. CONST. art. I, § 14; 42 PA. CONS. STAT. ANN. § 5701.
2. For bail considerations, a *capital offense* is any crime punishable by death, limited to first-degree murder. Commonwealth. v. Heiser, 478 A.2d 1355 (Pa. Super. Ct. 1984).
3. PA. CONST. art. I, § 13; PA. CONS. STAT. ANN. § 5701.
4. PA. R. CRIM. P. 4017(a).
5. PA. R. CRIM. P. 4004.
6. *Id.*

the proper amount for a pre-verdict bail, the court will consider the following defendant-relevant factors:

1. nature of the offense charged and any mitigating or aggravating factor that may bear on the likelihood of conviction and possible penalty;

2. employment history and current status and financial condition;

3. family relationships;

4. past and present residences;

5. age, character, reputation, mental condition, record of relevant convictions, and whether addicted to alcohol or drugs;

6. if previously released on bail, whether defendant appeared as required; and

7. any other facts relevant to whether the defendant has strong ties with the community or is likely to flee the jurisdiction.[7]

(B) Post-Verdict Bail

After a person has been found guilty of a crime, the court may set a new bail or may change the conditions of the previous bail. This may occur either before or after the person is sentenced.[8] If the person is convicted of a crime that could be punished by the death penalty, however, post-verdict bail will not be granted unless the person's motions for appeal are delayed for an extended period of time.[9]

---

7. Id.
8. PA. R. CRIM. P. 4010.
9. PA. R. CRIM. P. 4010(A)(1).

7.5

Competency to Stand Trial

It is an "absolute and basic condition of a fair trial" that a person on trial is mentally competent.[1] In general terms, the requirement of competency to stand trial demands that, at the time of trial, the defendant is able to comprehend that he or she is a defendant in a criminal trial and is able to cooperate with an attorney to build a defense.[2] A court-ordered competency evaluation must be conducted by at least one psychiatrist.[3] Other MHPs may have contact with a defendant declared not competent to stand trial, either during preliminary assessments or during court-ordered involuntary treatment. The court may order involuntary treatment for such a defendant if it is reasonably certain that the defendant will gain competency during treatment.[4]

(A) Legal Determination of Competency to Stand Trial

(A)(1) Test of Competency

Pennsylvania had adopted, in large part, the test for competency to proceed to trial established by the U.S. Supreme Court:

---

1. Commonwealth v. Hazur, 539 A.2d 451, 452 (Pa. Super. Ct. 1988); *See also* Pate v. Robinson, 383 U.S. 375 (1966).
2. *Id.*
3. PA. STAT. ANN. tit. 50, § 7402(e)(1).
4. PA. STAT. ANN. tit. 50, § 7402(b). *But see* Riggins v. Nevada, 504 U.S. 127 (1992) (violates due process to forcibly administer antipsychotic medication to pretrial detainee unless treatment is medically appropriate and, considering less intrusive alternatives, essential for detainee's safety or safety of others).

"Whether [the defendant] has sufficient present ability to consult with [a] lawyer with a reasonable degree of rational understanding—and whether [the defendant] has a rational as well as factual understanding of the proceedings."[5] The statutory language concerns whether the defendant is "substantially [ ]able to understand the nature or object of the proceedings against him or to participate and assist in his defense."[6] The tests for competency to stand trial focus on the mental state of the defendant at the time of trial, not at the time the alleged offense was committed (for those evaluations see chapter 7.7).[7] Further, under the competency test, a defendant may have a long history of mental illness, may carry a psychiatric diagnosis, and yet may be competent to stand trial.[8] It is not the nature of the mental illness that determines the defendant's competency; rather, it is the defendant's comprehension of the charges filed and ability to assist in a defense at the time of trial.[9]

Similarly, a defendant who cannot report information about the alleged crime because of amnesia may be competent to stand trial.[10] It is only when the loss of memory affects the defendant's capacity to understand the nature of the criminal proceedings or to assist in a defense that amnesia may result in a determination of not competent to stand trial.[11]

(A)(2) Raising the Competency Issue

At any stage of the criminal proceedings, the defendant, the defendant's attorney, the prosecuting attorney, or an official in charge of holding the defendant may raise concerns about the defendant's competency to stand trial and petition the court to order a competency evaluation.[12] The trial court may order a competency evaluation, either after an application for an evaluation or on its own, without a competency hearing.[13] If the defendant, or the defendant's attorney, challenges the order for a competency evaluation, the court must hold a hearing to determine whether there is a prima facie question of the defendant's competency.[14]

---

5. Dusky v. United States, 362 U.S. 402, 402 (1960) (*per curiam*).
6. PA. STAT. ANN. tit. 50, § 7402(a).
7. Commonwealth v. Knight, 419 A.2d 492 (Pa. Super. Ct. 1980).
8. Commonwealth v. Hazur, 539 A.2d 451 (Pa. Super. Ct. 1988).
9. *Id.*
10. Commonwealth v. Epps, 411 A.2d 534 (Pa. Super. Ct. 1979).
11. *Id.*
12. PA. STAT. ANN. tit. 50, § 7402(c). The U.S. Supreme Court has held that a defendant is constitutionally entitled to a competency hearing and does not waive the right to a hearing by failing to request one. Pate v. Robinson, 383 U.S. 375 (1966).
13. PA. STAT. ANN. tit. 50, § 7402(d).
14. *Id.*

(B) Competency Evaluations

When a competency evaluation is ordered by the court, the defendant is examined by a court appointed psychiatrist.[15] The evaluation occurs on an outpatient basis, unless the court has ordered the defendant to receive inpatient treatment.[16] The psychiatrist evaluates both the defendant's competency to proceed to trial and the defendant's capacity for the criminal responsibility associated with the crime (see chapter 7.9).[17] During the evaluation, the defendant has the right to have an attorney present and has the right to refuse to answer any question or to perform any test not agreed to before the start of the exam.[18] Information disclosed by the defendant during this exam can be used only as evidence of the defendant's mental status; it cannot be used as evidence against the defendant at any criminal proceeding.[19]

The psychiatrist who performs the competency evaluation must submit a report to the court,[20] which must contain

1. a diagnosis of the defendant's mental condition;

2. an opinion concerning the defendant's capacity to understand the nature and object of the criminal proceedings and to assist in a defense;

3. if requested, an opinion about the defendant's mental condition as it relates to criminal responsibility; and

4. if requested, an opinion about the defendant's capacity to have a particular state of mind, when it is necessary to prove a state of mind in a criminal case.[21]

The report of the competency evaluation is submitted to the court and is not confidential. The court may release the information contained in the report.[22]

If either the defendant or the commonwealth requests, the court may allow both a psychiatrist hired by the defendant and a psychiatrist hired by the commonwealth to attend the competency evaluation.[23] If a defendant is unable to afford a private psychiatrist and raises a substantial objection to the court-appointed psychiatrist's findings, the court will provide a reason-

---

15. PA. STAT. ANN. tit. 50, § 7402(e)(2).
16. *Id.*
17. *Id.*
18. PA. STAT. ANN. tit. 50, § 7402(e)(3).
19. *Id.*
20. PA. STAT. ANN. tit. 50, § 7402(e)(4).
21. *Id.*
22. Commonwealth. v. Rendick, 47 D. & C.3d 5 (Mercer County, 1987).
23. PA. STAT. ANN. tit. 50, § 7402(f).

able amount of money for the defendant to hire another psychiatrist.[24]

(C) Competency Hearing

The party requesting the competency hearing has the burden of proving by a preponderance of the evidence that the defendant is not competent to stand trial.[25] In all instances, the trial court decides the issue of the defendant's competency based on the evidence presented.[26] The final determination must be made within 20 days of the court receiving the psychiatrist's report, although the final determination can be delayed if the defendant asks for a continuance.[27]

(D) Disposition of Defendants Found Not Competent to Stand Trial

If a person is found not competent to stand trial, then all criminal proceedings against that person are suspended.[28] When the court determines that the person has gained competency to stand trial, the proceedings will resume.[29] If the court believes that because of the passage of time it would be unjust to resume the criminal proceedings, it may dismiss the charges against the defendant.[30] The criminal proceedings may not be suspended for a period of time that is longer than the maximum sentence the person could receive if convicted of the charges, unless the charges are first- or second-degree murder.[31]

After the court determines a defendant is not competent to stand trial and while the criminal charges are pending, the court may order the defendant to receive involuntary treatment on either an inpatient, partial hospitalization, or outpatient basis.[32]

---

24. *Id.*
25. PA. STAT. ANN. tit. 50, § 7403. The U.S. Supreme Court has held that states may presume defendants are competent and require them to bear the burden of proving incompetence, Medina v. California, 505 U.S. 437 (1992), but it violates due process for states to require defendants to prove competence by clear and convincing evidence. Cooper v. Oklahoma, 517 U.S. 348 (1996); Commonwealth v. duPont, 681 A.2d 1328 (Pa. 1996).
26. Commonwealth v. Knight, 419 A.2d 492 (Pa. Super. Ct. 1980).
27. PA. STAT. ANN. tit. 50. § 7402(g).
28. PA. STAT. ANN. tit. 50, § 7403(b).
29. PA. STAT. ANN. tit. 50, § 7403(e).
30. *Id.*
31. PA. STAT. ANN. tit. 50, § 7403(f).
32. PA. STAT. ANN. tit. 50, § 7402(b). *See also Riggins,* 504 U.S. 127, 132–138.

The treatment should include diagnosis, evaluation, rehabilitation, or therapy "designed and administered to alleviate [the] person's pain and distress and to maximize the probability of . . . recovery from mental illness."[33]

If inpatient treatment is ordered, the confinement cannot exceed a reasonable time necessary to determine whether there is a substantial probability that the person will become competent. During this period of hospitalization, the person must be evaluated by a court-appointed psychiatrist every 90 days to determine if the person is making progress.[34] If the court believes that the person will not become competent to stand trial, then the person must be discharged, unless confined under other provisions of the law, such as a civil commitment (see chapter 8.4).[35]

If the defendant is found not competent to stand trial and the court does not order inpatient treatment, the defendant will be released. As long as the criminal charges are pending against the defendant, however, the court may order a court-appointed psychiatrist to evaluate the person at least every 12 months.[36] When the psychiatrist determines that the person is competent to stand trial, the proceedings will resume within 90 days.

---

33. PA. STAT. ANN. tit. 50, § 7104. The treatment team, which is directed by either a physician or a licensed clinical psychologist, provides individualized treatment to those in need.
34. PA. STAT. ANN. tit. 50, § 7403(c).
35. PA. STAT. ANN. tit. 50, § 7403(d).
36. PA. STAT. ANN. tit. 50, § 7403(g).

Provocation

Expert psychological and psychiatric testimony is admissible at trial in provocation cases, but only for the limited purpose of deciding whether the person acted under a sudden and intense passion at the time of the offense.[1] Testimony addressing the person's psychological makeup and general ability to respond to provocation or stress is not admissible. The testimony must relate to the person's actual response at the time of the incident.[2]

A person who intentionally, knowingly, recklessly, or negligently (see chapter 7.7) causes another person's death is guilty of a criminal homicide, which is classified as either murder, voluntary manslaughter, or involuntary manslaughter.[3] If a person acts intentionally, in a willful, deliberate, or premeditated manner, to kill another person, the criminal charge is murder.[4] If a person kills another while acting under a sudden and intense passion, resulting from a serious provocation, the charge is voluntary manslaughter.[5] If a person responds to the provocation of another person, and in the process accidently kills a third person, the charge is also voluntary manslaughter.[6]

In the context of voluntary manslaughter, serious provocation is defined as "conduct sufficient to excite an intense passion in a reasonable person."[7] The test for serious provocation employs an objective standard.[8] The provocation must be of the sort

---

1. Commonwealth v. Stasko, 370 A.2d 350 (Pa. 1977).
2. *Id.*
3. 18 PA. CONS. STAT. ANN. § 2501.
4. 18 PA. CONS. STAT. ANN. § 2502.
5. 18 PA. CONS. STAT. ANN. § 2503(a)(1).
6. 18 PA. CONS. STAT. ANN. § 2503(a)(2).
7. 18 PA. CONS. STAT. ANN. § 2301.
8. Commonwealth v. McCusker, 292 A.2d 286 (Pa. 1972).

that a "reasonable man confronted with the same series of events would become impassioned to the extent that his mind was incapable of cool reflection."[9]

If a sufficiently serious provocation is established, the analysis turns to the person's response to the provocation. There are three relevant inquiries:

1. Did the defendant actually act in the heat of passion at the time the homicide was committed?

2. Did the provocation directly lead to the slaying of the person responsible for the provocation?

3. Was there insufficient "cooling time" thus preventing a reasonable person from using his or her "reasoning faculties" and "capacity to reflect?[10]

The case law indicates that a mere argument is not sufficiently serious provocation,[11] nor are words of provocation accompanied by a slight physical assault.[12] If the person retreats to a safe place, but later returns and kills the person, there is evidence of a sufficient cooling off period to allow a reasonable person to reflect on the provocation.[13]

The courts recognize a difference between the concepts of provocation and legal insanity, although both refer to the person's mental state at the time of the offense. (Legal insanity is discussed in chapter 7.9.)[14]

---

9. Commonwealth v. Eddowes, 580 A.2d 769, 772 (Pa. Super. Ct. 1990), *appeal denied*, 600 A.2d 951 (Pa. 1991).
10. Commonwealth v. McCusker, 292 A.3d 286, 290 (Pa. 1972).
11. Commonwealth v. Lassiter, 321 A.2d 902 (Pa. 1974).
12. Commonwealth v. Cisneros, 113 A.2d 293 (Pa. 1955).
13. Commonwealth. v. Eddowes, 580 A.2d 769 (Pa. Super. Ct. 1990), *appeal denied*, 600 A.2d 951 (Pa. 1991).
14. Commonwealth v. McCusker, 292 A.2d 286 (Pa. 1972).

Mens Rea

The minimum requirement for criminal liability is a voluntary act (or omission to perform a duty) that causes the criminal result. In addition, almost all crimes require the prosecution to prove that the defendant performed the act with *mens rea*—in other words, culpable state of mind. The purpose of determining a mental state is to distinguish between inadvertent or accidental acts and those that are performed with a "guilty mind." Each criminal statute defines the material elements of a criminal offense and the *mens rea*, or mental state, required for each element. Whenever the mental state of the individual is at issue, mental health professionals may testify about the person's mental state at the time of the offense.[1] See further discussion in chapters 7.8 and 7.9.

(A) Culpable Mental States

There are four culpable states of mind. Acts can be performed intentionally, knowingly, recklessly, and negligently. The statute defining the criminal offense will indicate which level of culpability is required for each material element of the offense. To be found criminally liable, the person must satisfy the required level of culpability for each material element of the offense.[2] The four mental states of culpability are defined as follows:

1. *Intentionally.* (a) It was the person's conscious object to engage in conduct of that nature or to cause such a result; and (b) if the

---

1. Commonwealth v. Walzack, 360 A.2d 914 (Pa. 1976).
2. 18 PA. CONS. STAT. ANN. § 302(a).

element involves the attendant circumstances the person was aware of the existence of such circumstances or believed or hoped that they existed.

2. *Knowingly.* (a) The person was aware that the conduct was of that nature or that such circumstances existed; and (b) if the element involves a result of the person's conduct, the person was aware that it was practically certain that the conduct would cause such a result.

3. *Recklessly.* The person consciously disregarded a substantial and unjustifiable risk that the material element existed or would result from his conduct. The risk must be of such a nature and degree that, considering the nature and intent of the actor's conduct and the circumstances known to him, its disregard involved a gross deviation from the standard of conduct that a reasonable person would observe in the actor's situation.

4. *Negligently.* The person should have been aware of a substantial and unjustifiable risk that the material element existed or would result from his conduct. The risk must be of such a nature and degree that the actor's failure to perceive it, considering the nature and intent of his conduct and the circumstances known to him, involved a gross deviation from the standard of care that a reasonable person would observe in the actor's situation.[3]

If the statute defining the criminal offense does not indicate the required mental state, any of the four levels of culpability will suffice to establish criminal liability.[4] Further, if the statute indicates the required mental state for the criminal offense in general but does not provide the required mental state for each material element of the offense, then the mental state for the criminal offense in general is required for each material element.[5]

The four mental states form a hierarchy of culpability, running from the highest level of culpability to the lowest level—intentionally, knowingly, recklessly, negligently. Along this hierarchy, a higher level of culpability may satisfy the required mental state when a lower level of culpability is listed in the statute. For instance, if the statute requires that a person act negligently with regard to a material element of the offense, criminal liability will be found if the person acts recklessly, intentionally, or knowingly;[6] if it requires the person to act knowingly with regard to a

---

3. 18 Pa. Cons. Stat. Ann. §§ 302(b)(1–4).
4. 18 Pa. Cons. Stat. Ann. § 302(c).
5. 18 Pa. Cons. Stat. Ann. § 302(d).
6. 18 Pa. Cons. Stat. Ann. § 302(e).

material element of the offense, then the element is satisfied if the person acts intentionally.[7]

Some criminal statutes require that the person act willfully. This requirement is satisfied if the person acts knowingly with respect to the material elements of the offense.[8] Other criminal offenses are defined as summary offenses and do not require a voluntary act or an accompanying mental state.[9] An example of a summary offense is a traffic ticket. Other crimes, usually those involving the regulation of businesses or dangerous instrumentalities, may require a voluntary act but no requisite mental state. These are known as *strict liability crimes.*

---

7. *Id.*
8. 18 PA. CONS. STAT. ANN. § 302(g).
9. 18 PA. CONS. STAT. ANN. § 305(b)(1).

7.8

Diminished Capacity

The term *diminished capacity* describes two different concepts. It may be used to negate the requisite *mens rea* of the crime, thereby completely exonerating the defendant of that charge. It may also be used as an affirmative defense to reduce the degree of crime for which the defendant may be convicted, even if the defendant's conduct satisfied all of the formal elements of a higher offense. The use of diminished capacity is strictly circumscribed. Where it is used, however, courts have allowed MHPs to provide relevant, but limited, information about an accused person's diminished capacity.[1]

(A) Legal Test of Diminished Capacity

The diminished capacity defense is very limited and generally is a defense to charges of first-degree murder.[2] *Murder of the first degree* is defined as "a criminal homicide . . . committed by an intentional killing."[3] To prove first-degree murder at trial, the prosecutor must establish that the accused person unlawfully killed another person, that the accused is not insane under the M'Naghten test (see chapter 7.9), and that the killing was done with malice aforethought.[4] The prosecutor must also prove that

---

1. Commonwealth v. Walzack, 360 A.2d 914 (Pa. 1976).
2. Commonwealth. v. Zettlemoyer, 454 A.2d 937 (Pa. 1982), *cert. denied,* 461 U.S. 970 (1983).
3. 18 PA. CONS. STAT. ANN. § 2502(a).
4. Commonwealth v. Weinstein, 451 A.2d 1344 (Pa. 1982).

the accused specifically intended to kill and acted with premeditation and deliberation.[5]

A defense of diminished capacity contests the accused's capacity to possess the particular state of mind required for first-degree murder.[6] Under this defense, the accused concedes criminal liability but argues that because of his or her mental condition he or she lacks the cognitive ability to form the specific intent to kill through premeditation and deliberation.[7] If this defense is successful, then the accused will not be convicted of first-degree murder but will be convicted of either second-degree murder or manslaughter.[8]

The testimony of an MHP related to diminished capacity is limited to the issue of the specific intent to kill.[9] Testimony is admissible only if it relates to whether the accused has a mental disability that affects his or her cognitive functions to a degree that precludes the ability to premeditate or deliberate about the killing.[10] The Supreme Court of Pennsylvania stated that proof of a below-average intellect alone is not sufficient for a diminished capacity defense to first-degree murder.[11] The Superior Court has ruled that testimony about the accused's schizoid personality disorder was irrelevant to the diminished capacity defense.[12] As a general rule, the court will reject testimony that addresses the accused's irresistible impulse (see chapter 7.9) rather than diminished capacity.[13]

(B) Intoxication and Diminished Capacity

Under the relevant statute, neither voluntary intoxication nor a voluntary drugged condition is a defense to a criminal charge, and evidence related to such a condition is not admissible.[14] Evidence of voluntary intoxication or a voluntary drugged condition is admissible at trial, however, if the evidence might reduce a charge of first-degree murder to a lower degree of murder.[15]

---

5. *Id.*
6. *Walzack*, 360 A.2d 914.
7. *Id.*
8. *Id.*
9. *Weinstein*, 451 A.2d 1344.
10. Commonwealth v. Terry, 521 A.2d 398 (Pa. 1987), *cert. denied*, 482 U.S. 920 (1987).
11. *Id.*
12. Commonwealth v. Davis, 479 A.2d 1077 (Pa. Super. Ct. 1984).
13. Commonwealth. v. Kenny, 474 A.2d 313 (Pa. Super. Ct. 1984).
14. 18 Pa. Cons. Stat. Ann. § 308.
15. *Id.*

When evidence of voluntary intoxication or drugged condition is admitted into a first-degree murder trial, its only effect is to establish that the voluntary condition so affected the accused's mental capacity that the accused was incapable of forming the specific intent to kill.[16] To be successful, the defense must establish that the accused was overwhelmed by the alcohol or drugs to the point of losing control of his or her faculties and sensibilities.[17] If a diminished capacity defense is successful, based on a voluntary intoxication or drugged condition, the crime of first-degree murder is reduced to second-degree murder. It is never reduced to manslaughter.[18]

In some states, a defense of involuntary intoxication is viable if the defendant can establish that the intoxicating substance was not ingested voluntarily but because of an overwhelming influence that precluded the exercise of independent judgment.[19] There is only one reported case in the commonwealth in which the involuntary intoxication defense was successful.[20] In all other cases, the Superior Court has acknowledged the involuntary intoxication defense as an abstract possibility, but the courts have never ruled explicitly on its viability.[21] The courts have expressly stated that an involuntary intoxication defense premised on the argument that the defendant suffers from chronic alcoholism and therefore is unable to control the ingestion of the intoxicating substance will not be accepted.[22]

---

16. Commonwealth v. England, 375 A.2d 1292 (Pa. 1977).
17. Commonwealth v. Breakiron, 571 A.2d 1035 (Pa. 1990), *cert. denied*, 498 U.S. 881 (1990).
18. *England*, 375 A.2d 1292.
19. Commonwealth. v. Butterfield, 17 Pa. D. & C.3d 62 (1980), (*citing* New Hampshire v. Plummer, 374 A.2d 431 (N.H. 1977)).
20. *Id.* In *Butterfield*, the defendant was convicted of driving under the influence of alcohol. In posttrial motions, the defendant successfully argued that the trial court should have considered his involuntary intoxication defense that the car he was driving had been painted 12 hours before his arrest and that his intoxicated state resulted from the involuntary ingestion of paint fumes from the car.
21. Commonwealth v. Griscom, 600 A.2d 996 (Pa. Super. Ct. 1991); Commonwealth. v. Kuhn, 475 A.2d 103, 110 (Pa. Super. Ct. 1984) (Montemuro, J., concurring) ("No Pennsylvania case has ever held that the defense of involuntary intoxication is a viable one").
22. Commonwealth v. Ellis, 581 A.2d 595 (Pa. Super. Ct. 1990), *aff'd* 626 A.2d 1137 (Pa. 1993); Commonwealth v. Kuhn, 475 A.2d 103 (Pa. Super. Ct. 1984) (plurality decision).

Criminal Responsibility

An early, yet still controversial, contribution of MHP expertise in the courtroom has been the evaluation of criminal defendants who plead not guilty by reason of insanity because of their mental state at the time of the offense. MHPs may evaluate defendants and testify about their psychological functioning at the time the criminal behavior occurred.

(A) Legal Insanity or the Not Guilty by Reason of Insanity Verdict

Pennsylvania adheres to the M'Naughten rule for legal insanity and criminal responsibility.[1] Under this standard, a defendant in a criminal trial will be relieved of criminal responsibility if the defendant proves by a preponderance of the evidence that he or she was legally insane at the time the offense was committed.[2] The M'Naughten test for legal insanity is defined as follows: "At the time of the commission of the offense, the actor was laboring under such a defect of reason, from disease of the mind, as not to know the nature and quality of the act he was doing or, if the actor did know the quality of the act, that he did not know that what he was doing was wrong."[3]

---

1. Commonwealth v. Heidnik, 587 A.2d 687 (Pa. 1991).
2. 18 Pa. Cons. Stat. Ann. § 315(a).
3. 18 Pa. Cons. Stat. Ann. § 315(b).

(A)(1) Burden of Proof

The not guilty by reason of insanity defense is an affirmative defense. That means it must be raised and proved by the defendant, not by the prosecution.[4] A defendant who intends to raise an insanity defense must provide the commonwealth with information concerning the nature and extent of the alleged insanity, the period of time during which the defendant suffered from the insanity, and the names and addresses of witness and experts whom the defendant plans to have testify at trial. This information must be delivered within 30 days of the defendant's arraignment.[5] At this stage, the court may order a psychiatric evaluation of the defendant, as described in chapter 7.5. This evaluation will be conducted by a psychiatrist and will address the defendant's mental condition in relation to criminal responsibility.[6]

(A)(2) Raising the Competency Issue

The issue of competency is typically raised by the defendant, who privately arranges for an MHP to conduct the evaluation or requests the court to appoint an expert to conduct the evaluation.

(B) Mental Examination

Once the issue is raised, the prosecution has the right to retain its own expert to perform a separate evaluation. In general, criminal responsibility evaluations relate to one of the following conditions: provocation (see chapter 7.6), the legal insanity defense (this chapter); a determination that the defendant is guilty but mentally ill (this chapter), or a diminished capacity defense (see chapter 7.8).

The determination of legal insanity may occur either at trial or at a separate hearing.[7] In insanity defense cases, expert testimony by MHPs is admissible at trial, or at the hearing, only as it is related to whether the defendant satisfies the M'Naughten standard for insanity.[8] The courts have ruled that neither voluntary intoxication[9] nor behavior resulting from a passive pathological

---

4. *Heidnik,* 587 A.2d 687; 18 PA. CONS. STAT. ANN. § 314(a).
5. PA. R. CRIM. P. 305 C(1)(b).
6. PA. STAT. ANN. tit. 50, § 7402(e)(4)(iii).
7. PA. STAT. ANN. tit. 50, § 7404. At such a proceeding any qualified expert witness, whether the prosecution's expert of the defense's expert, may testify. PA. STAT. ANN. tit. 50, § 7402 n.3.
8. Commonwealth. v. Faulkner, 595 A.2d 28 (Pa. 1991), *cert. denied,* 503 U.S. 988 (1992).
9. Commonwealth v. Plank, 478 A.2d 872 (Pa. Super. Ct. 1984).

state brought on by alcohol ingestion satisfies an insanity defense (see chapter 7.9).[10] In addition, courts are reluctant to accept an insanity defense argument when the defendant voluntarily engaged in activity that induced the mental state.[11]

(C) Not Guilty by Reason of Insanity

If the defendant is found not guilty by reason of insanity, the defendant will be acquitted of all charges. The acquittal reflects "a societal judgment as to the minimal mental capacity that must be possessed by the actor to be held criminally responsible for his acts."[12] After a verdict of not guilty by reason of insanity, however, the defendant may be subjected to involuntary treatment.[13] The involuntary treatment is not a mandatory result of an acquittal for lack of criminal responsibility.[14] There must be a separate hearing to determine whether the acquitted person is in need of treatment based on the standards for involuntary treatment listed in the civil statutes (see chapter 8.4).[15]

(D) Diminished Capacity and the Irresistible Impulse Test

As described in chapter 7.8 some states follow an irresistible impulse test for diminished capacity. The irresistible impulse test is similar to the not guilty by reason of insanity defense because the person may avoid criminal liability altogether.[16] For this defense to be successful, it must be proved that even though the person was capable of distinguishing between right and wrong and was fully aware of the nature and quality of the actions, the person was unable to refrain from acting.[17] Pennsylvania does not accept the irresistible impulse doctrine, and as such, MHPs can

---

10. Commonwealth v. Henry, 569 A.2d 929 (Pa. 1990), *cert. denied*, 499 U.S. 931 (1991).
11. *Id.*
12. Commonwealth v. Plank, 478 A.2d 872, 875 (Pa. Super. Ct. 1984) (quoting Commonwealth v. Hicks, 396 A.2d 1183, 1186 (Pa. 1979)).
13. PA. STAT. ANN. tit. 50, § 7406.
14. Commonwealth. v. McCann, 469 A.2d 126 (Pa. 1983), *rev'g*, 448 A.2d 1123 (Pa. Super. Ct. 1982). *But see* Jones v. United States, 463 U.S. 354 (1983) (standard for involuntary commitment after a not guilty by reason of insanity defense may be a lesser standard—in other words, a preponderance of the evidence—than clear and convincing standard for civil commitment).
15. PA. STAT. ANN. tit. 50, § 7406.
16. Commonwealth v. Walzack, 360 A.2d 914 (Pa. 1976).
17. *Id.*

not offer testimony related to a person's inability to control behaviors because of an irresistible impulse.

(E) Guilty But Mentally Ill

A defendant who unsuccessfully raises an insanity defense and subsequently is found guilty of the criminal offense may be found guilty but mentally ill by the jury.[18] For the guilty but mentally ill verdict, a mentally ill person is defined as "one who as a result of mental disease or defect, lacks substantial capacity either to appreciate the wrongfulness of his conduct or to conform his conduct to the requirements of the law."[19] This verdict does not relieve the defendant of criminal responsibility, nor is it intended to mitigate any punishment the defendant might receive.[20] The only effect of a guilty but mentally ill verdict is to trigger an inquiry at the time of sentencing to determine whether the defendant is mentally ill.[21] As a result, neither the commonwealth nor the defendant bears the burden of proving the defendant was mentally ill at the time of the offense.[22] The court may hear expert testimony from MHPs only after the defendant is convicted, but before sentencing, to determine mental illness (see chapters 7.10, 7.15).[23]

A person found guilty but mentally ill may receive any sentence that is appropriate for the crime for which that person was convicted.[24] However, the guilty but mentally ill defendant who is severely mentally disabled will receive whatever psychological or psychiatric treatment is indicated and is within available resources.[25] The commonwealth will pay for this treatment.[26]

When a person found guilty but mentally ill no longer needs treatment in an inpatient setting, the person will be returned to a correctional facility or county jail.[27] The releasing agency will submit a report to the correctional facility. This report must discuss the person's current condition and the reasons for discontinuing treatment, the course of treatment, the potential for recur-

---

18. 18 Pa. Cons. Stat. Ann. § 314(a).
19. Pa. Cons. Stat. Ann. § 314(c)(1).
20. Commonwealth v. Sohmer, 546 A.2d 601 (Pa. 1988).
21. Id.
22. Id.
23. 42 Pa. Cons. Stat. Ann. § 9727(a).
24. Id.
25. 42 Pa. Cons. Stat. Ann. § 9727(b)(1).
26. 42 Pa. Cons. Stat. Ann. § 9727(b)(2).
27. 42 Pa. Cons. Stat. Ann. § 9727(c).

ring behavior, the person's potential to be dangerous, and any recommendations for future treatment.[28]

As an alternative to serving the remainder of the criminal sentence in a prison, the person found guilty but mentally ill and released from treatment may be eligible for probation or parole under the same terms as other offenders (see chapters 7.12 and 7.18).[29] Psychological and psychiatric counseling may be a condition of release on probation or parole and failure to comply with these conditions could result in the person being returned to prison.[30]

---

28. *Id.*
29. 42 PA. CONS. STAT. ANN. § 9727(d).
30. *Id.*

7.10

Competency to Be Sentenced

As with competency to stand trial (see chapter 7.5), a person convicted of a crime will not be sentenced if that person is substantially unable to understand the nature of the proceedings or is unable to participate in the proceedings by assisting defense counsel.[1] For the procedures and requirements of a competency evaluation see chapter 7.5. In addition to conducting competency evaluations, MHPs may examine defendants with regard to conditions of sentencing (chapter 7.15) and competency to be executed (chapter 7.19).

---

1. PA. STAT. ANN. tit. 50, § 7402(a).

7.11

Sentencing

After a person is found guilty at trial, but before sentence is imposed, the sentencing judge may order a psychiatric or psychological evaluation of the defendant.[1] The purpose of this evaluation is to provide the court with information relevant to the person's final disposition and sentence.[2] The court may select any of the following:

1. probation,
2. monetary fine,
3. determination of guilt with no further penalty,
4. partial confinement, or
5. total confinement.[3]

The sentencing statutes suggest that while determining the appropriate sentence, the judge or jury should consider whether the imposed sentence is consistent with the needs of the community, the seriousness of the offense, and the rehabilitative needs of the individual.[4] MHPs have a role in informing the jury about the presence or absence of several of these aggravating or mitigating factors.

---

1. PA. R. CRIM. P. 1403(B).
2. PA. STAT. ANN. tit. 50, §§ 7406, 4410.
3. 42 PA. CONS. STAT. § 9721.
4. 42 PA. CONS. STAT. § 9721(b).

(A) Presentence Mental Health Examination

The court can order a presentence evaluation on either an outpatient or inpatient basis.[5] If the court orders an inpatient evaluation, the defendant is sent to an available clinic, hospital, institution, or state correctional diagnostic and classification center.[6] The defendant may not be held as an inpatient for more than 60 days[7] and the duration of the hospitalization is credited as time served on any sentence subsequently imposed.[8]

(B) Disclosure of Presentencing Evaluations

All presentencing psychiatric and psychological reports are confidential and are not included in the public record of criminal proceedings.[9]

(C) Sentencing Guidelines

Pennsylvania provides sentencing judges with specific guidelines to consider when deciding on a sentence for a person convicted of a crime.[10] These guidelines create a procedure that the judge must follow to determine the recommended sentence[11] and require the judge to issue a statement of the reasons for selecting a particular sentence.[12] The procedure requires the judge to consider the following issues:

1. defendant's prior criminal record,
2. recommended sentence range,
3. whether defendant is eligible for boot camp program or an intermediate punishment (discussed later),
4. any mitigating or aggravating circumstances, and

5. PA. STAT. ANN. tit. 50, § 7405.
6. PA. R. CRIM. P. 1403(B).
7. Id.
8. PA. STAT. ANN. tit. 50, § 7401(b).
9. PA. R. CRIM. P. 1404(a).
10. 204 PA. CODE § 303.1(a).
11. 204 PA. CODE § 303.2.
12. 204 PA. CODE § 303.1(h).

5. whether the defendant possessed a deadly weapon during the crime.[13]

Intermediate Punishment Sanctions
The sentencing judge also must consider whether the individual is eligible for intermediate punishment short of total confinement.[14] Intermediate punishment programs include

1. noncustodial programs that involve close supervision, but not housing, of the offender in a facility, including but not limited to intensive probation supervision, victim restitution or mediation, alcohol or drug outpatient treatment, house arrest and electronic monitoring, psychiatric counseling, and community service;

2. residential inpatient drug and alcohol programs based on objective assessments that the offender is drug or alcohol dependent or a residential rehabilitative center;

3. individualized services that evaluate and treat offenders, including psychological and medical services, education, vocational training, drug and alcohol screening and counseling, individual and family counseling, and transportation subsidies; and

4. partial confinement programs, such as work release, work camps, and halfway facilities.[15]

Aggravating and Mitigating Circumstances
The Code does not provide an extensive list of aggravating and mitigating circumstances for most convictions. For convictions involving illegal substances, the judge may consider the following factors in sentencing the defendant to the upper ranges:

1. drug was of exceptional purity (e.g., "crack" cocaine);

2. defendant was engaged in continuing series of violations of Controlled Substance, Drug, Device and Cosmetic Act;

3. defendant's violation was in concert with one or more other persons with respect to whom the defendant was supplier, occupied position of organizer, supervisory or other position of management;

4. defendant obtained or had obtained substantial income or resources from ongoing drug activities;

5. defendant involved juveniles in the trafficking or distribution of drugs; or

---

13. 204 PA. CODE § 303.1(a).
14. 204 PA. CODE § 303.2(4).
15. *Id.*

6. other facts that warrant sentence in the aggravated range.[16]

In determining whether a sentence within the lower range should be imposed for a drug conviction, the judge should consider

1. if defendant appears to have cooperated in the apprehension or prosecution of other violations of the Act or other criminal statutes; or

2. other factors that, in court's judgment, warrant a sentence within the mitigated range.[17]

In addition, if the court determines that a person convicted of a drug charge would benefit from treatment and the minimum sentence for the offense would be 6 moths or less, the court can order inpatient drug treatment.[18] In those instances, the court cannot order a period of treatment shorter than the recommended minimum sentence for the offense.[19]

Deadly Weapon Enhancement
If the judge concluded that the defendant possessed a deadly weapon during the commission of a criminal offense, 12 to 24 months are added to whatever sentence the judge imposed under the guidelines.[20]

Death Penalty Sentencing
Persons convicted of first-degree murder are sentenced to life in prison or death.[21] Whenever a person is convicted of first-degree murder the court must follow special procedures to determine the appropriate sentence. After the verdict the judge must hold a separate (bifurcated) sentencing hearing after which the jury decides whether the person should be given life imprisonment or death.[22] At the hearing the convicted person may present any evidence of mitigating circumstances and the commonwealth's attorney can present evidence of aggravating circumstances.[23] MHPs may testify at this stage of the hearing.[24] The judge must instruct the jury about the aggravating and mitigating circum-

16. 204 Pa. Code § 303.3(b).
17. 204 Pa. Code § 303.3(c).
18. 204 Pa. Code § 303(e).
19. *Id.*
20. 204 Pa. Code § 303.4(a).
21. Pa. Cons. Stat. Ann. tit. 18, § 1102(a). The U.S. Supreme Court has declared the death penalty constitutional as long as certain clear and objective standards for sentencing are in place. Gregg v. Georgia, 428 U.S. 153 (1976).
22. 42 Pa. Cons. Stat. § 9711(a)(1).
23. 42 Pa. Cons. Stat. § 9711(a)(2).
24. Commonwealth v. Faulkner, 595 A.2d 28 (Pa. 1991), *cert. denied,* 503 U.S. 988 (1992).

stances and explain that the commonwealth has the burden of proving all aggravating circumstances beyond a reasonable doubt but that the defendant need prove mitigating circumstances only by a preponderance of the evidence.[25]

When determining the sentence, the jury must sentence the person to death in two situations. First, if it finds at least one aggravating circumstance and no mitigating circumstances on a unanimous vote or, second, if it finds two or more aggravating circumstances that, when combined, outweigh any mitigating circumstances.[26] If neither of these conditions are met, the defendant is sentenced to life in prison.[27]

The only factors that can be considered aggravating circumstances in the context of sentencing someone to death are the following:

1. victim was public safety officer (or one assisting law enforcement officer), judge, or certain high state officials, killed in performance of his duties or as direct result of his official positions;
2. defendant was paid or was paid by another or had contracted to pay or be paid by another or had conspired to pay or be paid by another for the killing;
3. victim was being held by defendant for ransom or reward, or as shield or hostage;
4. victim died while defendant was hijacking an aircraft;
5. victim was prosecution witness to murder or other felony committed by defendant and was killed for purpose of preventing testimony against defendant;
6. defendant committed killing in perpetration of felony;
7. in commission of offense, defendant knowingly created grave risk of death to another in addition to victim;
8. victim was tortured;
9. defendant has significant history of felony convictions involving threat or use of violence to a person;
10. defendant was convicted of another federal or state offense;
11. defendant was convicted of another murder;
12. defendant was convicted of voluntary manslaughter;
13. defendant committed the killing or was accomplice in the killing during perpetration of felony listed in the Controlled Substance, Drug, Device and Cosmetic Act;

---

25. 42 PA. CONS. STAT. § 9711(c).
26. 42 PA. CONS. STAT. § 9711(c)(iv).
27. Id.

14. at time of killing, victim was or had been involved, associated, or in competition with defendant in sale, manufacture, distribution, or delivery of any controlled or counterfeit controlled substance in violation of the Act and defendant committed the killing or was an accomplice to the killing resulting from or related to that association, involvement, or competition;

15. at time of killing, victim was a nongovernmental informant or had provided law enforcement agencies with information concerning criminal activity and defendant committed the killing or was an accomplice to the killing in retaliation for the victim's activities; or

16. victim was a child under 12 years of age.[28]

The statutory mitigating factors are

1. defendant has no significant history of prior criminal convictions;

2. defendant was under influence of extreme mental or emotional disturbance;

3. defendant's capacity to appreciate criminality of his or her conduct or to conform that conduct to requirements of law was substantially impaired;

4. defendant's relative youth at time of crime;

5. defendant acted under extreme duress, although not such duress as to constitute excusable defense, or defendant acted under substantial domination of another person;

6. victim was participant in defendant's homicidal conduct or consented to the homicidal acts;

7. defendant's participation was relatively minor; or

8. any other evidence of mitigation concerning character and record of defendant and the circumstances of the offense.[29]

---

28. 42 Pa. Cons. Stat. § 9711(d).
29. Id.

7.12

Probation

After a person is found guilty of a crime the sentencing judge may elect to place the defendant on probation rather than impose a prison term.[1] MHPs may be asked to evaluate persons to determine whether probation is warranted.

Because probation is not an automatic right, the judge has the discretion to consider the character of the defendant, the circumstances of the case, the likelihood of the defendant committing another crime, and whether the public good demands imposition of a sentence of confinement.[2] More particularly, in choosing between confinement and probation, the judge may weigh the following factors:

1. defendant neither caused nor threatened serious harm;
2. defendant did not contemplate that the criminal conduct would cause or threaten serious harm;
3. defendant acted under strong provocation;
4. there were substantial grounds tending to excuse or justify the criminal conduct, though short of creating a defense;
5. victim of crime induced or facilitated its commission;
6. defendant compensated or will compensate victim for damage or injury sustained during crime;
7. defendant has no history of delinquency or criminal activity or has led law-abiding life for substantial period prior to present offense;

---

1. 42 PA. CONS. STAT. ANN. § 9721(a).
2. PA. STAT. ANN. tit. 61, § 331.25.

8. criminal conduct was result of circumstances unlikely to recur;

9. defendant's character and attitudes indicate little likelihood that criminal activity will reoccur;

10. defendant likely to respond affirmatively to probation;

11. confinement would entail excessive hardship to defendant or his or her family; and

12. such other grounds as indicate the desirability of probation.[3]

When probation is warranted, the period of probation may not exceed the maximum period of confinement that the judge could have ordered for the offense committed.[4] The judge may not order probation for conviction of first-degree murder.[5]

---

3. 42 PA. CONS. STAT. § 9722.
4. *Id.*; 42 PA. CONS. STAT. § 9754(a).
5. PA. STAT. ANN. tit. 61, § 331.25.

7.13

Dangerous Offenders

Some states allow for a criminal sentence to be increased if the defendant is a dangerous offender and poses a special threat to the community. Pennsylvania does not have a statute explicitly requiring enhanced sentences for dangerous offenders, although there is one applicable to "high risk dangerous offenders" (see chapter 7.14). A defendant's dangerous nature, however, might be considered as an aggravating circumstance by the sentencing judge, unless the death penalty is imposed (see chapter 7.11). The complicated sentencing guidelines are described in chapter 7.11.

Habitual Offenders

The law requires enhanced sentencing for offenders who are found to be "high risk dangerous offenders."[1] The court will presume that an offender is a high-risk dangerous offender if the offender was previously convicted of a crime of violence, and the previous conviction occurred within 7 years of the date of the commission of the instant offense, except that any period of time in which the offender was incarcerated or on probation or parole is not to be considered in computing the 7-year period.[2] The law defines a "crime of violence" as murder of the third degree, voluntary manslaughter, aggravated assault, rape, involuntary deviate sexual intercourse, arson, kidnapping, burglary of a structure adapted for overnight accommodation in which at the time of the offense any person is present, robbery, robbery of a motor vehicle, or criminal attempt, criminal conspiracy, or criminal solicitation to commit murder or any of the offenses listed.[3]

Before the hearing to determine whether an offender is a high-risk dangerous offender, the court may order a psychiatric or psychological examination of the offender.[4] At the hearing, the court shall consider, but not be limited to, such factors as:

1. age of the offender,
2. age of the victim,
3. use of illegal drugs or alcohol by the offender,
4. offender's prior criminal record,

---

1. 42 PA. CONS. STAT. § 9714.
2. 42 PA. CONS. STAT. § 9714(b).
3. 42 PA. CONS. STAT. § 9714(g).
4. 42 PA. CONS. STAT. § 9714(c)(3).

5. whether the offense involved multiple victims,

6. offender's failure to complete a prior sentence,

7. any mental illness or mental disability of the offender,

8. if the offense included attempted or actual sexual contact with the victim and if this was part of a demonstrated pattern of abuse,

9. if the offense included a display of unusual cruelty by the offender during the commission of the crime,

10. the nature and circumstances of the current offense,

11. the use of a deadly weapon, and

12. the impact of the current offense on the victim and the extent of injury caused to the victim.[5]

Second Violent Offense

If the offender successfully proves that he or she is not a high-risk violent offender, the law requires a minimum sentence of 5 years.[6] If the offender fails to prove by clear and convincing evidence,[7] however, that he or she is not a high-risk violent offender, the law requires a mandatory sentence of 10 years.

Third Violent Offense

If the offender is convicted of a third violent offense, the law imposes a mandatory minimum sentence of 25 years, but court has the option of imposing a life sentence without parole "if it determines that 25 years of total confinement is insufficient to protect the public safety."[8]

Maximum Sentence

If the offender is sentenced to a mandatory minimum sentence under this section of the law, the sentence cannot exceed twice the mandatory minimum sentence.[9]

---

5. 42 PA. CONS. STAT. § 9714(c).
6. 42 PA. CONS. STAT. § 9714(a)(1).
7. 42 PA. CONS. STAT. § 9714(c)(5).
8. 42 PA. CONS. STAT. § 9714(a)(2).
9. 42 PA. CONS. STAT. § 9714(a.1).

7.15

Competency to Serve a Sentence

A court-appointed committee containing at least one psychiatrist may evaluate a person convicted of a crime to determine if that person is competent to proceed to the sentencing phase of the criminal process (see chapters 7.5 and 7.14).[1] After the person is sentenced, however, Pennsylvania does not offer relief from the sentence because the person is mentally ill. Instead, if the person becomes severely mentally ill during the period of confinement, then proceedings similar to civil commitment hearings can be initiated just as if the person were not serving a criminal sentence (see chapter 8.4).[2]

Any person found to be in need of an inpatient examination or treatment while serving a criminal sentence will be transferred to a mental health facility (see chapter 7.17).[3] During the period of treatment, the mental health facility must take measures to maintain the person's status as an incarcerated individual, unless a release from the criminal sentence is secured during the treatment period.[4] When treatment is finished, the mental health facility must return the person to the responsible prison or to any other agency granted control over that person for the remainder of the sentence.[5] Any period of inpatient treatment at a mental health facility is credited as time served toward completion of the person's criminal sentence.[6]

---

1. Pa. Stat. Ann. tit. 50, §§ 7402(a) & (e)(2).
2. Pa. Stat. Ann. tit. 50, § 7401(a).
3. Pa. Stat. Ann. tit. 50, § 7401(b).
4. *Id.*
5. *Id.*
6. *Id.*

7.16

Mental Health Services in Jails and Prisons

The Pennsylvania Code, which lists the standards and requirements for jails and prisons, establishes the minimum requirements for medical and mental health services provided by each county prison. Although the Code does not delineate clear requirements for the state prisons, these institutions are required to establish procedures that guarantee each inmate access to health care staff and appropriate treatment for serious medical needs.[1] Presumably, these needs include mental health services as well.

(A) Medical and Health Services Required of County Prisons

Every person admitted to a county jail must undergo a physical examination and a mental health examination within 48 hours of admission.[2] The Code does not provide a list of professionals qualified to perform these examinations. Because county jails are required to provide access to MHPs, however,[3] such professionals do probably conduct some examinations.

---

1. 37 PA. CODE § 93.12.
2. 37 PA. CODE § 95.232.
3. 37 PA. CODE § 95.243(a)(1).

(B) Mental Health Services in County Jails

The Code recommends that each prison secure the services of a psychiatrist either through full-time employment or through a contract to provide needed services.[4] In any event, prisons are required to provide counseling services for inmates.[5] These services must include individual counseling, group counseling, vocational rehabilitation, social casework, and group work, which includes self-help groups such as Alcoholics Anonymous, psychological testing services, clinical psychology services, and psychiatric services.[6] Counseling services must be provided either by a full-time qualified counselor, through contracts with an outside agency, professional volunteers, or self-help groups.[7] Prisons also are required to provide medical detoxification and treatment programs for inmates physically dependent on alcohol or drugs.[8] All services must be supervised by a qualified counselor, preferably one who has at least a master's degree.[9] A person with a bachelor's degree in a behavioral science and who satisfies the minimum standards of the profession he or she is engaged in nevertheless can supervise the delivery of mental health services.[10]

---

4. 37 PA. CODE § 95.233(b)(3).
5. 37 PA. CODE § 95.243(a)(1).
6. *Id.*
7. *Id.*
8. PA. STAT. ANN. tit. 71, § 1690.106(a).
9. 37 PA. CODE § 95.243(a)(1).
10. *Id.*

7.17

Transfer From Penal to Mental Health Facilities

An incarcerated individual has access to a limited amount of mental health services while in a penal institution (see chapter 7.16). When the provided services are not adequate to meet an individual's needs, the Mental Health Procedures Act of 1976 permits the person to be transferred to a mental health facility. A transfer to a mental health facility can occur either through a voluntary request for treatment[1] or through commitment hearings leading to involuntary treatment.[2]

(A) Mentally Ill Inmates

When an incarcerated person desires mental health treatment, he or she can request a voluntary transfer to a mental health facility.[3] To be transferred, the person must understand the nature of voluntary treatment and must be examined by at least one physician.[4] The physician must certify that the person needs additional mental health treatment that the penal institution is not able to deliver.[5]

The second situation that leads to an incarcerated person's transfer to a mental health facility is triggered by a belief by an official at the penal institution that the person is severely mentally ill and needs additional treatment not provided by the host facility. In this case, officials at the penal institution initiate com-

---

1. PA. STAT. ANN. tit. 50, § 7407.
2. PA. STAT. ANN. tit. 50, § 7401.
3. PA. STAT. ANN. tit. 50, § 7407(a).
4. *Id.*
5. *Id.*

mitment proceedings similar to civil commitment hearings (see chapter 8.4).[6] If the hearing officer determines that the person is severely mentally ill and in need of treatment, a transfer to an appropriate mental health facility is ordered.[7]

When the person no longer needs the additional mental health treatment, he or she is returned to the sending penal institution. If the person's sentence has expired during the treatment period, however, or the person has secured release from custody through bail or other measures during this period, the person must be released.[8] As with voluntary treatment, the duration of time in involuntary treatment at a mental health facility is credited as time served toward completion of the person's criminal sentence.[9]

(B) Mentally Retarded Inmates

When a person who is serving a sentence in a penal institution suffers from mental retardation, the Mental Health and Retardation Act of 1966 allows for a transfer to a mental health facility after commitment proceedings, which may follow any of the procedures described in chapter 8.7.[10] If the court is satisfied that the person is mentally retarded and a commitment to a mental health facility is necessary, the court will order the transfer.[11]

---

6. PA. STAT. ANN. tit. 50, § 7401(a).
7. PA. STAT. ANN. tit. 50, § 7401(b). If the receiving facility is required to maintain custody and control of the transferred person, then the person cannot be sent to a Veteran's Administration Hospital. If no custody or control over the person is required, however, the person can be transferred to a Veteran's Administration Hospital.
8. Id.
9. Id.
10. PA. STAT. ANN. tit. 50, § 4411(b).
11. PA. STAT. ANN. tit. 50, § 4411(c).

7.18

Parole Determinations

Parole is a conditional release from confinement in a penal institution. It allows the convicted individual to serve the remainder of a criminal sentence outside of the penal institution, as long as the person adheres to certain parole conditions established by the parole board. The public policy behind the parole system is to provide a supervised structure for incarcerated individuals to rehabilitate, adjust, and restore themselves to the social and economic life and activities outside of the penal institution.[1]

Parole differs from probation in two respects. First, a person released on parole has received a criminal sentence and has served time inside a penal institution, whereas a person on probation has not been incarcerated. Second, a person who violates a condition of parole will be returned to prison to finish the remainder of the criminal sentence; a person on probation may receive a new sentence or another probationary term after a violation of probation. MHPs may evaluate individuals petitioning for release on parole or may encounter parolees who must seek treatment as a condition of the parole.

(A) Board of Parole

The Board of Probation and Parole is composed of five members appointed by the governor to serve 6-year terms. Each individual appointed to the Board must have at least 6 years of professional experience either in probation, parole, social work, or another related area, must have served 1 year in an administrative or

---

1. PA. STAT. ANN. tit. 61, § 331.1.

supervisory role, and must possess a bachelor's degree[2] or better. The Board has the exclusive power to review applications and to grant parole to all individuals sentenced to a maximum period of confinement of more than 2 years.[3] The Board may not grant parole to individuals sentenced to death or to individuals serving a life sentence.[4]

(B) Eligibility for Parole

The Parole Board has the authority to grant parole either on its own motion or when an inmate petitions the Board for a parole review.[5] In all instances, an inmate is not eligible for parole until he or she has served the minimum sentence imposed by the sentencing authority.[6] The Board may grant parole on its own motion if it believes the interests of justice require the inmate's release.[7] In making these determinations, the Board should consider the circumstances surrounding the crime committed by the individual, the person's character, mental characteristics and habits prior to the criminal offense, the conduct of the person while incarcerated, the person's physical and mental history during the confinement, the person's history of family violence, and the person's entire criminal record.[8] The Board should also consider any recommendations made by the trial judge and any statements made by the victim or by the victim's family.[9] Any victim or a member of the victim's immediate family must be notified of the inmate's parole hearing and given 30 days to inform the Board of an intent to provide a written statement about the parole considerations or to present testimony at the parole hearing.[10] The victim's report can include a statement addressing the victim's or the families' physical harm, psychological harm, emotional harm, or trauma experienced as a result of the crime.[11]

When an incarcerated person petitions the Parole Board for a parole hearing, the Board will establish reasonable rules for the prisoner, his or her attorney, family members, victims, and vic-

---

2. PA. STAT. ANN. tit. 61, § 331.2.
3. PA. STAT. ANN. tit. 61, § 331.17. In cases in which the person is sentenced to a maximum confinement of 2 years or less, the sentencing judge retains the authority to grant parole.
4. PA. STAT. ANN. tit. 61, § 331.21.
5. 63 PA. CODE § 63.1.
6. PA. STAT. ANN. tit. 61, § 331.21.
7. PA. STAT. ANN. tit. 61, § 331.22.
8. PA. STAT. ANN. tit. 61, § 331.19.
9. *Id.*
10. PA. STAT. ANN. tit. 61, § 331.22a.
11. *Id.*

tim's family members to present evidence at the hearing.[12] In reaching a parole decision, the Board should consider the same factors as when it reviews a parole decision based on its own motion.[13]

If the Board grants parole to the person, it has the power to establish general rules of conduct and specific conditions that the person must follow.[14] The general conditions of parole require that the person maintain regular contact with a parole officer, remain at the same residence and within an established region close to his or her residence, receive permission from the parole officer to move his or her residence or to leave the designated area, comply with all federal, state, and local laws, abstain from possessing or using narcotics and dangerous drugs, refrain from owning or possessing a firearm, refrain from assaultive behavior, and pay any fines or costs imposed by the court.[15] In addition to these general conditions, the Board may impose any specific condition it deems necessary, including mental health, drug, or alcohol treatment.

---

12. Pa. Stat. Ann. tit. 61, § 331.22.
13. Pa. Stat. Ann. tit. 61, § 331.19.
14. Pa. Stat. Ann. tit. 61, § 331.23.
15. 37 Pa. Code § 63.4.

7.19

Competency to Be Executed

There is no explicit statutory provision prohibiting the execution of a mentally ill or a mentally retarded person. In any event, the U.S. Supreme Court has decided that the federal constitution's prohibition against cruel and unusual punishment found in the Eighth Amendment bars a state from executing an 'insane" prisoner when mental illness prevents the prisoner from comprehending the implications of a death sentence or the reasons for imposing the death sentence.[1] In a separate case, the Court determined that the Eighth Amendment's ban on cruel and unusual punishment does not extend a total prohibition against executing mentally retarded individuals.[2] In this second case, the Court stated that mental retardation is a factor to be considered at the sentencing phase, when the sentencing authority can use its discretion to decide whether to impose a death sentence (see chapter 7.11).[3]

The Supreme Court of Pennsylvania has recognized a common law prohibition on executing "insane" individuals, defining *insane individuals* as those who are not able to comprehend their position or not able to make a defense.[4] The court has reexamined this issue in two cases. In the first case, a mentally ill person was sentenced to death, even after the sentencing jury found his mental illness to be a mitigating factor.[5] After reviewing the death penalty statute (see chapter 7.11), and the common law bar on executing "insane" prisoners, the court concluded that the death

---

1. Ford v. Wainwright, 477 U.S. 399 (1986).
2. Penry v. Lynaugh, 492 U.S. 302 (1989).
3. *Id.*
4. *See generally,* Commonwealth v. Moon, 117 A.2d 96 (Pa. 1955).
5. Commonwealth v. Fahy, 516 A.2d 689 (Pa. 1986).

penalty statute described a mental impairment as a mitigating circumstance but did not prohibit the jury from imposing a death sentence on a mentally ill person.[6] Further, the court stated that the common law bar against execution did not apply in the case, because the person was found competent to stand trial and to be sentenced.[7]

The ruling in the second case followed the previous case. Nevertheless, the court expressly allowed MHPs to testify about the person's mental condition at the sentencing phase.[8] Neither case addressed the issue of whether a person sentenced to death but who subsequently becomes severely impaired by a mental illness and does not understand the nature or implications of a death sentence at the time of the scheduled execution can be executed. In any event, Pennsylvania is compelled to follow the dictates of the Eighth Amendment, including the substantive and procedural rights granted in *Ford*.[9] Such rights allow a person on death row to obtain an appropriate evaluation by an MHP.

---

6. *Id.*
7. *Id.* The court's reasoning is faulty. The central issue concerning competency to be executed is whether the condemned person is competent at the time of the scheduled execution, not at the time of trial or sentencing.
8. Commonwealth v. Faulkner, 595 A.2d 28 (Pa. 1991), cert. denied, 503 U.S. 989 (1992).
9. 477 U.S. 399 (1986).

7.20

Pornography

It is unlawful to display any explicit sexual materials in or on a window, showcase, newsstand, display rack, billboard, display board, viewing screen, motion picture screen, marquee, or any other similar area displayed to the public.[1] In addition, it is unlawful to sell, lend, distribute, exhibit, give away, or show any obscene materials to any other person or to possess obscene materials for the purpose of providing them to another person.[2] It is also unlawful to manufacture or to prepare any obscene materials.[3] Advertising the availability and location of areas to purchase or receive obscene materials is also unlawful.[4] Producing, presenting, or directing an obscene performance is prohibited,[5] as is using a minor child to assist in any of the above unlawful actions.[6] MHPs knowledgeable about these issues may be asked to testify about whether challenged material meets the definition of obscenity or what the effects of sexually oriented material may be on minors.

Determining whether materials or performances are obscene, or explicitly sexual, depends on the definitions provided by the statute. In the statute,[7] explicit sexual materials are obscene materials and, in addition include

1. any picture, photograph, drawing, sculpture, motion picture film, videotape, or similar visual representation or image of a

---

1. 18 Pa. Cons. Stat. Ann. § 5903(a)(1).
2. 18 Pa. Cons. Stat. Ann. § 5903(a)(2).
3. 18 Pa. Cons. Stat. Ann. § 5903(a)(3).
4. 18 Pa. Cons. Stat. Ann. § 5903(a)(4).
5. 18 Pa. Cons. Stat. Ann. § 5903(a)(5).
6. 18 Pa. Cons. Stat. Ann. § 5903(a)(6).
7. 18 Pa. Cons. Stat. Ann. § 5903(c).

person or portion of the human body that depicts nudity, sexual conduct, or sadomasochistic abuse and that is harmful to minors; or

2. any book, pamphlet, magazine, printed matter however reproduced, or sound recording that contains any matter enumerated in paragraph 1, or explicit and detailed verbal descriptions or narrative accounts of sexual excitement, sexual conduct, or sadomasochistic abuse and that taken as a whole, is harmful to minors.

7.21

Services for Sex Offenders

Some states require all individuals convicted of sex-related crimes to serve part of their criminal sentence in a treatment center specially designed to evaluate and to treat habitual sex offenders.[1] Pennsylvania had such an act, known as the Barr-Walker Act. The Act, however, was ruled unconstitutional by the Supreme Court of Pennsylvania for failing to provide the necessary procedural safeguards for the convicted person.[2] Currently, there is no statute that requires individuals convicted of sex-related crimes to receive treatment.

Other areas of the criminal law have specific provisions for individuals convicted of sex-related crimes. For instance, any person taken into custody and charged with lewd conduct or a sex offense can be examined for a venereal disease by an appointed physician.[3] If the examination indicates the presence of a venereal disease, then the person shall be treated.[4]

In the criminal sentencing statutes, sex-related crimes such as rape and involuntary deviate sexual intercourse receive very high-offense gravity scores used in computing the recommended sentencing range (see chapter 7.11).[5] Further, convictions for rape or involuntary deviate sexual intercourse where the victim is either a minor under 16 years of age,[6] or an elderly person over 60

---

1. *See, e.g.,* N.J. STAT. ANN. § 2C:47-1 (requiring all persons convicted of aggravated assault, sexual assault, aggravated criminal sexual contact, or attempting any of these offenses to sentence of minimum of 10 days at Adult Diagnostic and Treatment Center).
2. Commonwealth v. Dooley, 232 A.2d 45 (Pa. 1967).
3. PA. STAT. ANN. tit 35, § 521.8(a).
4. PA. STAT. ANN. tit. 35, § 521.8(c).
5. 204 PA. CODE § 303.8(d).
6. 42 PA. CONS. STAT. ANN. § 9718(a).

years of age,[7] carry mandatory criminal sentences of at least 5 years.

Judges can order mental health treatment as a condition of probation (see chapter 7.12).[8] In cases involving sex crimes, the court may order treatment specially designed for sex offenders.

(A) Registration of Sex Offenders

After being released from prison or on commencement of an intermediate punishment or probation, all convicted sex offenders[9] must register a current address with the state police.[10] Registered offenders must notify the state police within 10 days of any change of residence, and the period of required registration is 10 years.[11] Failure to comply with the registration requirement is a felony in the third degree.[12]

(B) Sexually Violent Predators

If an offender will be subject to the registration law, the State Board to Assess Sexually Violent Predators and the trial court will presume that the offender is a "sexually violent predator." The law defines *sexually violent predator* as a person who has been convicted of a sexually violent offense (those that subject the offender to the registration requirement) as a result of a mental abnormality or personality disorder that makes the person likely to engage in predatory sexually violent offenses.[13] The court will order an assessment to be completed after conviction, but prior to original sentencing, to determine whether the offender is a sexually violent predator.[14] The assessment will be conducted by two members of the Board and will include consideration of such factors as

1. age of the offender;

---

7. 42 Pa. Cons. Stat. Ann. § 9717(a).
8. 42 Pa. Cons. Stat. Ann. § 9754(c)(3).
9. For purposes of this section of the law, a *sex offender* is a person who has been convicted of kidnapping a minor (except for kidnapping by a parent), rape, involuntary deviate sexual intercourse, aggravated indecent assault, prostitution and related offenses, spousal sexual assault, or indecent assault when the offense is a misdemeanor in the first degree). 42 Pa. Cons. Stat. § 97793(b).
10. 42 Pa. Cons. Stat. § 9793(a).
11. *Id.*
12. 42 Pa. Cons. Stat. § 9793(e).
13. 42 Pa. Cons. Stat. § 9792.
14. 42 Pa. Cons. Stat. § 9794(a).

2. offender's prior criminal record, sexual offenses, as well as other offenses;

3. age of the victim;

4. whether the offense involved multiple victims;

5. use of illegal drugs by the offender;

6. whether the offender completed any prior sentence and whether the offender participated in available programs for sexual offenders;

7. any mental illness or mental disability of the offender;

8. the nature of the sexual contact with the victim and whether the sexual contact was part of a demonstrated pattern of abuse;

9. whether the offense included a display of unusual cruelty by the offender during the commission of the crime; and

10. any behavioral characteristics that contribute to the offender's conduct.[15]

The court will conduct a hearing[16] on the issue and if it determines that the offender is a sexually violent predator, the offender's sentence is automatically increased to a life sentence;[17] if the offender is released on parole, the offender must comply with the registration requirements indefinitely.[18] In addition, any offender who is found to be a sexually violent predator is required to attend at least monthly counseling sessions in a program approved by the Board.[19] The offender is responsible for the costs of counseling unless the offender convinces the court that he or she is indigent.[20] One year after release from prison and in 5-year intervals thereafter, offenders who have been designated sexually violent predators may petition the original trial court for a reconsideration of the designation.[21] The court may request a new report from the Board and the court may terminate the offender's designation as a "sexually violent predator."[22]

Victim and Community Notification
When an offender has been designated a sexually violent predator, the local police will give written notice of the offender's name,

---

15. 42 Pa. Cons. Stat. § 9794(c).
16. 42 Pa. Cons. Stat. § 9794(e).
17. 42 Pa. Cons. Stat. § 9799.4(a).
18. 42 Pa. Cons. Stat. § 9795(a).
19. 42 Pa. Cons. Stat. § 9799.4(b).
20. *Id.*
21. 42 Pa. Cons. Stat. § 9794(f).
22. *Id.* The statute does not indicate what standards the court will follow in making these decisions.

address, offense, designation as a sexually violent predator, and a photograph (if available) to the victim within 72 hours of the original registration or any change of residence.[23] If the victim wishes to avoid notification, he or she can submit a written request to the local or state police.[24] In addition to victim notification, the police will also notify

1. neighbors of the offender;
2. the director of the county children and youth service agency of the county in which the offender resides;
3. the superintendent of each school district and the equivalent official for private and parochial schools enrolling students up through Grade 12 in the municipality;
4. the director of each licensed day care center and licensed preschool program in the municipality; and
5. the president of each college, university, and community college located within 1000 feet of the offender's address.[25]

Neighbors will be notified within 72 hours of registration or change of address. Others who are entitled to notification will be notified within 7 days of registration or a change of residence.[26] Members of the general public may obtain this information on request.[27]

---

23. 42 PA. CONS. STAT. § 9797(a).
24. Id.
25. 42 PA. CONS. STAT. § 9798(b).
26. 42 PA. CONS. STAT. § 9798(c).
27. 42 PA. CONS. STAT. § 9798(d).

7.22

Services for Victims of Crimes

The two principal areas dedicated to protecting and servicing victims of crime are found in the Basic Bill of Rights for Victims and the Crime Victim's Compensation Board, and these include provisions of mental health services to victims of crime, such as counseling to deal with the trauma of being a crime victim.

(A) Basic Bill of Rights for Victims

The commonwealth enacted the basic Bill of Rights "to ensure that all victims of crime are treated with dignity, respect, courtesy and sensitivity; and that the rights extended . . . to victims of crime are honored and protected."[1] The Bill of Rights covers all persons who are victims of crimes and who have reported the crime to law enforcement authorities within a reasonable period of time after the crime occurred or was discovered.[2] The reporting requirement is included to encourage crime victims to cooperate in the prosecution of crimes.[3] The Victim's Bill of Rights guarantees that crime victims will be given information about victim services, will be notified of significant actions and proceedings pertaining to their cases, will be allowed to be accompanied by family members during criminal proceedings, may submit comments to the prosecutor before any charges are dropped or reduced, may submit comments to the court before the defendant is sentenced, may receive restitution for their losses, may have their

---

1. PA. STAT. ANN. tit. 71, § 180-9.
2. PA. STAT. ANN. tit. 71, § 180-9.2.
3. PA. STAT. ANN. tit. 71, § 180-9.

property that was used as evidence returned to them, may submit a comment before the defendant is released from prison on parole or furlough or transferred to a mental health treatment facility, and may have assistance with the preparation of the required claim forms.[4]

(B) Crime Victim's Compensation Board

The Crime Victim's Compensation Board is composed of three full-time members appointed by the governor to serve 6-year terms.[5] This Board has the authority, among other powers, to hear and determine the legitimacy of all claims filed by crime victims and to order crime victims to undergo medical testing.[6]

To receive a claim from the Board, an eligible person must submit a written request within 1 year of commission of the crime, unless the Board specifically extends this time deadline.[7] If the Board approves the claim, then the eligible person can be reimbursed for out-of-pocket expenses incurred as a result of the crime.[8] *Out-of-pocket expenses* include the costs of medical care, psychological counseling, prosthetic devices, eyeglasses, corrective lenses, or dental devices that the victim required as a result of the crime.[9] The victim is not be reimbursed for any property damage or pain and suffering.[10]

The eligible person also can receive reimbursement for loss of earnings,[11] which includes the cash equivalent of 1 month's Social Security, railroad retirement, pension plan, retirement plan, disability, child support, or spousal support.[12] In all cases, the maximum award granted by the Board will not be more than $35,000,[13] nor will the Board award a claim if the total loss is less than $100.[14]

All service providers, including MHPs, who treat persons eligible for compensation from the Board must respond in writing and within 30 days after receiving a request for information from

---

4. Pa. Stat. Ann. tit. 71, § 180-9.3.
5. Pa. Stat. Ann. tit. 71, § 180-7.1.
6. Pa. Stat. Ann. tit. 71, § 180-7.2.
7. Pa. Stat. Ann. tit. 71, § 180-7.4(b).
8. Pa. Stat. Ann. tit. 71, § 180-7.9(b).
9. Pa. Stat. Ann. tit. 71, § 180-7.
10. *Id.*
11. Pa. Stat. Ann. tit. 71, § 180-7.9(c).
12. Pa. Stat. Ann. tit. 71, § 180-7.
13. Pa. Stat. Ann. tit. 71, § 180-7.9(b).
14. Pa. Stat. Ann. tit. 71, § 180-7.5(a).

the Board.[15] Any provider who fails to respond within 30 days may receive a civil penalty of $10 for each day the report is not submitted after the 30-day deadline.[16]

---

15. PA. STAT. ANN. tit. 71, § 180-7.19(a).
16. PA. STAT. ANN. tit. 71, § 180-7.19(b).

Voluntary or Involuntary Receipt of State Services

8.1

Medicaid

Medicaid[1] is a federally supported program under which each state provides direct payments to suppliers of medical care and services for eligible individuals. Eligible individuals include those receiving cash payments under the old-age assistance, aid to families with dependent children (AFDC), aid to the blind, and aid to the disabled programs. Thus, the benefits primarily go to elderly adults and children whose parents receive welfare. Others might also be eligible for medical assistance benefits. The Department of Public Welfare administers this program (see chapter 8.2).

---

1. 42 U.S.C. § 1396.

8.2

Medical Care Cost Containment

Medicaid benefits are provided to indigent people through the Medical Assistance Program, administered by the Department of Public Welfare.[1] This program covers both inpatient and outpatient mental health services.[2] Providers must be enrolled in the program to render services and must comply with applicable regulations.[3] Beneficiaries may receive laboratory and radiology tests, nursing services, physician services, social services, family planning services, prescription drugs, and inpatient and outpatient care.[4]

(A) Outpatient Psychiatric Treatment

The Medical Assistance Program covers medical and psychiatric services for the diagnosis and treatment of mental disorders provided at approved outpatient psychiatric clinics and partial hospitalization facilities.[5] To be eligible for payment, services at psychiatric clinics and partial hospitalization facilities must meet the following conditions:

1. a psychiatrist must be present to perform or to supervise the performance of all covered services;

2. psychiatric evaluations must be performed by a psychiatrist in a face-to-face interview;

---

1. PA. STAT. ANN. tit. 62, § 441.1.
2. 55 PA. CODE §§ 1151, 1153.
3. *Id.*
4. 55 PA. CODE § 1150.
5. 55 PA. CODE § 1153.12.

3. psychotherapy may be provided only by a member of the clinical staff;

4. psychiatric partial hospitalization services may be provided only by a clinical staff person;

5. diagnostic psychological and intellectual evaluations may be administered and interpreted only by a licensed psychologist or by a psychologist in preparation for licensure under the direct supervision of a licensed psychologist;

6. a psychiatric clinic medication visit may be provided only by a psychiatrist, physician, registered nurse, or licensed practical nurse;

7. within 15 days following intake, each patient in a clinic must be examined and initially assessed; and

8. a clozapine monitoring and evaluation visit may only be used for a person receiving clozapine therapy.[6]

(B) Inpatient Psychiatric Treatment

Recipients 21 years of age and younger and 65 years of age and older are eligible for medically necessary inpatient services provided by a participating inpatient psychiatric facility.[7] Recipients between the ages of 21 and 65 are eligible for up to 60 days of medically necessary inpatient services provided by a participating private psychiatric hospital within a benefit period.[8] A recipient's benefit period begins to run when the recipient has not received inpatient psychiatric services from an inpatient psychiatric facility or a public psychiatric hospital for at least 60 consecutive days.[9] Recipients of any age who are receiving psychiatric services in distinct psychiatric units of general hospitals are eligible for coverage of medically needy inpatient psychiatric services without regard to the benefit-period limitations.[10]

---

6. 55 Pa. Code § 1153.52(a).
7. 55 Pa. Code §§ 1151.21 and 1151.22.
8. *Id.*
9. *Id.*
10. *Id.*

8.3

Voluntary Admission of Mentally Ill Adults

The Mental Health Procedures Act[1] provides for the voluntary admission of mentally ill persons to facilities. MHPs are involved in this process both by evaluating the person for admission and by providing services within the facility.

(A) Admission

Voluntary admission may be requested by anyone who is 14 years of age or older, by the parents of someone under age 18, or by a guardian who has legal authority to seek admission.[2] When a hospital accepts a person between the ages of 14 and 18 for treatment, it must notify the parents or guardian who have the right to challenge the admission before a judge or mental health review officer within 72 hours of the admission.[3]

(B) Discharge

A person in voluntary treatment may withdraw at any time by giving written notice, unless he or she has agreed in writing at the time of his or her admission that release can be delayed following such notice for a period specified in the agreement, usually 72 hours.[4] The facility may file a petition for involuntary commit-

---

1. PA. STAT. ANN. tit. 50, §§ 7101–7503.
2. PA. STAT. ANN. tit. 50, § 7201.
3. PA. STAT. ANN. tit. 50, § 7204.
4. PA. STAT. ANN. tit. 50, §§ 7203, 7206.

ment during that 72-hour time period to have the person retained (see chapter 8.4).[5] When the 72-hour notice period applies, then, a voluntary admission is conditional on a commitment petition not being filed (see chapter 8.4).

---

5. PA. STAT. ANN. tit. 50, §§ 7301, 7302.

8.4

Involuntary Commitment of Mentally Ill Adults

The law pertaining to involuntary civil commitment concerns mentally ill adults as well as minors (see chapter 4.19). MHPs evaluate adults for commitment, testify in court about their findings, and provide services within facilities in which patients are committed. Physicians must be involved in the evaluation process, although other MHPs may assist.

(A) Emergency Commitments

The law provides an emergency procedure for involuntary hospitalization for a person who is severely mentally disabled and in need of immediate treatment. People are defined as *severely mentally disabled* when, as a result of mental illness, their capacity to exercise self-control, judgment, and discretion in the conduct of their affairs and social relations or to care for their personal needs is so lessened that they pose a clear and present danger of harm to others or to themselves.[1]

A clear and present danger of harm to others is shown by establishing that the person has within the past 30 days inflicted or attempted to inflict serious bodily harm on another and that there is a reasonable probability that this conduct will be repeated, unless the person was found incompetent to be tried or was acquitted by reason of lack of criminal responsibility on charges stemming from such conduct, in which case the determination or verdict must have occurred within the past 30 days.[2] A

---

1. Pa. Stat. Ann. tit. 50, § 7301.
2. Pa. Stat. Ann. tit. 50, § 7301(b)(1).

clear and present danger to self is shown by establishing that

1. within the past 30 days the person has acted in such manner as to evidence that he would be unable without care to satisfy his need for nourishment, personal or medical care, shelter or self-protection, and safety and that there is reasonable probability that death, serious bodily injury, or serious physical debilitation would ensue within 30 days without adequate treatment;
2. within the past 30 days the person has attempted suicide and there is a reasonable probability of suicide without adequate treatment; or
3. the person has substantially mutilated or attempted to mutilate himself or herself and there is a reasonable probability of mutilation without adequate treatment.[3]

Procedures
A physician or other responsible party may file a written application with the county administrator setting forth facts constituting reasonable grounds to believe a person is severely mentally disabled and in need of immediate treatment. In response, the county administrator may issue a warrant requiring an authorized person or any peace officer to take the person to the facility specified in the warrant for an emergency examination.[4] In addition, on personal observation of a severely mentally disabled person, a physician, peace officer, or other authorized person may take such person to an approved facility for emergency examination. The observer, from the time of arrival, must make a written statement setting forth the grounds for believing that the person needs to be examined. In either case, the receiving facility will examine the individual and determine whether or not to admit him or her for a treatment period not to exceed 120 hours.[5]

(B) Procedures for Extended Involuntary Emergency Treatment (Not to Exceed 20 Days)

Application for Extended Treatment
An authorized person from a mental health treatment facility may file an application for extended involuntary emergency treatment (not to exceed 20 days) for any person being treated pursuant to

---

3. PA. STAT. ANN. tit. 50, § 7301(b)(2).
4. PA. STAT. ANN. tit. 50, § 7302(a)(1).
5. PA. STAT. ANN. tit. 50, § 7302(a)(2).

the involuntary civil commitment procedures whenever the facility determines that the need for treatment is likely to extend beyond 120 hours. The application is filed in the Court of Common Pleas and must state the name of any examining physician, his or her opinion of the person's mental condition, and the grounds on which the treatment is believed to be necessary.[6] The petition must be filed in the Court of Common Pleas before the 120 hours allowed for an emergency commitment have elapsed.

Time Requirements for Hearings
The law requires that an informal hearing on an extended involuntary treatment application be conducted by a judge or mental health review officer within 24 hours after the filing of the application.[7] A mental health review officer is a member of the bar of the Supreme Court of Pennsylvania, and whenever possible should be familiar with the field of mental health.[8] When a hearing is conducted by a mental health review officer, the person who is subject to treatment shall have the right to petition the Court of Common Pleas for review of the certification.[9]

Informal Hearing on Extended Emergency Treatment Applications
At the commencement of the informal hearing, the judge or mental health review officer must inform the person of the nature of the proceedings. Information relevant to a finding of severe mental disability and the need for continued treatment must be reviewed. The person or his appointed counsel or representative may ask questions of the examining physician(s) and of any other witnesses and may present any relevant information. At the conclusion of the review, if the judge or the review officer finds that the person is severely mentally ill and in need of continued involuntary treatment, the person will be certified for further commitment. Otherwise, the judge will direct that the person be released from the mental health facility.[10]

Right of Petition for Review of the Certification
Where the certification hearing was conducted by a mental health review officer, the person committed for involuntary treatment may petition the court of common pleas for review of the certification. Unless a continuance is requested by the person's counsel, a hearing will be held within 72 hours. If the court determines that further involuntary treatment is necessary and required proce-

---

6. PA. STAT. ANN. tit. 50, § 7303(a).
7. PA. STAT. ANN. tit. 50, § 7303(b).
8. PA. STAT. ANN. tit. 50, § 7109(a).
9. PA. STAT. ANN. tit. 50, § 7109(b).
10. PA. STAT. ANN. tit. 50, § 7303(c).

dures were followed, it will deny the petition. Otherwise, the person will be released.[11]

Duration of Extended Involuntary Emergency Treatment
Whenever a person is no longer severely mentally disabled or no longer needs immediate treatment, or when 20 days have passed since the commitment, the person must be discharged from the mental health facility, unless within that 20-day period the person is admitted to voluntary treatment pursuant to Section 202 (see chapter 8.3) or the court orders involuntary treatment (see later in this chapter).

(C) Procedures for Court-Ordered Involuntary Treatment (Not to Exceed 90 Days)

A person who is severely mentally disabled and in need of treatment may be ordered by a court to undergo involuntary treatment on a determination of clear and present danger to self or others, as described under section (A), earlier in the chapter.[12]

Petition for Commitment
Where a petition is filed for a person already subject to involuntary treatment, the petitioner, at a court hearing, need only reestablish that the conduct giving rise to the initial commitment occurred and that the person committed still represents a clear and present danger to self or others. It is not necessary to show the reoccurrence of dangerous conduct, either harmful or debilitating, within the past 30 days.[13]

Filing Procedures
For those persons already subject to involuntary treatment, the county administrator or the director of the facility in which he or she is located must submit a form to the Court of Common Pleas setting forth the reasons that continued treatment is needed.[14] The form must include the name and opinion of the examining physician.[15]

---

11. PA. STAT. ANN. tit. 50, § 7303(g).
12. PA. STAT. ANN. tit. 50, § 7301.
13. PA. STAT. ANN. tit. 50, § 7304(a)(2).
14. PA. STAT. ANN. tit. 50, § 7304(b)(1)(2).
15. PA. STAT. ANN. tit. 50, § 7304(b)(2).

The procedures for initiating court-ordered involuntary treatment not to exceed 90 days for persons not already in involuntary treatment are somewhat more complex.[16] The county administrator must inform the person committed, his or her attorney, and all other interested persons of the filed petition along with an explanation of the proceedings.[17] The person committed is entitled to employ a physician, clinical psychologist, or other mental health expert to assist him or her in connection with the hearing. If the person committed cannot afford to hire one, he or she may apply to the court for financial assistance.[18] A hearing must be held not more than 5 days after the petition is filed.[19]

Requirements for the Hearing
The person being committed has the following rights with regard to his or her hearing:

1. the right to counsel and to the assistance of a mental health expert;
2. the right not to be called as a witness without his or her consent;
3. the right to confront and to cross-examine all witnesses and to present evidence in his or her own behalf; and
4. the right to request that the hearing be private.[20]

The hearing is conducted by a judge or mental health review officer and may be held at a location other than a courthouse when this appears to be in the best interest of the person being committed.[21] An official record of the hearing is made.[22] A decision must be rendered within 48 hours after the close of presentation of evidence.[23] The petitioner must prove by clear and convincing evidence that the person to be committed is severely mentally ill and in need of treatment.[24]

Decision of the Judge or the Mental Health Review Officer
The court may order the person being committed to receive inpatient treatment only if it is the least restrictive available alternative. Investigation of treatment alternatives must include consideration of the person's relationship to his or her community

---

16. PA. STAT. ANN. tit. 50, § 7304(c).
17. PA. STAT. ANN. tit. 50, § 7304(b)(3).
18. PA. STAT. ANN. tit. 50, § 7304(d).
19. PA. STAT. ANN. tit. 50, § 7304(b)(4).
20. PA. STAT. ANN. tit. 50, §§ 7304(e)(1)–(4).
21. PA. STAT. ANN. tit. 50, § 7304(e)(6).
22. PA. STAT. ANN. tit. 50, § 7304(e)(5).
23. PA. STAT. ANN. tit. 50, § 7304(e)(7).
24. PA. STAT. ANN. tit. 50, § 7304(f).

and family, the person's employment possibilities, all available community resources, and guardianship services.[25] A person may be ordered by a court to involuntary treatment for a period of 90 days. Persons may be subject to a treatment period of up to 1 year if they have been charged with specific crimes and are found to be either incompetent to stand trial (see chapter 7.5) or were acquitted because of lack of criminal responsibility (see chapter 7.9).[26]

(D) Medication Order

A petitioner for civil commitment may request the administration of medication if the person being committed is refusing psychotropic medication. If the judge first determines that the person meets the standard for commitment, the petitioner may then ask for a determination of incompetency and a substituted judgment order for medication (see chapter 3.7).

In an emergency situation, patients who have been committed involuntarily may be given psychotropic medication over their objection if necessary to protect the health and safety of the patient or others, but in other situations, various procedures must first be followed.[27] Patients who have been voluntarily committed may refuse psychotropic medications unless they pose an imminent threat of danger to themselves or others.[28] Electroconvulsive therapy, any experimental treatment involving risk to the patient, and aversive treatments may not be administered without informed consent.[29]

(E) Appeals

The law does not provide for an appeals process for persons involuntarily committed for fewer than 120 hours. A person who was originally involuntarily committed for fewer than 120 hours by a mental health officer, however, may petition the Common Pleas Court for a review of any decision to extend the involuntary commitment.[30]

---

25. *Id.*
26. PA. STAT. ANN. tit. 50, § 7304(g)(2).
27. Pennsylvania Department of Public Welfare. (1985, April 11). *Mental health bulletin.*
28. *Id.*
29. 55 PA. CODE § 5100.54 art. VI § 2.
30. PA. STAT. ANN. tit. 50, § 7303(g).

8.5

Voluntary Admission and Involuntary Commitment of Alcoholics

The law provides for both voluntary treatment and involuntary commitment of individuals who are disabled by alcoholism. Admissions and commitments to treatment facilities for chemical dependency are governed by the procedural provisions of the Mental Health and Mental Retardation Act of 1966.[1] MHPs may be part of a multidisciplinary evaluation and treatment team.

(A) Voluntary Admission

Alcoholics may apply for evaluation and treatment directly at any treatment facility. If the alcoholics are minors, their parents or guardians may apply.[2] Adults voluntarily admitted for alcoholism treatment may withdraw at any time. In the cases of minors, their parent or guardian may withdraw them from treatment at any time.[3]

(B) Emergency Admission, Detention, or Commitment

Alcoholics, who by reason of their acts or threatened acts, appear to be so mentally disabled as to be dangerous to themselves or

---

1. PA. STAT. ANN. tit. 71, § 1690.105; PA. STAT. ANN. tit. 50, §§ 4101–4426; PA. STAT. ANN. tit. 50, § 7102.
2. PA. STAT. ANN. tit. 50, § 4402(a).
3. PA. STAT. ANN. tit. 50, § 4402(c).

others and are in need of immediate care may be taken into custody for the purpose of examination.[4] On written application, a relative, guardian, friend, or other individual standing *in loco parentis* to the person believed to be mentally disabled, an executive officer, or authorized agent of a governmental or recognized nonprofit agency providing health or welfare services, or a police officer may take such person into custody.[5] The written application for admission must set forth the acts or threats that give cause to believe the person is mentally disabled and in need of immediate care. These acts or threats must be overt and must demonstrate a clear and present danger to self or others.[6] Any person so committed may be detained for a period not more than 10 days.[7]

(C) Involuntary Commitment

Any "responsible person" may petition the Court of Common Pleas to have an alcoholic involuntarily committed.[8] The petition must set forth the facts on which the petitioner bases his or her belief of mental disability (alcoholism) and the efforts made to secure examination of the person by a physician.[9] The court may then issue a warrant requiring the individual's presence at a hearing (to be held as soon as the warrant is executed).[10] After the hearing, the court may either order an immediate examination by two court-appointed physicians or order the commitment of the individual to a facility for a period not to exceed 10 days for the purpose of examination. Under appropriate circumstances, the court may order that the examination be accomplished by partial hospitalization.[11] Once the examination is complete and if it is determined that the individual is in need of care at a facility, the examining physicians or the director of the facility may notify the court of this finding.[12] The court may then order the individual to inpatient or outpatient care or partial hospitalization.[13]

---

4. Pa. Stat. Ann. tit. 50, § 4405(a).
5. Pa. Stat. Ann. tit. 50, § 4405(a)(1).
6. Pa. Stat. Ann. tit. 50, § 4405(a)(2).
7. Pa. Stat. Ann. tit. 50, § 4405(f).
8. Pa. Stat. Ann. tit. 50, § 4406(a)(1).
9. Pa. Stat. Ann. tit. 50, § 4406(a)(2).
10. Pa. Stat. Ann. tit. 50, § 4406(a)(3).
11. Pa. Stat. Ann. tit. 50, § 4406(a)(4).
12. Pa. Stat. Ann. tit. 50, § 4406(b).
13. Commitment of alcoholics charged with crimes is covered under Pa. Stat. Ann. tit. 50, §§ 4407 and 4408.

8.6

Voluntary Admission and Involuntary Commitment of Drug Addicts

The law permits both voluntary and involuntary admission of drug-dependent persons to facilities for treatment.[1] The procedure is the same as that described for alcoholics (see chapter 8.5).[2]

---

1. PA. STAT. ANN. tit. 71, § 1690.101; PA. STAT. ANN. tit. 50, §§ 4401–4426.
2. PA. STAT. ANN. tit. 50, §§ 4401–4426.

8.7

Services for People With Developmental Disabilities

The law provides various inpatient and outpatient services to persons with mental retardation through the Department of Public Welfare.[1] MHPs assist in providing evaluation and treatment services. As with mentally ill persons, services can be provided on a voluntary basis or through involuntary commitment. The Mental Health Procedures Act does not apply, however, to persons with mental retardation (see chapters 8.3 and 8.4). For these people, the applicable law is the Mental Health and Mental Retardation Act of 1966 (1966 Act).[2]

(A) Definitions

Mental retardation is defined as "subaverage general intellectual functioning which originates during the developmental period and is associated with impairment of one or more of the following: (a) maturation, (b) learning, and (c) social adjustment."[3] Under the 1966 Act, any person over 18 years of age may apply for voluntary admission or commitment to a facility for examination and treatment.[4]

---

1. PA. STAT. ANN. tit. 50, § 4101.
2. PA. STAT. ANN. tit. 50, §§ 4201–4426.
3. PA. STAT. ANN. tit. 50, § 4102.
4. PA. STAT. ANN. tit. 50, §§ 4402 & 4403.

(B) Voluntary and Involuntary Admission to Services

If the person to be admitted or committed is 18 years of age or younger, a parent, guardian, or individual standing *in loco parentis* to that person may apply for admission or commitment to a facility for examination and treatment.[5] Such a person also may be committed "involuntarily" over the objection of a parent, guardian, or person standing *in loco parentis*.[6] The procedures used for involuntary commitment of adults with mental retardation must be followed.

(C) Community Homes for Individuals With Mental Retardation

Community homes for mentally retarded persons are regulated for the protection of the individuals receiving their services.[7] The policy of the commonwealth is that community homes should develop programs that facilitate "normalization" for mentally retarded individuals so that these individuals can "live a life which is as close as possible in all aspects to the life which any member of the community might choose."[8] The regulations establish safety and treatment standards and enumerate the rights that must be afforded to individuals residing in these facilities.

Rights of the Individual
The regulations for community homes require that each individual residing in a facility, or the individual's parent, guardian, or advocate, if appropriate, be informed of the individual's rights on admission and annually thereafter.[9] Moreover, the regulations require that an individual be "encouraged to exercise his rights,"[10] including the rights to

1. not be neglected, abused, mistreated, or subjected to corporal punishment;
2. not be required to participate in research projects;

---

5. *Id.*
6. PA. STAT. ANN. tit. 50, §§ 4404–4406.
7. 55 PA. CODE §§ 6400.1–6500.203.
8. 55 PA. CODE § 6400.1.
9. 55 PA. CODE § 6400.31(a).
10. 55 PA. CODE § 6400.31(c)

3. management of one's own personal financial affairs;

4. participate in program planning that affects the individual;

5. privacy in bedrooms, bathrooms, and during personal care;

6. receive, purchase, have, and use personal property;

7. receive scheduled and unscheduled visitors, communicate, associate, and meet privately with family and persons of the individual's own choice;

8. have reasonable access to a telephone and the opportunity to receive and make private calls, with assistance when necessary;

9. have unrestricted mailing privileges;

10. be informed of the right to vote if of voting age and to be assisted to register and to vote in elections;

11. practice the religion or faith of the individual's choice; and

12. not be required to work at the home, except for the upkeep of the individual's personal living areas and the upkeep of common living areas and grounds.[11]

The regulations also require community homes to respect the individual's civil rights, including freedom from discrimination based on race, color, religion, creed, disability, handicap, ancestry, national origin, age, or gender.[12] Individuals residing in these facilities must be provided with the opportunity to lodge such complaints and they must be informed of their right to register civil rights complaints.[13]

Aversive Conditioning
Aversive conditioning, meaning the application of startling, painful, or noxious stimuli in response to maladaptive behavior, is prohibited in community homes for mentally retarded persons.[14]

Seclusion
Community homes for mentally retarded persons may not place an individual in a locked room. This includes a room with any locking device, such as a key lock, spring lock, bolt lock, foot pressure lock, or physically holding a door shut.[15]

---

11. 55 Pa. Code § 6400.33.
12. 55 Pa. Code § 6400.34(a).
13. 55 Pa. Code §§ 6400.34(b)(3–4).
14. 55 Pa. Code § 6400.198.
15. 55 Pa. Code § 6400.197.

8.8

Hospice Care

Hospice care provides psychological and physical support offered for terminally ill persons in their homes and inpatient facilities. Hospices attempt to enhance the quality of life of the patient during the terminal phase of his or her illness by providing care for physical needs through continued medical treatment and control of pain and other symptoms to allow the person to concentrate on other aspects of life. A complete program may consist of three phases: (a) home care with nursing, emotional, and religious support; (b) inpatient care with overnight facilities for the family; and (c) bereavement services for the family. MHPs may be involved in all three phases as a member of the support team.

Pennsylvania has no statute relating to hospice care. Regulations in the *Medical Assistance Manual,* which is part of the Pennsylvania Code, however, describe eligibility requirements for reimbursement and available medical assistance benefits for services.[1]

---

1. 55 PA. CODE §§ 1101.11–1251.81.

Appendixes

Table of Cases

References are to page numbers in this book.

Table of Statutes

References are to page numbers in this book.

Table of Rules of Court

References are to page numbers in this book.

Table of Administrative Rules and Regulations

References are to page numbers in this book.

Table of References to Constitution

References are to page numbers in this book.

Table of Other Authorities

References are to page numbers in this book.

Index

E

EDUCATIONAL SYSTEM
Services for gifted and handicapped children, 4.20
EMOTIONAL DISTRESS
As personal injury, 5.4
EMPLOYMENT DISCRIMINATION
Generally, 5.12
EMPLOYMENT SCREENING
Police officers, 7.1
EXPERT WITNESSES
Court rules, 6.2
On eyewitness identification, 6.9
Provocation defense, 7.6
Workers' compensation hearing, 5.2(C)
EYEWITNESS IDENTIFICATION
Expert testimony on, 6.9

F

FAMILY COUNSELORS
Licensure and regulation, 1.9
FOSTER CARE
Generally, 4.13
FREEDOM OF INFORMATION
Generally, 3.6

G

GIFTED/HANDICAPPED CHILDREN
Education for, 4.20
GUARDIANSHIP
For adults, 4.2
For minors, 4.11
GUIDANCE COUNSELORS
Confidentiality issues, 3.3(C)

H

HABITUAL OFFENDERS
Generally, 7.14
HEALTH MAINTENANCE ORGANIZATIONS
Regulation, 2.4
HOSPICE CARE
Generally, 8.8
HOSPITALS
Peer review, 3.9(A)
Quality assurance, 3.9
Records maintenance, 3.2(C)
Staff privileges, 2.7

HYPNOTISTS/HYPNOTISM
Courtroom use, 6.8
Licensure and regulation, 1.11

I

INCARCERATED PERSONS
Competency to be executed, 7.19
Mental health services, 7.16
Parole determinations, 7.18
Transfer to mental health facility, 7.17
INDIVIDUAL PRACTICE ASSOCIATIONS
Regulation, 2.6
INFORMED CONSENT
Generally, 3.1
Services for minors, 4.21
INSANITY
Civil liability and, 5.5
Legal defense, 7.9
Liability insurance and, 5.5(B)
INSURANCE
Insanity defense and, 5.5(B)
Reimbursement for mental health services, 2.9
State plans, 2.10
Workers' compensation, 5.2
INTEGRATED DELIVERY SYSTEMS
Regulation, 2.12
INVASION OF PRIVACY
Professional liability, 3.11(A)(2)

J

JURY SELECTION
Generally, 6.1
Right to waive jury trial, 7.2(D)
JUVENILE JUSTICE
Competency to stand trial, 4.16
Delinquency, 4.15
Nonresponsibility defense, 4.17
Transfer to stand trial as adult, 4.18

L

LAW ENFORCEMENT
Employment screening, 7.1
Rights of detained individuals, 7.2
LIABILITY OF PROFESSIONALS
Civil, 3.11
Credentialing boards, 3.13
Criminal, 3.12
Immunity, 3.9(B)

N

NONRESPONSIBILITY DEFENSE
Generally, 4.17
NURSES
Mental status, 5.1(A)(3)

O

OPEN MEETING LAW
Generally, 1.15

P

PARENTAL RIGHTS
Consent for minor's abortion, 4.22
Education of gifted and
handicapped children, 4.20(D)
Guardianship for minors, 4.11
Noncustodial parents, 4.23
Services for minors, 4.21
Termination of, 4.10
PAROLE
Generally, 7.18
PARTNERSHIPS
Regulation, 2.3
PATIENT RIGHTS
Access to records, 3.2
Admission and commitment of
alcoholics, 8.5
Admission and commitment of drug
addicts, 8.6
Developmental disability, 8.7
Involuntary commitment of
mentally ill adults, 8.4
Refusal of treatment, 3.7
Voluntary admission of mentally ill
adults, 8.3
PEER REVIEW
Hospitals, 3.9(A)
PENAL SYSTEM
See INCARCERATED PERSONS
PHARMACISTS
Mental status, 5.1(A)(4)
PHYSICIANS/PHYSICIAN
ASSISTANTS
Mental status, 5.1(A)(5)
POINT OF SERVICE PLANS
Regulation, 2.4(B)
POLICE OFFICERS
Employment screening, 7.1
POLYGRAPH TESTING
As legal evidence, 6.3

Licensure and regulation of
examiners, 1.12
PORNOGRAPHY
Generally, 7.20
PREFERRED PROVIDER
ORGANIZATIONS
Regulation, 2.5
PRETRIAL EVALUATIONS
Generally, 7.3
PRIVILEGED COMMUNICATIONS
Generally, 3.4
Reporting of adult abuse, 4.7(C)
Reporting of child abuse, 4.7(E)
PROBATION
Generally, 7.12
PRODUCT LIABILITY
Generally, 5.10
PROFESSIONAL CORPORATIONS
Regulation, 2.2
PSYCHIATRIC NURSES
Licensure and regulation, 1.3
PSYCHIATRISTS
Confidentiality issues, 3.3(A)
Licensure and regulation, 1.2
Privileged communications, 3.4(A)
Records maintenance, 3.2(B)
PSYCHOLOGICAL AUTOPSY
Evidentiary rules, 6.5
PSYCHOLOGISTS
Confidentiality issues, 3.3(A)
Licensure and regulation, 1.4
Mental status, 5.1(A)(6)
Privileged communications, 3.4(A)
Records maintenance, 3.2(A)
School, 1.7
Subdoctoral/unlicensed, 1.5
PUBLIC RECORDS
Access, 3.6

Q

QUALITY ASSURANCE
For hospital care, 3.9

R

RECORDS MAINTENANCE
Access to public records, 3.6
Generally, 3.2
Privileged communications, 3.4
Search and seizure of records, 3.5
REFUSAL OF TREATMENT
Generally, 3.7

About the Authors

Donald N. Bersoff (JD, Yale Law School; PhD, New York University) is director of the JD/PhD Program in Law and Psychology jointly sponsored by Villanova Law School and the Department of Clinical and Health Psychology at the Allegheny University of the Health Sciences. He has served as president of the American Psychology–Law Society and on the American Psychological Association's board of directors and its council of representatives. He was the APA's first general counsel from 1979 to 1990. He has taught at the University of Maryland Law School, the Johns Hopkins University, and Mansfield State University, among others, and has written more than 100 articles, chapters, and books on law, ethics, and psychology. He is the author of *Ethical Conflicts in Psychology,* published by the APA. In 1997 he was recipient of the Pennsylvania Psychological Association's Award for Distinguished Contributions to the Science and Profession of Psychology.

Robert I. Field (JD, Columbia Law School; MHP, Harvard School of Public Health; PhD, Boston University) directs planning and business development for primary care in the University of Pennsylvania Health System. For many years he practiced law with the Philadelphia firm of Ballard Spahr Andrews & Ingersoll, focusing on health care business arrangements. He has also done health policy research with the Institute of Medicine of the National Academy of Sciences and the Center for Law and Health Sciences at Boston University and has served as a consultant on health care issues to the Congressional Office of Technology Assessment and the RAND Corporation. He currently teaches health law at the Wharton School and Villanova Law School and is a Senior Fellow at the Leonard Davis Institute of Health Economics at the University of Pennsylvania.

Stephen J. Anderer (JD, Villanova Law School; PhD, Allegheny University of the Health Sciences) is an attorney with the law firm of Schnader Harrison Segal & Lewis in Philadelphia, specializing in domestic relations and mental health aspects of divorce, custody, and civil competency. He is the author of an influential monograph, *Determining Competency in Guardianship Proceedings,* published by the American Bar Association, and has given several talks on the presentation of direct- and cross-examination evidence in child custody cases.

Trudi Zaplac (JD, Villanova Law School) has completed a psychology internship at Norristown State Hospital, where she specialized in working with forensic and civilly committed patients. She is senior author of an article on mental patients' rights in *Psychology, Public Policy, and the Law,* and is scheduled to complete her PhD at Villanova/Allegheny University of the Health Sciences in December of 1998.

Agenda Games

How Today's High-Stakes Political Combat Works

Inaugural Edition

ISBN-13:
978-0615675435
(Midnight Whistler Publishing)

ISBN-10:
0615675433

For More Information Contact
Midnight Whistler Publishers
http://www.midnightwhistler.com
info@midnightwhistler.com

Agenda Games

How Today's High-Stakes Political Combat Works

by
B. K. Eakman

Midnight Whistler Publishers, since 1979

AGENDA GAMES

AGENDA GAMES

PREFACE

This book was initially conceived as a response to readers' requests for help in communicating effectively with local, state and federal representatives on complex issues. Concerns like national health care, the budget, energy policy, educational standards, foreign wars and job creation all have many aspects. Unfortunately, people today are awash in the nuanced language of attorneys, politicians and special interests. This makes it not only difficult for the layperson to comprehend any particular subject at hand, but to track news stories over time, and then link them to other, tangential topics that necessarily affect discussion.

Efforts to contact representatives for a one-on-one conversation are roundly discouraged, save for exceptionally wealthy individuals—and then only because such persons might be cajoled into donating tens of thousands of dollars. Anyone not belonging to that category can expect to encounter a phalanx of screening mechanisms—receptionists, "executive" and "legislative" assistants, and "contact me" forms on websites that require some 30-minutes' worth of menu options, as we will see in chapter 6. These mandatory website inputs are aimed more at identifying new campaign contributors than ascertaining a constituent's viewpoints. The "comments" box is calculated to discourage adding explanatory remarks. In any case, messages are reviewed by someone other than the intended recipient, and only rarely are passed along.

Today's political leaders are quite satisfied with this process. They are not keen on engaging in an exchange of ideas with those they pretend to serve. While their minions tweet, dig up dirt on

I

opponents for ad campaigns and help political marketing firms, legislators themselves are busy consulting with their speechwriters and practicing "position statements" that will sound good on the stump and in televised pseudo-debates. Such debates are typically moderated by TV commentators or news anchors—most of whom are more concerned with their own celebrity than the views of office-seekers.

Recognizing this sad state of affairs led to a re-examination of the book's purpose. In struggling to simplify concerns such as the health care bill, the federal deficit, foreign policy, climate debates and education, so that typical taxpayers could communicate knowledgeably with elected representatives, it became increasingly apparent that the voting public is being "played."

Moreover, the citizen has become a pawn in a high-stakes game of political maneuvering that has morphed from the competitiveness and rhetorical give-and-take of 40-plus years ago, to something more closely resembling combat, with countless new and old deceptive strategies continually being auditioned and evaluated for their mass appeal. Elections 1952 and 2012 are rather like the difference between the classic 1980s video game, "Pac-Man," and later concoctions such as "Grand Theft Auto." The old classic was challenging entertainment; the new renditions incorporate intimidation and are wholly calculated to make the players (as well as any onlookers) uncomfortable.

Pick any issue of political significance—education, for example—and you will find yourself awash in a high-stress, depersonalized battle. But it will be one that you, the ordinary "player," have virtually no chance of influencing one way or the other.

Meanwhile, the ever-expanding civil-service "machine" churns out a familiar hodgepodge of rules, regulations, controls, zealously guarding old turf, while greedily appending new offices, bureaus and directorates. States are tricked into "competing" for grants—

or risk losing *all* their federal funding.

Consequently, today's political contests bear no resemblance to the post World Wars I and II eras. Rather, there exists a calculated effort, by all sorts of demagogues, to sow dissention—to alienate, demoralize and, if possible, neutralize entire potential pools of voters, with all the negative energy such a scheme entails: coercion, ostracism, intimidation, loss of status or job, and outright censorship. In this scenario, the agenda becomes all-important; the individual recedes into expendability.

Suddenly, it became painfully clear that no matter how proficient the average, citizen becomes at recognizing professional agitators, rigged consensus-building, a "psychologically controlled" gathering, or even mastering the art of argument, events have moved to the point where once-cherished ideals, cultural norms, allegiances and beliefs have become liabilities in the eyes of the courts and the State—often with accompanying penalties and repercussions.

Thus the title of this book: *AGENDA GAMES: How Today's High-Stakes Political Combat Works*. Readers will notice something different in the format. Given this new era of publishing, in which people purchase books specifically for digital products like Kindle and Nook, and that people no longer wish to trudge to the library to access footnoted works or information, as many footnotes as possible are provided as links, which you can either click on, if your device is electronic, or type the link directly into your browser if you have the hard copy.

A special note of thanks goes to Simon Sebag Montefiore for his two watershed, historical tomes, *Young Stalin* and *Stalin: Court of the Red Tsar*. These can't-put-it-down works were particularly insightful in thrashing out the unique and distinctive reasoning behind Josef Stalin's ahead-of its-time approach to goading a far-flung populace into swapping one set of beliefs and values for another—long before modern "market research." Unlike the

III

heads of previous totalitarian regimes, Stalin figured out how to broker a mixture of charm, "rock-star" likeability, and intellectualism into what we would today call "regime change."

Many other authors, columnists, experts and organizational heads—all having expertise in their areas of specialization—provided clarity and context on topics ranging from health care to national security and budget issues, to molding public opinion. The stand-outs are discussed in text as well as in the **Acknowledgments**. The reader is strongly urged to access their works using the hyperlinks provided, directly if you can, or by typing the link into your browser.

Inasmuch as this book is largely about the strategies involved in maneuvering people and molding public opinion, a word must be said here about Daniel J. Flynn's work, *Intellectual Morons: How Ideology Makes Smart People Fall for Stupid Ideas* in 2004. In it, he articulates the process by which otherwise sensible individuals are manipulated into espousing delusional ideas, typically at the behest of a few charismatic political charlatans whose fortes lie in generating mass hysteria. He added considerably to an understanding of how the frenzy of emotion shuts down the intellect, subverting both historical context and real facts to the point where nobody cares.

Flynn's research dovetails nicely with Christopher Simpson's seminal 1994 work, *Science and Coercion: Communication Research and Psychological Warfare 1945-1960*, in which he exposes the details of a method well-known among the officers of the Second World War's old Office of War Information. These methods were passed along subsequent intelligence services, but are not understood by the general public. The technical name for it is "scientific coercion." Today, the Department of Defense spins it for the news media and political commentators as "perception management" (or PM), a topic this book explores in detail. Both Flynn and Simpson clarify the tactics of wartime psychology, and show they have been tweaked and applied more widely and deftly than ever before.

The biggest difference between the 1920s, 30s and 40s and today, of course, is the quantum leap in technology. Computerized surveys, polls, and market figures can measure approval or rejection by demographic subgroup quickly and accurately—or even arrange these data to deliberately mislead. Experts can apply an algorithm to the data and predict how future incursions on our freedoms might fare. Face recognition technologies, meanwhile, have come so far that a face can be selected from out of a crowd, matched with a name from a database, then cross-matched against other data-bases so that advertisers might market a product (or political message) to a single individual. Obviously, such capabilities were unavailable to wannabe dictators of an earlier era.

Ironically, the digital-age technologies upon which we depend, and even "love," are serving to accelerate the timetable required to fulfill a larger, overriding Agenda. The various "games" described in this book support this overarching Agenda.

What is this grander scheme? It is nothing less than a replacement of the Founders' vision of an independent, self-sufficient nation, based in individual resolve and grit, and minimal interference from government, with a super-State based in Old World notions of dependency, maximum government intrusion, crushing regulation and regimentation.

The purpose of this book, then, is to explain how all the new capabilities, when combined with older ones, can be made to work against an upstanding, law-abiding population on an individual level—all "seamlessly," as experts would say.

~

B. K. Eakman

INTRODUCTION

Milton Friedman, the great economist, once famously quipped: "If you put the federal government in charge of the Sahara Desert, in five years there'd be a shortage of sand."

The founders of our nation were all visionaries who, fortunately for us, were born around the same time. They no doubt had the same general thought. They were determined that America's federal government should have strictly limited powers. Their greatest fear was that somewhere down the road, when Americans had become more comfortable than watchful, that these limited powers would be played into something altogether different—not just bigger, but oppressive. They had "been there, seen that…".

The key to knowing when you're being "played"—politically speaking—is recognizing the signs that accompany an arrogant bureaucracy, one that is always trying to curry favor with the sitting administration, usually by going overboard with assigned duties. Another red flag is a president or high-level member of Congress who says something, with great conviction, to one audience, then turns around and declares the opposite to an interviewer weeks or months later ("political posturing"). Yet another bad sign is a town hall-style meeting which has been "packed" in order to build a predetermined consensus.

These and many other deceptive maneuvers signal that something is amiss. Even if you can't quite put your finger on it, and you're tempted to believe you're just overreacting or "being paranoid," your gut often tells you otherwise—especially if the politician is likeable. You could be wrong, of course—or you could be ignoring that inner discomfort at your peril.

A good political charlatan can pull off something like this—better yet, a group of them, with an axe to grind. It all looks remarkably real, until the "other shoe" drops.

The formula is recognizable once one knows what to look for. The same grandstanding and glamour that mesmerizes audiences, can be re-tooled in such a way as to, first build hopes, and then dash expectations. One could call it "deceit by crisis." Finally, out of nowhere, government gallops to the rescue and appears to save the day with unprecedented "reforms"—for example, bailouts of troubled industries (virtually nationalizing them), grand "stimulus" packages that bankrupt the country and tax burdens that somehow evade the term "tax." Then, there's the "disingenuous freebie"—a new take on Franklin Roosevelt's "chicken in every pot—recast, perhaps, as free birth control for all, which, for all intents and purposes, already exists for persons so inclined. Yet, such pronouncements never fail to woo the gullible and the greedy.

When we started hearing such dramatic rhetoric from the Obama administration beginning in 2009, some people were outraged and others thought him bold.

What almost no one mentioned was a certain sense of *déjà-vu*.

They should have.

Classes in world history should have jumped out at Americans in a gasp of sudden recognition. But then, most people alive today didn't really study world history. Rather, they sat through a bunch of courses nebulously referred to as "social studies," so nothing clicked...

The Obama administration, like many before it, came in promising an overhaul—a "transformation." Most folks took this to mean streamlined regulations, and more bang for the taxpayer's buck. They expected the U.S. military would move quickly out of the Middle East; that big-ticket entitlements like Medicare

VII

B. K. Eakman

(without being called, specifically, "socialistic"), would be more equitably distributed; that government investment (i.e. "taxpayer investment") in schools, energy production, medical research, and infrastructure projects would soar.

Things underwent a transformation, all right, but not in the way even Mr. Obama's supporters imagined. The newest generation (the "Millennials"), for example, did not expect to take on personal debts amounting to $100,000 or more for a college credential that often turned out to be meaningless as far as near-term employment was concerned. Even when opportunity knocked, it was more likely to be for an "internship," not a job offer—in other words, free labor. Young adults did not imagine that many of them would be moving back in with their parents—a reality that today applies to some 30 percent of individuals between the ages of 24 and 35.

Young parents and first-time home buyers did not anticipate that the American Dream of home ownership would vanish nearly overnight. Even an apartment, in our modern "condo-ized" era, came with stiff monthly "assessments," plus utilities, added onto the regular purchase price, unlike the owner-subsidized repairs-and-upkeep and one-time deposits (usually refundable upon moving) of their grandparents' day.

Budding entrepreneurs were stunned at the volume of regulations and paperwork associated with start-up costs—$1.7 trillion all told, according to Rep. Tom Price (R-GA). This meant smaller staffs and a trend toward part-time hiring to avoid at least some of the bureaucratic nightmares and benefit packages like annual leave and mandated health care coverage.

While ongoing disasters in the Middle East had many people thinking they understood the justifications surrounding the hikes in fuel costs and gas prices, they did not expect "conservation" efforts, which they initially supported, to merge with oppressive environmental and "climate change" polices. They didn't want to be dependent on that dastardly part of the world to light their houses, run their heaters and air conditioners, and fuel their vehicles—not when we had plenty of oil and gas right here in America, enough to last an easy thousand years, by which time some genius researcher would come up with something viable.

If, that is, U.S. regulators didn't kill all incentive for the next Bill Gates, Steve Jobs, Thomas Edison or Werner von Braun to roll up his sleeves and invent something!

People wanted real oil, mineral and coal exploration, not European-style gas prices (along with their teensy-weensy cars). Even the most liberal Americans drive SUVs, not automobiles the size of tricycles!

Initially, most Americans thought basic pollution-control efforts made sense. No one wanted to ruin the bays in which they fished, or to contaminate the air so badly they had to wear masks. But they didn't anticipate being saddled with year after year of *pro forma* vehicle inspections, long after they were actually needed, or mercury-laden light bulbs that required special disposal when they failed—predictably, far short of the bulbs' advertised lifetime.

Despite the warning signs from the 1980s on, following the Libyan-initiated terrorist attack on Pan Am Flight 103 (a.k.a. "the Lockerbie incident"), American travelers were on the same page with government's call for security. But they were thinking "real security risks," not themselves! So they were ill-prepared for the new round of insults that awaited them at airports under the Transportation Security Administration. Although TSA employees took on the trappings of law enforcement agents—and brooked no interference—technically, they had no credentials in law enforcement! Americans were shocked when even justifiable complaints against agents were brushed aside.

The income tax structure, instead of being simplified, went way beyond the average adult's capability to comprehend it. Together with the many savings plan options (401K, rollovers, 529 plans, etc.), younger adults, having had virtually no preparatory courses either in high school or college to help them cope, struggled to decipher the ins and outs of Social Security, Medical Savings Accounts, Federal Insurance Contributions Act (FICA) taxes, and Payroll taxes. Their eyes glazed over, even though they knew they were probably paying far more than they actually owed.

More worrying was the risk of being victimized by crime. To hear and read the news, the crime rate was down; yet the likelihood of being assaulted or burglarized in real-world terms had risen—thanks to offenders with long "rap sheets," who never seemed to serve out their sentences. Neighborhoods once deemed very safe had reached a point where potential buyers shied away and law-abiding folks moved away—which, again, meant more money for a better area or a "gated community." Then, there were all the gadgets that had to be purchased as safety precautions. And Neighborhood Watch committees, which carried their own risks—à la the Trayvon Martin debacle. Everyone was on edge, for Lord's sake! Where on earth were the police? Couldn't the nation's leaders relate to that?

Americans have always known we had a multiethnic country, and even a multiracial one, and most had long ago made peace with that. If Barack Obama said he was born in Hawaii, or even had said that his parents weren't legally married at the time of his birth, the majority would have been willing to give the man the benefit of the doubt and move on. But when he started spouting nonsense like America having "57 states" or "hundreds of national parks" (we have 58), it went a bit beyond a slip of the tongue.

Suddenly, people started wondering: Just where was the President really born, and who *really* mentored the President's meteoric rise to fame back in Chicago?

As for "green energy," well, everybody liked lush hills and landscapes. But all too soon they realized that "go green" didn't mean that. It was just a slogan to drum up support for doing with less and paying more. And where was the infrastructure Mr. Obama had promised? Weren't all those "revenue cameras"—the ones that were purportedly for traffic safety—supposed to be going into the revamping of America's 1940s-era power lines and sewer systems?

Then there were was illegal immigration, the strain on our nation's schools and hospitals, alien criminal enterprises setting up shop on the land of murdered Southwestern ranchers, and, as a "last straw," America's embattled border agents allegedly being tasked with aiding and abetting gun-running operations to foreign drug cartels. The flip side was that we were nearly all immigrants—many of our forebears running away from hellish lives. What happened to legal immigration, Ellis Island, and sponsorship laws?

Suddenly, Americans had visions of Iran's entire Revolutionary Guard walking through!

What were our nation's leaders thinking?

In the Internet-Tweeter Age, there is the tendency to push even well-schooled individuals into a sound-bite mentality—meaning that today's news (and often people's views) typically reduced to less than one sentence.

Increasingly, average citizens are losing patience, and in their angst the ability to articulate the core beliefs that underlie the issues about which they feel so strongly take a hit, whenever taxpayers try to contact their local, state or federal representative. As citizen debate diminishes, the cognitive processes that once accompanied weighty matters are compromised. This flies in the face of our Founders' vision for the nation.

The term "information overload" doesn't begin to describe the plight of committed citizens yearning to take back the reins of their country and be actively consulted in decision-making— whether in their communities or at the state, regional or national level. Instead, they are met with dinner-interrupting "cold calls," surveys, blogs, quickie "click-on"- polls, and "chat rooms"—all provoking their understandable ire to demonstrate their anger by clicking *yes* or *no*, *like* or *don't like*—and to do so RIGHT NOW.

It's almost as if the American people have been complicit in their own destruction. They "follow" people on Twitter—from the living room on into the bathroom—but they can't (or maybe the proper term is "are not allowed to") follow a train of logic regarding the policies their government is handing down: pieces of legislation under feel-good titles that seem always to incorporate words like "freedom."

Has "freedom" turns out to be a façade? And just when the Obama Administration was promising the real thing!

Welcome to the *Agenda Games*.

~

Agenda
Games

How Today's High-Stakes Political Combat Works

by

B. K. Eakman

ISBN-13:
978-0615675435

ISBN-10:
0615675433

For More Information Contact
Midnight Whistler Publishers
http://www.midnightwhistler.com
info@midnightwhistler.com

Midnight Whistler Publishers – since 1979

AGENDA GAMES

What They're Saying:

As Mrs. Eakman perceives, "health care reform" is not about health but about the agenda. She shows how, in many ways, the ongoing transformation is destroying the spirit of medicine.

Dr. Jane Orient, M.D. Executive Director of
American Assoc. of Physicians and Surgeons

Reading *Agenda Games* left me speechless while giving me a voice! Speechless because frankly I don't know how Beverly does it! Using dazzling scouting skills, she identifies and tracks down each footprint left by a political gamesman. She shows us where they've been, then points out where they're headed. *Agenda Games* gave this reader voice enough, to "head 'em off at the pass!" Whether she realizes or not, Beverly has started the posse that will rescue America.

Roni Bell Sylvester, president and co-founder, LawUSA

Beverly Eakman has created a powerful and eye-opening primer on how politics really is played, and how it can play out. Her book focuses on nine major legislative arenas that critically impact our election process —and our way of life!

Paul Driessen, syndicated columnist and author

PREFACE

This book was initially conceived as a response to readers' requests for help in communicating effectively with local, state and federal representatives on complex issues. Concerns like national health care, the budget, energy policy, educational standards, foreign wars and job creation all have many aspects. Unfortunately, people today are awash in the nuanced language of attorneys, politicians and special interests. This makes it not only difficult for the layperson to comprehend any particular subject at hand, but to track news stories over time, and then link them to other, tangential topics that necessarily affect discussion.

Efforts to contact representatives for a one-on-one conversation are roundly discouraged, save for exceptionally wealthy individuals—and then only because such persons might be cajoled into donating tens of thousands of dollars. Anyone not belonging to that category can expect to encounter a phalanx of screening mechanisms—receptionists, "executive" and "legislative" assistants, and "contact me" forms on websites that require some 30-minutes' worth of menu options, as we will see in chapter 6. These mandatory website inputs are aimed more at identifying new campaign contributors than ascertaining a constituent's viewpoints. The "comments" box is calculated to discourage adding explanatory remarks. In any case, messages are reviewed by someone other than the intended recipient, and only rarely are passed along.

Today's political leaders are quite satisfied with this process. They are not keen on engaging in an exchange of ideas with those they pretend to serve. While their minions tweet, dig up dirt on opponents for ad campaigns and help political marketing firms, legislators themselves are busy consulting with their speechwriters and practicing "position statements" that will sound good on the stump and in televised pseudo-debates. Such debates are typically moderated by TV commentators or news anchors—most of whom are more concerned with their own celebrity than the views of office-seekers.

Recognizing this sad state of affairs led to a re-examination of the book's purpose. In struggling to simplify concerns such as the health care bill, the federal deficit, foreign policy, climate debates and education, so that typical taxpayers could communicate knowledgeably with elected representatives, it became increasingly apparent that the voting public is being "played."

Moreover, the citizen has become a pawn in a high-stakes game of political maneuvering that has morphed from the competitiveness and rhetorical give-and-take of 40-plus years ago, to something more closely resembling combat, with countless new and old deceptive strategies continually being auditioned and evaluated for their mass appeal. Elections 1952 and 2012 are rather like the difference between the classic 1980s video game, "Pac-Man," and later concoctions such as "Grand Theft Auto." The old classic was challenging entertainment; the new renditions incorporate intimidation and are wholly calculated to make the players (as well as any onlookers) uncomfortable.

Pick any issue of political significance—education, for example—and you will find yourself awash in a high-stress, depersonalized battle. But it will be one that you, the ordinary "player," have virtually no chance of influencing one way or the other.

Meanwhile, the ever-expanding civil-service "machine" churns out a familiar hodgepodge of rules, regulations, controls, zealously guarding old turf, while greedily appending new offices, bureaus and directorates. States are tricked into "competing" for grants—or risk losing *all* their federal funding.

Consequently, today's political contests bear no resemblance to the post World Wars I and II eras. Rather, there exists a calculated effort, by all sorts of demagogues, to sow dissention—to alienate, demoralize and, if possible, neutralize entire potential pools of voters, with all the negative energy such a scheme entails: coercion, ostracism, intimidation, loss of status or job, and outright censorship. In this scenario, the agenda becomes all-important; the individual recedes into expendability.

Suddenly, it became painfully clear that no matter how proficient the average, citizen becomes at recognizing professional agitators, rigged consensus-building, a "psychologically controlled" gathering, or even mastering the art of argument, events have moved to the point where once-cherished ideals, cultural norms, allegiances and beliefs have become liabilities in the eyes of the courts and the State —often with accompanying penalties and repercussions.

Thus the title of this book: *AGENDA GAMES: How Today's High-Stakes Political Combat Works*. Readers will notice something different in the format. Given this new era of publishing, in which people purchase books specifically for digital products like Kindle and Nook, and that people no longer wish to trudge to the library to access footnoted works or information, as many footnotes as possible are provided as links, which you can either click on, if your device is electronic, or type the link directly into your browser if you have the hard copy.

A special note of thanks goes to Simon Sebag Montefiore for his two watershed, historical tomes, *Young Stalin* and *Stalin: Court of the Red Tsar*. These can't-put-it-down works were particularly insightful in thrashing out the unique and distinctive reasoning behind Josef Stalin's ahead-of its-time approach to goading a far-flung populace into swapping one set of beliefs and values for another—long before modern "market research." Unlike the heads of previous totalitarian regimes, Stalin figured out how to broker a mixture of charm, "rock-star" likeability, and intellectualism into what we would today call "regime change."

Many other authors, columnists, experts and organizational heads—all having expertise in their areas of specialization—provided clarity and context on topics ranging from health care to national security and budget issues, to molding public opinion. The stand-outs are discussed in text as well as in the **Acknowledgments**. The reader is strongly urged to access their works using the hyperlinks provided, directly if you can, or by typing the link into your browser.

Inasmuch as this book is largely about the strategies involved in maneuvering people and molding public opinion, a word must be said here about Daniel J. Flynn's work, *Intellectual Morons: How Ideology Makes Smart People Fall for Stupid Ideas* in 2004. In it, he articulates the process by which otherwise sensible individuals are manipulated into espousing delusional ideas, typically at the behest of a few charismatic political charlatans whose fortes lie in generating mass hysteria. He added considerably to an understanding of how the frenzy of emotion shuts down the intellect, subverting both historical context and real facts to the point where nobody cares.

Flynn's research dovetails nicely with Christopher Simpson's seminal 1994 work, *Science and Coercion: Communication Research and Psychological Warfare 1945-1960*, in which he exposes the details of a method well-known among the officers of the Second World War's old Office of War Information. These methods were passed along subsequent intelligence services, but are not understood by the general public. The technical name for it is "scientific coercion." Today, the Department of Defense spins it for the news media and political commentators as "perception management" (or PM), a topic this book explores in detail. Both Flynn and Simpson clarify the tactics of wartime psychology, and show they have been tweaked and applied more widely and deftly than ever before.

The biggest difference between the 1920s, 30s and 40s and today, of course, is the quantum leap in technology. Computerized surveys, polls, and market figures can measure approval or rejection by demographic subgroup quickly and accurately—or even arrange these data to deliberately mislead. Experts can apply an algorithm to the data and predict how future incursions on our freedoms might fare. Face recognition technologies, meanwhile, have come so far that a face can be selected from out of a crowd, matched with a name from a database, then cross-matched against other data-bases so that advertisers might market a product (or political message) to a single individual. Obviously, such capabilities were unavailable to wannabe dictators of an earlier era.

Ironically, the digital-age technologies upon which we depend, and even "love," are serving to accelerate the timetable required to fulfill a larger, overriding Agenda. The various "games" described in this book support this overarching Agenda.

What is this grander scheme? It is nothing less than a replacement of the Founders' vision of an independent, self-sufficient nation, based in individual resolve and grit, and minimal interference from government, with a super-State based in Old World notions of dependency, maximum government intrusion, crushing regulation and regimentation.

The purpose of this book, then, is to explain how all the new capabilities, when combined with older ones, can be made to work against an upstanding, law-abiding population on an individual level—all "seamlessly," as experts would say.

~

INTRODUCTION

Milton Friedman, the great economist, once famously quipped: "If you put the federal government in charge of the Sahara Desert, in five years there'd be a shortage of sand."

The founders of our nation were all visionaries who, fortunately for us, were born around the same time. They no doubt had the same general thought. They were determined that America's federal government should have strictly limited powers. Their greatest fear was that somewhere down the road, when Americans had become more comfortable than watchful, that these limited powers would be played into something altogether different—not just bigger, but oppressive. They had "been there, seen that...".

The key to knowing when you're being "played"— politically speaking—is recognizing the signs that accompany an arrogant bureaucracy, one that is always trying to curry favor with the sitting administration, usually by going overboard with assigned duties. Another red flag is a president or high-level member of Congress who says something, with great conviction, to one audience, then turns around and declares the opposite to an interviewer weeks or months later ("political posturing"). Yet another bad sign is a town hall-style meeting which has been "packed" in order to build a predetermined consensus.

These and many other deceptive maneuvers signal that something is amiss. Even if you can't quite put your finger on it, and you're tempted to believe you're just overreacting or "being paranoid," your gut often tells you otherwise—

especially if the politician is likeable. You could be wrong, of course—or you could be ignoring that inner discomfort at your peril.

A good political charlatan can pull off something like this —better yet, a group of them, with an axe to grind. It all looks remarkably real, until the "other shoe" drops.

The formula is recognizable once one knows what to look for. The same grandstanding and glamour that mesmerizes audiences, can be re-tooled in such a way as to, first build hopes, and then dash expectations. One could call it "deceit by crisis." Finally, out of nowhere, government gallops to the rescue and appears to save the day with unprecedented "reforms"—for example, bailouts of troubled industries (virtually nationalizing them), grand "stimulus" packages that bankrupt the country and tax burdens that somehow evade the term "tax." Then, there's the "disingenuous freebie"—a new take on Franklin Roosevelt's "chicken in every pot—recast, perhaps, as free birth control for all, which, for all intents and purposes, already exists for persons so inclined. Yet, such pronouncements never fail to woo the gullible and the greedy.

When we started hearing such dramatic rhetoric from the Obama administration beginning in 2009, some people were outraged and others thought him bold.

What almost no one mentioned was a certain sense of *déjà-vu*.

They should have.

Classes in world history should have jumped out at Americans in a gasp of sudden recognition. But then, most people alive today didn't really study world history. Rather, they sat through a bunch of courses nebulously referred to as "social studies," so nothing clicked...

The Obama administration, like many before it, came in

promising an overhaul—a "transformation." Most folks took this to mean streamlined regulations, and more bang for the taxpayer's buck. They expected the U.S. military would move quickly out of the Middle East; that big-ticket entitlements like Medicare (without being called, specifically, "socialistic"), would be more equitably distributed; that government investment (i.e. "taxpayer investment") in schools, energy production, medical research, and infrastructure projects would soar.

Things underwent a transformation, all right, but not in the way even Mr. Obama's supporters imagined. The newest generation (the "Millennials"), for example, did not expect to take on personal debts amounting to $100,000 or more for a college credential that often turned out to be meaningless as far as near-term employment was concerned. Even when opportunity knocked, it was more likely to be for an "internship," not a job offer—in other words, free labor. Young adults did not imagine that many of them would be moving back in with their parents—a reality that today applies to some 30 percent of individuals between the ages of 24 and 35.

Young parents and first-time home buyers did not anticipate that the American Dream of home ownership would vanish nearly overnight. Even an apartment, in our modern "condo-ized" era, came with stiff monthly "assessments," plus utilities, added onto the regular purchase price, unlike the owner-subsidized repairs-and-upkeep and one-time deposits (usually refundable upon moving) of their grandparents' day.

Budding entrepreneurs were stunned at the volume of regulations and paperwork associated with start-up costs— $1.7 trillion all told, according to Rep. Tom Price (R-GA). This meant smaller staffs and a trend toward part-time hiring to avoid at least some of the bureaucratic nightmares and benefit packages like annual leave and mandated health care coverage.

While ongoing disasters in the Middle East had many people thinking they understood the justifications surrounding the hikes in fuel costs and gas prices, they did not expect "conservation" efforts, which they initially supported, to merge with oppressive environmental and "climate change" polices. They didn't want to be dependent on that dastardly part of the world to light their houses, run their heaters and air conditioners, and fuel their vehicles—not when we had plenty of oil and gas right here in America, enough to last an easy thousand years, by which time some genius researcher would come up with something viable.

If, that is, U.S. regulators didn't kill all incentive for the next Bill Gates, Steve Jobs, Thomas Edison or Werner von Braun to roll up his sleeves and invent something!

People wanted real oil, mineral and coal exploration, not European-style gas prices (along with their teensy-weensy cars). Even the most liberal Americans drive SUVs, not automobiles the size of tricycles!

Initially, most Americans thought basic pollution-control efforts made sense. No one wanted to ruin the bays in which they fished, or to contaminate the air so badly they had to wear masks. But they didn't anticipate being saddled with year after year of *pro forma* vehicle inspections, long after they were actually needed, or mercury-laden light bulbs that required special disposal when they failed—predictably, far short of the bulbs' advertised lifetime.

Despite the warning signs from the 1980s on, following the Libyan-initiated terrorist attack on Pan Am Flight 103 (a.k.a. "the Lockerbie incident"), American travelers were on the same page with government's call for security. But they were thinking "real security risks," not themselves! So they were ill-prepared for the new round of insults that awaited them at airports under the Transportation Security Administration. Although TSA employees took on the trappings of law enforcement agents—and brooked no interference—technically, they had no credentials in law enforcement! Americans were shocked when even justifiable complaints against agents were brushed aside.

The income tax structure, instead of being simplified, went way beyond the average adult's capability to comprehend it. Together with the many savings plan options (401K, rollovers, 529 plans, etc.), younger adults, having had virtually no preparatory courses either in high school or college to help them cope, struggled to decipher the ins and outs of Social Security, Medical Savings Accounts, Federal Insurance Contributions Act (FICA) taxes, and Payroll taxes. Their eyes glazed over, even though they knew they were probably paying far more than they actually owed.

More worrying was the risk of being victimized by crime. To hear and read the news, the crime rate was down; yet the likelihood of being assaulted or burglarized in real-world terms had risen—thanks to offenders with long "rap sheets," who never seemed to serve out their sentences. Neighborhoods once deemed very safe had reached a point where potential buyers shied away and law-abiding folks moved away—which, again, meant more money for a better area or a "gated community." Then, there were all the gadgets that had to be purchased as safety precautions. And Neighborhood Watch committees, which carried their own risks—à la the Trayvon Martin debacle. Everyone was on edge, for Lord's sake! Where on earth were the police? Couldn't the nation's leaders relate to that?

Americans have always known we had a multiethnic

country, and even a multiracial one, and most had long ago made peace with that. If Barack Obama said he was born in Hawaii, or even had said that his parents weren't legally married at the time of his birth, the majority would have been willing to give the man the benefit of the doubt and move on. But when he started spouting nonsense like America having "57 states" or "hundreds of national parks" (we have 58), it went a bit beyond a slip of the tongue.

Suddenly, people started wondering: Just where was the President really born, and who *really* mentored the President's meteoric rise to fame back in Chicago?

As for "green energy," well, everybody liked lush hills and landscapes. But all too soon they realized that "go green" didn't mean that. It was just a slogan to drum up support for doing with less and paying more. And where was the infrastructure Mr. Obama had promised? Weren't all those "revenue cameras"—the ones that were purportedly for traffic safety—supposed to be going into the revamping of America's 1940s-era power lines and sewer systems?

Then there were was illegal immigration, the strain on our nation's schools and hospitals, alien criminal enterprises setting up shop on the land of murdered Southwestern ranchers, and, as a "last straw," America's embattled border agents allegedly being tasked with aiding and abetting gun-running operations to foreign drug cartels. The flip side was that we were nearly all immigrants—many of our forebears running away from hellish lives. What happened to legal immigration, Ellis Island, and sponsorship laws?

Suddenly, Americans had visions of Iran's entire Revolutionary Guard walking through!

What were our nation's leaders thinking?

In the Internet-Tweeter Age, there is the tendency to push even well-schooled individuals into a sound-bite mentality—

meaning that today's news (and often people's views) typically reduced to less than one sentence.

Increasingly, average citizens are losing patience, and in their angst the ability to articulate the core beliefs that underlie the issues about which they feel so strongly take a hit, whenever taxpayers try to contact their local, state or federal representative. As citizen debate diminishes, the cognitive processes that once accompanied weighty matters are compromised. This flies in the face of our Founders' vision for the nation.

The term "information overload" doesn't begin to describe the plight of committed citizens yearning to take back the reins of their country and be actively consulted in decision-making—whether in their communities or at the state, regional or national level. Instead, they are met with dinner-interrupting "cold calls," surveys, blogs, quickie "click-on"- polls, and "chat rooms"—all provoking their understandable ire to demonstrate their anger by clicking *yes* or *no*, *like* or *don't like*—and to do so RIGHT NOW.

It's almost as if the American people have been complicit in their own destruction. They "follow" people on Twitter—from the living room on into the bathroom—but they can't (or maybe the proper term is "are not allowed to") follow a train of logic regarding the policies their government is handing down: pieces of legislation under feel-good titles that seem always to incorporate words like "freedom."

Has "freedom" turns out to be a façade? And just when the Obama Administration was promising the real thing!

Welcome to the *Agenda Games*.

~

Chapter 1:

REGIME CHANGE COMES TO AMERICA

It's midnight in America. Does anybody know where our country went?

From pundits to porters, people from all walks of life are noticing an uncomfortable shift in government priorities. From federal agency decrees, to Appeals Court verdicts to high-profile U.S. Supreme Court decisions an increasing contempt for the rights of average citizens is evident. Many of the issues in dispute are quite different from one another; and yet...there is an elusive similarity to all of them—primary among them being a demand for "compliance." Failure or outright refusal to "comply" comes with untenable fines and nonstop harassment by officials.

Establishing a Base of Core Support

Before there can be anything approaching "regime change," as we like to call it today, there first must be a significant base of enthusiasts and followers open to new attitudes. The first new outlook to be inculcated involves the *role* of government. A second centers on the *apparatus* (tools and tactics) of government. An apparatus, in this context, includes bureaucrats, police, teachers and professors, journalists, and other public "servants"—the old Soviets had a more definitive term for it: *apparatchiks*—all of whom must are willing, at least at the outset, to look the other way when something doesn't sound quite right, and carry out the wishes of an elite inner circle or ruling class. Only later can entertainers and leaders of various associations and trade organizations be galvanized to further support.

Investigative "Punts"

Two indications that regime change is underway—occur when both agencies tasked with investigative oversight and media "watchdogs" decline to "dig" for information and/or report findings to the people. This is a particularly crucial when something looks "fishy" to begin with (for example, in the brouhaha over Mr. Obama's birth certificate), or when too many contradictory facts from highly credible sources emerge to discredit a government policy initiative (as in the copious global-warming scandals).

In the case of the now-infamous Barack Obama birth certificate: It only became an issue when Mr. Obama delayed over what is normally a simple request. It took many months, and a direct challenge by hotel magnate and television personality Donald Trump, of all people, before Barack Obama finally forked over a document to "prove" he really was an American citizen. Everyone sighed in relief and moved on, except for a few cranks (ridiculed as "birthers"), who scratched their heads and asked why the math didn't add up and why the terminology used on the long-lost certificate was not in keeping with the era of his birth.

The U.S. Supreme Court was correct in its refusal to hear the birth certificate challenge in June 2011. The job of the High Court is to determine constitutionality—which had already been established (that one must be a native-born U.S. citizen to become President of the United States). Whether Barack Obama's birth certificate legitimately actually met those standards was a question for the *Justice Department*, not the Supreme Court—and before he was elected, not after.

Four issues should have been examined by Justice:

1. Why does the Obama birth certificate refer to Barack Obama as "African-American," when that term hadn't been coined in 1961, the year of his birth? In 1961, "people of color" were still called "Negroes," regardless of mixed race.

2. Why does the certificate say Barack Obama's father was born in Kenya, when the nation of Kenya didn't exist until 1963, two years *after* President Obama's birth, and a full 27 years after his *father's* birth? The country was known instead as the "British East Africa Protectorate."

3. Why does the birth certificate give the location of his birth as "Kapi'olani Maternity & Gynecological Hospital," when it was *1978* that the place was renamed to reflect that, when two other hospitals merged?[1]

4. How does one square Mr. Obama's book, *Dreams from my Father*, in which he takes pains to say how proud he was of his father fighting in World War II, with his father's date of birth on the certificate, about 1936? This dates, even if off by two or three years would have made his father somewhere between three and 10 years old in the Second World War?

The Justice Department and the major media dropped the ball on these questions, which are critical, not only to presidential eligibility, but to national security—calling into question the integrity of the Justice Department as a cabinet-level agency (more than justified, as we will see in chapter 5), the state of American journalism, and Mr. Obama's reticence to produce a measly birth certificate.

---

[1] See: http://www.kapiolani.org/women-and-children/about-us/default.aspx and
http://www.kapiolani.org/women-and-children/about-us/default.aspx

Military Options v. Internal Destabilization

Today, a strong, obedient military alone is not enough, by itself, to assure long-term "staying power" for aspiring control freaks and wannabe dictators, particularly in industrialized societies still thought of as "the free world." Given today's high-tech, explosive devices, purely military campaigns cannot control such societies successfully without inflicting permanent and unsustainably costly damage that is counterproductive both to the occupying elite and to the land-mass itself. Any halfway logical usurper today expects that that a conquered people and the ground they stand on will be useful. Rendering the country unlivable for the foreseeable future is not the option it was in the 1930s and 40s. Only an irrational enemy (e.g., the fanatical terrorists of 9/11) will pummel their quarry (and maybe themselves) to death.

This leaves some other, less physically destructive, mode of coercive acquisition as the only alternative. In other words, a logical foe would assume control by regulatory and psychological means, if possible.

A more subtle approach to regime change, especially from within, is *destabilization*. This occurs when a series of calamities is engineered, behind the scenes, all designed to require circumvention of whatever liberties exist—as an emergency measure, of course—so as to *appear* to fend off impending disaster.

Meanwhile, loyalties to family, friends, community and employers are deftly shifted to the State. With the benefit of today's marketing and promotional know-how, targeted to specific demographics, the ensuing chapters will show how nearly everyone falls for the ruse, regardless of educational or socio-economic status—from eager young university students and intellectuals with multiple Ph.D.'s to common laborers.

Deceit by "Crisis"

Rahm Emanuel, the early-on Chief of Staff to Barack Obama, cynically quipped in 2009: "You never want a serious crisis to go to waste." He couldn't have described an "agenda game" in action more succinctly.

Given today's sound bite era, or Age of the Tweet, young adults and middle-age citizens are more vulnerable than ever to the kind of distracting and exaggerated messages that pass for news. Oversimplifications are delivered to tired audiences as serious solutions for complex problems.

The Random-Killer Crisis.- For an example of how "crisis opportunism" plays out in real time, take the Aurora, Colorado, movie theater killings on July 20, 2012. In this latest version of the random-shooter rampage[2], the alleged perpetrated was a man costumed for a role of "the Joker" from the new, violent Batman film, *The Dark Knight Rises*. Subsequent newscasts, of course, were quick to highlight legislators' calls for more gun control laws—even though all the background checks in the world would still have allowed the primary suspect, James Holmes, to obtain weapons ranging from assault rifles to bombs. He used the latter to booby-trap his apartment.

But government is more interested in abridging the people's right to bear arms—i.e., the right to self-defense—that it is in real-time crime control. So, pseudo-solutions are passed along to consumers of TV news by "info-tainers"—news anchors who are trained to make issues either palatable or entertaining, depending on the issue they are "selling." News anchors today are mostly wannabe celebrities who follow a script, delivering it in a pleasant, or righteously indignant, voice, depending on the impression their "betters" wish to transmit.

---

2   See: http://www.washingtonpost.com/national/health-science/james-eagan-holmes-held-in-colorado-shooting/2012/07/20/gJQA213UyW_story.html

Thus, virtually any news item can be made into a "crisis" that accommodates a greater agenda.

This is what Rahm Emanuel was alluding to in his wisecrack about never letting a crisis go to waste. It's an "old standby" tactic that, in the long term, trivializes critical problems.

A wholly different problem was discovered in the aftermath of the Aurora, Colorado, theater-shooting: the suspect was as an ardent fan of violent video games. But the media only mentioned this in passing. That somebody would play out a drama featuring random killings in a *theater*, dressed in *costume*, speaks volumes to the issue of violent video gaming, not guns. Yet, bans on "assault weapons," handguns, and even more aggressive screening of schoolchildren for any views that could be stretched into a definition of "mental illness" were the topics of legislative debate.

Budget Crisis Backpedaling.- This nation has not had a federal budget for three years running. We've had Budget Control Acts (which failed to control the budget), "budget resolutions," "budget deals," and various games, like the "Payroll Tax Holiday," but no actual budget passed by Congress, as required by law.

The troubling trend began in 1999. There was also no federal budget in fiscal years 2002, 2003, 2005 and 2007—and now for three years straight. This, and Mr. Obama's spending spree, spurred a "Budget Crisis."

Only one man dared to roll up his sleeves in 2012 and declare "Enough!": House Budget Committee Chairman Paul Ryan (R-WI.). He was the only man in Congress still uttering the "s" words on the House floor—"supply-side." His pitch to balance the budget shocked even his own party—enough so that some Republicans actually criticized him, either for not cutting enough, such as unloading an agency or two, or for proposing massive changes to "untouchable" entitlements like Social

Security and Medicare, a cap on federal spending and lower tax rates across-the-board. Always happy to shoot themselves in the foot in the name of "compromise," these Republicans joined Democrats by asking where Ryan's economic principles lay— *with Jesus, or Ayn Rand*! (The American Civil Liberties Union wisely stayed mum on that one!)

Once Mr. Ryan was tapped by then-presumptive presidential nominee Mitt Romney (R-MA) as a vice-presidential running mate, Republican critics stifled a collective "oops" and hoped no one recalled their jeer.

Ryan was savvy enough to recognize that in an ongoing climate of entitlement fixation, no agencies were going to be cut, whether his proposed "Path to Prosperity" passed or not. But no major entitlement should be "raided" to fund another, either, as Mr. Obama did with Medicare to fund ObamaCare.

Thus, Ryan would have to come at the budget mess from another direction, knowing that changes to big-ticket entitlements, spending caps and lower taxes had all been bandied about before, with little to show for it.

The big Welfare Reform Act of 1996, for example, as well as prior efforts under Ronald Reagan, both in California and on a national scale during Reagan's presidency, resulted in significant short-term decreases in welfare rolls—but not long-term ones.

There's a good reason for that: No matter what proposals are passed by Congress in one administration, they can be undone by the next. Worse are the deceptive and imaginative ploys that government uses to rob from one money pot (such as Social Security) in order to refurbish another. This game, played at the expense of the electorate, is sometimes little more than a colorful form of bribery: Congress (or even an agency, through the grant process) will fund some Senator's or Representative's pet project so that he or she can look good to the folks back home; in return, that member of Congress quietly agrees to cast an affirmative vote on a controversial bill, or maybe even to co-sponsor a proposal.

But every now and then a diligent politician comes along who is rightly put off by the increasing culture of dependency that has been allowed to take root. Rep. Ryan was one such man. He dared to challenge majority bureaucratic wisdom—always focused more on its own expansion than the nation's financial health. For that, he was quickly labeled a "Game-Changer" in 2012 by Democrats and liberal Republicans—as someone who would threaten the "social safety net." Rahm Emanuel's quip was invoked: A crisis did not go to waste.

Low Voter-Turnout in Local Races

Local election races, in particular, for years have met with decreasing voter turnout, with most people thinking that national elections are quite enough, thank you. The old saying that "all politics is local" may be true, but not enough to keep unscrupulous candidates from padding their résumés at the local and state level, when no one is alert, before moving onto the national stage with high-name recognition.

Apathy, disillusionment, and finally a sense of futility and alienation have come to characterize local American campaigns, especially in an off-year. By the time a national election comes along, people wonder why they feel out-maneuvered. News accounts to the effect that a candidate has won 52 percent of the vote disguise the fact that the actual number of votes cast, as compared to the census count, remains small.

Such a population is ripe for "regime change."

Diversion, Distraction and Displacement

Three threads run through nearly all agenda games: diversion, distraction and displacement. The first two, *diversion* and *distraction*, are like a conjurer's trick. The magician forces the audience to look at his right hand so they will miss what's really going on with his left. The "audience" can comprise any major faction of the populace—the media, parents, teachers, religious leaders, medical professionals, etc. In matters of public policy, these factions will, in turn, help the magician sidetrack the attention of other individuals.

The third thread is *displacement*. Most people do not recognize that loyalty to family, religion, friends and associates have more to do with whether or not attitudes, principles and ideals are handed down through successive generations than the attitudes, principles or ideals themselves. Transfer, or *displace*, the old loyalties, and once-cherished values and beliefs can soon be swayed toward opposing attitudes held by special interests. Such "interested parties" typically operate behind the scenes, but exercise enough clout to manipulate political leaders at the top. With surprising swiftness, long-accepted viewpoints, concepts and norms become liabilities and disappear, at least out in the open.

That's what "kills" once-cherished beliefs and values. As soon as people feel threatened—and that need not be interpreted as "bodily harm," but rather just enough discomfort to feel the need to hide an honest opinion—they are already losing control and accelerating regime change. In a constitutional republic, some may rush to the supposed safety of the ballot box to vote their true beliefs, as we do in America, but then turn around and say something different in conversation or an e-mail.

Most people quickly figure out what is politically correct and what isn't, and recognize a "sacred cow" topic—such as race or homosexuality. What people don't know is exactly *when* a certain expression or remark will suddenly become *verboten*. That's when things get dicey. Somebody—let's call him "Mr. Smith"—seizes upon a statement, or maybe an e-mail, then circulates it. Turns out that Mr. Smith is privy to the inner circle and knows the timing is right make an issue of this e-mail or remark. The State and its acolytes then back up the anonymous Mr. Smith, and loudly denounce the comment he has circulated—calling it offensive, or hateful, or obstructionist, or inappropriate, or (worst case scenario) mentally deranged.

This launches a new psychological environment of political intimidation.

A climate of intimidation doesn't just happen. It is carefully set it up, as we will see in the following three case studies, linked to the Community Standards Game. The first order of business by the Left is to always confirm the indebtedness of institutions that are key to its agenda. These institutions must be linked in some way to the federal government, either through direct funding, maybe a grant, to remain in good standing. That way, any *interruption* of funding, or penalties and fines, can be held over the head of, say, a university or a television station. Pressure on these agencies will then rein in any miscreants— and seal their fate.

Case Study I: The "Slut" Word

Rush Limbaugh, the radio shock-jock icon for the conservative side, was lambasted in March 2012 for calling free-contraceptives advocate, Sandra Fluke, a "slut" on the air. Liberals, who mostly heard about the comment second-hand, as they rarely listen to Mr. Limbaugh, demanded that the Federal Communications Commission order the station to take him off the air.

Never mind the organized "Slut-Walks" of the previous summer, convened by groups of young women wearing even less than "hooker-chic." They had marched along downtown streets in cities, ridiculously advocating against rape by exposing their bosoms and derrières. They enjoyed their romp without a comparable outcry—except by a few "prudish" conservatives who were ridiculed and dismissed.

Mr. Limbaugh predictably apologized for the "slut" word, as conservatives always take the bait.

Lost in the furor was the fact that community standards everywhere once shunned the term "slut" as vulgar, no matter who used it or why. Somewhere in the 1970s, it became trendy to be shocking. Mr. Limbaugh, born in 1951, was among the first-wave of Baby Boomers who, political viewpoints notwithstanding, became the beneficiaries of sixties- and seventies-era provocation. They saw their job as a call to knock down barriers—community standards of decency and tact.

As a result, both sides, from so-called "far-right" to "ultra-left," began waging a war of "can-you-top-this."

For example, one "pro-life" faction countered "pro-choice" advocates with posters showing dead or dismembered fetuses, and put on at least one show-stopping exhibition at a Washington-area subway station: A huge, white billboard covered in red splatter, made to look like blood, bearing a single caption in large letters that read **VIRGIN IS NOT A DIRTY WORD**.

About that time, a left-leaning Hollywood machine started churning out movies like *American Pie*—all centered on losing one's virginity, with none of the sensitivity associated with 1940s or 50s coming-of-age stories, but rather more on the order of *Animal House*.

Case Study II: Mocking "Bourgeois" Values

The *Smothers Brothers Comedy Hour*, featuring folk singing, comedy duo Tom and Dick Smothers, delivered the opening salvo in challenging what Josef Stalin would have pejoratively described as "bourgeois values." In the late 1960s, the pair served up not only oppositional, then-counterculture politics, but also launched the battles over so-called censorship.

The Smothers Brothers were among the first in a long line to use comedy (in the form of cleverly written ridicule) as a platform for politics. In the process, they mocked standards of acceptable good taste.

In hindsight, it is ironic to see rebroadcasts of their old sketches celebrating the hippie drug culture, interspersed with material opposing the war in Vietnam and deriding religious values. The drug culture, of course, has become so politically incorrect students are treated like criminals for carrying an aspirin.

One standard sketch on the Smother Brothers' show featured comedienne Leigh French, who created the recurring hippie character, Goldie O'Keefe. She would parody afternoon advice shows for housewives in a segment called "Share a Little Tea with Goldie." It was actually a glorification of mind-altering drugs. This helped stoke the fires of rampant substance abuse—and ultimately fulfilled the purposes of those who would, many years later, regiment society and waste tax dollars in a fruitless, let's-pretend War on Drugs.

The real came in 1969, when the duo tried, yet again, to push the boundaries of acceptable (read *establishment*) speech on TV. For failing to supply a review tape to CBS editors on the Wednesday prior to the show's air date, they were thrown off the air.

According to pundits, all the Smothers Brothers wanted was to provide a prime time forum on television for the perspectives of a disaffected and rebellious youth movement "deeply at odds with the dominant social order." If anyone had bothered to analyze the expression "dominant social order," it would have been revealing. The social order was "dominant" only if the standards of taste were, in fact, societal norms ("*givens*") held by a majority of Americans!

Most of the "disaffected" youths (i.e., by definition, a statistical minority) were not "deeply at odds" with much of anything, except maybe being drafted. Mostly, they were looking to put a thumb in the eye of the parents whose largesse paid for their *faux* outrage.

Even though the Smothers Brothers didn't use four-letter words or show vomit on their broadcasts, they set the tone for later TV offerings that did. It wasn't even the fact that they lampooned a few political issues. So did Bob Hope, after all. The difference was their clear intent to offend—the very opposite of Bob Hope. The Smothers raised insolence to the level of an art form—thereby creating a new standard for mass entertainment.

Today a much older Tom Smothers extolls the virtues of PBS as "family entertainment" In at least one pledge drive he said that PBS was the only station he let his children watch. If true, the two hypocrites should have been awarded an Emmy for "Most Useful Idiots."

Perhaps it is unsurprising that in their old age, the pair has set up a web site to endorse folk singer Pete Seeger—a self-admitted, card-carrying Communist—for the Nobel Peace Prize.

Case Study III: Censoring an American Icon

On February 15, 2012, long-time conservative commentator, author and former presidential contender, Patrick Buchanan, was dismissed from MSNBC—essentially for stating the same views he had espoused since the 1970s. Although Mr. Buchanan was the token conservative on an otherwise liberal network, his name-recognition was so high that sacking him was a creepy reminder of old Stalinesque intimidation process. In effect, Mr. Buchanan, as well as his audience, were being censored *for resisting the Party Line.*

Once a nation starts down this road, it is very difficult to reverse, especially once a majority of the media is onboard. While there was yet some pretense of divisiveness between candidates over various issues in Election Year 2012, the almost paranoid trend across the political spectrum not to "offend," or deviate from the State-endorsed view, should have been instantly recognizable.

In practically no time, anyone still holding to what Stalin would have dubbed "bourgeois" (traditional) ideas—for example, traditional marriage, or home schooling, or English as the official language of the U.S.—is marginalized as pariahs if they dare to say so in public.

The Seductive State

It was none other than Josef Stalin who coined the term "politically reliable" to describe persons who could be counted on to be loyal to, and acceptant of, State intrusion. Those who openly held to what were formerly mainstream, or "bourgeois," standards were marked as "politically *un*reliable"—and subsequently deemed a "security risk."

If this is beginning to sound familiar, it should!

Today Americans have merely renamed the term— "political correctness." But political correctness is morphing into *political reliability* with every year that passes. Grownups and young people alike are growing accustomed to—and even acceptant of—a Stalinesque style of harassment and repression: loss of status, careers, pensions, and even entrance into a career path, such as journalism or teaching. Individuals who dare to cross the State in a public way are headed for trouble.

Founders' Worst Nightmare Becomes a Reality

Joseph Stalin's appearance exemplified the fears outlined by the Framers of our Constitution in their letters back and forth, all collected into the Federalist Papers. They worried that average people would not be sophisticated enough to see through a charlatan—or to handle democracy. So, they opted for a republic over a pure democracy, mainly to avoid the emergence of a "mobocracy" led by some unscrupulous insurgent or malcontent.

Still, there were those who argued that the common tradesman, farmer or laborer—which would necessarily comprise the majority—could not be expected to hold onto the reins of a representative democracy, either. Thus: the three independent branches of government and a system of "checks and balances."

However, this concept came with a certain understanding— not articulated in the Constitution per se, but certainly in their deliberations: Underlying their entire model of governance was an assumption that the fledgling nation would continue on a path of a *shared* body of *common knowledge* (incorporated into their notions about literacy), as well as the cohesiveness of explicit moral principles (i.e., religious upbringing). These were prerequisites, even if the details of both education and religion were not the proper prerogatives of government. John Adams explains (emphasis mine):

> Because we have no government, armed with power, capable of contending with human passions, unbridled by morality and religion…, [a]varice, ambition, revenge and licentiousness would break the strongest cords of our Constitution, as a whale goes through a net. **Our Constitution was made only for a moral and religious people. It is wholly inadequate to the government of any other.** *--from John Adam's letter to the Officers of the First Brigade of the Third Division of the Militia of Massachusetts, 11 October 1798*

So, Adams and several other Framers clearly had qualms about future waves of newcomers to our shores who might not share any of their values. They figured, at least in the short term, that they could keep government from dictating, say, Presbyterianism or Catholicism, and from determining the exact content of each child's curriculum (and, by extension, every youngster's upbringing). This was all to the good. But, the question was, would it be enough to safeguard the Republic over the long term?

Adams' fears turned out to be warranted, but it took over 200 years to become evident.

The Framers' wise decision to leave the details surrounding education and moral imperatives to the states, localities and individual families provided a wedge opening for the enemies of freedom.

Beginning with post-World War II schoolchildren, the Baby Boomers, progressive trendsetters in education and childrearing began transmitting the notion that popularity and group-accommodation trumped everything else, whether in the classroom or on the playground. Youngsters interpreted this to mean that striking good looks, combined with the right mix of brashness, boldness and amenability were the tickets to popularity (later dubbed "self-esteem").

The Answer Is Tweeting in the Wind

All this was very cute—until it wasn't. As Boomer children became older adolescents, they over-interpreted the message, as adolescents typically do. They took personal appearance, brashness, boldness and amenability to new heights to secure more of these fine feelings of self-esteem until it turned into smug arrogance. Simple "attractiveness" morphed into ostentatious exhibitions of crudity, immodesty and vulgarism; brashness reinvented itself as open defiance of traditional norms and contempt for good manners, à la the Smothers Brothers. Boldness devolved into gaudy and shameless displays of bad taste. Amenability (likeability) took an odd left-turn into group-think and, finally, into anonymity. Suddenly, acceptance of the crowd became more important than any particular individual, save for the occasional charismatic leader.

This was the kind of thinking that produced the Tate/LaBianca murders, orchestrated by Charles Manson in August of 1969. Manson virtually hypnotized his drug-addled "flock" into committing gruesome and senseless stabbings. One victim, Sharon Tate, was two weeks away from giving birth. Manson, now 77 years old, is still unrepentant and in prison.

Parents and adult authority figures quickly lost control, having bought in to the media's mantra about a "Generation

Gap." Old loyalties to family, church and community shifted under the weight of interventionists and opportunists who seduced young Americans both for monetary profit (Boomer kids were nothing if not flush with cash)—and for foot soldiers in a different kind of war of acquisition, always in the name of some grandiose cause for which high-school and college-age youths hadn't the benefit of any context.

This had consequences for a representative democracy: The ideals of independence, self-reliance and self-sufficiency were stood on their heads. It challenged the family unit in ways that were central to the American way of life, destabilizing the nation.

Regime Change Rising

The face of "regime change" is now upon us full force. Almost daily, we read and hear reports further confirming usurpation of the public trust.

For example, the government now decides the number of children permitted in home day care facilities. Most states require in-home day cares to be licensed; that is, to be "in compliance" with county regulations. Of course, these regulations do not really emanate from any particular county, even though that may be what it looks like on the form to the untrained eye. Rather, it is part of a national movement to get children into government-sponsored "early childhood" programs that will leave behind the element we used to think of as "the home." That way, toddlers can be introduced to the preferred attitudes of the State without interference from parents, whose typical lack of expertise in behavioral psychology makes them unfit, in the eyes of "child experts," to satisfy the emotional and intellectual needs of their offspring.

Any excuse to further this cause is good enough. Government wants home providers to go out of business; that is

17

the point of the exercise. Sometimes it uses "zoning laws," as in Fairfax County in Virginia,[3] or maybe government subsidies, initially aimed at "at-risk" children.

The Pass-Through Dollars Trap.- A favorite scheme is to get local and state governments "hooked" on federal greenbacks via the "pass-through dollars" trap.

Long-time education columnist Robert Holland explains, by way of illustration, how even before the release of the Obama Administration's so-called Common Core of Standards for the nation's public schools, the states were being pressured to commit to phony benchmarks if they wanted to "compete" for a share of $4.35 billion "Race to the Top" funds, monies that were set aside from the rest of the federal "stimulus" package.

Education is certainly not alone in falling for the pass-through dollars trap. The housing sector and the banking sector, among others, exercise their own variations on the same pattern.

Of course, state and local governments are always assured, early on, that any federal standards will be purely *voluntary* and *determined by the states*. But voluntary measures quickly morph into "compliance regulations." The individual states (and their tax bases) become reluctant clients of the U.S. Government—"customers" (that's what federal agencies actually call them) who find themselves plowing through three levels of government—local/county, state and federal bureaucracies—only to learn they have no say.

The GSE Trap.- Another example, which most people aren't aware of, is something called *government sponsored enterprises* (or *GSEs*). These are quasi-federal institutions—privately held corporations (at least at the outset), but with *public* purposes, disingenuously created by the U.S. Congress to reduce the cost of capital for certain borrowing sectors of the

---

[3] http://www.washingtonpost.com/local/dc-politics/in-fairfax-hundreds-of-home-day-cares-may-be-forced-to-trim-enrollments/2012/07/28/gJQABI3mGX_story.html

economy. Members of these sectors include students, farmers and homeowners. The now-infamous—since the housing market meltdown—Fanny Mae (Federal National Mortgage Association) and Freddie Mac (Federal Home Loan Mortgage Corporation), for instance, were originally established to help people realize the American dream of home ownership.

GSEs carry the implicit backing of the U.S. government from the get-go, even though they are not *direct obligations* of the feds. That's the disingenuous part, this particular wording. What happens is that the indirect shoring up of these "private" institutions—which Congress, don't forget, actually created, together with government incentives and supports—over the years amount to creating a federal agency without *officially* creating one (yes, you read that right). This helps government further its various concealed agendas without being quite so blatant about it.

Unfortunately for taxpayers, this means that GSEs eventually tend to require more investment than they can secure on the open market, and so, like Fannie Mae and Freddie Mac in 2008, they wind up in federal takeover status (obliquely referred to as "being placed into *conservatorship*").

The upshot is that, today, way too many institutions cannot operate without Big Government's investment and/or its seal of approval. These include even some household-name businesses and organizations that depend upon government *contracts* or *grants* for their continued existence.

A Piecemeal Approach to Dependency

Whether you call it "pass-through money," "technical assistance," or "competing for government funding," the end-game is dependency. Eventually, scores of accompanying strings are attached—from "equal opportunity" paperwork, to recycling constraints and energy-related mandates—thus forcing any company, corporation, or even a local sheriff's department receiving small law-enforcement subsidies, are maneuvered into adopting whatever positions the political elites at the top happen to want. So, if recipient institutions and organizations want to *maintain legitimacy* and *assure an uninterrupted flow of federal funding*, they will comply, and do so enthusiastically.

Mandatory sexual harassment workshops for employees; posters offering free "mental health counseling"; compulsory removal of any icon deemed religious: All entail losing some portion of states' rights and, with it, individual liberty.

Moreover, highly charged political games—agenda games—are being played out before our eyes. Taken together, they comprise a gauge of how much "weight" government can throw around before it is met with a significant backlash. None of the issues, from the perspective of government bureaucrats and socialist-statist advocacy groups, are actually about the subject one sees in the news media.

In other words, day care restrictions are not really about caring for children. ObamaCare is not about anybody's health. The Confederate flag is not *verboten* out of any concern for racial issues. The abortion furor is not about family planning, the health of the mother or the welfare of babies. Bailouts of giant business sectors, along with various "stimulus" packages, are not about jump-starting the economy. Nobody is actually "competing" for anything in "Race to the Top" education funding. So-called "cap-and-trade" legislation is not about carbon footprints; even carbon footprints are not about carbon footprints! And global-warming (a.k.a. "climate change") is not about the environment or saving the planet.

What these issues *are* about is the State being closer to dictating decisions that used to be the prerogatives of private individuals. Somehow, Americans are failing to make this distinction.

Once the State has given its tacit approval (or disapproval) to certain actions and/or attitudes, it has, in effect, endorsed the kind of "new thinking" that an earlier generation would have instantly recognized as power plays. Subsequent demands usually follow in rapid succession: a mandate, followed by the force of law, which in turn brings penalties for "noncompliance"—along with intimidation.

The psychology of the American populace today appears to be such that, as long as people aren't being lined up before firing squads, they will accept abuse of their freedoms piecemeal.

~

CHAPTER 2
THE HEALTH CARE GAME

> Your Children's children will live under communism without a shot being fired...You Americans are so gullible. No, you won't accept Communism outright; but we'll keep feeding you small doses of Socialism until you will finally wake up and find that you already have Communism.... We won't have to fight you; we'll so weaken your economy, until you fall like overripe fruit into our hands. **--Nikita Khrushchev, 1959**

There's a reason why health care tops the Agenda Games list! It has all the elements of high-stakes political combat: diversion, distraction, displacement, intrigue, pressure to shift loyalties, attempts to alter the U.S. Constitution, crisis-engineering, attacks upon individual and state prerogatives, *uber*regulation, and bureaucratic nightmares!

With the U.S. Supreme Court having upheld the constitutionality of ObamaCare (a.k.a. the Patient Protection and Affordable Care Act, or PPACA) on June 28, 2012, the federal government effectively nationalized health care and set what was once called "socialized medicine" in stone. Included were an individual and an employer penalty for refusing to "play" the game. This makes U.S. health care the poster child for all the other Agenda Games we will examine in this book. Readers will encounter many of the same "moves" (strategies and maneuvers) over and over; only the contexts will be different. Once they start to seem familiar, that is when grassroots organizations can begin to take evasive actions to neutralize these "games" and put forth in their stead ideas more deserving of popular support.

The High-Stakes Principle

There high-stakes principle on the health care decision mirrors the combat positions on other issues: Is the U.S. Constitution meant to be taken at its word, or not? Stated another way: Does the Constitution limit the powers of the federal government to those expressly delegated to it? Or can politicians, lawyers and agency heads expand and interpret the Constitution to death, treating it as "an evolving document"?

The Supreme Court Justices, in a predictably narrow 5-4 decision, decided on the latter, which opens the door to justifying just about anything a sitting Administration, or even Congress itself, wishes to do.

On the ObamaCare question, the Justices had to juggle four issues: the constitutionality of the individual mandate; the ability to seek legal redress for a tax not actually levied; whether an individual-mandate provision could be considered in isolation from the rest of the health care package; and ObamaCare's concurrent requirement for states to expand their Medicaid coverage.

The Supreme Court's choices were: to uphold the law; strike down the law; strike down just the "individual mandate" portion; strike down only the part that would allow Congress to withhold federal Medicaid funds from states that refused to comply with ObamaCare; or punt. The latter means that the Justices could have waited until the individual mandate was supposed to take effect, in 2014, arguing that they had to see how it actually worked first. This would have been seen, of course, as giving the President a free pass (almost an endorsement) for the 2012 election, which is probably why they didn't choose to defer.

The Chief Justice's Encoded Message

For years, watchdog organizations on both sides of the political aisle have observed that Supreme Court judges, as well as many cabinet appointees, seem to ease their agencies leftward once they are in power, even if they are "conservative" at the beginning. The Supreme Court's healthcare decision provided that extra little nudge to the Left: impunity.

Chief Justice John Roberts appears to have been sending conservatives—and, indeed, all Americans—a reluctant, but potent, encoded message, when he tacked on this comment to the majority opinion for the High Court:

"It's not our [the Court's] job to protect people from the consequences of their electoral choices."[4]

Conservative news outlets picked up on the comment to slam it as a cop-out; liberals cited it to confirm their own support for the Court's decision. But nobody really looked at Roberts' comment in light of his *other* decisions, or saw it for the optional statement that it was. If they had, they might have taken the trouble to read between the lines.

Yes, "conservative Justice Roberts no doubt "went rogue"—and in a very astonishing way—as author and columnist John Scalzi contends in a July 3, 2012, online column. But, who knows the pressure Judge Roberts may have been facing, given that he did the unthinkable: *rewrite* a portion of the healthcare law! Supreme Court justices do not write or rewrite laws. If a rewrite is necessary, the Court sends it back to Congress. It is Congress that writes legislation.

What Justice Roberts is telling us is that the fire has hit the proverbial fan in American politics; that we have dallied with socialism, under the cover of either "bipartisanship" or

---

[4] Chief Justice John Roberts, writing the majority opinion in <u>National Federation of Independent Business v. Sebelius</u>, upholding the constitutionality of PPACA (a.k.a. "Affordable Care Act," or "ObamaCare"), June 28, 2012.

"compromise," for way too long, and it's time now to either reverse course at election time or just shut up.

The High Court's move was unexpected because:

(1) Throughout the congressional hearings on ObamaCare (whether lawmakers read the bill or not), those pushing it emphasized how the individual mandate was *not* to be taken for a tax on Americans. If so, the Supreme Court could have handed the bill back to Congress and told legislators to rewrite it if they expected ObamaCare to fly.

(2) After the Court's decision, in an interview with George Stephanopoulos, Mr. Obama was pressed on the issue of whether the law is, or is not, a tax. Mr. Stephanopoulos even quoted the dictionary definition of "tax," and pointedly asked the President to explain how it *wasn't* a tax. Mr. Obama derisively brushed off Stephanopoulos, as if the Clinton-era White House communications director-turned-news journalist was naïve to imagine that words used in legislative language bore any relation to their dictionary definitions!

Health Care as a Government Interest

Because so many tactical strategies were involved in the rush to impose this radical legislation, ObamaCare stands as a uniquely "teachable moment."

This wasn't the first effort to bring in universal, nationalized health coverage under the banner of "reform." Thanks to a lack of any meaningful chronological history in today's classrooms, few Americans are aware that two of the original proponents of universal health care were Republican Presidents Theodore Roosevelt, who advocated for it in 1912, and Richard M. Nixon, whose efforts prompted the Health Maintenance Organization (HMO) Act in 1973. The HMO Act is somewhat of a puzzle for a president so outspokenly opposed to socialism.

In 1993 came the infamous (and failed) "HillaryCare." It parallels ObamaCare in many respects. In the 20 years between Nixon's HMO Act and the Clinton Administration Health Security Act, big-player political combatants became more aggressive. Activist organizations, and finally the U.S. government itself, had become well-practiced in the art of *perception management*, a strategy we shall take up in more detail later.

The endless repetition of buzz-terms like "health care," for example, serves to distract the population from the realities of political combat. Health care is played out in the *Name* of Health Only. Barring a sudden epidemic or pandemic, the government **does not care about anyone's health**. Socialized medicine, whether in the context of the 1993 HillaryCare, or the modern-day Affordable Care Act ("ObamaCare"), is a tool—a means to increased government control (through regulation), intrusiveness into individual lives, and redistribution of wealth.

The Hook of "Health"

A compromised, top-heavy Government utilizes what appear to be critical issues—health, budget, national security, crime, education, the environment—as a "hook" on which to hang its real agenda.

The pejorative label HillaryCare came about because it was an overt attempt to nationalize medicine. Then-First Lady, Hillary Rodham Clinton, spearheaded a health care task force at the behest of her husband, President Bill Clinton.

Events surrounding this fiasco are instructive for their now-familiar sticking points:

- both an employer and an individual mandate;
- hidden costs of "universal coverage," especially onerous to small businesses;

- secretiveness at the top (i.e., not the "government transparency" promised); and
- duplicity among the power brokers (lobbyists, legislators and insurance companies, all trying to have it both ways, to cover their bases).

These are typical hallmarks of high-stakes political combat: compromising the self-determination of individuals and small businesses, hiding real costs, launching secret meetings, and enlisting power brokers to get a piece of the action. There is always a lot of talk, of course, about cost-cutting, but precious little about quality, and even less about personalization—things that once set this nation apart.

For comparison purposes, it is worth the reader's time to revisit the high points of HillaryCare to better recognize the tactical maneuvers made to "sell" ObamaCare. For readers who wish to satisfy themselves as to the uncanny similarities between the two, an excellent online reference guide exists: "Timeline of the Clinton Era Health Care Debate," put together by the Jim Lehrer News Hour staff for PBS. It was also consolidated for a documentary entitled *The System*.[5]

Mr. Obama, and his unprecedentedly powerful Health and Human Services Secretary, Kathleen Sebelius, made use of the "reform" tactic in a way that a student of political science might recognize—an outrageous free-contraceptives mandate, which we shall examine in detail further on in this chapter ("Obama's High-Stakes Gamble to 'Protect' Women").

Meanwhile, it is important to understand that in today's political setting, reform movements are "hooks." These hooks never go away; they just keep reappearing—sometimes under a more appealing title, or under a subsequent administration, or perhaps with a change of high-profile backers. The core supporters of the "reform" in question stay pretty much the

---

[5] http://www.pbs.org/newshour/forum/may96/background/health_debate_page1.html and http://millercenter.org/public/debates/healthcare .

same, but they exert their influence behind the scenes, away from media scrutiny.   George Soros, for example, is a high-profile name as a hedge-fund management billionaire, but few recognize him as the long-term financial force behind a young Barack Obama, just starting out in Chicago politics.

Since the mid-1980s, Soros has used his immense wealth to help reconfigure the political landscapes of countries worldwide—in some cases playing a key role in toppling regimes that had held the reins of government for years, even decades. Even in the United States, a strong case can be made for the claim that Soros today affects American politics and culture more profoundly that any other living person.[6]

The hallmark of "reform" is to take what was merely an important issue into full-blown-crisis mode. Once a critical mass is reached—i.e., most of the voting public is thoroughly disgruntled about the issue in question—the sitting administration gallops in with a "reform" *initiative* (sometimes labeled a *compromise* or an *accommodation*), and pretends to save the day. All the individual has to give up for this *faux* stability is a bit more self-determination.

Changing Perceptions About Medical Care

"Health care reform," in the generic sense, is built around the notion that everyone has a "right" (a constitutional right!) to access quality, affordable health care *without regard for their ability to pay*.

The problem is, somebody *does* have to pay.

There have always been individuals who, for one reason or another, either put off seeing, or cannot afford to see, a doctor. Prior to about 1940, consulting a doctor for every little sniffle was considered bad form. Absent today's smorgasbord of antibiotics, X-rays, probes, blood workups and so on, a person of character learned to "suck it up," as the expression goes

---

[6] http://www.discoverthenetworks.org/individualProfile.asp?indid=977 .

today. Of course, waiting often came with consequences. But many senior citizens now in their 80s and 90s will tell you that the "grin and bear it" mentality is still strong among most people of their generation.

In their day, however, doctors and hospital staff took more of a personal interest in the patient. The bill typically came in the mail as one inclusive sum. To illustrate the difference in quality of care that sum bought, let's take an average, middle-class, married woman giving birth in 1946, in any city about the size of Washington, D.C.

First, she was sent to labor in a private room, unless she came in as an emergency patient. If the birth was difficult (last-minute Caesarian Sections were not yet possible), then she might stay hospitalized for 10 days or so, with a nurse available to give her a sponge bath, help her with the bathroom right away, gently show her how to tend her newborn if she was a first-time mom, and even give her a rubdown with perfumed lotion. (This author ought to know; one such woman was my mother.)

Compare that with today's typical fare. First-time moms are placed in a ward with a bunch of screaming women, without privacy, in all stages of labor. Many foul themselves, and there is not much they can do. Some are given spinal injections to numb the pain (which was not available in the 40s), and sometimes husbands are present throughout, if they can stomach the ordeal and have had a bit of training.

Whether the delivery is difficult or not, the woman is discharged long before the stitches have healed in a very delicate area. But it's up to mom to practically stand on her head to keep the area clean. (Today's readers supposedly want "reality"; so this is it!)

First-time mothers go home scared to death that they will be too weak, that they will drop their baby, pop their stitches, get an infection, and so on. The pain medicine has worn off; they have a bad headache and their whole body hurts; and a crying baby makes it worse. Mom may even be nauseated. Too bad. If she's nursing, she cannot take most medications.

In other words, it's not much like the TV version. Certainly there is no rubdown from the nurse armed with sweet-smelling lotion.

The bill, when it comes, arrives in dribs and drabs: The anesthesiologist's bill here, the obstetrician's bill there, the neonatal bill in another envelope, the hospital bill separately, and maybe three months later, a bill from an aide who helped the obstetrician. Oh, and another bill for any non-surgical medications dispensed over the day or two mom was there.

Prior to the 1950s, charity cases were handled by, well, charities. If a doctor knew the patient, and the community was fairly small, he shaved a few dollars from the bill, and neighbors and the church usually pitched in to cover the rest, usually without much profit to the doctor or the hospital. But wealthier patients often added a few dollars more to their bill, not because they had to, but because they knew it might come in handy when needy folks fell ill. Today, one cannot on the occasional philanthropist. Philanthropy today is more about grandstanding than quiet good deeds.

As technological marvels like CAT scans, MRIs, sophisticated laboratory equipment and "replacement therapies" increasingly became "givens," health evolved into a business rather than a "calling." Much of the personalization disappeared. Not surprisingly, that tended to make people— including those *not* accustomed to being "charity cases"—wind up waiting too long to seek medical attention.

Medical professionals and tech support staff who see guts and blood every day inhabit a completely different world, no matter how many TV dramas like *Grey's Anatomy*, *House* and *ER* have tried to desensitize the masses to gore. People still feel very queasy about own their bodies being poked, stabbed, probed and "prepped." Many of these queasy folks are the same ones who land in high-priced emergency rooms once they become too incapacitated to function, and with no primary-care doctor who can be consulted by ER staff.

What many ER patients discover when they hobble in is a backlog of generational welfare cases. In the interest of "fairness," they have to wait their turn behind at least the most life-threatening cases. They sit, pace or lie down beside noisy youngsters and indigent parents with communicable colds and flu—people who *routinely* use emergency rooms as their primary care office with no intention of paying for services.

Many uninsured, but working, patients who put off their symptoms die, whether they waited out of queasiness or concerns over out-of-pocket costs. Ever the optimists, they discover to their horror that they cannot access care because they can't get to a *primary* health care provider, much less a *specialist*, in time to save their lives.

The insured ER patient is better off than that, but still has to fill out innumerable forms that should already be in the system, such as address, phone numbers, Social Security number, birth date, known allergies, and a laundry list of previous surgeries, diseases and so on that all waste valuable time. They are usually asked the exact same questions again once they are lucky enough to get face time with a nurse's aide. If the insured patient comes in unconscious and on a stretcher, of course, he or she may get basic treatment, but until that insurance card shows up, the person is just another body in a backlog of cases.

That is why primary care is considered the most cost-effective way to provide individuals with the information and referrals they need to stay healthy. Of course, people become inconveniently sick outside of the business hours of 9 a.m. and 4:30 p.m. on weekdays, so, once again, they are told to go to the ER. But at least there is a point of contact, a primary-care physician, out there somewhere for consultation, and that's what turns just another human body into a real person.

When those not covered by insurance, and not linked to any primary-care physician, are hospitalized for what would normally be a treatable illness (had it not been exacerbated by waiting), he or she becomes an "indigent" patient—unless, of course, the patient can produce his checkbook or Medicare card on the spot. The costs to care for the indigent are sometimes subsidized by a few doctors who make a practice of donating a certain number of hours, weekly or monthly, to such cases, or by charities that give regularly to hospitals (usually religious charities)

But ever since hospitals became huge conglomerates competing for federal and foundation grants—not to mention the requirement for whiz-bang technologies just to pass muster—individualized attention has declined. This is a causative factor in the number and frequency of frivolous lawsuits.

Grants monies come with their own down-sides. A cancer wing, for example, may get grants based on how many patients they put on chemotherapy or radiation therapy. That being the case, they will try to talk as many patients as they can into these gruesome ordeals, even if the tumor appears to have been safely removed or, on the other side, if the cancer has spread so that the prospects for a good outcome are bleak. Many patients do not want—or even need—these treatments; yet, this author has seen persons badgered to death (literally) into suffering through what are, in reality, still experimental treatments—and horrendously expensive. Patients who refuse chemotherapy and radiation frequently get better on their own once a tumor is removed, and live long, fruitful lives with no further treatment necessary and no further cancer incidents. Many who have the treatments, on the other hand, die of the treatment or from a damaged immune system before they ever have to worry about another cancer.

All that said, health care *has* become an issue—as in "a major expense"—in a way that it was not in Theodore Roosevelt's day when he first broached the subject of universal coverage in 1912. But thanks to the above factors, plus 30 years of disastrous policy decisions not generally associated with medicine—coddling of illegals, generational welfare, out-of-control entitlement programs, contrived doctor shortages, etc.—medical expenses now consume a major part of the individual and family budget, surpassing even a mortgage. Thus, did health care morph into a full-blown crisis.

Remember the game: (1) Create a crisis, then (2) impose "reform." So, let us examine both the *pro* and the *con* side of universal health care.

A Case For *Government-Subsidized Health Care*

Those who supported Medicare, the failed HillaryCare, and now ObamaCare do so because they argue that "the market" doesn't work for health care.

Donna Dubinsky, an occasional columnist and chief executive of the software company Numenta, makes a convincing argument when she points out that if you want to join a health club, no one is going to turn you away, whether you are ill, obese or whatever. Yet, health insurers can and do. Or, take burial services, she says: Everyone, after all, will die at some point, so "no seller of [burial] services will turn you away."

Ms. Dubinsky reasons that if the market worked, the same would apply to health care. At some point, everybody gets sick or is injured, too.

But, she points out: In the absence of U.S.- government *subsidized* health care, insurers are mainly interested in selling to healthy people. They turn prospective purchasers away for any number of reasons.

In passing, she questions why government hasn't simply passed a law "requiring insurance companies to accept all applications." She answers her own question: That would not work, she says, because with only sick people seeking insurance, and healthy people waiting around until they become ill or injured, just the knowledge that coverage was assured would bring the health insurance "market" to a standstill. The program would become impossible to administer and overwhelmingly expensive.

Moreover, Dubinsky alleges that the only "rational business model" is to spread the risk. Forcibly spread it. Dubinsky bases her logic on the idea that the average person will not do the sensible thing—avail themselves of health insurance while they are young and healthy, knowing that, of course, nobody is healthy 100 percent of the time. Therefore, she says, health care does not itself to a market-based approach. She insists that a government-subsidy approach, while not perfect, is "the best shot we have."

Others on the *pro* side of government-subsidized health care debate agree. They point out that as recently as the 1960s and 70s, most couples with a middle-class income, or slightly above, were in no danger of losing everything with one major illness. By the 1990s, all that had changed, including for the insured. Even with no major outstanding debts—say, a mortgage, a car loan or unpaid credit card purchases—a major illness can quite literally wipe out a family's nest egg and throw them into debt. If one has children or aging parents, the problem grows exponentially.

Take, for example, a young woman's kidney stone operation, complicated by intestinal dysfunction. While her interrelated conditions may be curable, they will require a series of "fixes."

Similarly, suppose an accident results in a person's jaw being cracked and loss of several teeth, requiring two years of surgery since not everything can be done at once. The jaw has to be set (wired shut), which means at least eight weeks for healing; adjacent teeth may have to be extracted, and bone grafts done. These grafts may not "take" the first time around, which means a re-do, with four months more of healing time before implant can be surgically inserted.

Here's what will happen with the insurance for our accident victim. The regular medical insurance will try to claim that the entire procedure is a dental issue and will decline to cover it. The dental insurance company will complain that the jaw was the problem and that, therefore, medical insurers should cover it. Back and forth it will go, endlessly, with a brand new piece of paper each time requesting "more information" (which is never enough). Every new graft, every temporary prosthetic and every anesthetic will be questioned. Bottom line: about $100,000 out of pocket for the patient, most of it not reimbursed.

As for young woman with the kidney stones, it will be messy and excruciating. Even so, pain medicines will meanwhile be questioned *ad infinitum* (the pain of a kidney stone is said to be worse than being in labor). The ordeal will be hugely expensive and time-consuming, with constant monitoring to avert infection. For this patient, the out-of-pocket expenses won't kick in until she realizes, belatedly, that she has used up all her insurance for the year, having signed up for the "standard" option because she was still young.

Moreover, only top-tier health-insurance investors get anything out of this scheme.

Elderly parents, aged 75 or older, generally do not have insurance because in their work days it either wasn't available, or most people just didn't think about it. In fact, most folks believed they had enough money to pay for their medical needs as they got older. And until about 1980, they did.

Moreover, proponents of subsidized health care argue that freak accidents and illnesses happen all the time, and one never knows; thus, it is better to spread the risk (actually, the *wealth*, via taxes) around so that average people wouldn't lose everything. They could get on with their lives, make money, be productive—even start paying taxes again.

Case **Against** *Government-Subsidized Health Care*

The greatest argument against government-subsidized anything, is that bureaucrats focus on costs and abstractions, not on actual people. National security, under that argument, lends itself to government oversight because of the immensity of defending the country, but as we know from experience with the Transportation Security Administration, once security concerns trickle down to common citizens, abuses start occurring and perspective disappears when it comes to respecting the individual. Virtually anything can be done to individuals in the name of "security."

So, what distinguishes health care, by definition, is its very personal nature, and that makes for a poor fit with decision-makers being thousands of miles away.

The following attempts by the federal government to institutionalize universal health care are, in themselves, proof that the government is not up to the job—even if the "health" of the individual really was a government priority, which it isn't.

Act I: Medicare

Senior citizens were the first demographic to be seen as at risk. Costs had risen to the point that seniors who thought they were set for life—no mortgages or car payments, children grown and employed—had a rude awakening, especially widows. The Golden Years seniors believed they had coming became less "golden" in an era when a couple of illnesses could wipe out their savings. Costs were passed along to their grown children, who had family obligations of their own.

So, in 1965 Congress created Medicare under Title XVIII of the Social Security Act to provide health insurance to people age 65. The Act was made responsible for determining Medicare eligibility and processing premium payments.

It was among the first hints that Social Security—the original "safety net" for the elderly—would require enormous influxes of cash once it was forced to handle a massive health program. For that reason, the SS# (an unfortunate acronym), became a *de facto* national ID. It was required every time you registered with a doctor's office, had lab work done, or were admitted into a hospital. From there, the SS# became compulsory for every type of document—medical or not.

Act II: SSDI, Medicaid, SCHIP, and CLIA

Medicare morphed—big time! In 1972, it was expanded to include younger people with permanent disabilities, individuals who received Social Security Disability Insurance payments, and those who had end-stage renal disease. Congress expanded Medicare again in 2001 to cover persons with amyotrophic lateral sclerosis (ALS, or Lou Gehrig's disease).

Today, the Centers for Medicare and Medicaid Services (CMS), which is a component of the Department of Health and Human Services (HHS), administers Medicare, Medicaid, the State Children's Health Insurance Program (SCHIP), and the Clinical Laboratory Improvement Amendments. Together with the Departments of Labor and Treasury, CMS also implements the insurance provisions of the Health Insurance Portability and Accountability Act of 1996 (HIPAA). That's the program which pretends to assure individual privacy, but doesn't; a virtually unread document every patient signs in order to pick up a prescription or see a new doctor. It is a paperwork nightmare that keeps family members from providing or receiving information that might help their loved ones.

Even the original proponents of Medicare, like the late President Lyndon B. Johnson, never imagined that Americans might lose the liberty even to *pay* for better medical care on their own dime. Medicare's ever-expanding boards, committees, vested interests, rules and new regulations (like

HIPAA), over the years has created a culture of de-personalization.

So, while those who insist "there is no health-care crisis" are mistaken indeed, that does not change the fact that government is now able to use the *hook* of health care to advance an agenda of a different sort.

Act III: HillaryCare

One of the more significant facets of the aforementioned HillaryCare in 1993 was the way in which the health insurance industry started playing both sides of what it assumed would be an inevitable government takeover (nationalization) of medicine.

On May 28, 1993, Bill Gradison, the head of the Health Insurance Association of America (HIAA), wrote to the First Lady, ostensibly to support "universal coverage." But he also used his letter to complain about Mrs. Clinton's public attacks on the health insurance industry for "price-gouging, cost-shifting and unconscionable profiteering"—all of which, no doubt, carried a kernel of truth. According to the aforementioned Lehrer/PBS "Timeline":

> [Gradison was] playing a double game. He wanted to diminish public support for a Clinton plan that might adversely affect the [insurance] industry, yet he also wanted to appear accommodating so that he would have input into in the reform bill, which he expected to pass.

This move has "agenda game" is written all over it. Although HillaryCare did not pass, the Clinton Administration laid the groundwork for what would come two decades later. It was the first aggressive attempt to socialize medicine, complete with accusations of internal disloyalty, closed meetings, "private negotiations," withholding White House logs, and professional stakeholders playing both sides of the fence. These maneuvers are eerily reminiscent of the internal power struggles that characterized the Stalinist regime, not the heated debates of the Framers of our U.S. Constitution, as outlined in the Federalist Papers.

As with ObamaCare, "employer mandates" and "individual mandates" were both bandied about during the HillaryCare debates, but health care and the costs associated with it had not yet reached "critical mass." Also, Americans were not as acclimated to socialism as they are today—whether it goes by that label or not.

To forestall a government takeover of medicine, the Health Insurance Association of America launched an advertising campaign against HillaryCare. The signature line from the now-classic Harry and Louise ads was: "They choose, you lose"—*they* meaning the government. HillaryCare got two thumbs down from just about everybody except the most left-leaning of the Clinton White House advisers—such as Ira Magaziner—and some far-left members of Congress.

The National Federation of Independent Business (NFIB) also knew a job-killer when they saw one, particularly the idea of an "employer mandate." The organization launched thousands of "Alerts" to owners of small businesses and conducted seminars nationwide. This time, the NFIB won. Twenty years later, small businesses would be in the position of paying a penalty, or "tax" for their trouble.

Act IV: ObamaCare

The same charges levied in 1993 against HillaryCare were the essentially the same as those against ObamaCare in 2012: Firms with 50 or more employees face a pseudo-tax penalty of between $2,000 and $3,000 *per worker* for failing to offer what the government considers "adequate and approved" medical insurance under ObamaCare.

Even though the U.S. Senate passed the Patient Protection and Affordable Health Care Act (a.k.a. "ObamaCare") in 2009, and the U.S. House in 2010, various states, numerous organizations and even individual citizens, started filing lawsuits in federal court challenging ObamaCare's constitutionality. In January 2012, two of four federal appellate courts had upheld it; a third declared the individual-purchase mandate unconstitutional, and a fourth ruled that the federal Anti-Injunction Act prevented the issue from being decided until taxpayers begin paying penalties for not purchasing health insurance in 2014.

The U.S. Supreme Court agreed to review the lawsuits beginning with *Florida v. HHS* (U.S. Dept. of Health & Human Services) March 2012. This was the very eventuality Mr. Obama had already been dreading for months. With a straight face and considerable *chutzpah*, Mr. Obama taunted the judges (via the media), saying that the High Court, with its "unelected judges," would be taking an "unprecedented, extraordinary step" if it overturned his health-care scheme, since it was enacted by "a strong majority of a democratically elected Congress."

Obama Reveals Disdain for the Constitution

Those Americans who took the trouble to listen up in their high school government class, were stunned that the same man who was once touted as "the smartest giant in town," was belittling Supreme Court judges for being "unelected" (as if he didn't know the Constitution was written that way), and talking as if striking down legislation passed by Congress was something unusual (it's what the Supreme Court does). For more than 237 years Supreme Court judges had been declaring laws passed either by Congress or the state legislatures unconstitutional whenever a valid challenge was issued. Indeed, the only thing "rare and unprecedented" was for a sitting president to comment on a Supreme Court case while the justices were still deliberating it!

ObamaCare had only cleared the House by *seven votes*, even though Democrats held a majority. In the Senate, the measure barely avoided a filibuster.

Congress Reveals Disdain for Its Job

Many members of Congress admitted they had really never read the text of ObamaCare before they passed it. At about 2,000 pages, the legislative monstrosity was 360 percent longer than the epic novel, *War and Peace*, and 2½ times as long as the Bible. Little wonder that former House Speaker Nancy Pelosi demurred in 2010: "We have to pass this bill [ObamaCare] so that you can find out what is in it, away from the fog of the controversy."

This isn't the first time laws have been passed largely unread by legislators, both at the federal and the state level (an example of the latter is a bill related to mental health screening of schoolchildren in Illinois). That most laws today are written, not by our elected representatives, but rather are drafted by lawyers and lobbyists, is one problem. Pressure to get a piece of legislation passed before the public gets wind of it, is another. One of our Constitution's Framers, James Madison, anticipated this very situation when he wrote in Federalist Paper #62:

> It will be of little avail to the people that the laws are made by men of their own choice if the laws be so voluminous that they cannot be read, or so incoherent that they cannot be understood.

Obama's High-Stakes Gamble to 'Protect' Women

With increasing rumblings of major lawsuits against ObamaCare in the wake of the Affordable Care Act's 2009-

2010 passage in Congress, the administration needed to come up with a whopping distraction to deflect public attention away from the constitutionality question. On January 20, 2012, Barack Obama, with the aid of Kathleen Sebelius, his appointed Secretary of the U.S. Department of Health and Human Services, came up with one: a "reform" mandate to "ensure women's access to reproductive health."

This proposal brought new meaning to the term "risky sex." The measure promised free contraceptives of every type and description: Depo-Provera injections (typical cost: approximately $600 a year); diaphragms (about $70 annually); sterilizations (a.k.a. "Band-Aid surgery" and vasectomies); and even free condoms. Obviously vasectomies and condoms apply to males, not females, but it was "sold" as part of the package to protect women's reproductive health nevertheless.

Thus the Obama administration set the terms of debate and the parameters of public perception—the two keys in any agenda game. Predictably, the proposal caused an uproar. Both fiscal and social conservatives—took the bait—hook, line and sinker.

The Logic Behind the Contraception Ploy

Many sensible people would ask: If Mr. Obama was truly worried about his signature legislative achievement coming under such heavy fire that it reached the U.S. Supreme Court and risked being overturned, then why would he suddenly launch a proposal for free contraceptives, something that was *sure to cause a furor*? Wouldn't this be political suicide?

Not if you think like a "community organizer" in the Marxist vein, which is exactly how Barack Obama had been groomed to approach politics back in Chicago! Indeed, this is *exactly what Barack Obama wanted*: everybody squabbling over the contraception mandate. It's the old conjurer's trick, again. Make your audience look at this outrageous mandate so they will miss the more important misuse of the Constitution going on under their noses. If they were thinking about the morality and the cost of employers assuring free contraceptive services, they wouldn't be paying attention to ObamaCare's use of the Commerce Clause!

Could the President and the HHS Secretary, working together, somehow ward off lawsuits against ObamaCare and finagle acceptance of the whole health care package *by appealing to women*?

The only way to find out was to try. The idea that the measure might be seen as "sanctioning promiscuity" did not faze them.

Although birth control is typically considered an elective "treatment" that most health insurers do not cover, the new spin as "preventative medicine" was untested in the courts. The Obama Administration argued that contraception was less expensive than an unplanned pregnancy or an abortion—to which the Catholics hooted, "What about 'morning-after' pills[7]?"

While the new mandate did take care to exempt churches and houses of worship *per se*, it did not exempt **employees of religious institutions**, such as Catholic and Baptist hospitals; religiously funded K-12 schools and colleges; and charities that are part of a *religious mission*, at least on paper for income-tax purposes.

Brilliant Risk, Or Fool's Errand?

"The Obama administration," announced Richard Land, president of the Ethics and Religious Liberty Commission of the Southern Baptist Convention, and his colleague Barnett

---

[7] Emergency Contraceptive Devices, or "ECPs," and all the variations on what is popularly known as "Plan B" ("RU 486," "Ella," etc.) are thought to be dual-purpose abortifacients, because they can interrupt pregnancy *after* conception has occurred, the window of time between intercourse and conception being extremely short.

Duke, vice president of the Baptist Ethics Commission, "has declared war on religion and freedom of conscience. We consider this callous requirement by the Obama administration to be a clear violation of our nation's commitment to liberty of conscience and a flagrant violation of our constitutional protection to freedom of religion."

Messrs. Land and Duke assured the Administration and the nation that Baptist institutions 'will not comply' with the Obama mandate requiring religious institutions to cover various birth-control devices in their health-insurance programs. The Catholics were even more livid, especially when they understood that the "morning-after" pill would be included.

Oh, dear.... How was the Administration going to play this?

On the one hand, the contraceptive mandate *was* a clear slap at religion, particularly the Christian religion, which still reflects the largest body of believers in America, if one were to do an actual head count. As if that weren't enough, it dealt a blow to the very concept of a free, ***personal conscience***, whether in the context of religion or not, because even in these sex-obsessed times, the general public still makes a passing show of disapproving casual sex and keeping government out of the bedroom. Add to that, the fact that free birth control for everybody, in an era when even marriage itself is being disparaged, is almost a sales pitch for promiscuity.

So, again, the question becomes: Why jeopardize the entire ObamaCare package, as originally written, over a new contraceptives measure that was bound to trigger a controversy?

The answer is that the diversionary tactic had to be outrageous if it was going to work—something that the administration could string out long enough to detract from the *Florida v. HHS* hearings once they started.

The "Accommodation" and "Clarification".- Mr. Obama didn't have long to wait for a lawsuit to make its way through the federal appeals process and on to a U.S. Supreme Court challenge. With less than a month away from Supreme Court hearings, the White House needed to "up the ante" on the distracting birth-control controversy. On Friday, February 10, 2012, Barack Obama feigned an "accommodation." Journalists, pundits and commentators covered the stern-faced Mr. Obama as he announced a "revised" policy.

In a tortured statement which took obfuscation to new heights, the President explained that he and Secretary Sebelius had reworked the mandate so that it would "protect religious liberties" (a ridiculously disingenuous notion) as well as secure a woman's **access** to contraception (which every woman in America already had!). The revised wording now required that *employers* provide female workers *access* to free "preventive care" services, but that (now, read this carefully), religious **employers** would *not* have to cover birth control for their employees. Instead, insurance **companies** would be responsible for providing free contraception.

Huh?

Well, let's quote directly from the White House statement. Maybe that will clear things up: Under the revised policy, women would still have:

> ...free preventive care that includes contraceptive services no matter where she works.... The new policy ensures that women can get contraception without paying a co-pay and fully accommodates important concerns raised by religious groups by ensuring that objecting non-profit religious employers will not have to provide contraceptive coverage or refer women to organizations that provide contraception.... [It] also ensures that if a woman works for religious employers with objections to providing contraceptive services as part of its health plan, the religious employer will not be required to provide, pay for or refer for contraception coverage. [Instead], "her insurance company will be required to *directly offer* her contraceptive care free of charge.

Still don't get it? Don't feel badly; it's all part of the game.

Let's take a clinical approach to this mumbo-jumbo (since we're on the topic of medicine anyway):

First of all, the insurance company will have to increase insurance *premiums* to any Catholic, Baptist or other religious hospital, school or charity in order to *cover the cost* of contraceptives. As indicated earlier on, somebody always has to pay…. Hence, the Catholic (or other religious) hospital, university or charity ultimately will *still be paying* for contraceptive coverage for its employees. Government may well be the new Almighty, but it still cannot force insurance carriers to pay for something without any premiums.

As for hospitals, religious or not, most are *self-insured*. So, hospitals may contract out the *paperwork*, meaning that hospital staff, *per se*, do not have to take the time to figure out all those medical codes, collate the charges, get invoices inside the envelopes and in the mail. But hiring a company to do paperwork is *not* the same as paying **premiums** for medical services, "preventive" or otherwise. As columnist Jonah Goldberg put it: "A Catholic hospital would still pay for services; there just wouldn't be a line item for it in the monthly insurance bill."

Moreover, the White House made no accommodation whatsoever! The Administration didn't "shift" any costs; it simply "laundered" the paperwork, so to speak, and allowed the public to jump to erroneous conclusions based upon most people's ineptitude for gobbledygook.

As one wag put it in a blog on Fox News' website, the logic behind the whole accommodation sounded "a little like mandating Jews to simply slaughter and provide pork in their hospitals but not necessarily eat it themselves."

By February 15, HHS Secretary Sebelius was again pretending to quell criticism by telling reporters that self-insuring church-affiliated employers would be exempted from the contraceptive-coverage mandate. That failed to mollify anybody very much. Under intense questioning by Senator Orrin G. Hatch (R-Utah), Mrs. Sebelius admitted she hadn't consulted with the Catholic bishops (or apparently any other clergy) before releasing the ever-evolving "new" versions of the mandate. She said she didn't know whether the President had done so, which most congressional colleagues took to mean "no."

Long into the following week, the decibel level of commentators, editorial writers and bloggers were, if anything, more shrill and strident. One headline screamed that there was "no end in sight" to the arguments and counter-arguments over the contraceptives mandate, "revised" or not.

So, the whole scheme was unraveling, right? Surely, people were figuring it out. And when they did, wouldn't they be really, really mad? Was a measure that required first "accommodation," then "clarification" really worth it?

The Commerce Clause Conundrum.- Constitutionalists who refused to be drawn into the free contraceptives debate were banking on the Commerce Clause as the downfall of ObamaCare. They were in for a rude awakening, but essentially, they were right. Mr. Obama's version of socialized medicine, unlike HillaryCare, *forces private individuals to **buy** something. Congress colluded in the deception by taking the bold step of enacting ObamaCare under the U.S. Constitution's Commerce Clause*—something that, unfortunately, had been watered down repeatedly by precedents set during previous cases already reviewed by the U.S. Supreme Court.

As originally written, the Commerce Clause gave Congress power only "to regulate Commerce with foreign Nations, and among the several States, and with the Indian Tribes." In other words, the Framers were trying to prevent the states from establishing trade barriers *against each other*.

Chip Mellor, president and General Counsel of the Institute for Justice, was among the first to highlight the pivotal role the Commerce Clause played in ObamaCare. He also called attention to an even sneakier move that most other analysts missed in Congress' 2010 passage of ObamaCare: a backdoor attempt to increase its power over individuals by *compelling* them to perform an activity that would necessarily entail federal oversight. In effect, Mellor writes, Congress was telling the public: "We are going to force you to engage in commerce so we can regulate you."

In a brilliant piece for *Forbes* magazine's February 13, 2012 issue, Mr. Mellor explained how the Commerce Clause operated precisely the way the Framers wrote it—until 1938, which was during America's first liberal-left administration, the popular "Depression-wartime" presidency of Franklin D. Roosevelt. That was when, writes Mellor, the U.S. Supreme Court decided the case *Wickard v. Filburn*, which "effectively amended the Constitution by turning the Commerce Clause into an affirmative grant of federal authority allowing Congress to regulate *any economic activity that has a 'substantial effect' on interstate commerce* [emphasis mine]."

Mellor goes on to explain how this innocuous-sounding decision (at least as far as the public understood it) actually gave a tremendous boost to federal agencies looking to extend their regulatory tentacles into as many realms as possible—"the environment, energy, civil rights, transportation and education."

Congressional authority got another boost from the Commerce Clause under George W. Bush's administration in 2005. It was then that the Court upheld the Controlled Substances Act in *Gonzales v. Raich* and allowed "prosecution of a cancer patient who used homegrown marijuana, which was [then] legal under California law."

You can hold any views you like on the dubious benefits of marijuana, but that is not the point. "The four justices who dissented [in that case] viewed this expansion of Commerce

Clause power as an unprecedented violation of federalism and the eradication of any line between federal and local authority," writes Mellor.

That is why, from a political gamesmanship viewpoint, *the "preventative reproductive health care" ploy was no risk whatsoever to the Obama administration. It was a throwaway issue because the Commerce Clause had already been expanded.* For the High Court to overturn its own rulings would be awkward, to say the least. President Obama and HHS Secretary Sebelius were betting, therefore, that the Affordable Care Act would not be stopped from the Commerce Clause angle. They were right. It wasn't.

This is a game the Left is very, very good at.

By the time the Supreme Court began oral arguments in the constitutionality of ObamaCare in March 2012, the news media realized they had been sidetracked and started focusing on the Commerce Clause. The contraceptives mandate was now treated more as a side dish, not the main course. Lawyers and lawmakers could hardly pen op-eds fast enough to argue the constitutional questions. If government could bring in socialized medicine under the benign-sounding moniker, Patient Protection and Affordable Care Act, then it could pursue federal powers that went *way* beyond health care, which is why both the Clinton and Obama administrations were so hot to do it.

Even though George W. Bush said he was utterly opposed to nationalized health care, his administration, too, sought to broaden federal health care via a senior citizen drug benefit ("Medicare Part D"). This, added to the Controlled Substances Act, had the effect of "growing" the government and negatively impacting the decision-making power of the individual.

As Justice Clarence Thomas famously put it in his dissenting opinion (*Gonzoles v. Raich*): "If the majority [in favor] is to be taken seriously, the Federal Government may now regulate quilting bees, clothes drives, and potluck suppers throughout the 50 States."

Justice Thomas was more right than he knew. Today, the State is in the process of regulating children's lemonade stands—applying hidden pressure on the individual states, such as New York and Maryland. New York fined a little girl and her parents $50 for not "registering" a lemonade stand, and Maryland levied a fine of a whopping $500 for the same. Once the "bugs" are out of this outrageous infringement of individual rights, such registrations will go national and the Feds can take regulation of neighborhood activities—"quilting bees, clothes drives, and potluck suppers"—to new heights, all in the name of "commerce."

Why more conservatives, in a Republican Bush administration, didn't balk back when the Controlled Substances Act was being debated and the *Gonzales v. Raich* case was being decided shows just how carefully the Left gauges its timing in promoting a statist agenda.

George W. Bush: Culpable or Clueless?

The Left knows good and well that most conservatives and traditionalists are troubled by talk of legalization of mind-altering drugs, including marijuana. Aging Boomers (George W. Bush included) remember all too well the volatile Aquarius Culture: "drugs and sex and rock 'n' roll," hippies and Flower Children of the 1960s and 70s. Later, in their adult years, saner heads among that generation worked to save themselves and their families from cars filled with recreational drug-users and downright addicts driving the wrong way down the same highways as older and wiser folks on their way home from work.

What they never imagined was that laws like the Controlled Substances Act, supposedly aimed at taking irresponsible potheads off the streets, would come back to bite them at the pharmacy! In seemingly no time at all, every person in America became suspect if he or she expected anything stronger than aspirin when they went home from surgery. Even the most reputable physicians and surgeons suddenly were afraid to prescribe any pain killer for more than a couple of days for fear that the Drug Enforcement Agency (DEA) would question their judgment and revoke their license, just to prove it could.

Like so many agencies in modern times, the DEA was on a "high" of its own. Ironically, it failed utterly in its stated mission to end, or even to stem, illicit drug use and addiction, much less curtail purchase of truly dangerous substances, such as heroin and crack cocaine; or to stop the flow of precursor ingredients from entering the country. If anything, the situation is worse than before there *was* a DEA.

George W. Bush actually created several openings for the Left, other than the Controlled Substances Act. Intentionally or not, he increased the ability of government to intrude into individual lives and the costs to government of health care.

Mr. Bush overhauled the way in which Part A and B of Medicare were processed and created a new Health Savings Account (HSA) statute in 2006 that replaced and expanded the previous Medical Savings Account law, by expanding allowable contributions *and employer participation.*

While some viewed the latter as a good thing—giving individuals a tax-incentive to save for unexpected medical emergencies—it also made for additional complexity and provided a wedge opening for the Left to force the involvement of employers, almost as if to prepare them for mandated coverage under a future Obama administration. But with some 12 million Americans enrolled in HSAs after a decade, providing much-needed relief for those educated enough to take advantage of it, public objections waned.

But President Bush's most damaging overstep went virtually unnoticed by the press and the public: He rammed a radical mental health screening mandate through the House Appropriations Committee in 2004. The bill came with the astounding misnomer: the New Freedom Initiative.

Is Everybody Nuts—Or Is It Just the President?

The New Freedom Initiative was a plan to screen the entire U.S. population for mental illness and provide a cradle-to-grave continuum of services for those identified as mentally ill or at risk of becoming so. Under the plan, the school would become the hub of the screening process, not only for children, but for their parents and teachers. There was even a component aimed at senior citizens. Initially, the project was so hush-hush that two officials were sacked for speaking to the press about it.

The "Trial Balloon" Game

Mr. Bush had set this up while still the Governor of Texas. This precursor endeavor, the Texas Medication Algorithm Project (TMAP), was a "trial balloon," which means a start-up venture (usually confined to one town or state) to assess the amount and type of resistance to an idea.

TMAP started in 1995 as an alliance of individuals from the pharmaceutical industry, the University of Texas, and the mental health and corrections systems of Texas. Eventually, the New Freedom Commission on Mental Health designated TMAP a "model" *medication treatment plan*, whereupon George W. Bush, as President instead of Texas governor, instructed more than 25 federal agencies to develop a nationwide "implementation plan."

TMAP was funded via a Robert Wood Johnson Foundation grant—and several drug companies that stood to gain billions of dollars. The Robert Wood Johnson Foundation is the philanthropic (read: *public relations*) arm of the Johnson & Johnson medical-supply/household-products empire.

TMAP promotes the use of newer, more expensive antidepressants and antipsychotic drugs. For that reason, the Commission's nationwide version of the proposal sent up red flags in the Pennsylvania Office of the Inspector General. OIG employee Allen Jones blew the whistle when he revealed that key officials had received money and perks from drug companies with a stake in TMAP. Some members of the New Freedom Commission had served on advisory boards for the same pharmaceutical companies whose products were being recommended. Other members had indirect ties to TMAP. Jones was sacked for speaking to the *British Medical Journal* (BMJ) and *The New York Times*.

So much for free speech! This was not exactly the stuff of a national security breach—or was it?

"TMAP," said Jones, "arose during a period of decreased Food and Drug Administration (FDA) oversight and vastly increased sophistication in pharmaceutical industry marketing practices. These practices aggressively pursued favorable public and professional 'opinion' through media promotion and biased reporting of drug trial results."

TV Pushes Trendy Drugs

Most people can remember a time when prescription drugs were not advertised over the air waves. Simple over-the-counter remedies, such as the various brands of aspirin, were advertised, but not prescription-strength drugs. Not until after TMAP, that is. Between 1995 and 1999 the use of antidepressants for 7- to 12-year-olds increased 151 percent—and 580 percent for children under six, *with some as young as five committing suicide*.

The issue of coercive child-drugging in public schools eventually caused such a public outcry that the U.S. House of Representatives passed the Child Medication Safety Act in May 2003, to prevent schools from intimidating parents into drugging their youngsters as a condition of attending school. But it was too little too late, as teachers merely referred naughty and underperforming children to "counselors," who referred them to psychiatrists, as a condition of returning to the classroom. Most of these children came back with prescriptions for psychiatric drugs—to aid their concentration, to prevent fidgeting, to handle shyness.

This sort of misuse of prescriptive medicine undercut parents and all adults genuinely interested in instilling the concept of self-discipline in children. The psychopharmaceutical industry, meanwhile, went on a marketing binge. Suddenly, ads were pitched hyping one psychiatric drug after another. Soon, both children and adults were being prescribed virtual psychiatric cocktails—stimulants, anti-depressants, anti-anxiety medications, tranquilizers—all based on the notion that there was an imbalance of brain chemicals, such as serotonin or dopamine.

But whenever anyone tried to nail down the correct, natural amount of these brain chemicals—i.e., the range for "normal"—they were rebuffed. This should have been a red flag to the Food and Drug Administration that something was "off," that there might be ulterior motives at work. These drugs, of course, had to be covered under health insurance plans, even though most—especially antidepressants—were of questionable value. Even the advertisements for them pitched the now-familiar phrase "if your antidepressant alone is not enough…"

Catch-22 for Drug-Makers and Takers.- Even the suggestion of mental illness is a career-stopper. It is a recipe for losing all credibility. It goes without saying that such a stain on a child's permanent record could be a life-altering event, one that the student might not even know about until he volunteers for the military, or fills out an application for college, or seeks a job involving certain levels of security. Many former students find themselves inexplicably turned down. For example, some young men applying for the Marine Corps found that a drug like Ritalin on their record of prescribed medications, even for a short length of time in their past, could be grounds for rejection.

The Witch-Hunt Begins.- TMAP opened the floodgates for invasive, psychological questionnaires everywhere—schools, job applications, and more. For example, an applicant for a plainclothes position in California became a key figure in a class-action suit against Target stores. Apparently, the application form asked personal questions in such a way that a candidate was placed in a Catch-22 situation. No matter how the questions were answered, it could be interpreted as a proclivity for being dishonest. But as Alan M. Dershowitz, a Harvard law professor explained for a 1990 *Parade* magazine article: "Truly honest people reveal proclivities, [and therefore] have to fail the test."

By the time TMAP had morphed into the New Freedom Initiative, psychological questionnaires had become the opening salvo for marginalization of political opponents. Psychotropic drugs became a cottage industry—and government expense. The boost President Bush may have imagined Republicans would gain from the wealthy pharmaceutical industry abruptly turned into something quite different.

"Denial of Coverage" Gets Enhanced Definition

The closer one examines the Obama administration's Affordable Care Act, the more surprises one encounters. One is the Independent Payment Advisory Board.

Most people know that once they reach age 65 they get a Medicare card from the government, which then becomes the primary insurance. Whatever insurance one already carries becomes the secondary insurer—unless one declines Medicare Part B, which applies specifically to physician services, but not hospitals. Hospitalization has become enormously expensive, so most folks do not decline Part A, unless they are wealthy enough to locate one of the elite hospitals that don't accept Medicare patients. At issue, then, is what happens when coverage for a particular procedure is denied. One may be covered, technically, but both Medicare and the private insurance carrier can still deny payment, especially in-patient care.

Here's how this plays out in real time: A 72-year-old woman in Texas had emergency surgery to remove her gall-bladder. Such operations are performed in a hospital and are covered by Medicare.

The woman's daughter, meanwhile, was 3,000 miles away and could not get to Dallas to care for her mother until two days later. Having talked to the surgeon and fully expecting her mom to be discharged *after* the plane had landed, the daughter was shocked to get a call from the Dallas apartment manager later that afternoon saying that her mother was home and in bed. A family friend had taken her mom home, but had had to leave soon thereafter.

The daughter immediately dialed her mother's number, and listened to the same incoherent ramblings she'd heard just a few hours after her mother's surgery in the hospital.

Here was an elderly patient with tubes still sticking out of her (which needed regular emptying and cleaning), all alone in her room. Furious, the daughter called the doctor and was told that Medicare rules dictated that a patient with that particular surgery (now reduced to a code number on a piece of paper) can only be held for a certain amount of time. The doctor explained that he could lose his license unless he abided by the rules. The daughter reminded him that she had offered to pay for any extra time in the hospital. The doctor responded that *there was no option for paying extra for lengthier hospital care under the rules.*

This brings new meaning to "denial of coverage." It's not how most people think of that term.

The daughter ended the conversation with the thinly veiled threat that if her mother fell on the way to the bathroom in her present condition, he'd have more to worry about than his license. To his credit, the doctor personally called his patient early the next morning to be sure she was okay. The daughter hired some help via long distance and arrived a few hours later. She cleaned tubes, administered medication (including injections of blood thinner), fixed something her mother could eat, brought in a potty chair for next to the bed, scrubbed vomit, and all the things which, back in 1960, hospital staff would have done as post-operative care.

This incident occurred in 1997. It is much worse today. Certain surgeries, such as repairing a badly torn rotator cuff (on the shoulder), including insertion of biodegradable anchors to hold everything in place, is done on an out-patient basis. Neither Medicare nor most private insurance plans pay for that type of surgery to be done in a hospital, much less keep the patient overnight, as it is considered "routine." Turns out, this is probably the most painful type of orthopedic surgery there is, much worse than knee replacements.

When it is already established that the patient cannot tolerate pain medications taken by mouth, or that complications like a propensity for blood clots exist, and that the patient will likely be vomiting all night, complete with a useless arm—well, that's too bad. The patient can get up and go to the ER. Even if one offers to pay the *difference* to be in a properly staffed hospital, the answer may be "no," the carrier will not pay. The insurance company is willing to risk paying for an emergency room visit. The "rules" are....

With these real-life scenarios in mind, consider the eye-opening article written on March 6, 2012, for the *Washington Times* by Dr. Jane Orient, executive director of the Association of American Physicians and Surgeons. In it, she addresses the issue of "death by Medicare rationing," especially as it applies to the Independent Payment Advisory Board. Citing "the absolute power that is vested in an unaccountable 15-member oligarchy," she wrote:

> The key, unasked question which Congress, Medicare and the AMA [American Medical Association], are trying to duck, is whether Americans have the right to spend their own money to obtain necessary, lifesaving care, even if "covered" (but denied) by insurance. Or must they be at the mercy of the Centers for Medicaid and Medicare Services, the Department of Health and Human Services, Blue Cross or other insurer, the Independent Payment Advisory Board or its successor?

Well, surely, you say, there's an appeal process. But Dr. Orient soon disabuses us of that notion: "[T]here is no point in investing years and millions of dollars in taking the Board's decisions to the Supreme Court. Congress has ruled out any review of its *diktats*, either administratively or judicial." ObamaCare, of course, is now cast in concrete. All the talk about repealing ObamaCare after the U.S. Supreme Court has already decided the case belongs in Fantasyland.

Dr. Orient goes on to discuss the complex details of the Medicare Payment Review Commission and its Resource-Based Relative Value Scale, which physicians must adhere to. Imagine: a "value scale" placed on a living, breathing human being! How many people even know such a thing exists?

Dr. Orient further explains how the AMA actually "owns the [medical] codes that determine whether Medicare can pay for a procedure." Then, there's "the AMA/Specialty Society Relative Value Scale Update Committee, which determines how Medicare values shall be divided." After reading about all these "value scales," it is an open question as to whether the individual patient is any longer valued at all.

Business Community Throws In the Towel

With the Supreme Court having upheld ObamaCare and new "tax" penalty soon to be levied on entrepreneurs and small businesses, many company heads realized that, unlike with HillaryCare in 1993, this time they had lost. Even before the

Supreme Court decision, a May 3, 2012, *Washington Times* editorial was saying that 2014, when the tax/fine penalty kicked in, "businesses are likely to find it more cost-effective to pay the government penalty than to provide insurance to their employees."

Small business owners stood to lose millions or even face bankruptcy—especially those with fewer than 50 employees. Few small businesses can withstand a whopping $2,000 to $3,000 *per worker* for so-called "noncompliance." A figure that large would have to be passed along to consumers. This, in turn, would affect shareholders and investors in the form of lower profits.

Added to the predictable avalanche of new regulations and paperwork, business leaders could foresee that the government takeover of health care would erode any capital that might otherwise go into investment, new jobs or pay increases.

"ObamaCare has already generated some 10,000 pages of rules and regulations," wrote Steve Forbes in his December 2011 editorial for *Forbes Magazine*, also before the 2012 Supreme Court decision. It didn't take a brain surgeon to figure out that entrepreneurs would start depending more on part-timers, to whom the new mandate did not apply.

Many business heads started downsizing. Others closed up shop, stopped expansion projects, or declined to start up new firms at all, leaving other countries to take advantage and fill the gap.

The "Wellness" Game

The objective of any debate about health care today boils down to *cutting costs*. In patient terms, this increasingly means keeping a sick individual out of the hospital and only briefly in counsel with a physician. The whole emphasis on "wellness" is phony, as pre-emptive treatment for major health problems down the road are no longer covered—usually with the excuse that they are "unnecessary."

For example, when a patient complains of limb or joint pain, even clear X-ray evidence that the limb or joint in question is malformed or deteriorating frequently is not acted upon, or "covered." Some five years later, corrective treatment either comes too late or is hideously expensive compared to what it would have been when the patient first complained.

The "complete patient workup" may translate to check-marks being placed beside a laundry list of illnesses, past surgeries and known allergies. But even though it is technically easier than ever before to cross-check these findings via computer, both for accuracy and implications, this is rarely done, in the name of cost-cutting.

In an op-ed for *The Washington Times* by Dr. Richard A. Armstrong, chief operating officer of Docs4PatientCare, revealed on February 15, 2012, that Mr. Obama's Affordable Care Act "rewards physicians for skimping on treatment."

> The law promotes a 'new' model, the Accountable Care Organization (ACO), in which an entity that covers a specified number of Medicare patients is given a fixed pot of money. …if the doctors can provide care for less than what is in the pot over a defined period, they get to share the leftovers. If, however, the doctors overspend the pot, they are financially liable for the consequences.

Dr. Armstrong discovered this "sleight of hand" in an article published in the *Journal of the American Medical Association* (JAMA) by lead author Dr. Ezeliel Emmanuel. It seems that in the article, Dr. Emmanuel (a bioethicist, of all things) was actually trying to persuade private-practice physicians that they would, in Dr. Armstrong's words, "enjoy expanded autonomy and greater liberty under the new act [ObamaCare]."

Welcome to the "new ethics" of modern medicine.

The Food Police

Every first Lady, of course, has to have a gimmick, and Michelle Obama's is obesity. Not satisfied with having schools teach about the major food groups and their merits, she "evolved" her cause into nightmarish quest to inspect school lunches. Indeed, the food police at one school recently examined the contents of a pupil's lunch sack and, finding a nicely wrapped turkey sandwich, compliments of mom, threw it out in disgust and exchanged it for, of all things, chicken nuggets—which, last anyone heard, contained the dreaded "f" word: **f-r-i-e-d**. Who knows? Maybe the food police boil them. Plain. Without salt.

Often wrong but never in doubt, progressives and do-gooders develop amnesia about the past 40 years of regulatory activism. Even when progressives get it wrong, they never recant.

Something *Stalinesque* in the Air

Whether the government chooses to fixate on sugar, trans-fats, obesity, substance-abuse, contraceptives, health-insurance mandates, Medicare, mental-health screening, the mom-packed lunch sack, or outright denial of treatment, we see the same agenda game at work: *health* in the service of bigger, more intrusive, government.

That said, perhaps it is appropriate to end this chapter with an observation made by the aforementioned Dr. Jane Orient (American Association of Physicians and Surgeons) toward the end of her column on Medicare and the Independent Payment Advisory Board. She noted, chillingly, that "when Josef Stalin decided to starve the Ukraine, he confiscated all the food…or destroyed it. He made it a crime to buy, sell, or exchange things for food. [So,] the vast majority simply perished of deprivation—the ultimate consequence of socialism."

Apparently, more than one author senses something *Stalinesque* in the air.

~

CHAPTER 3
THE BUDGET GAME

...if I were the federal government, assuming you could wave a magic wand and pull everybody together, [I'd] pass a law letting immigrants come in as long as they agreed to go to Detroit and live there for five or 10 years. *--New York Mayor Michael Bloomberg, on* **Meet the Press,** *promoting the idea of immigrant "savants" jumpstarting the American economy by starting businesses here.*

Barack Obama spent his first term "transforming" America with an agenda of redistributionist economics and government–controlled health care. The nationalization of health care was at the top of his to-do list because he figured that once this largest sector of the economy was under federal control, then bailouts for other large-sector items, such as the housing, auto and banking industries (all calculated failures thanks to bad policymaking over the years) would encounter less resistance and hasten America's move into European-style socialism.

This view, unfortunately, is restricted to Obama administration liberals or leftists. European-style socialism has had advocates on both sides of the political aisle for a long time. Ambassador Gerald P. Carmen, a former chairman of the New Hampshire Republican Party during the Reagan years, pointed out in a January 30, 2012, piece for *The Washington Times*: "The cocktail party set [as far back as the Reagan Administration] thought capitalism was the past and socialism the future...."

Meanwhile, the United States had not had a federal budget, as required by law, for three years running. The lack of a federal budget for that length of time comes with distinctive consequences: Without itemized priorities and financial stability, a nation can be derailed and "turned." When long-existing procedures and guidelines no longer apply; when kickbacks, waste and institutionalized fraud become the orders of the day; when high unemployment, marketplace uncertainty, and a dwindling base of general business activity become increasingly permanent features on a nation's landscape, that country is easy pickings for regime change—which means a whole lot more than getting a new president.

The once-mighty economic engine that characterized our country—the lone symbol of individual opportunity in a world geared toward group goals—is stagnating. The Baby Boomer generation was the last to be able to aspire to the living standards of their parents—and even they were in for a reality check once they became middle-aged. Even with good, professional jobs, those of the sixties-generation Boomers who had had the benefit of private schooling, for example, suddenly discovered that the cost of the same schools were out of reach once they sought to enroll their own children. Poor policy decisions in the service of a socialist agenda, snowballed over the years—at a time when the United States was surrounded by terrorist regimes, infiltrated with "civilized jihadists," overrun with taxpayer-funded lobbyists for Big Government projects, a sputtering Federal Reserve, a European economy in shambles, and a U.S. regulated beyond what the entrepreneur could bear. Today, the U.S. stands at a juncture in time when we can least afford more failed entitlement programs, redundant projects, and far-fetched experiments: $16 trillion in debt, no federal budget for three years running, stripped of its AAA rating except for <u>Moody's</u> and <u>Fitch</u>), jobs escaping overseas, and college grads who get internships instead of entry-level jobs and then move back in their parents.

Thus, it is appropriate here to take on the complex topics related to the federal budget and the American economy. Having addressed health programs like Medicare and

Medicaid—together with all their various spinoffs (e.g., the State Children's Health Insurance Program, etc.)—we know that these programs are projected to grow faster than the economy overall because the population is both aging and increasing. The "Medicare Part D" drug benefit alone—part of President George W. Bush's Medicare Modernization Act of 2003—was projected to cost some $549.2 billion between 2006 (the first year the program started paying benefits) and 2015. With ObamaCare now deemed constitutional, that figure will be a drop in the bucket.

Economic Illiteracy

Barring some calamity—say, war or a life-altering birth defect—a person's financial independence is the result of responsible and intelligent decisions.

It would be helpful in discussing the national budget and debt, if all Americans had at least a passing familiarity with the terms and realities associated with basic economics, as well as some knowledge of the rules and regulations the President and Congress are expected to follow in hammering out the nation's budget each fiscal year.

Unfortunately, our nation's public schools, and even many private ones, do not teach the most elementary terminologies that govern financial matters, much less transmit economic legislative history. As for college graduates, unless they majored in economics or business, they have only the haziest grasp of fiscal realities.

Consequently, increasing numbers of Americans today believe *self-sufficiency* is unattainable (if not downright mean-spirited) and have replaced it—subconsciously, at least—with ethics like "interdependency" and "free-market socialism." The latter is an oddball combination of extreme regulation, high taxes, large entitlement expenditures—but with a robust stock-market! Such an ambiguous core belief system makes it easy to for the Left to sell the notion, for example, that the main drawback of Rep. Paul Ryan (R-WI) as a vice-presidential candidate was that he would trash the nation's "social safety net," or Joseph Biden's goofy claim to a majority-black audience in Virginia on August 14, 2012, that relaxing some regulations on Wall Street "[is] going to put y'all back in chains." ("Y'all"? A fellow from Delaware? How patronizing…)

The trouble is, most Americans, regardless of ethnicity, wouldn't bother to read what Ryan actually said, or what Republicans proposed regarding Wall Street, even though accessing such statements and obtaining a liberal, centrist and conservative analysis on the issues has never been easier.

A Minimal Economic-Knowledge Base

To thrive in a market-based, free-enterprise society such as ours, every high school graduate should have at least a passing understanding of terminologies such as: *annuity*, appropriation, *capital asset*, *commodity*, *Consumer Price Index*, *deficit*, *default*, *fiscal year*, *Gross National Product*, *Gross Domestic Product*, *inflation*, *mandatory versus discretionary spending*, *prime rate*, *purchasing power*, *recession*, and *thrift industry*.

At minimum, all college graduates, whatever their major, should be familiar with the terms *budget authority*, *balance of payments*, *bracket creep*, *Bretton Woods System*, *capital gains*, *capital stock*, *central versus commercial bank*, *Continuing Resolution*, *deficit* (the six types), *derivatives*, *debentures*, *dollar value* (including *weak dollar* and dollar collapse), *intangible asset*, *price earnings ratios*, *stagflation*, and *trust*.[8]

Unfortunately, most young adults are doing well to balance their checkbook, as these topics are not deemed a priority either in high schools or undergraduate college programs.

---

[8] Definitions and explanations related to all terms can be accessed via http://www.answers.com, http://www.investopedia.com/terms or http://www.investorwords.com.

Without a common base of economic knowledge, it is nearly impossible to comprehend the dangerous game our nation's leaders are playing in busting the federal budget and turning what should be a national strength into an Achilles heel.

When it comes to how our nation's economy is supposed to work, the most frequent response, especially among younger adults is something along the lines that "America is based on free enterprise which means you can buy and sell what you want."

Such a statement is all well and good, but it does not explain why the fiscal year is different than a calendar year; it does not clarify why government cannot "create" jobs or wealth; it does not elaborate on anything related to a "trade deficit."

The freedom to "buy and sell what you want" fails to distinguish between a **budget resolution** and a **continuing resolution**—the latter having become, since 1974, the largest part of the "game" known as the Federal Budget. While most people know what an "asset" is, per se, when they hear the term "net asset value," their eyes glaze over. And we haven't even gotten to "capital*ism*" versus "capital*ization*" yet.

A survey by the Council for Economic Education (CEE)/State Farm Insurance found that in 2010:

- Only 19 states required the testing of student knowledge in Economics, four *fewer* than in 2007.

- The number of states that required students to take an economics course as a high school graduation requirement increased from 17 in 2007 to 21 in 2009—less than half of U.S. schoolchildren.

- The number of states that required students to take a personal finance course (or personal finance included in an economics course) as a high school graduation requirement increased from seven in 2007 to a measly 13 in 2009.

- Only five states required entrepreneurship to be included as a component of a high school course in 2009, up from just three in 2007.

Such lack of information has ramifications at election time—as well as for personal financial independence. A nation's voting public is operating from a position of weakness when a whole range of news items is lost on the majority of citizens: for example, reports (pro or con) relating to Goldman Sachs,[9] government bailouts,[10] deficits and the Gross National Product,[11] subprime lending and mortgages,[12] the excesses[13] of Fannie Mae and Freddy Mac, hidden taxes[14] the so-called housing "bubble,"[15] and the projected costs of ObamaCare.

America once encouraged small businesses, but unfortunately not business acumen. Some learn the financial ropes to invest their money in something more lucrative than a bank savings account, but they still remain hazy as to the *rationale* behind free-market economics—as well as their opposites, like socialism. Most schools do not require, for example, a study the two "biggies" of economic theory: free-market icon, Milton Friedman[16] or John Maynard Keynes (Keynesian) post-World War II economic model.[17]

---

[9] http://financial.washingtonpost.com/custom/wpost/html-qcn.asp?dispnav=business&mwpage=qcn&symb=GS&nav=el)

[10] http://www.economicpolicyjournal.com/2010/04/will-they-print-money-to-bailout-cities.html

[11] https://www.pay.gov/paygov/forms/formInstance.html?nc=1271991815942&agencyFormId=23779454

[12] http://www.calculatedriskblog.com/2010/05/965-of-mortgages-backed-by-government.html

[13] http://searchfinancialsecurity.techtarget.com/definition/Dodd-Frank-Act and http://www.thefiscaltimes.com/Articles/2012/08/14/Why-Ryan-Wants-to-Dump-Fannie-and-Freddie.aspx#page1

[14] http://www.heartland.org/full/27485/Regulation_The_Huge_Hidden_Tax_We_Pay_for_Government.html)

[15] http://www.huffingtonpost.com/2010/05/03/greenspan-wanted-housing_n_560965.html)

[16] http://en.wikipedia.org/wiki/Milton_Friedman

[17] http://en.wikipedia.org/wiki/Keynesian_economics

The Sky That Fell: Obama's Debt Ceiling

Congress established an "out" of sorts on spending about the time the U.S. entered World War I, giving the federal government approval for most types of borrowing—as long as the total was less than an established limit, called a *debt ceiling*. Ironically, this was aimed at allowing for more flexibility, so that Congress would not have to specifically approve additional borrowing each time something important came up. Until recently, the Treasury has never been unable to make payments as a result of reaching the debt limit.

But today the U.S. has long since broken the $14.3 trillion National Debt Ceiling. With the national debt at about $16 trillion, every U.S. citizen (based on the latest census figure of upwards of 313 million people) owes $50,823.[18] The U.S. borrows some 43 cents for every dollar it spends, and that spending amounts to approximately $1 trillion per year more than we take in.

Unfortunately, as per the Government Accountability Office: "The debt limit does not control or limit the ability of the federal government to run deficits or incur obligations. Rather, it is a limit on the ability to pay obligations already incurred."[19]

As a result, the liberal-left has called for the debt ceiling to be abolished, while fiscal conservatives have redoubled their efforts to enact a constitutional amendment to balance the budget. As of August 2012, the U.S. Senate had still refused to raise the debt ceiling—meaning the government could default on its obligations, which would be unprecedented in American history and create more chaos in the global market.

To pay off the existing $16 trillion, even over 20 years, means the government would have to cut at least two-thirds

---

[18] http://www.brillig.com/debt_clock/ as of Aug. 15, 2012
[19] Government Accountability Office (February 22, 2011). "Debt Limit: Delays Create Debt Management Challenges and Increase Uncertainty in the Treasury Market"

from the elusive annual federal budget. There is plenty to cut, but the vested interests in agencies nobody needs and livelihoods spent in busywork make cuts nearly impossible. Take, for example, the following absurdities, just a few among hundreds of similar tax-dollar sprees. (Some of these were especially selected for their obscure titles, meaning you have to look them up even to know what they are for, or they sound like something they are not):

- Federal properties the government does not make use of -- $15 billion total savings.
- Death gratuities for Members of Congress. Exact amount unknown.
- Mohair Subsidies -- $1 million annual savings.
- Presidential Campaign Fund -- $775 million savings over ten years.
- USDA Sugar Program[20] -- $14 million annual
- Title X Family Planning -- $318 million annually. Subsidies to the U.N. Intergovernmental Panel on Climate Change -- $12.5 million annual savings.
- Department of Energy Grants to States for Weatherization[21] -- $530 million annually.
- Fund for Ireland -- $17 million annually.
- Legal Services Corporation (free legal aid to those "eligible" while average people pay a fortune) -- $420 million annually.
- Hope VI Program (public housing via HUD-- $250 million annually.
- Biofuel subsidies, including corn-based ethanol fuel[22] and "cellulosic ethanol" (which doesn't exist commercially) – set at $400 billion between 2008 and 2022.

---

[20] This product of the 1981 Farm Bill, consists of a domestic commodity loan program that sets a support price (loan rate) for sugar and establishes an import quota system that restricts foreign competition and ensures a high domestic price for sugar. Instead of a more stable sugar economy, the result is higher prices for everything that contains sugar.

[21] This is not an infrastructure program.

- Duplicative education programs – some 68 at about $1.3 billion annually
- HHS Fatherhood Initiative -- $75 million annually
- Claims Resolution Act of 2010[23] -- $150 million annually.
- Economic Development Administration[24] -- $293 million annually.
- National Organic Certification-Share Program[25] -- $56.2 million annually.
- Ready to Learn TV Program -- $27 million savings.

Some administrations have tried overhauling agencies—meaning they shut down various bureaus *within* agencies. But, then, they always create new bureaus and offices. This means, basically, shifting employees around while trying to close out certain jobs as employees retire (called *attrition*).

Over the past 25 years, even when conservatives manage to pick up enough seats to predominate in the state legislatures or win a few governors' races, it usually reflects a temporary disillusionment on the part of cash-strapped voters rather than a commitment to turning the leftist tilt of government. So, even if something like Paul Ryan's "Path to Prosperity" and the proposed cuts listed above by Republicans were to be pushed, or if Mr. Romney makes good on his promise to build a new mentality in government, it is no longer enough to replace one face at election time with another. The special interests have dug in their heels.

As soon as the newer face becomes too familiar, as inevitably happens, then next time around there is an even harder turn toward the Left, followed by more "pork" spending,

---

[22] With the Midwestern drought of 2012, the price of our best *food* crop, corn, will now rise precipitously and permanently with the redirection of a food crop into questionable biofuel efforts.

[23] For "healthy marriage promotion": Yep, the same marriage that is now on the chopping block as the definition of "marriage" changes.

[24] Not actually for economic development in the usual sense: It's a public works and job training since 1965 bill that started under Johnson Administration

[25] "Organic" has become a slogan that translates mostly to higher prices, not "safer food."

more regulations, more restrictions and taxes—almost as if to "make up for" years when conservatives were in office.

A 2011 report in *The Washington Times* carried an inset showing the last few election cycles for one state in which Democrats controlled both houses of the state's legislature with the exception of one election cycle, when Republicans happened to win control. The inset showed the tax bite *increasing* with each successive cycle of Democratic rule, then went down slightly under the lone Republican administration. But once the Democrats regained control, one could see that an even larger-than-usual rise in taxes occurred—*almost exactly enough to "make up for" the one cycle when Republicans were in power.*

One can see the scenario repeating on a national level. One administration "sets up," as it were, the next, always promising a turn-around. The general public, with its short-lived memory and basic inexperience on economics, plays hopscotch, ever more leftward.

Playing Dodge-Budget

The annual federal Budget has become a game in its own right. It's aimed, as all games are, at expanding government. In this regard, the federal budget is in a league by itself: It allows Congress and the President to fuel dependency *and* intrude into people's lives simultaneously!

In every election cycle, sectors of the population that are up-for-grabs hear what their "betters" *think* they want to hear. Thus, one Continuing Resolution after another aimed at avoiding a "shutdown of the federal government" like one engineered in 1995 by then-House Speaker Newt Gingrich under the Republican Party's Contract with America to counter Bill Clinton.

Gingrich thought he had public support for this hardball tactic. What he didn't count on was the strength of unionized government (their paychecks above all else!) and the public's shift in values—namely, convenience over principle. If people couldn't get into their favorite museum, that was a disaster!

The debacle pretty much finished Gingrich as an effective leader, but it proved that Americans as a whole had already moved to the Left, whatever else they might say in polls and surveys.

With the Obama administration, it was one gimmicky sound-bite after another: the Penny Plan, the Buffett Rule, the Payroll-Tax Holiday, Too Big to Fail, and more. Nobody really won, of course. Costs were neither cut nor saved; rather, they were shifted around, with new entitlements—and debt—piled on.

The Payroll Tax Game.- In the months leading up to the 2012 primary season, the President and Congress lathered up the media with arguments over a "payroll tax cut." Practically no one realized that this was a calculated move by Democrats to exploit a bad economy, mark their territory, and at the same time, manage to score brownie points with the public. Republicans, of course, took the bait, which temporarily deflected attention from the lack of a federal budget.

The first problem was that too few understood the term "payroll tax" as such. They knew it as "withholding tax."

A payroll tax is your contribution to Social Security and Medicare: 15.3 percent of your salary, up to a pre-determined limit, half of which is paid by your employer. Payroll taxes are the taxes withheld by an employer from an employee's paycheck. It covers the appropriate amount of federal and state taxes as well as the FICA (Social Security) tax.

These taxes are held "in trust" and submitted *on behalf of* the employee to the various entities above on a quarterly basis. It is this sum that is determined by the amount of deductions you claim on your W-4 Form. If too much tax is collected, you will receive a refund at the end of the year after filing a tax return. If not enough taxes are paid, a debt is owed by the employee to the IRS and/or at the end of the year.[26] Many people pay more in payroll taxes than they do in income taxes.

What? How's *that*?

That is the reason so many people were confused by the term. According to the Glossary in *Moneychimp*, the payroll tax isn't a true "tax" in the sense that *it is not supposed to be a source of revenue for the government*; rather, it's *supposed* to be a contribution to an account that you'll be entitled to withdraw at a later date, from benefits (if they happen to still be around).

For that reason payroll taxes generally aren't included in discussions about cuts. The only way you can get a cut in your "contribution" is to (a) accept a corresponding cut in benefits, (b) have your benefits subsidized by somebody else, or (c) reform the system.

Got it? Team Obama didn't think you would, so he proposed:

Payroll Tax Holiday.- This so-called "cut" to the payroll tax began in 2011 by taking money from the Social Security system—again (remember… "Robbing Peter to pay Paul"). The "cut" reduced the Social Security withholding rate from 6.2 percent to 4.2 percent. The idea was that people *would eagerly spend this money instead of saving it, thereby spurring the economy with increased demands for goods and services.* This, of course, is the reverse of supply-side logic. It is demand-side logic for spurring a floundering economy.

Retailers and other companies were expected to respond by increasing production—and by hiring employees. But by the end of the year, the economy was not only still sluggish, but unemployment was still around 8.3 percent.

Actually, in real terms, unemployment was higher than 8.3 percent. If you add in the percentage of people who had thrown

---

[26] http://wiki.answers.com/Q/What_is_payroll_taxes#ixzz1svWXsqao.

in the towel along with the underemployed (contract workers, part-timers, etc.), then the figure hovers around 20 percent.

Some lauded Mr. Obama's payroll tax-cut idea because it appeared that the government was "allowing" people to keep more of their own money (how kind!). But upon closer examination, the temporary nature of the "holiday" was not exactly an inducement for people to splurge on high-ticket items like cars and homes.

As Paulette Minter, a finance-investing columnist, put it in a February 7, 2012, article for the *Washington Times*: "The classic way to increase productivity is to innovate, or develop new technologies that allow us to produce the same product or service at less cost." Handing out dollars in the hope that people who are already "maxed out" will spend even more, instead of saving, is not even a responsible idea.

Thus the five-month argument, which ended with the Republicans caving, as usual, on a revised gimmick:

The Payroll Tax Cut Compromise.- This "deal" to extend the 2011 Payroll Tax Holiday from 2011 was shot down in February 2012. However, it was axed, the deal renewed the 2-percentage-point payroll tax cut for 160 million U.S. workers through the end of 2012. For a family earning $50,000 a year, the cut supposedly would "save" them $1,000 annually—and would "save" the economy even more if they spent it!

The $150 billion package also would renew expiring jobless benefits for millions of long-term unemployed <u>and</u> prevent a steep pay cut for doctors treating elderly Medicare patients. (Team Obama likes to bundle as many "benefits" together as it can get away with.) Never mind that Mr. Obama's insistence on the short-term payroll tax cuts *raised Social Security's 2011 deficit to $148 billion*, the second-largest single-year decline since 1983. Thus, no gain here…

So, Mr. Obama got by, sort of, with one more game, figuring, as always, that because the majority of Americans understand so little about the economy, he would be able to play it as "more money in people's pockets," and pick up votes. Republicans who went along also decided that sticking to their principles on spending cuts wouldn't make a lot of difference in a climate of ignorance about national finance. If they were going to stick their neck out, it would be on a battle that would give them more bang for the, er, buck.

The Buffett Game.- Billionaire investor/elitist and ardent Obama supporter, Warren Buffett, feigned shock in March of 2012 that his secretary paid more in taxes than he did. Whereupon, he proffered a plan that would require individuals earning $1 million or more a year to pay at least 30 percent on their income taxes. Congressional tax analysts, however, estimated that this would only bring in only about $31 billion over 11 years. It would barely make a dent federal budget deficit projected for the same timeframe.

A February 14, 2012, *Washington Times* editorial aptly pointed out that even if the President managed to raise taxes on businesses and "the wealthy" to 100 percent, that would still not be enough to overtake the red ink on Medicare alone. Mr. Obama had already proposed increasing the tax on capital gains to 30 percent—a job-slayer.

Predictably, the Senate, including one Democrat, blocked the Buffett Rule legislation on April 16, 2012.

Deficit Versus Debt

The above discussions may produce some confusion concerning *debt* and *deficit*. Accessing this particular distinction online, not to mention the actual numerical figures for the Obama administration, is guaranteed to drive the reader crazy. So, the following provides a simplified, if "quickie," explanation.

The federal **deficit** and the federal (a.k.a. *national*, or *public*) **debt** are two different things. They are not synonymous.

Budget deficit is an annual number reflecting the budget passed by Congress minus the revenues (mostly taxes) received by the Government (except that Congress has not passed a budget in over three years, which complicates matters). The national debt is the current sum of these annual budget deficits.

What happens is that <u>cumulative</u> <u>annual</u> budget deficits become the ***national debt***. As of August 13, 2012, the **National Debt** stood at just under $16 trillion—an unprecedented figure. Mr. Obama's 2012 budget *proposal* (not passed) would have added another $6.4 trillion to that debt over 10 years. However, he had already run up about $5.1 trillion in debt during his first term.[27] This averages out to $4.2 billion of additional debt per day.

The term *deficit* is typically used to indicate a shortfall in revenue, or the amount by which the federal government's total budget outlays (expenditures) exceed their total receipts (income) for a fiscal year.

The <u>government budget deficit</u> is of various types (for expanded definitions, see the website in the footnote[28]):

- <u>Deficit spending</u> -- spending money the government does not have
- <u>Primary deficit</u> -- the deficit derived after deducting the interest payments
- <u>Structural and cyclical deficit</u> -- parts of the public sector deficit
- <u>Income deficit</u> -- difference between income and payouts
- <u>Trade deficit</u> -- when the value of imports exceed the value of exports

---

[27] http://www.washingtonpost.com/blogs/fact-checker/post/obama-and-the-national-debt-the-latest-crossroads-gps-ad/2012/06/06/gJQAAmjOJV_blog.html

[28] For additional information on most of them a concise source can be found at http://www.answers.com/topic/measures-of-national-income-and-output#ixzz1su3vf HQr.)

- <u>Balance of payments</u> deficit -- when a tally of government payments are negative

The **deficit** for 2012 was projected to be $1.5 trillion.[29] On February 13, 2012, Mr. Obama touted his second-term plans for a ludicrous $4 trillion deficit "reduction." But his proposed budget hikes told a different story—another $350 billion of *additional* stimulus spending, to try to spur job growth one more time!

A "Stimulating" Flop

The American Recovery and Reinvestment Act of 2009 (ARRA), also commonly referred to as "The Stimulus" or "The Recovery Act," was Barack Obama's response to the late-2000s recession. It was signed into law on February 17, 2009 at a price tag of $829 billion (later revised upward to $831 billion) with the promise of jumpstarting the economy, making infrastructure improvements, and maintaining some 3.5 million jobs over ten years. The Labor Department took $495,000 of the stimulus funds to pay a public relations firm to run TV ads on at least two cable channels hyping the administration's "green training" via Job Corps and "environmentally friendly" initiatives.[30] But since the ads generated no new jobs, and aired on stations that were more Obama-friendly than job-friendly, they were seen as an agenda game by such watchdog organizations as the Taxpayers Protection Alliance.

The stimulus not only failed to jumpstart the economy, but unemployment rose and green programs flopped. So far, no new or improved roads, bridges, power plants or other infrastructure enhancements can be tied to stimulus funds. At least $1 million

---

[29] http://www.americanthinker.com/2012/08/debt_drag.html and http://www.usgovernmentdebt.us/us_deficit composite
[30] http://wizbangblog.com/2012/08/23/obama-stimulus-bucks-paid-for-advertising-on-msnbc/ and http://www.washingtontimes.com/news/2012/aug/21/stimulus-funds-spent-obama-ads-olbermann-maddow/

in stimulus funds went overseas via an FCC contract[31] to London—another attempt at a "partnership" that created no U.S. jobs.

By late August 2012, every news outlet was wringing its hands over whether or not the economy was going to fall off a "fiscal cliff" by January 1, 2013. Between the Obama administration's reckless spending spree, the new health care law ($22 billion in new taxes for ObamaCare), and several kinds of tax relief provisions set to expire, Congress was being admonished to "do something"—anything!

Paradoxically, if defense spending was cut—always a favorite target of Democrats and left-leaning liberals—the economy would lose more than a million private-sector jobs, according the National Association of Manufacturers,[32] compromising the economy *and* national security. If Defense spending was increased—well, the economy couldn't afford it! Catch-22.

The stimulus was supposed to save existing jobs and create new ones almost immediately, in addition to stopping further economic deterioration. Secondary objectives included providing temporary relief for those most impacted by the recession, and investing in infrastructure, education, health, and "green" energy.

Just what category the online soap opera, "Diary of a Single Mom," fell under is anyone's guess. But according to a top news story in the *Washington Times* in December 2011 by Jim McElhatton, the $1 million in stimulus money for that brainstorm "came through an award by the Department of Commerce to One Economy Corporation...to help boost broadband Internet service in underserved areas across the country." A spokesperson for the corporation claimed such

---

[31] http://www.politicollision.com/story.php?title=fcc-sent-stimulus-funds-to-london-no-jobs-created-

[32] http://www.washingtonpost.com/business/capitalbusiness/dont-push-our-economy-off-a-fiscal-cliff/2012/07/13/gJQAb18tmW_story.html

programming would help provide an incentive (as if anybody needed one) "for people to connect to the Internet."

About the only thing the stimulus package *did* stimulate was the national debt.

Solar Power Sputters.- In keeping with Mr. Obama's commitment to invest in alternative energy sources and "go green," one need look no further than three solar equipment companies— Abound Solar in Colorado, a $400 million stimulus–funded failure that filed for bankruptcy; and Solyndra LLC and SunPower, both based in California, and specializing in solar panels and related equipment. Solyndra received $528 million in stimulus loans; SunPower got $1.2 billion.

Solyndra went bankrupt, was raided by the FBI, and left hundreds of thousands of dollars' worth of mess behind, including chemicals and lead-contaminated equipment. SunPower's stimulus "investment," according to the Department of Energy's website, was to help build the California Valley Solar Ranch in San Luis Obispo County, a project that would have created only 15 permanent jobs (about $80 million in tax money for each job!).

SunPower apparently was already receiving capital from private investors. Shortly after the "conditional" stimulus, a French energy giant, Total, bought a majority ownership in SunPower and extended a $1 billion credit line to the company. Somehow, SunPower managed to lose $150 million during the first half of 2011, with a debt nearly 80 percent higher than the market value of *all* its outstanding shares. At this writing, the company faces a class action lawsuit by investors who claim it made false public statements.

The solar firm fiascos were dubbed "Solargate."

High-Speed Bullet Trains Shot Dead on Arrival.- Then there was the proposed network of high-speed trains! What few train projects Mr. Obama managed to launch by 2012, according to the Federal Railroad Administration's High Speed and Intercity

Passenger Rail Program, produced just 130 rail cars. The project stalled over design and testing issues. What's more, even the fastest ones were _not_ high-speed, nor were they based on anything remotely resembling the "green energy" Mr. Obama touted as part of his shtick. Instead, if they run at all, they will use diesel fuel.

According to an April 25, 2012, *Washington Times* editorial, the 25-year project is looking more and more like a "bait-and-switch" gimmick aimed at transferring massive amounts of cash "for inner-city pork projects."

Green Jobs Leave Home Without Us- Meanwhile, ABC News found that 80 percent of the $2 billion set aside in the stimulus package for "green jobs" *had gone overseas*, to countries like China, Spain and South Korea. (So much for American jobs!)

Unsurprisingly, by late 2010, the administration had lost its appetite for "green energy" and "environmentally friendly" start-ups.

A Case Against Tax-Subsidized "Investing".- Blog columnist Rob Port argues against government "investing" tax money in the private sector, saying "if the investment is lost, we all lose because it's our tax dollars." He notes that "when the government invests it's usually based on...how politically popular that company is, like being a 'green' company."

Of course, research and development ("R&D") is a time-honored use of tax dollars, as one never knows when a new technology or innovation might prove to be a world-changing discovery like electricity or integrated circuitry. But, then, that's why there is a budget—to categorize and *cap* expenditures each year for such things as R&D.

"Too-Big-to-Fail"

Some people find it difficult to comprehend how a house they bought in 1984, during the Reagan Administration for $190,000, which, if they sold it today, would be way outside their own budget at $840,000—a 442 percent increase—represents a "collapse" in the housing market. So, let's back up and come at it from simpler, if humorous, angle.

Mortgage in the Doghouse.- Let's say your local bank provides a mortgage loan to Rover, Spot, Buckles and Sheba. Sheba passed away four years ago, but no matter, her application got approved anyway. As payments on these loans get further behind, they go into a big bag labeled "p_ _p," because no way are these pups going to come up with the payments, eager and lovable as they may be. In the same bag are also hundreds of other unpaid, risky housing loans. This is called "bundling."

Eventually, banks realize they need funds to pay off the bad debts, so they hand the bag over to two ***quasi-federal, government sponsored enterprises (GSEs)*** called Fanny Mae (Federal National Mortgage Association) and Freddie Mac (Federal Home Loan Mortgage Corporation), originally established to help more potential buyers realize the American dream of home ownership. Anxious to be perceived as compassionate and relevant, Congress pushes Fannie and Freddie to cut buyers more slack and approve even more high-risk loans.

Banks, for their part, see no down side as long as they are receiving government "incentives" and/or subsidies, in addition to the money they are receiving good loans to high-quality, low-risk buyers.

So Fannie and Freddie buy up these bags of "p_ _p," because that frees up capital for banks to make more loans. Mind you, Fannie and Freddie have no idea what they are going to do with these enormous bags from thousands of lending institutions like yours, but that's what the federal mandate calls for.

In a few years, a terrible stench becomes noticeable everywhere. In 2008, this stench is dubbed "the subprime mortgage crisis." Turns out the federal government had provided supports of one kind or another for years to Fannie and Freddie (beginning in the wake of the Savings and Loan crisis of 1992). But by September 2008 the awful smell resulted in an official takeover of these GSEs to "ensure their financial soundness" through a guaranteed, steady infusion of Treasury funds.

In other words, the government took on increased deficits, which means taxpayer liability. At some point (like after a national election) this equates to higher taxes, inasmuch as government never cuts its spending enough to amount to anything.

As for Rover, Spot, Buckles and Sheba: Well, since Sheba passed away, she gets home free...so to speak. But Rover's meager position as household guardian is jeopardized with his master's death. Spot is retired as Therapy Dog due to the economic downturn and small-business layoffs, and Buckles is looking for new Search and Rescue work. So, with virtually no collateral, they lose their doghouses. Charities that would have helped the poor dears are struggling under the weight of over-regulation and fewer donations on the part of budget-conscious individuals. Unless grateful families take them in, they will be homeless.

Bad Policy, Compromised Regulators.- This is essentially the agonizing situation for all the parties concerned today—from individual banks, to charities, to former home owners. Even the Federal Reserve admits that the net exposure of the entire housing/mortgage debacle to taxpayers would be difficult to determine.

Because of cumulative bad policy-making on the part of Congress, a system evolved which allowed financial institutions to make loans and pass them along to somebody else (or another institution). This means that the loan you got in 1984 for a $190,000 house could be "bundled" with other loans and sold as a package. If the quality—or risk factor—associated with some of the buyers in that "bundle" is unknown, it calls into question *the quality of the whole package.*

The result is that, over the years, financial institutions could make money by granting questionable loans and passing the problem along to someone else to worry about. Predictably, a lot of bad loans got into the system.

When the economy as a whole started having problems, people with questionable loans could no longer make their payments. Foreclosures resulted. This put additional houses on the market that otherwise would not have been there, and drove prices down. Once many people reached a point where they owed more money than their houses were worth, this dumped even more houses on the market, and the cycle started repeating itself.

Unfortunately, that didn't stop government from establishing even more agencies to "help" people stay in houses they couldn't afford, among them, the **Home Affordable Modification Program (HAMP)**. HAMP's website explains that all they have to do is "qualify" or "be eligible."

The words "qualify" and "eligibility" carry positive connotations. Everyone wants to "qualify" or "be eligible" for something! In keeping with America's course toward socialism and rewarding laziness, being unemployed, or unable to read or write passably helps assure "eligibility" for many types of government handouts. The costs, of course, are passed along to taxpayers.

HAMP came under yet another program, the **Making Home Affordable Program**, created by the Financial Stability Act of 2009, which established the disastrous Financial Services

Oversight Council (FSOC) in 2010, with Rep. Barney Frank (D-MA) and Sen. Christopher Dodd (D-CT) posturing as "regulators."

Federal regulators have *not* been successful in putting the brakes on excessive speculation. In fact, the same regulators were at the helm of three major baking crises over the past 40 years, and the 2010 <u>Dodd–Frank Wall Street Reform and Consumer Protection Act</u>, offered nothing new in all its 2,500 pages.

In fact, one could probably not have picked worse legislators to pen such an Act.

In his role as chairman of the Senate Banking Committee, Sen. Dodd proposed a program in June 2008 that would assist troubled sub-prime mortgage lenders such as Countrywide Financial in the wake of the U.S. housing collapse. *Condé Nast Portfolio* reported allegations that in 2003 Dodd had refinanced the mortgages on his homes in Washington, D.C. and Connecticut through Countrywide Financial and had received favorable terms due to being placed in the "Friends of Angelo" VIP program, so named for Countrywide CEO Angelo Mozilo. Dodd received mortgages from Countrywide at allegedly below-market rates on both homes, even though he could well afford the standard rate.

Apparently, Dodd had not disclosed the below-market mortgages in any of financial disclosure statements he filed with the Senate and Office of Government Ethics since obtaining them in 2003.

But, of course, he is a left-leaning Democrat, so he just got a tsk-tsk.

Predictably, Dodd denied rumors that Fannie Mae and Freddy Mac were in financial crisis. He described the firms as "fundamentally strong," saying they were in a "sound situation" and "in good shape."

As for Rep. Frank, while the ranking minority member on the Financial Services Committee in 2003, he stated: "These two entities ... are not facing any kind of financial crisis.... The more people exaggerate [accounting] problems, the more pressure there is on these companies, the less we will see in terms of affordable housing."

That was the same year Rep. Frank gave his infamous "dice roll" comment: "I do not want the same kind of focus on safety and soundness [in the regulation of Fannie Mae and Freddie Mac] that we have in the Office of the Comptroller of the Currency and the Office of Thrift Supervision. I want to roll the dice a little bit more ... towards subsidized housing."

Subsidized housing is pure socialism.

Wheeling and dealing, secret emergency meetings, and inconsistent decision-making characterized Sen. Dodd's and Rep. Frank's attempts at oversight. Eventually, it was determined that Freddie and Fannie needed a bailout.

The **Financial Stability Oversight Council (FSOC)**, established by Title I of the Dodd–Frank Act, was touted as being bigger, with more resources and power to forecast meltdowns, address regulatory breakdowns and provide early warning signs of impending bankruptcy. But for all the hype, the FSOC didn't manage any of these. MF Global, a financial institution under FSOC oversight, filed for bankruptcy on October 28, 2011. No "early warning system" there!

Moreover, these two liberal Democrats, both with their own high-profile ethics challenges, did much to exacerbate the housing downturn, had little understanding of the pitfalls associated with quasi-governmental agencies like government–sponsored enterprises (GSEs), and seemed, for all their much-ballyhooed smarts, to be clueless. Easy federal credit and weakening of mortgage credit standards is what caused the mortgage crisis and led to the subsequent wholesale financial crisis. Pressure on Freddie and Frannie to buy, bundle and guarantee ever-riskier loans to the less-affluent resulted in taxpayers having to fork over some $145 billion into the failed mortgage giants, thus undercutting the general standard of living.

Back to the Budget

Barack Obama did submit a budget to Congress in March 2012, but it was so outlandish, even his own party rejected it out of hand. Mr. Obama's budget) projected that the national debt would continue to rise in 2013, and reach a whopping $25.9 trillion in 2022. According to CBS White House correspondent, Mark Knoller, even by Mr. Obama's own estimates, the national debt would top $20 trillion in 2016.

Of course, Democrats dissembled and pretended to take it seriously, [33] but surprisingly, they also refused to come up with an alternative plan. Democratic Majority Leader Harry Reid insisted that it would be "foolish" for his party to do a budget. Just about the time a budget was actually due on April 15, Democratic Budget Committee Chairman Kent Conrad was reportedly forced *by his own party* "to cancel what would have been the first committee votes on a budget resolution in more than two years," according to Senator Jeff Sessions (R-AL).

A federal budget is not optional, as per the 1974 Congressional Budget Act. It cannot be filibustered.

Tax policy, of course, is at the heart of any budget debate. It includes *mandatory spending*, *entitlement spending* and *discretionary spending*, which are too lengthy to cover in a thorough way. These are three of those basic terminologies all voters should know. Suffice it to say, tax revenues have declined significantly due to a severe recession and counterproductive tax policies, while expenditures have expanded for entitlement programs, reckless projects, ongoing wars, unemployment insurance and what is termed *"safety net*

---

[33] (For a humorous, easy-to-understand take on the nation's budget woes, read Joseph Curl's classic column, "Econ 101 for Dummies," published September 19, 2011, in the *Washington Times* at http://www.washingtontimes.com/news/2011/sep/18/curl-econ-101-for-dummies/?page=all.)

spending,"[34] which includes more than the common, well-known entitlements.

U.S. debt now exceeds 100 percent of the nation's Gross Domestic Product. Federal budget records show the national debt once topped 121 percent of GDP at the end of World War II (1946), a relatively small $270 **b**illion dollars. A post-war economic boom followed—mostly because the heads of big American companies were turning out bombers and other armaments. They placed factories on empty prairie fields. After the war, those same factories got an extreme makeover, turning out new marvels for American consumers. With saner heads at the helm of the nation's economy, the $270 billion debt was quickly retired.

By contrast, even with our "shock-and-awe" technologies for the Gulf War, there was no comparatively massive manufacturing buildup—and what there was could not be easily retooled for consumer markets. Our manufacturing capability has gradually disappeared overseas.

Below, in a nutshell, are the steps typically taken in the lengthy process of creating a budget, compliments of an online table from the National Volunteer Fire Council's website.[35] Although it's dry reading, every American should visit this site to see the long version. Doing so enables one to grasp the enormity of what the absence of a budget means. Is the nation moving ever closer to a day when the lack of a budget is perpetual? If three years without a budget were to turn into five or six, congressional leaders or the President could make that an excuse to declare a state of emergency, initiating a chain of events that would bring America down.

---

[34] http://www.usatoday.com/news/politics/story/2012-02-02/safety-net-programs/52939824/1

[35] (http://www.nvfc.org/resources/legislativeaffairs/take-action/the-federal-budget-process-fact-sheet/).

The Budget Calendar Summary

Before the 1st Monday in February	President transmits proposed budget to Congress
Six Weeks Later	Congressional committees report budget estimates to Budget Committees
April 15	Action to be completed on congressional budget resolution
May 15	House consideration of annual appropriations bills may begin
June 15	Action to be completed on conference committee reports
June 30	Action on appropriations bills to be completed by House
July 15	President transmits Mid-Session Review of the budget
October 1	New Fiscal Year begins

The Continuing Resolution Game

If the budget process is not completed by October 1 (the fiscal year deadline), a "Continuing Resolution" (CR) to extend current funding for government operations must be passed and signed by the President to avoid a government shutdown. These days, Continuing Resolutions tend to go on "autopilot," as Stanford's Hoover Institution fellow Deroy Murdock put it in a piece that appeared in the *Washington Times* April 23, 2012. This has become a game to avoid the law requiring a federal budget. There was a CR in 2001, 2002, 2003, 2007, 2008, 2009, 2010, 2011 and 2012.

Six shutdowns occurred between fiscal year 1977 and 1980, ranging from eight to 17 days, according to the Congressional Research Service. From fiscal year 1981-1996, nine shutdowns occurred, none lasting more than five days. But the Gingrich-led shutdown, the second one that year, stretched for 21 days, the longest in U.S. history. Some 284,000 federal employees were furloughed, along with an untallied number of federal contractors. All of the federal employees wound up paid, but a few contractors did not.

It will be interesting to see if Republicans ever seriously attempt that game again.

The $250,000 Question

Back when the spotlight was on the "middle class" throughout Campaign 2008, candidate Barack Obama (and others) kept fixating on a figure that supposedly distinguished the middle class from the wealthy—$250,000. The term "middle class," consequently, has become muddled. This first became noticeable when the late Tony Snow stepped down from his position as President George W. Bush's press secretary, explaining that he simply "cannot make it on $168,000 a year." The comment didn't play well in Peoria.

Confusion as to exactly what constitutes "middle class" is due in part to a media that downplays the enormous wealth enjoyed by former chief executives of bankrupted companies; special-interest moguls; lobbying giants; and too many Members of Congress, like former House Speaker Nancy Pelosi (between her husband and herself, the couple was raking in some $400 million a year at the time).

Sarah Palin used the term "middle class" interchangeably with "working class." The latter actually equates to "blue-collar." The usually astute columnist Thomas Sowell, in rightly criticizing the State Children's Health Insurance Program (SCHIP in one of his columns, charged that some people who qualified for the program were making "as much as $80,000"— the implication being that a couple making $80,000 is well-off financially. The SCHIP may well be another redistribution-of-wealth entitlement, but $80,000 in the 2000s is not "well-off."

It isn't so much that the gap between rich and poor is widening, as that the middle class can no longer buy what it could afford without difficulty just three decades ago. The terms "inflation rate" and "purchasing power" fail to capture the plight of middle-class wage-earners.

So, let's give it a try here:

Humble Oven Meets Drippy Faucet.- Take, for example, the humble oven in your kitchen and the new energy-efficient furnace in your basement. Both incorporate a sophisticated array of computer chips, electronics and digital equipment. When something goes wrong, the entire "mother board" must be replaced on both of these big-ticket items. It's not just a question of replacing a selector switch or thermostat like it was 40 years ago. So, the cost of an oven repair comes to $800 - $1,000, unlike the $100 that was quoted by a now-retired repairman as having been a top figure in the 1950s, 60s and 70s.

Built-in obsolescence means that small appliances, from clock-radios to coffee pots, must be regularly replaced because they are similarly outfitted with chips and digital electronics and, therefore, are *not worth* the cost of repair. Many such appliances, in fact, are sealed units, meaning they cannot even be opened for repair.

Now consider the drippy bathroom faucet. Whereas in 1972, you would have purchased a 50-cent washer and screwed it into the spout yourself, today one cannot purchase that sort of washer, much less a mere handle or spout; you must purchase an entire assembly. So when people finally replace bathroom fixtures, they often spring for something attractive. Not "upscale," because anything with porcelain or embedded colors typically runs between $400 and $950. By contrast, a "plain vanilla" faucet at the hardware store costs between $75 and $140, but unless it is going in the basement, most people want something a little prettier.

So, let's settle for "attractive." Your cost will be between $220 and $380. You purchase the set, which comes with directions, and go home.

Next, you attempt to get your old faucet out. You likely discover that at least one of the handles is "frozen" in place by hard water deposits. That means it cannot be unscrewed (thus the dripping), and will require either a saw, or removal of the sink from the wall to "un-stick" it. Unless you call a professional, you will probably chip your sink and perform other collateral damage that sets you back hundreds of dollars. You may already have wasted a day searching for the "attractive" faucet (because everything in your price range is conveniently out of stock). You are in no mood to go on another expedition to replace your sink.

So, you hire a handyman or plumber and pay him another $200. Your "attractive" faucet has now cost you some $420. That is close to the cost of private school tuition for an entire year of the 1960s!

Figures like these are not reflected in annual inflation statistics or the Consumer Price Index. Food, gas and housing prices are the primary focus of such statistics, which are only somewhat offset by lower electronics and computer prices—cell phones with "apps," plasma TVs, etc.

Computer Crazy.- No matter what business you are in, if you are among the demographic known to economists as upper-middle, middle-middle, or lower-middle class, you must own at least one personal computer (a laptop usually), and probably a handheld planner with "apps." Without these, you cannot—you will not—function as a professional. Every company or service is programmed to urge logging onto its web site for information. Computer ownership is *presumed*, just like the seat belts in your car, whether you want them or not.

The working-class and unskilled labor sectors have some leeway on these points, but not much. That is because the "less fortunate" tend to operate on a kind of barter system. A buddy "fixes" the neighbor's car so that it will pass inspection, with the promise of a return favor when needed. Working-class inspectors are not so picky with this neighbor, unlike the fellow who drives up in a suit and tie.

In any case, your word processor is the key(board) to your continued existence as a professional. However, the software for it is outdated two years from time of purchase, if not before. Upgrades are expensive, time-consuming, and glitch-laden. They require an ever-increasing array of software packages. Yet, as a professional, your letter, document and business card are all expected to be error-free. No old-fashioned "white-outs," erasures, or correction-tapes.

The "less fortunate" are under no such constraints to "stay in business."

"Spam" (much of it blatantly pornographic) and identity theft require a plethora of encryption packages, "firewalls," parent controls, and virus protectors—which, of course, are additional expenses. Going wireless requires more outlays for conversion.

Caller-IDs are becoming a must-have for every telephone to avoid the scores of computerized robo-callers soliciting "on behalf of" various causes, surveys or services. Thanks to computerized soliciting, the national no-call registry was dead-on-arrival. The "less fortunate," of course, do not receive so many nuisance calls, and the exorbitantly wealthy have many "someone-elses" to answer their phones. An answering machine, of course, is embedded into telephones, so nobody has the option of bypassing that cost.

There are no "freebies" for middle-class wage-earners and no way around the additional taxes to support institutionalized "equality." Trouble with heating costs? Government rushes to provide a handout to the "less fortunate." Never mind that the recipients' children are cavorting down the street with a Bluetooth in one ear, an iPod ear-bud in the other, and a new iPad in a backpack.

Kid Stuff.- In 2010, the Department of Agriculture released the latest figures on the cost of raising a middle-class child to age 18—yes, the Department actually specified "middle-class"! The total, including child care, medical expenses, public education, transportation, food, housing, clothing, and miscellaneous expenses (a cell phone with "apps"?) was $226,920. The annual figure for a middle-income, two-parent family ranged from $11,880 to $13,830—depending on the child's age.

Now, for a reality check:

If you expect your child to be accepted at a good college without having to take remedial courses (see chapter 7), a private school is your best "accredited" option. But unlike in the 1950s, 60s and 70s, private schooling today is typically out of reach for middle-class families. It is noteworthy that most privately schooled youngsters the 50s and 60s generation could not manage it for their own youngsters, even with steady, professional jobs.

Here's the math:

A typical secular, private day-school in the Washington, DC Metro area costs $18,000 - $22,000 per year, per pupil. In greater New York City, the figure is higher; in the heartland and Southwest (where any exist), costs are lower. Where private schools are fewer, waiting lists are longer. Parochial schools are cheaper, but most accredited ones are Catholic. Obviously, not everyone is Catholic. Non-accredited means universities ignore them. So, the Washington, DC, Metro area, with its hundreds of options, serves as a baseline.

Let's say you have two children and make a high-range middle-class wage of $200,000 a year. You have no additional large assets, such as a house paid for by your parents as a wedding gift. You do not have employer-provided transportation, or a top-drawer insurance plan like members of Congress. Your net worth consists mostly of basics, and you earned them yourself. You took the trouble to understand the employee-health programs, mutual funds and pension options, but that's about it.

How much do you need to send your child to a private day school (forget boarding)?

2 kids x $20,000 average annual tuition
x 12 years = $480,000

But, you're not through yet. There are books; annual donations (expected); clothes (no jeans or T-shirts); and field trips—all requiring hefty, out-of-pocket expenses.

So, let's make round off that $480,000 to $500,000 for two youngsters. (Over the course of 12 years, even $275,000 *per child* is not a stretch.) Three children bring the total to $720,000. You have federal, state, county, property and sales taxes; a mortgage; food; auto-maintenance and inspection; breakdowns of appliances; insurance premiums; non-covered outlays for orthodontics and dental work; aging parents; occasional trips to the beach; and a pet. Your various savings plans are non-liquid assets. How far do you think $200,000 a year will go?

Suppose you decide against private education and opt for home-schooling. Well, that is ideal, but you have to be highly organized, committed to keeping a schedule, willing to endure constant oversight by the state—and either be "up" on every subject area or know someone who is. And one of you will not work outside the home.

As for public schooling? Well, if you are willing to accept that parents' rights stop at the schoolhouse door, maybe you can handle that. You will have zero control as to the prevailing moral and political climate, and neither teachers nor administrators are likely to back you up if push comes to shove. Hooker/jailhouse-chic will be the standard dress, and parents who are not politically and socially liberal will be treated as morons ("breeders and feeders"). This will send a message to your child, who will react, in turn, by questioning your authority and balking at your rules.

At some point, you probably will have to shell out for a private tutor. Thanks to the chaotic school environment, the risk of violent assault at a public school will be higher—despite invasive pat-downs, metal detectors and police on rooftops.

The irony in all this, however, is that the privately schooled pupil expects to maintain the *lifestyle* their parents have exposed them to over the course of 12 years! Thus, again, a Catch-22. Your choices are to dump your youngsters into a cesspool of culture rot from preschool through 12th grade at the government school, or to sow the primary years with something more rigorous, principled and academic. Either way, you are likely to suffer financial consequences when you need your children's help in your "golden" years. Young grads today tend to get internships, not entry-level jobs that pay well enough to live on their own. So, likely as not, *they'll still be living with you.*

College Bound (Literally)

When Boomers were starting out, one didn't require a university degree to secure a good job. Bill Gates dropped out of Harvard, remember? Steve Jobs didn't get a college degree. Individual initiative, experience, merit and commitment were valued more than a framed piece of paper.

Today, that framed piece is a necessity—several pieces, preferably: graduate and post-graduate. The exceptions are entertainers and sports figures, which is why so many young people take the gamble. Most don't make it and have no backup plan if they decide to throw in the towel on celebrity.

In the 1960s, college students could work their way through college packing sandwiches for vending machine companies, collecting garbage for the county, becoming crop-dusters and salespersons in the summers—all to afford a state college, which was nominal compared to private universities. The August 20, 2012, edition of *Forbes* magazine ran a cover story,

"The Only Colleges That Matter," debating whether any but the 50 top (expensive) colleges are worth the trouble.

Wise parents in the 1960s and 70s, who could easily have sent their children to college, often compelled their heady young high school graduates to get a job, as a reality check. Good plan. Understanding what jobs were available *without* a college degree was more important than subsidizing four years of frat parties and husband-hunting.

Working-class families, of course, had no choice but to tell their kids to go to college on their own dime.

Today, youngsters trying to pay their own way to those 50 top colleges (and many others) wouldn't earn enough to pay tuition, let alone books, dorm fees, mandatory cell phones and transportation.

One reason is that many of the students attending college via government loans and freebies should not be there. Remedial classes are standard fare at most colleges and universities, again helping prices to rise. In fact, most colleges and universities today receive federal or state monies, directly or indirectly.

In the 1950s and 60s, grocery stores were not the size of football fields, pharmaceuticals and dry cleaning were delivered for a small price, and kids didn't need chauffeuring to so many after-school activities. That meant fewer trips in the car, so most families had, and needed, only one. Now a family needs two cars to get anything done, and they cost the price of two 1960s-era houses. Dilapidated highways, traffic cameras, speed bumps and other nuisances ensure that your commute is as costly as possible.

The "Soak-the-Rich" Gambit

Obviously, exorbitant wealth (meaning hundreds of millions of dollars, not a couple of million) makes grocery shopping, pharmaceutical or dry cleaning delivery and long commutes non-issues. Multi-millionaires just hire personal assistants and chauffeurs.

Long security lines at the airport? Jet-setters charter a flight, or use a private plane. Power outage? Several backup generators kick in. Check overdraft? The bank will access other accounts. Spam? Let the secretary deal with it. Painful medical condition? Forget haggling over painkillers or satisfying DEA requirements or divulging embarrassing details one might not want in the newspaper. A "quiet word" with the doctor will suffice—or a quick trip outside the country.

Long waiting lists for a private school? No need to navigate the maze of Mickey Mouse exercises like writing an essay on "what I like best about my child." No forking over financial and employment histories. Extreme wealth allows one to donate substantial sums to the institution of choice *prior to any mention about enrollment, then hiring someone to give Billy or Suzie an "aptitude test."* Voilà, done!

Cap-and-trade, airport pat-downs, and other nuisance regulations? The Al Gores, Nancy Pelosis, Theresa Heinzes and Barbra Steisands of the elite won't stand for it. Al Gore and his entourage bypassed airport security lines; Nancy Pelosi demanded a chartered jet. When you own a house in Maui, an apartment in New York and a villa in France, it's easy to be generous with other people's money.

All this is why so many voters, being products of America's schools and universities, have come to cast a jaundiced eye upon the whole "capitalist system." Of course, they don't specifically pick on the above names because they are leftists of the favored elite. Still, average people have made the mental leap toward socialism that Nikita Khrushchev taunted us with in 1959. What most who use the term "capitalism" don't know is that it was coined by communists as a pejorative to describe a free-market system!

But even if one acknowledges a certain advantage among the perpetually wealthy—what used to be called "old money"—

and a penchant among a few such families (like the Kennedys and the Bushes) to turn themselves into political dynasties, it doesn't make sense for a nation to wage war on people above a certain arbitrary income level. Many countries have tried that approach, and found both their people and their country poorer for the effort.

The bottom line is that people with money create jobs—the good jobs, the jobs with benefits and insurance, paid annual leave, sick days and pensions.

The Framers of our Constitution looked around at other systems of government before they selected one based on individual opportunity and free markets. They decided that even if a few scoundrels made it big, the nation itself was better off with an unencumbered chance to be upwardly mobile than with a controlled economy. They would have been horrified by wage and price controls, rent controls, and other socialistic schemes that end up facilitating class envy.

One could argue for hours as to what figure constitutes "rich": $250,000; $500,000; $5 million; $100 million?

A better question is: How far does the money go? What is the *purchasing power*? Baby Boomers who, as teenagers, paid $20.00 for an item would pay $145.65 for that same item today. That represents a 628.2 percent inflation rate. This represents the enormous jump in *inflation* since 1965.

David Malpass, in explaining the dollar's value collapse in an article for *Forbes*, December 5, 2011, describes how, especially in the 1970s, the "rich" were able to do well: In large part, he says, they protected themselves from the weak dollar." Furthermore, he explains, "[w]hen growth is fast the incomes of the poor go up as the incomes of the rich go up even more. When growth is slow or negative, the real incomes of the poor go down the most. Income disparity widens most when the dollar is weak...." Thus the need to understand these terms.

One reason the exceptionally wealthy can retain so much of their income and become even wealthier is that they know the financial rules. They use many of the same methods middle-class wage-earners do to protect, or "shelter," their own assets: long-term capital gains, mortgage interest deductions, and retirement savings plans. The difference is, the very wealthy have more capital to do it with—their houses and properties are worth more; their sales from investments, such as stocks and bonds, are larger; the money they can set aside for retirement earns more interest.

Another approach to wealth is the "step-up" asset. Basically, it allows one to pass along assets—such as a business, stock or antiques that have grown in value over the years—so that the inheritor saves capital gains taxes. Phrased another way, with a step-up, the value of the asset is determined to be the higher market value *at the time of inheritance*, not the value at which the original party purchased it. Investopedia[36] explains it like this:

> In most cases, when an asset is passed on to a beneficiary, its value is more than what it was when the original owner acquired it. The asset therefore receives a step-up in basis so that the beneficiary's capital gains tax is minimized—because it is not based on the increase in value from the original purchase price.

This is **_not_** the same as a "tax loophole," although that is what the leftist media and candidates like the public to believe. The *step-up basis* is quite legitimate.

For example, say your father purchased a house for $40,000 in 1975 and he left it to you upon his death, at which time it was worth $200,000. For tax purposes, the house would receive a step-up *in basis* on the day he died. *Basis* is the operative word here. If you hold onto it, and don't sell, you pay no taxes on it, as this is viewed as *unrealized gains*. Your *basis* is the current market price of $200,000.

Now, if you turn around and sell ("dispose of") the house for, say, $300,000, you would be taxed on what you sold it for

---

($300,000) minus the basis ($200,000). So *you would be taxed only on $100,000*—your profit *after* the step-up in basis.

Without this step-up basis, you would have been taxed on $260,000; that is, the *difference* between what your father originally paid for the property ($40,000) and what you sold it for ($300,000). According to IRS rules, you saved on *capital gains taxes*.

Donald Lambro, columnist and former *Washington Times* chief political correspondent points out that "[b]illionaires and millionaires benefit from a lower capital gains tax because almost all of their income comes from capital investment in our economy."

The difference between rich versus poor is not so much about amounts earned or inherited, but an *understanding* of economics—something too many people never learned and don't take the trouble to study.

Many multi-millionaires and billionaires start out as small entrepreneurs. They have to learn enough to make a success of their companies, which in turn enables them to hire scores of employees.

Take, for example, J. Willard Marriott. At age 27, he and his young son, Bill, turned a Washington, D.C. root-beer stand into a chain of family restaurants. So successful was the father-son team, that they tried the motel business, founded Marriott Corporation and eventually presided over the worldwide Marriott hotel empire, which included restaurants, hotels, resorts and two theme parks.

Steve Jobs pioneered the personal computer and the desktop publishing revolutions in his 20s, without finishing college or getting a business degree. Jerry Yang and David Filo founded the Yahoo search engine as young graduate students. But these people were once economic neophytes. Beyond the innovations that sparked their success, they had to learn how finance works in order to grow their businesses. Only *after* they understood the economic ropes themselves could they trust their judgment to hire loyal accountants to handle taxes and benefits for their employees.

Some newcomers to celebrity—for example, in the entertainment and sports industries—realize (usually through their agents) that they, too, must hire this kind of expertise, inasmuch as they often come into money nearly overnight. Having never learned anything about free-market economics, and without enough time for a learning curve, some get ripped off by their managers and/or unethical financial planners. Unless they remain "stars" over a long period, these celebrities may never recover enough to build a second career or retirement.

Name-recognition alone is not necessarily enough long-term. Without means, it is that much harder to put out feelers for a second career, such as sports commentator. With no financial plan, multimillion-dollar sports icons, for example, never find their way back to the kind of lifestyle they briefly enjoyed.

All good leftists and liberals, Mr. Obama included, give the obligatory "soak-the-rich" message somewhere in their campaign repertoire. Otherwise, they cannot sustain the mantra that the "rich"—wherever that cut-off line begins—do not pay "their fair share." To curry favor with media moguls, today's "celebrity culture" jumps on the bandwagon. But columnist Donald Lambro obtained the following figures from the horse' mouth: Internal Revenue Service (published April 27, 2012, in The *Washington Times*):

- The top 5 percent of income earners paid 58.7 percent of the federal income taxes collected.
- The top 10 percent paid 70.5 percent.
- The top 25 percent paid 87.3 percent.
- The top 50 percent paid 97.7 percent.

And guess what? Approximately 46 percent of American households *paid no federal income tax in 2011*, according to a study published by the Tax Policy Center (affiliated with the Urban Institute and Brookings Institution). The Center explains that "provisions in the tax code, such as the personal exemption, the standard deduction, and various other tax credits and preferences," had reduced millions of Americans' tax liability to zero.

The upshot of the "haves versus have-nots" debate is that many individuals inappropriately blame "the system" because the Left can bamboozle them into thinking free-market economics is to blame for their lack. Some leftists even argue that people shouldn't *have* to learn any rules; that income should be guaranteed. This condescending argument implies that only "high-IQ" people can master the basics.

Poor education concerning economic matters produces such misguided reactions as the "Occupy" movement, and other monetary-policy protests. Simply shouting slogans condemning Wall Street, denouncing the world's banking industry and carrying signs decrying "corporate welfare" are of value only to professional opportunists who thrive on dissension, chaos, rebellion and conflict.

Moreover when lawmakers make war on small-scale entrepreneurs (via regulations) and punish "the wealthy" (via taxes), they essentially succeed in shooting the middle and lower classes in the foot.

The Economy As a Political Event

The economy of a nation is, in many respects, a political event. Inflation, the national debt, the prime interest rate—none of these can be fully understood without invoking a political dimension. Nothing exemplifies this truth more than the volatile eras when the most damage to this nation was done—a time when U.S. Baby Boomers were coming of age and launching their careers: the Lyndon B. Johnson, the Richard M. Nixon and the Jimmy Carter Administrations.

The variously named "Peace and Love," "Flower Power," and "Peter Pan" generations were in for a reality check. By the time most of them "got it," the economy had taken a nosedive, privacy was toast, wars had been lost, opportunities had come and gone, and where in heck was their Social Security check? Their world had been made safe for Enron and Bernie Madoff, but not for the American Dream.

Johnson's "Great Society" Boondoggles

President Lyndon B. Johnson got the ball rolling in the Boomers' college years with the Great Society programs. He believed in greatly expanding the role of government, especially in education and health care, as poverty-reduction measures. Today, we see these policies as a continuation of Franklin D. Roosevelt's New Deal, which ran from 1933 to 1935.

President Johnson's Office of Economic Opportunity (OEO) was the agency responsible for administering most of the War on Poverty programs; among them, Volunteers in Service to America (VISTA), Job Corps, Head Start, Legal Services and the Community Action Program. Directors of the OEO included Sargent Shriver, Bertrand Harding, and (surprise!) even Donald Rumsfeld, who later oversaw the Gulf War under the Republican George W. Bush Administration. So, here was an indication that socialism might be gaining traction; party affiliation, per se, was vanishing as a dependable barometer of either socialistic or free-market inclinations.

President Johnson's "War on Poverty" speech was actually delivered during a time of recovery (the poverty level had already fallen from 22.4 percent in 1959 to 19 percent in 1964 when the War on Poverty was announced). That is why it was justifiably viewed by critics as an effort to get the United States Congress behind social welfare programs as part of a new move toward a socialist state. Economists like free-market icon Milton Friedman, predicted that Johnson's policies would have a negative impact on the economy because of their interventionist nature. Adherents of the Friedman school of thought recommended that the best way to fight poverty was not through government spending, but rather, through economic growth.

In the decade following the 1964 introduction of the War on Poverty, with its huge entitlement programs, poverty rates in the U.S. did drop a bit further, but it also created the concept of generational welfare—a permanent underclass that passed along the welfare mentality from parents to children, with no intention of climbing out of that cycle. The work ethic plummeted; illegitimacy became institutionalized.

Add to that, many other high-dollar programs, most of which expanded over the years after Johnson's presidency to the present time; among them, Medicare, Medicaid, the Elementary and Secondary Education Act of 1965, the Higher Education Act of 1965, the National Endowment for the Arts, National Endowment for the Humanities and the Supplemental Nutrition Assistance Program. Johnson's Community Action Program launched a multitude of radical activists that drew in hard-core Marxist coordinators and negatively impacted our country's value system.

We see the results today in Barack Obama, former "community organizer" in Chicago, backed by billionaire leftist George Soros, and mentored directly or indirectly by self-described communist revolutionary and "school reformer," Bill Ayers, who participated in the bombing of public buildings.[37]

---

[37] The former left-wing radical-turned conservative intellectual Sol Stern, who "studied Mr. Ayers's work for years and read most of his books," once summarized: "Calling Bill Ayers a school reformer is a bit like calling Joseph Stalin an agricultural reformer...." He further predicted: "The media mainstreaming of a figure like Mr. Ayers could have terrible consequences for the country's politics and public schools."

Then, there were the expenses associated with President Johnson's expansion of the Vietnam War, which he viewed as a "police actions," and had no intention of "winning" in the sense of clearly defined objectives. This made it enormously difficult and costly for his successors to pre-empt an attack on our nation.

President Johnson's OEO launched Project Head Start as an eight-week summer program in 1965. The project was designed to help end poverty by providing preschool children from low-income families with a program that would meet emotional, social, health, nutritional and psychological needs. Head Start became a sacred cow, despite its generally dismal results. But anyone who challenged it became automatically a "racist." This set the course for political correctness and all the bureaucracies that support it.

President Johnson's 1964 Civil Rights Act sounded a well-deserved death knell for "Jim Crow," at long last welcoming African-Americans who longed for full assimilation into the American culture. But the Act, coupled to the Great Society programs, helped shift the nation toward welfare dependency, spurred riots and generated disrespect for law and order at the hands of professional provocateurs with their own game plan. This was extremely costly to cities and states (most of which never recovered), and eventually impacted the economy at the federal level.

President Johnson also announced a project to follow children from the Head Start program in 1967. Project Follow Through, the largest educational experiment ever conducted, created new categories for "disadvantaged" and "at-risk" youth, which, unfortunately, spilled over beyond its immediate objectives, with "social skills" training minorities were believed to require in order to gain independence and to qualify for long-term jobs and success. The down side was that social engineering pretty much replaced "social skills" and, again, laid the groundwork for agencies that specialized, basically, in expensive regulatory measures to assure political correctness.

Johnson's Job Corps continues to help 70,000 youths annually at some 120 centers throughout the country. Besides vocational training, many Job Corps also offer General Education Development (GED) programs to help get students into college—*whether they are college material or not*. This, of course, helped push college tuitions into the stratosphere.

Ultra-Anti-Socialist Leaves Legacy of...Socialism

The next political event came with Richard M. Nixon's administration. Despite Nixon's vehement opposition to communism and socialism, political pressure to coordinate fiscal and monetary policies was inescapable. The advice Mr. Nixon took along these lines was a disaster. President Nixon even wound up imposing wage and price controls in August, 1971. The 90-day "freeze" was unprecedented in peacetime

The 90-day "freeze" turned into nearly 1,000 days of measures known as Phases I-IV. The attempt to dampen inflation by calming inflationary expectations with price and wage "freezes" was a monumental failure, but contributed to the nation's penchant for socialistic responses to economic woes all the same.

Richard Nixon left the White House in response to the Watergate fiasco—an agenda game played to the hilt by the media, which hated and completely out-maneuvered Nixon. While President Nixon was certainly no saint, and out-of-his league on economic matters, he had no idea how impenetrable and proficient the leftist media had become in taking out those viewed as a threat to its leftist agenda. Seemingly, Nixon had handed the Left everything it could have wanted: socialistic wage and price controls, founding of the Environmental Protection Agency (an outgrowth of his speech in 1970), civil rights successes that exceeded Lyndon Johnson's[38] even allowing Saigon to fall. But the Left played its decades-old payback threat to the hilt for Nixon's nabbing Alger Hiss as a spy (confirmed with the opening of KGB files after the demise of the Soviet Union), as well as for winning against the Left's favorite senatorial candidate, Helen Gahagan Douglas (1950 in California). He would be hounded unmercifully, no matter what he did in office.

Gerald R. Ford took over—for only a little over a year—until a left-leaning, virtually unknown governor from Georgia, Jimmy Carter, came out of nowhere to win the subsequent election.

Carter Succumbs to OPEC Blackmail

The first two years of Carter's Administration saw the nation's economy growing by an average of 3.4 percent (which is consistent with the historical average). The economy seemed to be heading for recovery from the severe 1973–75 recession during the Nixon-Ford administrations. But the second two years were marked by double-digit inflation, coupled with very high interest rates, oil shortages, and slow economic growth. As inflation and interest rates veered upward, economic growth, job creation, and consumer confidence fell.

But the real disaster occurred with the sudden doubling of crude oil prices by the Organization of Petroleum Exporting Countries (OPEC), the world's leading oil exporting cartel. This spurred inflation until it hit 13.5 percent in 1980. It was a wake-up call that the Middle East was going to be trouble.

OPEC is a permanent, intergovernmental organization, created at the Baghdad Conference on September 10–14, 1960, by Iran, Iraq, Kuwait, Saudi Arabia and Venezuela. The five founding member nations were later joined by nine other countries, most of them hostile to the U.S.

---

[38]   http://hnn.us/articles/5331.html

OPEC's influence on the market was such that member nations believed they could use oil as a weapon against Israel and the West. They started playing that game card during the Yom Kippur War by implementing oil embargoes against *any* country seen as a "friend" of Israel, thereby launching the 1973 oil crisis. So acute were the shortages that they initiated a shutdown of one of the premier refining facilities, which in turn led to a lawsuit against the company that year by our Federal Government.

As OPEC members still collectively hold some 79 percent of the world's crude oil reserves and 44 percent of the world's crude oil production, this gives them considerable control over the global market. The best response to OPEC's blackmail would have been to exploit and develop our own resources, which would have sent a message and possibly nipped Middle Eastern extremism in the bud. But of course we didn't.

Instead, we emboldened not only OPEC, but its more fanatical and terror-sponsoring elements. Meanwhile, Nixon's EPA had morphed into a leftist powerhouse that today is bringing America down almost single-handedly through its hostility to energy products from fossil fuel to light bulbs (see chapter 8).

The sudden shortage of gasoline as the 1979 summer vacation season began exacerbated President Carter's problems. Upon bungling a hostage rescue mission in Iran, Mr. Carter's tenure came to symbolize incompetence, a label he has since tried to rectify with humanitarian exercises—some of them misguided, some of them not.

Carter, like Nixon, asked Congress to impose socialist-style price controls on energy, medicine, and consumer products, but he was unable to secure passage, as Congress had already "been there and seen that" under Nixon. Congress decided that socialism would be "getting no respect," at least for a while.

Carter was forced to run against Ronald Reagan based on a record of *stagflation*. Predictably, he lost.

Reagan Launches "Supply-Side" Economics

President Reagan proved to be a Milton Friedman free-market advocate and pushed a "supply-side" economic recovery program that worked, at least in the short run. Even so, socialistic programs were again rammed down America's throat, with the excuse that the inner cities were being ignored. And Reagan discovered, to his surprise, that he couldn't shut down the Education Department behemoth; the Left was already too strong and left-wing special interests virtually owned it. Despite increased government funding under left-wing Democrats, most urban areas remain cesspools of mismanagement, crime and educational disaster.

Since the Reagan years, the Left has controlled the nation's agenda; no traditionalist or conservative has been able to completely surmount the leftist Wall of Confrontation, regardless of any credentials or merit, whether under the mantle of Republican, Democrat, Libertarian, Tea Party, Constitutionalist or Independent.

With that, the whole climate of the economy changed. If a proposed initiative or policy contained so much as a hint of traditionalism, it was blocked and its advocates marginalized. Gains of the Reagan era were undone. *Uber*regulation and political correctness became the orders of the day. Regimentation was in; Reagan's *"Morning in America"* was out.

No Business Like Your "Own" Business?

The snowballing damage of socialistic economic policies piled up. Business practices sought to get around a laundry list of draconian regulations. A favorite tactic became using contract workers and "franchising" businesses to so-called independent owners. That way, large companies can make the actual number of personnel in their operations seem smaller and maximize their profits. But unscrupulous heads of such operations often fool franchisers—especially immigrants and the less educated—into paying enormous fees for start-up costs and the high-recognition name of the lead company, leaving them with debt and little or no profits. These "pseudo-owners" become responsible for everything which, only a decade or so ago, would have been paid for by the larger entity.

One illustration of this sort of operation is the popular airport van service, SuperShuttle. Emma Schwartz, Center for Public Integrity, provided an eye-popping example in a special report on April 20, 2012.[39] Her account of what happened at SuperShuttle can only be described as legal exploitation.

Thirteen years ago, she writes, the drivers were all salaried employees, with sick leave, worker's compensation, annual leave and most of the usual advantages of being salaried personnel. The company also was responsible for providing a fleet of well-maintained vans, gas, inspection fees, and so on.

Then everything changed. Today, drivers must first pay a huge "franchise fee" up front to "buy in" to the company. They must either purchase or lease their own van at huge interest rates. They must pay insurance premiums; maintain vehicles; purchase their uniforms, pay for maintenance, inspections and cleanup. On top of that, there's a weekly "system fee."

Schwartz described a sickening list of fees: fees for customer discounts, fees from third-party websites (that advertise their services), fees associated with company revenue-sharing. By the time these "independent owners," are finished, she says, most are so indebted to the company, they can't even think about job-hunting.

And that's not the end of it! Log onto Schwartz's article (see separate footnotes, previous page and the other sites below)

---

[39] http://emmarschwartz.com/2012/04/23/supershuttle-drivers-say-they-face-tough-times-under-firms-franchise-system/

and see how much "entrepreneurs" pay since the European giant, Veolia Transportation, acquired SuperShuttle in 2006![40]

If this the form entrepreneurship is taking, the upwardly mobile American entrepreneur, especially the neophyte newcomer, will be history.

Foreign Investors Take on U.S. National Debt

While the Chinese, Japanese and other foreigners own substantial amounts of America's debt, it's really Americans who hold most of it. As of July 2011, Americans still "owned" most of the nation's debt.

But according to Business Insider, in July 2011 America already owed foreigners about $4.5 trillion in debt. Of course, Americans owed America even more, some $9.8 trillion—but that's not the issue here.

Business Insider is a project of *The Global Public Square*, containing insights from CNN's Fareed Zakaria and leading journalists at *Time* and CNN, among others. Amar C. Bakshi, editor, writer and producer, provided a breakdown detailing the *total amount* and percentage of our nation's debt that was held by foreign entities in 2011. China, for example, was holding 8 percent, or $1.16 trillion; Hong Kong (now under China's rule) 0.9 percent, or $121.9 billion.

Why is this troubling?

Just this: If we are going to borrow money from China, and allow China to invest heavily in our country, as well as dump thousands of its underpriced goods into our nation in a way that undercuts similar products made by American workers, then we shouldn't be surprised when China intimidates us on other levels. The United States can expect pressure to accept China's

---

[40]http://www.supershuttle.com/Portals/0/App_Images/SuperShuttleRelease1.pdf and http://www.ripoffreport.com/limousine-services/super-shuttle-veolia/super-shuttle-veolia-transport-aapa3.htm

increasingly menacing military buildup—not to mention its sales of nuclear technology to Iran.[41]

The same can be said for dependence on Middle Eastern oil. Here we are trying to discourage a saber-rattling Iran from developing nuclear weapons, and attempting to deter the Taliban, Hamas, Hezbollah, and other fanatical Islamic radicals in that part of the world from exporting terror to our country. Yet, we not only pour money into Pakistan, whose regime has sentenced (and is probably torturing) the physician, Shakil Afridi, who helped our Seal Team 6 find (via DNA evidence) the hidden residence of Osama bin Laden,[42] but we pump up Middle Eastern economies by failing to develop our own plentiful energy-producing resources.

When discussing foreign "investment" in our country, that may mean buying up part of our debt, building "cultural centers," purchasing skyscrapers and shopping malls, or flooding our markets with poorly constructed and/or underpriced goods so that American entrepreneurs can't compete. The latter could arguably be construed as an attack upon our country, but the much-lauded government hype about "our global marketplace" has caused modern Americans not to pay attention to the labels on the goods they purchase.

According to an entity called Team Aguilar's Real Estate Blog, which specializes in real estate news, the federal government actually foreign investment into U.S. real estate. Foreign ownership of U.S. property has never been higher.

State and federal legislators believe foreign investment is a positive influence on a depressed real estate market here. On February 26, 2012, Team Aguilar's Real Estate Blog revealed that, in "an effort to encourage international interest in U.S. real estate, Senators Charles Schumer (D-NY) and Mike Lee (R-UT)

---

[41] http://www.fas.org/sgp/crs/nuke/RL31555.pdf and
http://www.gertzfile.com/gertzfile/ (Aug 7, 2012).
[42] http://now.msn.com/doc-who-helped-us-nab-bin-laden-sentenced-for-treason?_p=34308553-1114-4920-a8ed-438187bbe6c1

introduced Visa Improvements to Stimulate International Tourism to the United States of America, or VISIT USA Act."

But this Act is not about sightseeing (emphasis mine below):

The bill aims to encourage *foreign home ownership* by offering overseas buyers and their families *residential visas for buying at least $500,000 worth of real estate anywhere in the United States.* The bill also removes red tape for foreign investors and reduces the waiting time for visa applications for qualified applicants who have passed all the necessary background checks.

Given that the TSA and Homeland Security can't vouch for "necessary background checks," even for Americans with Top Secret clearances, it is laughable to imagine that the background checks of foreigners will somehow be more rigorous.

Real estate investment works both ways, of course. For example, most of the major U.S. hotel companies have expanded into Europe, but privately, typically not at the behest of the federal government.

Lesson of the Economy Debacle

Lost in the general angst is that the State—i.e., Big Government—now has another toe-hold in all 52 states and every community that has a mortgage-lending bank. One can barely take in the enormity of the convoluted connections and interconnections the private sector, local governments, and state entities have with the federal Government.

All this constitutes a warning: A floundering economy without a federal budget for three years straight is national suicide. In an atmosphere of market instability, joblessness, congressional opportunism, and repressive regulation, it is easy to incite incoherent, even violent, action among people (think today's Occupy crowd ten years down the road) who are basically ignorant concerning the topic of their collective fury—

that is, individuals who have no context in which to address economic issues.

~

CHAPTER 4
The NATIONAL SECURITY GAME

Those who would give up essential liberty to purchase a little temporary safety deserve neither liberty nor safety. --**Benjamin Franklin, Framer of the Constitution, 1776**

Given our gover nment's success so far at intimidating its citizens into acquiescence via such agencies as the Transportation Security Administration (TSA), the Drug Enforcement Administration (DEA), the Environmental Protection Agency (EPA) and the variously named Child Protective Service (CPS) agencies over the course of the Clinton, Bush II, and Obama Administrations, the Left is poised to pour it on even thicker.

Today, Americans are bombarded with a cornucopia of legislation aimed at increasingly sophisticated data collection and "interventions." Information sharing since 9/11 has become pervasive, but much of it has little to do with the terror attacks that provoked it. That means most data is fair game: medical, social, and legal records; SmartCards that make surveillance and tracking easy; and social-media networks on the Internet. Fortunately, high-tech prying into homes and offices, using lasers and thermal sensors, is not as widespread—yet—but the technologies are maturing.

Three major news sources in May 2012 alone pointed to high-tech "drones," also known as "eye-in-the-sky," unmanned aerial vehicles (UAVs) set to deploy over the U.S. cities by the year 2020. Most Americans have heard of these drones, or UAVs, but thought they were used solely for tracking terrorists in the Middle East, Africa and other foreign military targets. An article by author-educator Charles Scaliger in *The New*

American[43] disabuses us of that notion. He revealed that these drones are capable of zeroing in on a plot of land as small as a person's backyard.

The same month, an editorial in the *Washington Times* (May 22) made reference to the same topic. Following up a Fox News report, it pointed to full-sized versions like the Reaper, which is armed not only with cameras, but Hellfire missiles. For now, smaller versions of these, without the missiles, are being planned to cover the 50 states.

Both publications alluded to a target figure of some 30,000 for deployment, but a top-tier source who wishes to remain unnamed, says that figure is unlikely, given the cost of such a number—and the risk of collisions with other high-altitude aircraft. Nevertheless, "eyes" over the American landscape appears to be in the works. As everyone has seen with the TSA, whenever the people give government an inch, sooner or later, it takes a mile. With Americans' Second Amendment right "to keep and bear arms" ever on the proverbial chopping block, any move in this direction would put an already overbearing Big Government on the path to establishing a once-dreaded, comprehensive surveillance state. The more random mass shootings, as in the Aurora, Colorado, theater; at the Sikh Temple[44] in Milwaukee, Wisconsin; and at the Family Research Council office building in Washington, D.C. (in July-August 2012), the closer such an eventuality becomes.

"Forward," ho!

With further revelations in May 2012 that foreign terrorists really do hide explosives not only in their underwear, but inside bodily orifices, travelers started bracing for random body-cavity

---

[43] http://gunnyg.wordpress.com/2012/05/15/the-surveillance-state-knowing-every-bit-about-you-by-charles-scaliger/

[44] Sikhism has its roots in 15th-century India, not related to Islam, with faith in *Waheguru*. It is the fifth-largest organized religion with approximately 30 million adherents worldwide.

searches, given that a U.S. Supreme Court ruling only a month before allowed guards to routinely strip-search individuals for even minor transgressions (like traffic offenses) whenever they are detained or arrested.

Typically, contentious directives like this begin with officials testing the waters at select locations to gauge public resistance. If opposition is isolated or low, then the new protocol is expanded to other locales. If the indignation is still deemed "manageable," then what might otherwise be seen as an enormous breach of citizens' rights is pushed forward. Sometimes the push results in a Supreme Court challenge; but, with even that possibility on the table, officials and lawmakers usually try to make sure the timing is in their favor, to coincide with some well-publicized, violent attack.

The April directive on strip searches for minor offenses gave government a huge green light to push forward. Just as editorials began alerting Americans to this affront and condemning it, proponents of the practice were conveniently accommodated with news of a second, more sophisticated, underwear bomb plot than the one first attempted in 2009—which turned out to be headed up by a double agent working for Britain's MI-6 secret intelligence service and the CIA *along with Saudi Arabian intelligence assets.*

Interesting, then, that Team Obama chose "Forward" as the new catch-phrase (replacing "change" and "hope") for Campaign 2012. Did they figure that most of the public, being poorly schooled and distracted with other matters, wouldn't recall the same slogan used as the frontispiece of numerous other socialist and Marxist campaigns, both here and abroad? For example:

- U.K. Socialist Party: **"The way FORWARD for anti-capitalism"**
- Communist Party, India: **"FORWARD Communist Party"**

- South African Communist Party: **"FORWARD to Socialism!"**
- Democrat Socialist Perspective (Australia): **"Socialism — the way FORWARD !"**[45]
- General Marxist: **"FORWARD to the Socialist Revolution!"**[46]
- Socialist Workers Party: **"Discussing the way FORWARD for Occupy"**[47]
- Communist China (circa 1970s): **"The Great Leap FORWARD"**[48]

What National Security Is—and Isn't

National Security encompasses six facets:

- **intelligence gathering:** data-collection, spying
- **investigation:** research, inquiry and analysis
- **prevention:** pro-active measures to pre-empt attacks, illegal immigration, infiltration and border patrol
- **counteraction:** non-military counter-measures such as economic sanctions, intended to thwart actions harmful to the U.S. or its citizens
- **military response:** defense and interdiction
- **foreign policy:** economic sanctions, negotiation, humanitarian aid

The U.S. Constitution requires government to provide for the common defense and general welfare. (The term "welfare" actually belongs in the context of national security activities, not entitlements.) The six undertakings associated with national security are supposed to be accomplished without trampling the

---

[45] http://www.dsp.org.au/
[46] http://www.Marxist.org
[47] www.socialworkers.org/conference
[48] Coined by Mao Tse-tung (Zedong) and unveiled Jan. 1958 as part of the Second Five-Year Plan

rights of either the 50 states or individual citizens. Sadly, our nation's leaders and those appointed to head the various agencies tasked with safeguarding the country are moving ever farther in the other direction.

Already, legal precedents citing an individual's right to "a reasonable expectation of privacy" have been thrown to the wind. The same goes for "probable cause." Popular television shows like *NCIS*, *NCIS Los Angeles*, *Hawaii Five-O*, the various *CSI* series and *The Mentalist* are normalizing—even popularizing—the newest generation of whiz-bang "crime-fighting" gadgets. But many of them grossly undermine or violate individual rights, especially when used in combination:

- RFID-based tracking devices (like EZ-Pass, Sun-Pass and other remote toll-sensors)
- dual-use revenue-surveillance cameras with real-time zoom-in capability
- innovative voice-recognition technologies that can isolate one person's words, even in a crowd of other voices
- biometric identifiers, such as retina and hand-scanners
- automated license-plate readers
- multi-use panel antennas
- sanctioned hacking for financial transactions

And there are more. Thanks to satellites and an Interpol-on-steroids mindset, much of these data can be transmitted worldwide (and even be reassembled in different formats later).

The War on Terror generated by the attacks of September 11, 2001, aggravated existing frustrations on the part of law enforcement officers, corrections personnel, prosecuting attorneys and committees on Capitol Hill. Agencies like the TSA, DEA, and EPA were all launched to much fanfare. But, for reasons we will be examining in this chapter, they mostly failed in their primary missions to forcefully and convincingly constrain the "bad guys."

In their frustration, officials turned to easier prey—the nation's good citizens. It's rather like a doctor faced with an elusive diagnosis for a patient who keeps getting worse, despite medicine's best efforts. Finally, in exasperation, he blames the patient. The analogy changes for left-leaning control freaks, however, when targeting average citizens becomes an obsession.

These frustrations had roots going back to the unsuccessful War on Drugs, a task which took domestic crime to a new level, which required merging the resources of the federal government with those of state and local law enforcement. That had its advantages—but also came with big disadvantages.

Notice that "crime-fighting" is not among the list above detailing the six facets associated with national security. Domestic crime-fighting, as we knew it pre-1960s, came under—and should have stayed under—the label of *criminal justice*. But with the War on Drugs, government began looking at national security through the lens of local and state law enforcement.

This view explains, in large part, why they started losing at both—a problem that will become increasingly clear in chapter 5: "The Justice Game." While it is true that there is some overlap, as in the case of arms smuggling, which often involves both foreign and U.S. players heading interconnected crime organizations, there needs to be a clearer distinction between the investigation of (and penalties for) national security offenses as opposed to various crimes listed under the FBI's Uniform Crime Report[49]—whether the crime is violent or nonviolent. As it is, the United States is failing to significantly deter either terror or crime, while our jails and prisons multiply and continue to overflow with repeat offenders.

---

[49]   www.fbi.gov/about-us/cjis/ucr/ucr

Intelligence-Gathering and Investigation

Nothing exemplifies the lack of delineation between crime-fighting and national security better that our approach to intelligence-gathering and its subsequent investigation. Intelligence-gathering has become a helter-skelter activity that reeks of desperation, rather than the focused, cautious targeting of enemy organizations and individuals one would expect from a superpower

As it stands today, 90-year-old disabled ladies in wheelchairs and toddlers traveling with Mommy are more likely to be targeted for investigation than a young male from Nigeria with a false passport, a backpack and no luggage, going through airport security. As a result, liberties detailed in our Bill of Rights are being replaced with the only illusion of safety, while respect for government and law enforcement plummets among the general public. This is not a recipe for success.

Legislative Launchpad for the Snooper-State .- Although surreptitious attempts by government to see how far they might be able to take warrant-free snooping on citizens had been quietly pursued for years in the 1960s and early 1970s, the Foreign Intelligence Surveillance Act (FISA) in 2008 was the first overt assault on privacy. Initiated under the George W. Bush ("Bush II") administration, it allowed spy agencies to eavesdrop on terror suspects (and inevitably other suspected criminals) by modernizing a 30-year-old piece of legislation with the same name.

The original FISA, in 1978, was a reaction to revelations that government had been engaging in an enormous amount of unauthorized spying during the 60s and 70s. So, Congress decided to provide a legal framework to rein in foreign-intelligence investigations. The 1978 version, according to the Electronic Frontier Foundation (EFF), created a warrant procedure for foreign-intelligence activities, so that there would no longer be any surveillance without court oversight.

But the bulk of that oversight disappeared with the Bush II administration's overhaul of the Act in 2008. His version of FISA also provided phone companies *immunity from prosecution* for aiding the administration's warrantless wiretap program following 9/11 terrorist attacks (in chapter 5 we will see just how pervasive federal immunity has become.)

The President shrewdly declined to rename FISA, adding only the words "Amendments Act of 2008." A brand new designation probably would have brought unwanted attention to FISA from privacy advocates and, ultimately, from the public. So it was left at the "FISA Amendments Act of 2008," and hardly anybody noticed until May 9, 2012, when FBI Director Robert S. Mueller III, urged Congress to reauthorize it in the wake of the new-and-improved supposed underwear bomb plot that conveniently coincided with the expiration date of Bush II's amended FISA bill.

No one will ever know, of course, whether the May 2012 plot was engineered internally, so as to generate legislative support for even more offensive searches than the full-body, X-ray scanners and intimate pat-downs already in place, and to ensure reauthorization of FISA 2008.

Initial news stories had it that there had been a second, more sophisticated incident that improved upon the well-publicized 2009 underwear bomb device. But mere days afterward the Associated Press revealed (May 7, 2012 that the individual at the center of the plot was there work of the aforementioned double agent.

What is significant, is that Mr. Mueller cited the need for reauthorization of the Bush-era FISA not only in the context of international terrorism, but due to "the threat from homegrown violent extremists."

Read the last three words of that quote again. Director Mueller is not talking about individuals like John Phillip

Walker Lindh—the bright, but directionless product of trendy 1980s parenting, who got involved with hip-hop lyrics, changed his name to a Muslim one, and literally packed his bags and went off to "find himself" among foreign terrorists. Lindh went on to receive training at both an Al-Qaeda training camp in Afghanistan and with Harkat-ul-Mujahideen, an internationally designated terrorist organization based in Pakistan, so he has every reason to be designated a terrorist.

But the neither the "terrorist" nor "homegrown violent extremist" label apply to persons such as Arizona shooter Jared Lee Loughner, Virginia Tech killer Seung Hui Cho, Aurora theater suspect James Holmes, or Sikh Temple mass-murderer Wade Michael Page. Like the Columbine kids in 1999 and several subsequent copycats, these persons went on shooting sprees but *were unconnected to politics or to terrorist organizations*.

Loughner shot Arizona Rep. Gabrielle Giffords in 2011 outside of a Safeway in Tucson, for no particular reason, killing six (including a little girl) and maiming 14. Seung Hui Cho,[50] fell through the cracks of an, as-usual, clueless mental health system, and inexplicably opened fire in 2007 at Virginia Tech in Blacksburg, Virginia, killing 32 and injuring at least 17 others. Suspect Holmes seems to have been play-acting, when he killed 12 (including a 6-year-old) and wounded 58, and Wade Michael Page was seeing a psychiatrist who was already in trouble for writing herself prescriptions in 2005—Lord knows what sort of psychiatric cocktail she may have given him. So, to append the terms "terrorist" and "violent extremist" to these people confuses the issue for national security purposes.

Of course, that is precisely why government does it—to confuse. Terminology, as we shall see further on, is not to be confused with dictionary definitions in today's agenda games.

Mr. Mueller knows that his use of the term "extremist" will not apply to the nutty "die-in" protesters who played dead

---

[50] http://www.nytimes.com/2007/04/16/us/16cnd-shooting.html?pagewanted=all

outside the building that held the Group of Eight (G-8)/NATO summits in Chicago in May 2012; or, to Gay Pride paraders stopping traffic with giant, paper-mâché penises and decked out in tutus; or to global-warming alarmists armed chiefly excessively loud vocal chords; or to "Slut Walkers"-gone-topless to protest rape; or to the "Occupy" movement's conscientious squatters defecating in New York City's Zuccotti Park. None of these goofballs are they considered "extremists" by government standards, only nuisances

Yet, average Americans going about their business are viewed as hate-criminals and terrorist-wannabes, all potential "extremists," especially if one of them happens to take vocal exception to a growing list of politically correct causes and clichés.

So, the kinds of power plays exemplified by FBI Director Mueller's anxious call for reauthorization of the FISA Amendments Act of 2008 is an effort to "morph" existing legislative authority and sets the stage for the future administrations to take even greater license.

Predictably, overstepping authority has been increasingly ignored as increasing numbers of terror cells are uncovered within our borders (thanks in part to years of lax immigration/student visa-overstay policies). Just as sleeper agents were uncovered in droves during the Cold War era, sleeper/terror cells, especially those associated with Al Qaeda, have been discovered in Texas, Oregon, California, Arizona and Minnesota, to name just a few.

The difference between the two cell networks is that America's liberals ridiculed any mention of communist sleeper cells, despite the damage they did, particularly among naïve college-age youth ("Awww! You got another Commie hiding under your bed?"). But now-grown-up liberals and ex-hippies today expect government to remove these cells—without too much "police harassment," of course, might be taken as an insult by Muslims and produce more terrorist attacks.

Intervention Games.- The unsurprising rise in domestic outbreaks of mass violence that got lumped together with foreign terrorism was a result of encouragement by the Department of Homeland Security (DHS). That's how little elementary-school pranksters mock-hollering "bang-bang!" while pointing a half-eaten chicken wing at a teacher or classmate during lunch got suspended for uttering a "terrorist threat."[51] It's why straight-A middle-schoolers carrying aspirin or Ibuprofen got strip-searched under idiotic "zero tolerance" policies originally aimed at illicit narcotics.[52]

While government was finding ever more inventive ways to eavesdrop on adults, any parent who listened in on their children's telephone conversations was labeled confrontational, overzealous and "authoritarian." During the 1970s, 80s and 90s, parents who questioned their youngsters about their friends, their whereabouts or choices of clothing were labeled by psychologists as "interrogators," "overprotective" and "inflexible." Checking under a youngster's bed or in the closet for "contraband" such as illicit drugs, inappropriate literature or weapons was considered—of all things—an affront to a child's privacy!

Moreover, parents were encouraged *not* to "parent," but rather to leave that task to professional interventionists (i.e., psychiatrists/therapists). Incredibly, these "child experts," as they became known, began looking to psychotropic drugs when their talk-therapy programs didn't work.

The trend toward mind-altering drugs, of course, made a laughingstock of the already failed War on Drugs. Previously unheard-of rates of suicide and mass violence coincided with the movement toward psychiatric medications. The giveaway clue that ulterior motives might be afoot was right in the box inserts that came with the drugs—information stating that *no*

---

[51] http://www.neoflux.com/content/horrible/
[52] http://www.nytimes.com/2009/06/26/us/politics/26scotus.html

one knew exactly how these new substances worked (or didn't work, as it often turned out).

It somehow escaped officials that psychologists were undermining parental guidance with the government's help, and seeding the culture with increasingly permissive childrearing advice over a period of four decades. Government bought into, and legitimized, the intervention of psychiatrists in schools, and looked to them as the "experts" on childrearing. One result was draconian child "protection" laws.

The new cottage industry of "mental health" eventually embarked on a mission of its own. First, they decreed old-fashioned discipline *verboten*—the kind typically dispensed by parents pre-1960. Thus, the childhood cliquishness and bullying of yesteryear had, by the late 1990s, taken a more vicious turn. Psychiatric "wisdom" over the years also advised that kids *not* stand up for themselves when being bullied or even attacked outright, as with punches or pushes. Instead, the advice was strictly pacifistic (just walk away, or laugh it off, or find a nearby adult to interfere).

Out-of-control gangs and teenagers in general, resulted in a variety of deadly acts that came with ever-more sophisticated weaponry.

Nevertheless, entire curricula were built around something called "conflict resolution," which taught that every child who snatched another's toy could be "negotiated" with, as if they were diplomats working out an arms treaty.

Such approaches rarely worked, of course; and they resulted not only in emboldening the schoolyard (or Internet) bully, but actually conditioning youngsters for an adult world in which good citizens routinely serve as doormats for vicious thugs, rapists, burglars, illegal immigrants—and an overstepping government!

Our grandparents would be shocked today to see how oblivious their progeny have become to the dangerous patterns emerging. Outrage, quite simply, is being stigmatized as "anger issues"!

The Perfect Storm for Cyber-Spying.- By 2008, the perfect storm was in place to push for unprecedented acceptance of warrantless searches and spying activities—a crime rate so staggering that older inmates were terrified by newcomers to the nation's jails and prisons. The War on Drugs had resulted only in more illicit drugs, many of them (or their precursor ingredients) brought into this country from foreign smugglers. Somehow, government officials thought to make war on the users—mostly the young—but the smuggling countries got more or less a free pass.

Meanwhile, the first World Trade Center parking garage attack in 1993 in New York (killing six and injuring more than 1,000); the 1996 Khobar Towers attack in Dhahran, Saudi Arabia, where American soldiers were stationed, and the TWA Flight explosion later that same year; the 1998 bombing of U.S. embassies in Kenya and Tanzania; and the 2000 attack on the USS Cole—all went unpunished, and were treated as a loose network of gangsters. The nation's most critical intelligence assets went unused,[53] while Bill Clinton was taken up with various scandals—so-called Filegate, Monica Lewinsky, Whitewater, the Kathleen Wiley allegations, and so on

Add to that, the spectacular rise of the Internet. It took less than 15 years to enable everyone—from the novice to the technology-obsessed—to make use of complex research tools to obtain news, communicate with others locally or globally, order products, contribute to causes and play games. Of course, there were downsides: unwanted solicitations, scams that managed to elude even the best detection software, and, of course, information-overload.

---

[53] http://www.nationalreview.com/articles/218683/facts-about-clinton-and-terrorism/byron-york

Businesses and government agencies suddenly had a whole new set of headaches—corporate spying via computer, cyberattacks, and massive breaches by hackers. As nearly everything became computerized, with no manual back-up in place, it suddenly occurred to anyone with a grain of sense that the entire country could be shut down overnight without actually killing anybody.

This insight sent proponents of cyber-spying into overdrive. The expense involved in safeguarding information was enormous, but a breach could be disastrous. National security and defense agencies started hyperventilating: They had a near-constant battle on their hands, above and beyond "worms": cyberattacks like "Stuxnet" in 2010, then "Flame" in May 2012. Embarrassingly behind the curve, government had to hire its *own* hackers simply to comprehend new cyber-technologies like "fuzzing"; software flaws like "zero days" (and "zero-day hunters"); a new kind of computer-manipulation satirically labeled "social engineering." The most recent coup for the bad guys? The surreptitious control of a computer system, undetectable by the victim, called "pwns."[54]

Meanwhile, patients couldn't worry about government: They had enough on their hands trying to safeguard their health records amid a flood of data breaches in May 2012 (not to mention trying to comprehend gobbledygook-ridden computerized bills and insurance co-pays). Beleaguered consumers labored in vain to discern legitimate from illegitimate promotions amid an avalanche of illicit "cookies" placed onto their computers. Then there was protection of one's children from smut and online perverts. Writers, songwriters and playwrights threw up their hands trying to protect their copyrighted works. Inventors and research firms agonized over how to safeguard their intellectual property rights: All these

---

[54] June 3, 2012, article in *The Washington Post*, by Tobert O'Harrow, Jr., "Cyberspace The Fragile Frontier" http://www.washingtonpost.com/investigations/understanding-cyberspace-is-key-to-defending-against-digital-attacks/2012/06/02/gJQAsIr19U_story.html

factions were suddenly at risk of a whole now kind of "prying eyes" no one could have imagined a mere 20 years earlier.

As Rutgers University student, Tyler Clementi, found out belatedly, these "eyes" could be placed surreptitiously in one's room or on one's computer and viewed from miles away. Clementi committed suicide when he discovered a web camera had been placed in the room to spy on his love life.

A 13-year-old Missouri girl, Megan Meier, committed suicide after the mother of a former friend spearheaded the idea of putting up the fake profile of a fictitious 16-year-old boy and proceeded to carry out a months-long campaign of harassment.

New terms suddenly entered the global lexicon: "spyware," "cyber-spying," "cyber-bullying," "webcam," and more. Privacy advocates had their hands full even explaining to young people what the term "privacy" meant! Whether a target was domestic, foreign or personal—suddenly none of that mattered so much. Momentum was building simply for government simply to "do something."

The "Perfect Storm" for government cyber-spying had been created! Finally, federal authorities would have virtual *carte blanche* to conduct warrantless searches anytime, anywhere. A reauthorized FISA was "in the bag."

Tracking Versus Eavesdropping

In a column for United Liberty's online journal, Doug Mataconis explains that although "police are tapping into the locations of mobile phones thousands of times a year, the legal ground rules remain unclear, and federal privacy laws written a generation ago are ambiguous at best."

Even though the Supreme Court had already nixed the administration's effort to allow warrantless installation of GPS trackers on automobiles in the landmark case, United States v. Jones, the Obama administration pursued cell-phone tracking in its stead. It was as if the *Jones* decision was irrelevant. Thus, law enforcement and the wireless industry, with few exceptions, continued to collude in the practice of warrantless surveillance.

In reality, *Jones* was sort of irrelevant. Tracking a cell phone can reveal far more information than merely following a car. Jim Harper, a policy scholar at the Cato Institute, explains that this is precisely why the Fourth Amendment protections should be extended to cell phone records, even if they are held by a third party[55]:

> Incredibly deep reservoirs of information are constantly collected by third-party service providers today. Cellular telephone networks pinpoint customers' locations throughout the day through the movement of their phones. Internet service providers maintain copies of huge swaths of the information that crosses their networks, tied to customer identifiers. Search engines maintain logs of searches that can be correlated to specific computers and usually the individuals that use them. Payment systems record each instance of commerce, and the time and place it occurred. The totality of these records are very, very revealing of people's lives. They are a window onto each individual's spiritual nature, feelings, and intellect. They reflect each American's beliefs, thoughts, emotions, and sensations. They ought to be protected, as they are the modern iteration of our "papers and effects".

This is exactly what government always wanted (Hitler would have thought he'd gone to Heaven!), and it speaks to the whole rationale behind early efforts at school-based data collection (see chapter 7 and two books on the subject by this author).

Unfortunately, it gets worse. Without saying it in so many words, Mr. Harper is basically talking about the government employing military-style "psy-ops" tactics within U.S.

---

[55] http://www.cato-at-liberty.org/the-government-can-monitor-your-location-all-day-every-day-without-implicating-your-fourth-amendment-rights/

boundaries. A *Washington Times* editorial noted on May 9, 2012:

> Today's privacy invasions aren't about tangible results. In February, President Obama signed the Federal Aviation Administration reauthorization bill into law, which includes a provision promoting the widespread use of military-style drones on U.S. soil. The Department of Homeland Security already has been handing out taxpayer money like candy for purchase of these high-tech spy machines.

No "Reasonable Expectation of Privacy".- In February 2012, the Justice Department filed a brief with the U.S. Court of Appeals for the 5th Circuit arguing that "the government had the right to gather 60 days' worth of tracking information from a cellphone without a warrant issued on probable cause." This was reported in several news articles, including the *Washington Times*.

Two months later, the results of a coordinated FOIA request were released that found law enforcement officials throughout the country were routinely obtaining cell phone location tracking information using various methods and semi-legal standards. Much of this information was being obtained without a search warrant.

Again, United Liberty's Doug Mataconis weighed in, saying that the Obama administration was arguing that warrantless tracking is okay because Americans enjoy *no such thing* as a "reasonable expectation of privacy. Justice Department lawyers insisted that "a customer's Fourth Amendment rights are not violated when the phone company reveals to the government its own records."

Mataconis quotes Kevin Bankston, an attorney at the aforementioned Electronic Frontier Foundation. He contends that "[i]f the courts do side with the government, that means that everywhere we go, in the real world and online, will be an open book to the government, unprotected by the Fourth Amendment."

The Cyber Intelligence Sharing and Protection Act.- The Cyber Intelligence Sharing and Protection Act (CISPA) is probably the most dangerous and precedent-setting of all the cyber-bills to come along so far. It will allow companies to bypass all existing privacy laws to spy on communications and pass sensitive user data to the government.

On April 26, 2012, the House of Representatives voted to pass CISPA, and its backers included some Republicans plus the conservative Heritage Foundation. As of May 2012, it was still under debate in the Senate. Lee Tien, Senior Staff Attorney for EFF, vehemently objected to CISPA, alleging that CISPA gives the federal government further unchecked powers of intrusion into everyone's private life.

The stated purpose of CISPA is to "allow elements of the intelligence community to share cyberthreat intelligence with private-sector entities and to encourage sharing of such intelligence." But given the license habitually taken with definitions of terms, who is to say just what might be considered "cyberthreat intelligence"—an e-mail condemning same-sex marriage? A parent arguing against suspension of her child over an aspirin tablet as part a school's "no tolerance" policy? Even the definition of "share" has morphed so that it now means "to routinely pass along."

Citizens have good reason to worry. Inimitable and renowned columnist, Wesley Pruden (and former editor-in-chief of the *Washington Times*, reported May 29, 2012, on a little-known project of the Department of Homeland Security's National Operations Center: collecting "suspicious" words into document called the Analyst's Desktop Binder.

The existence of this reference guide was discovered, writes Pruden, only because a hearing before one of the House subcommittees wanted to understand "how analysts monitor newspapers, magazines, Internet sites and social networks.

They're looking for 'comments that "reflect adversely" on the government'."

Some of the words, such as "attack" or "terrorism," while applicable, perhaps, are also part of everyday conversation. Focus resources on them is probably a waste of time and money. But the list apparently goes from the marginally applicable, to the absolutely ridiculous. Just a few of the many Pruden listed: *grid, bridge, delays, Mexico, tornado, tsunami, forest fire, airplane* and *subway*—which probably means this book is now in real trouble, given that it is critical of government and uses every single one of these terms!

But jesting aside, the list becomes serious business on social networks, discussed further on in this chapter. Both here at home and internationally, social networks are being monitored by employers and government entities.

If America's pretentious and overlapping criminal justice system cannot keep even known criminals with long "rap sheets" out of circulation, how can we trust Big Government's 16-agency intelligence community to deal effectively with terrorism and illegal immigration? The *Washington Post* reported in July 2010,[56] the size of the U.S. intelligence community is in the vicinity of 1,271 government organizations and 1,931 private companies, employing "nearly 1.5 times as many people as live in all of Washington, D.C.

Tom Davis, writing in United Liberty Online, allows that, technically, CISPA might result in the government obtaining information that it can actually use to detect threats and potentially do some good. "But at what expense?" he asks. He answers his own question when he quotes Benjamin Franklin, who pre-empted the question over 200 years ago: ***"Those who would give up essential liberty to purchase a little temporary safety deserve neither liberty nor safety".***

---

[56]   http://projects.washingtonpost.com/top-secret-america/articles/a-hidden-world-growing-beyond-control/

"Net Neutrality".- Even though the 2010 mid-term elections indicated that voters were growing unhappy with an intrusive, overbearing government, including so-called network neutrality, Mr. Obama nevertheless tried to pressure the Federal Communications Commission (FCC) into imposing congressionally rejected net-neutrality regulations.

In the FCC's first attempt to enforce a "net neutrality" policy, the agency issued an order precluding Comcast from interfering with subscribers' use of peer-to-peer software. In making its case, the FCC cited the Communications Act of 1934.[57] The FCC alleged that Comcast's method of bandwidth management breached federal policy. Comcast complied with the order, but appealed the decision.

On April 6, 2010, a federal appeals court ruled against the FCC in *Comcast v. FCC*. The court determined that FCC lacked the authority to force Internet service providers to keep their networks open to all forms of content—thereby denying the agency's status as "watchdog of the Internet" (whew!) under the cover of the Communications Act of 1934.

That pretty much took the starch out of the legislation introduced in June 2010 by Senators Joe Lieberman (I-CT) and Susan Collins (R-ME) in another misguided effort to combat cyber-warfare and terrorism, the *Protecting Cyberspace as a National Asset Act* (or PCNAA). The proposed legislation (S.3480/H.R.5548) was also supported by many congressional and foundation heavyweights.

Protecting Cyberspace as a National Asset Act.- According to the online journal, *Raw Story,*[58] among other sources like Newsmax,[59] critics said PCNAA would allow the president to disconnect Internet networks and force private websites to comply with broad cybersecurity measures. Future U.S.

---

[57] http://en.wikipedia.org/wiki/Communications_Act_of_1934
[58] http://www.rawstory.com/rs/2011/01/24/power-shut-internet-court-oversight/
[59] http://www.newsmax.com/GroverNorquist/Norquist-ATR-PCNAA-Internet/2010/06/18/id/362423

presidents would have those same powers passed along, of course. Under this act, wrote Grover Norquist, president of Americans for Tax Reform, "private businesses would be forced to comply with 'emergency decrees'. Additionally, any company that:

> ...relies on the Internet, the telephone system, or any other component of the U.S. information infrastructure would be subject to command by a new National Center for Cybersecurity and Communications (NCCC) that would be created inside Homeland Security.

Thus, yet another new bureaucracy aimed at national security and intelligence-gathering (there are already more than 50, all with multiple departments and sub-agencies), would be launched.

The bill was subsequently revised, but still gave the president a so-called Internet "kill switch" during times of emergency. Again, civil liberties advocates were concerned that it would give Mr. Obama, as well as any future presidents, the ability to shut down parts of the Internet *without any court oversight*, given any loose definition of "emergency."

Clearly irritated, Lieberman and Collins argued that the president already had "nearly unchecked authority" to control Internet companies because of the 1934 FCC law. But that was a pre-World War II *radio* emergency law—which possibly could have been stretched to include TV, except that television wasn't consumer-ready yet. The law stated that in wartime, or in a "state of public peril or disaster or other national emergency," the president may "authorize the use or control of any...station or device." It didn't say the president could just shut it down.

As one legal observer put it on May 25, 2011:[60] "If the President happens to be trailing in the polls in late October

---

[60] http://internetattorneysassociation.org/president-internet-kill-switch/

2012, would websites critical of his policies be shut down because of the "emergency" need for him to win re-election? ... This isn't picking on the current Oval Office occupant. Would you trust this power in the hands of any single politician without immediate real checks on that power?"

Thus, the federal appeals court ruling in *Comcast v. FCC* was appropriate and timely, what with the flurry of legislative proposals designed to regulate (and tax) the Internet. Somebody has to pay for the extra bureaucracy, after all, and who better than the users?

Despite the Obama administration's agenda games for control of the Web, and even despite the obvious abuses of the Internet, there are still way too many terms left undefined. Terms like "emergency" can be twisted against law-abiding Internet users.

But the game, as always, is to keep bills like this returning again and again, until the U.S. Supreme Court either rules on the issues or refuses to review a lower court's decision.

The broader concerns surrounding proposals like PCNAA and CISPA go back to the Law of Unintended Consequences. Protecting the legitimate expectations of ownership and intellectual property carry the ring of objectivity; brokering an agreement with service providers and search engines to block entire domains is seen as overkill. Government agencies themselves have yet to determine the thin line between online thefts, threats, scams and spams, and free expression. Only one thing is certain: Once Big Government (much less the United Nations) gets a toe-hold on the Internet, then everything is subject to "noncompliance" penalties, just as it has been with everything Big Government touches.

Social Media and Data-Sharing.- The Department of Homeland Security (DHS), like other federal law enforcement and intelligence gathering agencies, is increasingly turning to social networks such as Twitter and Facebook to keep ahead of the latest terror suspects and a range of other threats. Too few in Congress are concerned about how the practice, called "social media monitoring" is morphing—and the "chilling effect" this soon may have on online speech. More and more, private opinions are being taken for crimes in-the-making—"hate" crimes, threats against specific groups or organizations and other dangers to society.

For example, just hours after Jared Lee Loughner shot Arizona Rep. Gabrielle Giffords outside of the Safeway in Tucson, a collection of his online data was circulated by DHS among various federal law enforcement agencies. It was the first time DHS had collected and *disseminated personally identifiable social-media information to other federal agencies.*

Worse, it was implied to the press that Loughner's actions were the result of a hostile political environment spearheaded by conservative radio talk show hosts. Not liberal or leftist talk show hosts, not in-your-face gossip-mongers or late-night impresarios—but conservative broadcasters. When it turned out that Loughner did not have any political affiliations, pundits backpedaled and left it at "a climate of incivility."

But for anyone paying attention, the handwriting was on the wall—post anything on a social media network that runs contrary to the "prevailing wisdom," whatever that may be at the moment, and more than your career may be toast.

Both the *Washington Post* and *Forbes* magazine carried reports in 2011 pointing to governmental and corporate snooping into social media networks. Melissa Bell, in writing for the *Washington Post* ("Online exploits can derail hiring") explains how companies "regularly run quick Google searches to vet applicants...." Since September 2011, she says, a California-based firm by the name of "Social Intelligence Corporation has been contracting with corporations across the country to institute standard social media background checks—*with the blessings of the federal government.*" [Emphasis mine]

Kahmir Hill weighed in around the same time as Melissa Bell with a headline in *Forbes* asking "Will Facebook Destroy

Your Job Search?" Hill also focused on Social Intelligence Corporation with the news that in June of 2011: "the Federal Trade Commission dropped an investigation into the…company, determining that it complies with the Fair Credit Reporting Act and is free to scour publicly available material."

Anything relating to race, religion, sexual orientation, health or marital status, is of course fair game, but the twists these searches have taken should shock even those who shrug off privacy concerns. In her article, Hill points to one job applicant "who was designated racist for joining the Facebook group [called] 'I shouldn't have to press 1 for English. We are in the United States. Learn the language'."

This hugely impacts other organizations, such as U.S. ENGLISH, Inc., the nation's oldest and largest citizens' action group, launched "to preserve the unifying role of the English language in the United States"? It was founded in 1983 by the late Senator Samuel I. Hayakawa, an immigrant of Japanese descent born in Vancouver, Canada. The current chairman, Mauro E. Mujica, is also an immigrant-- from Chile. He arrived in 1965 to study at Columbia University and says that while learning the language was hard for him, he is "perfectly bilingual today." Today, U.S. ENGLISH has 1.8 million members nationwide.

If merely posting statements in favor of the English language is now considered "racist" or "hate speech," then it took *less than 30 years for our government to cast a patriot as an Enemy of the People.*

That sounds more like Josef Stalin's Russia than Abraham Lincoln's America!

Global Surveillance and the U.N.

Nearly everyone is familiar with "secure" and highly sensitive government laptops inexplicably disappearing, along with Social Security numbers and even more highly sensitive information. Sometimes they find the negligent employee or even a motivated culprit, sometimes not. But once personal information, officially sanctioned or not, is zapped around the world to parties unknown, it is effectively out of everybody's ability to control it.

International, like national, attempts to control the Internet as a vehicle to worldwide surveillance are growing. For example, the *Washington Times* carried a brief report stating that in the United Kingdom, "[a]n official with Britain's Internet Service Providers' Association says the government is preparing proposals for a nationwide electronic surveillance network that could potentially keep track of every message sent by any Brit to anyone at any time." This, despite a public outcry in that country against a similar plan in 2008!

Again, rejected proposals just keep reappearing.

Not to be outdone, the United States is building an "enormous and secretive new facility…in Bluffdale, Utah, [that] will give the NSA (National Security Administration) unprecedented resources for monitoring electronic communications and transactions both at home and abroad." A cover article in the May 21, 2012, issue of *The New American* ("Knowing Every Bit About You" by author/educator Charles Scaliger), shows three artists' renderings of the so-called Utah Data Center being erected "in the shadow of the Wasatch Mountains…[that] will occupy more than a million square feet when it becomes operational sometime [in 2013]. Apparently, it is based on the "total information awareness" concept of Reagan-era vintage (which got a black eye from the public at the time). It is preparing to bring together the vast network of databases that already exists today, ostensibly so that every "suspicious" credit card transaction, social network post, airline ticket purchase, Internet search, and so on, can be cross-matched and analyzed

Most people, including this author, assumed that since all local, state and federal computers can, in effect, "talk" to each other, computers having been made compatible and data- input methods standardized, there was no need for one huge, central Big Brother computer. We were wrong. Inevitably, it had to happen, as encryption, decryption, compaction and sheer computing power advanced.

In another troubling development, an October 16, 2011, article in the *Washington Times* entitled "Alarm in Germany over police spying via computers," featured a report from Berlin. Michael Birnbaum wrote:

> Police departments in Germany are using powerful computer programs via cameras to monitor activities, often looking directly into people's faces reminiscent of the Nazi police state. One can be unknowingly transmitting a snapshot every 30 seconds when a laptop is connected to the Internet. This follows a 2008 ruling by Germany's high court to allow government to monitor e-mail and Internet telephone conversations with a warrant.

Americans typically think of Germany today as a success story, having shed its dictatorial roots and gotten its economic house in order against all odds, including the sudden absorption of the old Communist-dominated eastern bloc that had not known a free market in decades.

But the capitalistic façade of Chancellor Angela Merkel's Germany disguises a smoldering, increasingly vocal, socialistic undercurrent. In May 2012 hundreds of reasonably well-dressed 20- and 30-somethings held an anti-capitalism demonstration in Frankfurt to demand an end to so-called austerity measures that had come with Europe's debt crisis.

Younger Germans, like those of so many other nations, have become attached to their social programs, extensive even by U.S. standards. According to a March 2012 report at *EurActiv.com*, French and German socialists have been trying hard to create a common front "against the centre-right's current management of Europe."

In another development, Angela Merkel's Christian Democrat Party is being challenged by a new "Pirate Party," which is advocating Internet freedom and "transparency" in government. For the fourth time, it has captured seats in Germany's state assembly. While the "Pirate Party" is riding the populist wave along with the rest of Europe, its members are committed left-wingers with a bent toward the European Union (EU). This necessarily entails some degree of loss of German sovereignty, as pro-EU views displace it).

As Merkel's government struggles to accommodate—and even court—less democratic regimes, such as Russia, the recent deployment of powerful surveillance equipment hints at what is to come, perhaps sooner rather than later.

The Infrastructure Protection Gambit

Anybody who has ever faced a computer breakdown at the prescription counter or grocery store knows that there is no manual backup system and that everybody leaves the store without their parcels and must return later. Imagine that situation on a grander scale. So, the infrastructure argument is not without merit. But it amounts to another wedge opening for international control freaks.

Turns out that Russia, China, Uzbekistan and Tajikistan had already thought of that. In 2011, they cobbled out a resolution for the U.N. General Assembly that called for giving individual countries the right to control the Internet. The benign-sounding moniker was *The International Code of Conduct for Information Security* (ICCIS). Unsurprisingly, Mr. Obama and Congress approved the resolution, though saner heads eventually seem to have prevailed—this time.

U.N. control over the Internet is not off the table, however. While the ICCIS may have gotten the cold shoulder from certain quarters for a while—mainly because some of the worst authoritarian regimes specifically submitted it—Congress, at this writing, is still considering either this, or a version of this amendment to the 1988 International Telecommunication Regulations. It could yet give the U.N.'s authoritarian bloc most of what it wanted.

If Congress continues to allow some of the worst human rights abusers on the planet to be involved in "protecting" cyberspace, as if the U.N. were an extension of Interpol—the damage to our economy, our privacy, our defense capabilities and our sovereignty would be immense. Countries like China that now tightly control the Internet, and even allies like Great Britain, which is nibbling around the edges, are inviting the nightmare of aggressive, global surveillance.

The Odds of Personal Surveillance

So does all this mean that every e-mail to your son or daughter, every communication between friends and employers (and even the occasional hidden mistress) are now automatic fodder for government agencies?

Probably not—unless a country's leaders already have effective totalitarian control of a nation, or nations.

Practically speaking, there is more than enough data out there for information-sharing purposes right now. These data can, without any further enhancements to the Internet, be cross-matched and analyzed in all sorts of ways. So, the short answer to the question of pervasive surveillance is: "need to know."

Who needs to know? Maybe nobody. But if you run for public office, if you are being considered for government appointment or other influential position, or if you are already in a position of leadership and make the mistake of uttering a politically incorrect remark—then there are potentially a lot of people who will "need to know." Your e-mails, your bank accounts, your credit information, particulars about your health and your medical prescriptions are then up for grabs. This information can, and already has been, in many cases, scrutinized, analyzed and cross-referenced for any possible negative connotation. And there's nothing you can do about it—except, if you have the money and the connections, you can hire a hacker of your own to "launder" or delete information from various databases: a very tall order.

The down-the-road worry is that the proliferation of new spy software, marketed under-the-table by foreign countries, may make its way into hands that could launch a worldwide surveillance race (rather like the old "arms race").

Consider the British-designed cyber-package called FinFisher, sold through a German company, Elaman, which, in turn, was marketed to government security officials who were told it could be covertly installed on' computers by exploiting security lapses in the automated update procedures. When it was discovered during the overthrow of the Egyptian President Hosni Mubarak that his government had purchased a license and a contract to run the FinFisher software, people got a reality check regarding the danger of covert spy software.

FinFisher is not the only package on the international market. India, Brazil, Russia, and China are all in the cyber-spy sales business, with other countries moving in on the market. Incredibly, even those countries that control their own Internet tightly, like China, stated award-winning journalist Shaun Waterman, in a special report[61] to the *Washington Times*, "market a package to the rest of the world called Internet Watcher…."

China claims, writes Waterman, that the product "can decrypt the secure Web connections used by Hotmail and Gmail email systems so users' accounts can be monitored." This package, he states, is sold through "China Top Communications, a government-owned company based in Beijing."

[61] http://www.washingtontimes.com/news/2011/dec/5/surveillance-tools-not-just-for-spies-anymore/?utm_source=RSS_Feed&utm_medium=RSS

With enough fingers in the same cyber-surveillance pie comes the potential of conflicting influences—not to mention potential windfall profits and blackmail. Just as modern film editors can keep those parts of footage that producers like, and consign those portions that don't pass muster to the cutting-room floor, so can end-users of high-tech software gizmos apply the same "creativity" to political opponents, "undesirables," and public officials. They can use the technologies to marginalize candidates in the media, and neutralize whistleblowers before they ever reach the public square. They can fake pictures, letters, certificates and either malign of promote those who might be popular with the public. By the time a victim (or a challenger, for that matter) gets around to launching a lawsuit, the damage is done; events move on and any "evidence" (such as it is) is corrupted by high-tech computer experts so as not to be viable in a court of law.

Cyber-tools like Internet Watcher (and there are others out there) are essentially unregulated—for which one can be thankful, or not—but, in the wrong hands, it threatens an already highly sophisticated psycho-political world in which adversaries are easily confused with allies.

No wonder, then, that Big Governments everywhere lick their considerable chops. Today, the individual citizen's slim hold on personal information is in trouble.

Intelligence Ops and Prevention Measures

A significant part of national security involves prevention, and that entails pre-empting threats gathered through intelligence (human and otherwise) and connecting the dots through analysis. A pre-emptive model was established during the Second World War. In hindsight, the Nazi regime's uniquely systematic and vile targeting of Jews, along with Adolf Hitler's rise to power, were seen as preventable. Every subsequent administration, therefore, and especially the Defense

Department, has taken pains to identify tyrants before they assume enough power to become a threat to this country or her interests and allies.

Unfortunately, those efforts have largely failed. One reason is our understandable moral distaste for assassinations. Killing, in the context of a declared war, is one thing; slaying tormenters, tyrants and oppressors in the name of pre-emption is viewed by most Americans as simply murder. So, we try to remove them by getting their own people to do the job. Sometimes that works, and sometimes it doesn't.

Given that Americans see it as a moral imperative to "neutralize" wannabe Hitlers, this presents a predicament—playing "cop" to the world and bringing to "justice" hundreds of tyrants who abuse their own people. The United States may, or may not even have a direct national security interest in the target country. The dilemma posed by our self-imposed, double-edged ethic is visible in random signs placed on American's lawns: "Save Darfur," "Never again," "War is not the answer," "End the Misery: Stop Human Trafficking," "Support our troops," "Think outside the bomb," etc.

The same people who camp out across from the White House to protest military involvement; participate in "die-ins" at the G-8/NATO summits, as they did the weekend of May 19, 2012, in Chicago; and go ballistic over the killing of civilians in Afghanistan; nevertheless expect the next Hitler or bin Laden to be intercepted before another Holocaust can take shape.

The upshot is that the U.S. has left in place the most ruthless dictators imaginable, even after we knew what they were capable of—e.g., Soviet dictator Josef Stalin; Cambodia's genocidal Pol Pot (a.k.a. Saloth Sar); North Korean dictators Kim Il-sung and Kim Jong-il; Cuban revolutionary Fidel Castro; China's inhumane Chairman, Mao Tse-tung (Zedong); Haitian tyrant Jean-Claude "Baby Doc" Duvalier; Romanian despot Nicolae Ceausescu; sadistic child-soldier recruiter and Liberian president Charles Taylor (educated in America, no less!); Iranian president Mahmoud Ahmadinejad (according to photos, among the hostage-takers in the 1979 U.S. Embassy takeover); and until the invasion of Iraq in 2003, its torture-for-kicks oppressor, Saddam Hussein.

Of these, at least seven were a direct threat to American citizens and/or American interests. Any one of the 10, however, would happily have followed in the footsteps of Hitler, not only invading their neighbors (which several of them actually did), but eagerly overthrow Western democracies.

The 2010 killing of Osama bin Laden notwithstanding, more than enough terrorist leaders and suicide bombers exist to continue attacking innocent civilians. But just as Americans have no stomach for pre-emptive assassinations, they also have no tolerance for racial and/or ethnic profiling. Again, a Catch-22.

Government knows that to maintain any semblance of credibility, it must be seen as being proactive in defending citizens and the nation. Unable to "take out" rogue dictators before they become news items, and having failed to make a significant dent in global terrorism so that Americans feel safe, our government is randomly targeting its own populace—half out of frustration, and half due to a now-insatiable appetite for control, aided and abetted by an increasingly permanent bureaucratic class whose livelihoods depend on it. Most infamous among the agencies supporting these elite *apparatchiks* is the Transportation Security Administration.

Conditioning Americans to Accept Regimentation

ABC World News with Diane Sawyer scooped[62] the media on April 24, 2012, with Jim Avila's interview of Kip Hawley, the head of the TSA between 2005-2009. At long last, a person as close to the horse's mouth as it comes stated bluntly that, in ABC's words, "most of those lines that we dread are a waste of time."

---

[62] http://abcnews.go.com/US/tsa-head-stop-searching-knives/story?id=16202126

Jim Avila said: "The man who helped build the TSA...says the system is broken and TSA should stop looking for weapons that cannot penetrate the post-9/11 fortified cockpit door." Avila added that, according to Hawley, "the TSA is sitting on important technology that screens liquids for explosives and could, as soon as tomorrow, allow passengers to carry everything from water to shampoo, through security and onboard."

Recent events, of course, show that while passengers are not fooled by this game of "let's pretend" on the TSA's part, they have grown oddly acquiescent and more fearful of their government. This is a dangerous trend, as throwing the weight of government around has always been a precursor to a police state—and it is looking more and more like work in progress, right here at home.

How did this happen? The answer is a careful, step-by-step program of psychological conditioning, alluded to previously, but in a new package called "perception management" (or "PM"). Forty years ago, psychologists and psychiatrists tended to work in dedicated clinics or private practice. Now they are mainstays of corporations, schools—and government.

The Roots of "Perception Management".- It is interesting that two of the best-known and most popular writers of political and/or futuristic thrillers, David Baldacci and the late Michael Crichton, came to very similar conclusions about the biggest threat to citizens worldwide—and did so quite independently of each other. In the course of research for their novels, they stumbled onto such a troubling insight that both were moved to pass it along to their audiences. Baldacci wrote an Author's Note to readers in his 2008 book, *The Whole Truth*:

> **...a major untruth can be established so quickly and overwhelmingly across the world that no amount of digging by anyone after the fact can make a dent in the public consciousness that it isn't actually true at all.**

He was describing something called "perception management," which you can find on the Department of Defense's website. This brand of "molding public opinion" has become key part of intelligence operations and will be discussing in some detail.

The late mega-novelist Michael Crichton, knowingly or not, referred to the same strategy in a September 2003 speech to The Commonwealth Club:

> **The greatest challenge facing mankind is...distinguishing reality from fantasy, truth from propaganda. ...[I]n the information age (or...the disinformation age), we must daily decide whether the threats we face are real, whether the solutions we are offered will do any good, whether the problems we're told exist are in fact real....**

If you "Google" *Department of Defense + Perception Management*, you will find PM characterized as "actions to convey and/or deny selected information..., to influence...emotions, motives, and objective reasoning...ultimately resulting in foreign behaviors and official actions favorable to the originator's objectives. [P]erception management combines truth projection, operations security, cover and deception, and psychological operations."

The *Wikipedia* definition of PM adds the "imposition of falsehoods and deceptions," seen as important to getting "the other side to believe what one wishes it to believe."

So, PM functions, in effect, as a euphemism for *molding public opinion*—a psychological conditioning ("psy-ops") program that can be disseminated through the media and by other means, against any target, including one's own people. That means information warfare—and anybody is fair game.

Baldacci and Crichton both were troubled by speed at which an untruth could be institutionalized—which always seemed to be legitimized by popular and trendy sources. At that point, regardless any proof to the contrary has little chance of altering the mistaken view.

That is how PM works, and we can thank World War II behavioral scientists working with both the allied <u>and</u> axis powers for discovering the techniques of the game; among them: "mass neurosis," "cognitive dissonance," "artificial disruption," "involuntary attention," "superimposing value structures," and other complex approaches. So, while psychiatric drugs may be of questionable value, these strategies work just fine!

It has been behavioral scientists and their later enablers in the marketing and advertising industries (where psychology is the major course of study), who made perception management the force that it is today. John Rawlings Rees, a British Brigadier General helped pioneer what was called "military psychiatry" in the 1940s. He once bragged that he could turn an adult population into the equivalent of "neurotic little children." He became the founding president of the <u>World Federation for Mental Health</u> (WFMH) and ran the Tavistock Clinic (a.k.a. the Tavistock Institute for Mental Hygiene). His goal was to ensure "that psychiatry permeate every [informational] activity of national life."[63] International life, too, if possible.

He and colleagues, Drs. Brock Chisholm[64] and Ewen Cameron[65] of Canada, eventually got their wish: via their WFMH organization's formal consulting status to the United Nations and pushed by the National Education Association (which also to pains to get the U.N. involved with America's education programs via UNESCO).[66] Readers can tell by dates

---

[63] From Rees' speech, "Strategic Planning for Mental Health," delivered to the Annual Meeting of the National Council for Mental Hygiene in 1940.
[64] See his 1946 speech to the WFMH reprinted in Psychiatry Magazine.
[65] "The Building of the Coming world Order," speech aired by the Canadian Broadcasting Corp., May 5, 1946.
[66] *Education for International Understanding in American Schools*," National Education Association, 1948.

on the footnotes that the major parties involved all promoted their mutual thesis around the same time.

High on Rees and his colleagues' to-do list was to ensure that school curriculum ditched the traditional focus on excellence and academics, to concentrate on an agenda of socialization and PM. Their socialization model was taken from John Dewey—but WFMH was more interested in the child's "belief-system."

So, as post-war Boomers moved into college in the 1960s, America saw a volatile change in the traditional mores. That belief system—what Lenin and Stalin would have labeled "new thinking"—still holds sway atn most government agencies, as their directors and chiefs are now of an age when they would have cut their teeth on this "new thinking" as schoolchildren.

By indoctrinating post-war Boomers early on, perception management (or PM) morphed into a psychological force to be reckoned with. Thus began the agenda game known as "behavior modification." To modify anyone's behavior, educators and pollsters must first find out what people are thinking and document (collect) it. Only then can the opinion-molders (perception managers) set about changing "offending" (politically incorrect) attitudes.

Take, for example, an expression nobody hears much anymore, but folks used to hear with regularity: "rugged individualism." Rugged individualism encompassed a range of characteristics—independence, self-sufficiency, thinking for oneself. In the 1970s, the axe was laid to all three. Negative terminologies like "loner" and "misfit" redefined the individualist. "Independence" was scrapped for interdependency, self-sufficiency for redistribution, and "thinking for oneself" was equated with intolerance. Today, any close reading of the newspaper reminds us daily that the "loner" requires psychiatric intervention, and maybe drugs as well.

Eventually, the new wisdom became ingrained; people become accustomed, or conditioned, to notions that would have been unacceptable just a few years before. Such are the facts behind Baldacci's and Crichton's ruminations.

To help things along, something known as "Fusion Centers" have been established by the federal government and placed around the country.

Fusion Centers.- Most people are probably not familiar with the term "Fusion Center." They think of fusion as a nuclear-energy technology. But "Fusion Center" in an intelligence context refers to information-sharing centers, created under a joint project between the Department of Homeland Security and the U.S. Department of Justice's Office of Justice Programs between 2003 and 2007. It works in partnership with the CIA, the FBI, the U.S. Military, and, of course, DHS and the Justice Department. The underlying aim is surveillance and threat assessment.

Guidelines for fusion centers were separated into three phases: law enforcement intelligence, public safety, and, significantly, the private sector. The *Fusion Center Guidelines: Law Enforcement Intelligence, Public Safety, and the Private Sector*, covering all three phases, is now complete and available, according to a U.S. Department of Justice website.[67]

Predictably, these Centers got out of hand and fell into what is referred to as "mission creep." Mission creep is defined by *Wikipedia* as: "the expansion of a project or mission beyond its original goals, often after initial successes.... [I]t is usually considered undesirable due to the dangerous path of each success breeding more ambitious attempts, only stopping when a final, often catastrophic, failure occurs."

Agencies like the TSA is part of that "mission creep."

Background of TSA.- December 1972, the FAA gave the airlines one month to begin searching all passengers and their bags. The effort was more or less random and of little or no noticeable

---

[67]http://www.it.ojp.gov/default.aspx?area=nationalInitiatives&page=1181

inconvenience to passengers. The next big wave of security measures came more than 15 years later. Just before Christmas 1988, a bomb onboard Pan Am flight 103 over Lockerbie, Scotland, killed 270 people. The separate airlines hired contractors to perform the task, which was more irritating than inconvenient, as people could no longer easily take hang-up bags onboard, especially ones containing expensive formals or tuxedos that were hard to pack to avoid having them pressed at one's destination. Instead, they had to be crammed through a narrow space before passing to a conveyor belt, or be hand-checked by not-so-gentle, minimum-wage personnel.

In the wake of the September 11, 2001, terror attacks, security became federalized via the TSA, which answered to the DHS. These personnel approached their task as law enforcement officers, but without any such credentials. They failed to catch virtually any actual terrorists—mostly because they were forced to abide by the rules of political correctness that precluded their focus on the typical profile of past terrorists (male, olive-to-dark skin, ages 19-41).

So, officials concentrated their energies on conditioning the public to accept invasions of privacy without probable cause. Passengers themselves became the ones who noticed suspicious activity and turned in perpetrators, several of whom turned out to be terrorists.

This situation resulted in loss of respect for law enforcement and a dislike of airline companies (although airlines per se were only trying to accommodate government *diktats*). Soon, free-world populations everywhere were so conditioned to government intervention and overkill that they didn't know where to direct their ire.

As for terrorist organizations, it became a game to "one-up" the TSA. The more obstacles they introduced to air travelers, the more ways terrorists found to circumvent them.

Spectacular TSA Failures.- The summer of 2011 wasn't a good one for the TSA. While Lena Reppert, the 95-year-old wheelchair-bound U.S.-born woman with terminal cancer, was being humiliated into removing her soiled adult diaper by TSA agents in Florida on her final trip home to die, a male Nigerian-American (dual citizenship), was casually frolicking through airport security checkpoints all across America — on stolen boarding passes, with only a university ID card, on flights that didn't even correspond to the destinations on the boarding passes.

All three network newscasts led with the TSA's botched apprehension of Olajide Oluwaseun Noibi on June 30. It was also covered by several major dailies and wire services. Dribs and drabs emerged until reporters had unravelled what may well be the most audacious and blatant example of double standards ever played out in the name of "security" since the TSA's inception on November 19, 2001.

But falling so close to the July 4 holiday, relatively few people noticed. ABC World News' George Stephanopoulos called the debacle a "stunning breach of security at one of America's busiest airports."

Noibi's first trip on June 24 took him from New York to Los Angeles. Even after a flight attendant with Virgin Airlines Flight 415 noticed, and alerted authorities to the disparities in responding to an unrelated complaint from passengers, the "Keystone Kops" in charge didn't bother detaining him. Instead, Noibi sashayed out of the airport and proceeded to try his luck again five days later, on June 29, when he booked a flight from L.A. to Atlanta.

Even then, he was *charged only with being a stowaway*! In a July 1 Associated Press story, reporter Jeff Wilson quoted Los Angeles FBI agent Laura Eimiller as saying that the reason Noibi wasn't immediately arrested after landing in L.A. was that *"beyond traveling without a ticket there was no immediate threat."*

Maybe Noibi should have been wearing a diaper, like Mrs. Reppert—or maybe had a urine bag attached to his thigh, like bladder-cancer survivor Thomas Sawyer, whose aggressive patdown by TSA agents in November 2010 caused his clothes to be drenched.

On July 1, Andrew Blankstein and Howard Blume provided further insights into the Noibi fiasco in the Los Angeles Times. Apparently, authorities were first alerted to Noibi by the flight crew of Virgin America Flight 415 *two full hours after the plane departed.* Then, fellow passengers complained of the man's body odor and asked to be re-seated. That's when a flight attendant asked Noibi for his boarding pass and saw that it was from a different flight and *in someone else's name.* She alerted authorities, while "Noibi went back to sleep" in his cushy, first-class, leather airline seat. But instead of arresting Noibi, the "politically reliable" FBI and TSA agents allowed him to exit the airport.

In the New York Times, Joseph Goldstein revealed more: The FBI "caught up to" Noibi at LAX on June 29, just as "he was trying to talk a Delta Air Lines agent into letting him get on a flight to Atlanta." But rather than being hauled away as a flight risk for proffering fraudulent papers to a federal agent, he was arrested merely as "a stowaway"—even as authorities were discovering "over 10 boarding passes" in other people's names *inside his luggage.*

In a follow-up piece, Goldstein reported that when Noibi landed in Los Angeles, the FBI interviewed him, did conduct a background check, and examined his luggage. The bureau decided he did not pose an immediate threat and let him go, ostensibly because they knew that Noibi would be traveling on June 29 from a reservation he had made in his name for Atlanta. Except he never actually purchased a ticket! "At 6 a.m. June 29, federal agents were on hand to watch Mr. Noibi try to persuade a Delta employee to let him board the Atlanta-bound flight. The employee rebuffed Mr. Noibi repeatedly, at which point the authorities arrested him...." Yet, according to Noibi's lawyer, these same officials decided the allegations against him were "at the lower end of the continuum of seriousness."

Thank heavens he wasn't a white female, 90-something, and in a wheelchair!

The Atlanta Journal-Constitution's Christopher Seward noted that FBI spokeswoman Eimiller could not confirm "why Noibi was travelling to Atlanta other than to say he may have family [there]."

May have? The elderly Mrs. Reppert *definitely* had family where she was going, but, of course, a woman who is ill and in her 90s is an easier mark.

See SPOT Run.- The saying goes that the classic definition of insanity is "to keep on doing the same things and expecting different results." So, surely the psychologists employed by the TSA for its behavioral detection program (SPOT) must be familiar with the expression.

SPOT stands for Screening Passengers by Observation Techniques. It works so well that on May 21, 2010, it was reported that at least 16 people later linked to actual terror plots sailed right past the agents! It seems the TSA instituted the program "without first validating the scientific basis for identifying passengers in an airport environment," according to the Government Accounting Office (GAO).

Chalk up another "win" for psychiatry!

Even so, BDOs (behavioral detection officers) continue to be deployed to sniff out anger, irritation, and annoyance of people going through airport-screening lines, a scheme reminiscent of both Soviet- and Nazi-style intimidation. Nabbed individuals typically miss their flight and/or are denied boarding.

Around the USA with the TSA.- Additional TSA failures abound:

Also in May 2010, Faisal Shahzad, a native Pakistani who admitted training in bomb-making at a terrorist camp run by militant Islamists, planted a car bomb in Times Square. He was arrested only *after* he had boarded Emirates Flight 202 to Dubai, final destination Islamabad, Pakistan, a notorious hot-spot. Shahzad had been placed on the "No Fly List" earlier in the day, but the airline *didn't check the list* either when Shahzad made his reservation, when he purchased the ticket, or when he boarded.

On February 26, 2011, a man slipped past TSA security screeners at JFK Airport and boarded a plane with three box cutters—discovered only after a flight attendant *saw them fall out of his bag*. The TSA was created as a reaction to the 9/11 attacks, *which began with box-cutters*. Yet, passenger Eusebio D. Peraltalajara, was *not charged with any crime*.

A white Anglo male, on the other hand, caught carrying so much as a pen knife, is subject to lengthy harassment.

Other box-cutter incidents include two men already on a flight from Chicago to Amsterdam in August 2010. They were casually questioned after it was discovered that their checked luggage contained *a cell phone taped to a Pepto Bismol bottle, box-cutters, and a knife*.

And who can forget Richard Calvin Reid, a.k.a. "the Shoe Bomber," the proud-of-it member of al-Qaeda? He attempted to down American Airlines Flight 63 in-flight by detonating explosives hidden in his shoes in December 2001. Again, passengers discovered and subdued him.

Ever since, U.S. citizens have paid homage to Reid by removing their shoes in phony TSA "security" lines.

The first infamous underwear bomber in 2009, Umar Farouk Abdulmutallab, another native Nigerian and open defender of the Taliban and al-Qaeda, tried to bomb Northwest Airlines Flight 253 on Christmas Day 2009. He was apprehended not by the TSA, but rather was reported *by his own father a full 35 days before the fact*, to two CIA officers at the U.S. Embassy in Abuja. Acting on the report, Abdulmutallab's name was added to the 550,000-name "U.S. Terrorist Identities Datamart Environment"—a database of the U.S. National Counterterrorism Center. *But his name never made it to the 4,000-person "No Fly List."*

Even DHS Secretary Janet Napolitano admitted the system "failed miserably."

In a now-familiar scenario, it was the passengers, again, who apprehended Abdulmutallab and took him down. They heard popping noises, smelled a foul odor, and saw Abdulmutallab's trouser leg and the wall of the plane on fire.

No wonder former TSA head Kip Hawley says the TSA is "broken"!

Moreover, the TSA's successes can be counted on fingers, and don't amount to much even then. The cost? An estimated $7 trillion.

Body-cavity searches anyone?

"Actionable Intel" Versus Harassment

The United States is awash in blame games—television commentaries, newspaper editorials and opinion pieces. Missing from these debates is any reference to the difference between **data collection** and "**actionable information, or 'intel'.**" Columnists and commentators—even Members of Congress who serve on the Intelligence Committee—don't bring this up. They chalk lapses up to a "failure to connect the dots."

Our computers are bursting with collected data—from every imaginable source. The sheer scope of *what* we collect is breathtaking.[68] Value-and-lifestyle data (VALS), religious preferences, political opinions (or anything that might point to such), medical trivia (up to and including the condition of your

---

[68] http://www.beverlye.com/vs1208.pdf

child's gums), magazine subscriptions, favorite shops and all sorts of other minutia could easily be used to build citizen dossiers. The point of this exercise is to "predict" what a person might do in response to some "stimulus" or crisis. But this prediction requires "longitudinal tracking" over *years*, and most of it seems to be focused on American citizens. It is not set up to catch terrorists.

The larger questions become, then: (a) *Who* is doing these analyses? And (b): *How* is all this data "crunched" so that "dots" which might point to a terror attack can be separated and acted upon?

The answer to the first question is primarily "behavioral scientists" (Ph.D.-level psychologists) with concurrent degrees in statistics, and maybe some background in intelligence, making it easier for them to get a Top Secret or higher security clearance.

The answer to the second question is that data tends to be a hodge-podge of unrelated actual facts and "factoids" (a term coined by renowned Norman Mailer to mean purportedly solid information posing as actual facts). If there is a "rap sheet" for a juvenile offender then yes, it *might* get transmitted to prospective employers, college admission offices or airline security. But, bet on bureaucratic incompetence and inaccuracies every time.

We have all seen how this works: A person with a long criminal record is released and goes on to commit another horrendous crime (see next chapter for specific cases), while a student or journalist with politically incorrect opinions gets nailed, with his or her career in ruins and an enormous fine.

Look at it this way: Remember those pesky word problems you were made to solve in school math classes? They were the bane of every kid who ever had trouble with math. The key was not how good you were at memorizing theorems, algorithms, or solving equations. Success boiled down to *ignoring* the *irrelevant* data and keying in on the information you actually needed. (Most teachers didn't explain that little tidbit, so clueless pupils were left to muddle through.)

But the same applies to identifying terror suspects. When irrelevant data are collected, and the wrong people analyze it, good information winds up in the wrong agency's lap.

Whether some celebrity takes Viagra onto an airplane, with or without his name on the prescription bottle, is *not* "actionable intel" and wastes precious resources. Taking aim at plastic eating utensils and forcing women to cram their cosmetics into tiny plastic baggies are actions that reflect desperation and do not inspire confidence.

Moreover, if the only way the TSA can "get a grip" is to literally grope Americans, government is inviting terrorists to have another "go" at us.

The Pre-Screening Gambit

Apparently, some travelers are more equal than others. A *Washington Post* article April 22, 2012 ("Express screening hinges on a fragile trust"), explained how the TSA is considering a program called Pre-Check for "safe" passengers in a belated "intelligence-driven, risk-based approach to security," wrote columnist Christopher Elliott.[69] However, according to Elliott, the government doesn't have to say why you were, or were not, selected for this new program, if you happen to apply.

Furthermore, if you try to get an answer, "you might find yourself in a bureaucratic labyrinth from which there is no escape." Could it be, then, that the political elite and big campaign donors will be the ones who get around TSA's phony security measures, as they largely do already?

So far, Pre-Check sounds about as credible as the now-defunct CLEAR® air traveler program. CLEAR® started in 2005 and shut down in 2009—after some 250,000 travelers had paid

---

[69] http://www.airliners.net/aviation-forums/general_aviation/print.main?id=3287608

nearly $200 a year for a detailed background check so they wouldn't have to put up with TSA security lines. The program had promised to speed a flier past the rigmarole, but basically all it did was hire agents to smile brightly, put the passenger's "special" VIP card ("Verified Identity Pass") into a reader at a designated kiosk, *then direct the unsuspecting sap to another line where TSA staff did what they always do.*

The high-tech VIP identification card carried a passenger's fingerprint or iris image. Passengers were encouraged to pay for additional years at a slight discount (especially when the program first opened), to avoid having to go through more background checks. But four years later, when the program closed—guess what? Travelers who had signed on couldn't get their money back. That part definitely wasn't, er, "clear."

As for their data? Well, it's somewhere in cyberspace!

Counteraction and Military Response

The now-infamous "Fast and Furious" scandal headlined in every news outlet is an outgrowth of U.S. incompetence on immigration and security issues but it comes under the heading of counteraction and military response—or at least it should. Unfortunately, border control and illegal immigration, contrary to reason in an age of foreign terrorism, is addressed pretty much like the War on Drugs, with similarly ineffective results,

Border Insecurity and Indifferent Immigration Policy

The alleged direct involvement of our own Attorney General, Eric Holder, in a gun-running operation that helped arm Mexican drug cartels is just one more breach in what is already a policy-driven national security disgrace. The whole episode was made possible because the United States has played long and loose with border control and illegal immigration— creating, in effect, a dual non-policy that was bound to blow up in our faces sooner or later.

The nation's porous borders took front and center stage beginning soon after the terror attacks of 9/11 in 2001. Ten years later, it was clear our nation's leaders lacked the political will to stem illegal immigration or provide even a halfway credible approach to border security—any border, not just the one in the South.

Each day brings instant-replays of the gory results of our government's inaction. In every report, we see an escalation of violence—either from foreign mafia, who deal in everything from "protection" rackets, to drugs, to human trafficking, or from drug-related gang wars that have moved from border towns and farms onto our side of a "Swiss-cheese" fence, and from there into urban U.S. cities nationwide.

The Southwest is sustaining terrible damage in both loss of life and property. Foreign thugs, primarily from Mexico, scare away or kill American ranchers and their livestock, then used the stolen land to establish safe-houses on American soil for various noxious enterprises—ranging from drug smuggling to sex slavery.

In the process, these thugs have created something else: "safe-*routes*" and gateways that could be used to transport enough rudimentary materials to carry out a limited radiologic, biologic or chemical terror attack capable of killing thousands within minutes. Given the similarities in outer appearance of many natives of South America and Middle Easterners, even profiling probably would not improve the chances apprehending an actual terrorist.

Making the U.S. Safe for WMD's.- Evidence of corruption and collusion is pervasive, although that is only part of the problem.

In a coup for incompetence, state and national leaders are quibbling over the definition of "bridge"—narrow metal footpaths on either side of our all-but-useless $2.4 billion border fence that provide easy passage for illegal immigrants and smugglers without their even getting wet as they cross the Rio Grande.

Alicia A. Caldwell explained in her report to the *Washington Times*[70] that "they are not called *bridges*, but rather 'grade control structures'… built in the 1930s to stabilize and prevent a shift during high river flow." These footpaths, or whatever one wishes to call them, now accommodate any terrorist who might cross over.

A Hudspeth County's Sheriff, Lt. Robert Wilson, noted that "a terrorist could pass through here with weapons of mass destruction and be in the United States and up on the interstate and gone in a short time."[71] Reporter Alicia Caldwell adds that there are always fresh sneaker tracks on the structures, indicating they're being actively used as passageways into the U.S.

A 2010 GAO Report identified other vulnerabilities at our borders. One report, compliments of the Terrorism Committee of the National Association of Chiefs of Police, concluded that terrorists were sauntering through most of the covertly tested ports of entry using counterfeit identification! Undercover agents examined ports of entry—by air, sea, and land, wherever international travelers can legally enter the United States. These undercover investigators "made 42 crossings with a 93 percent success rate," revealed Jim Kouri in an article for NewsWithViews.[72]

In all four states on the northern border (Washington, New York, Michigan, and Idaho), three states on the southern border (California, Arizona, and Texas), and two other states requiring international air travel (Florida and Virginia), government inspectors apparently were accepting oral assertions and counterfeit identifications provided by GAO undercover investigators as proof of U.S. citizenship and allowed them to enter the country.

---

[70] http://www.washingtontimes.com/news/2010/aug/19/unguarded-border-bridges-could-be-route-us/?page=1

[71] http://homelandsecuritynewswire.com/footpaths-across-rio-grande-allow-easy-route-us

[72] http://www.newswithviews.com/NWV-News/news188.htm

Meanwhile, Fox News' Jana Winter in a report April 19, 2011, interviewed Arizona's Cochise County Sheriff, Larry Dever. He confirmed that the federal government was, and perhaps still is, pursuing a no-apprehension policy for illegals who crossed the border.

Subsequent to the Fox News exclusive[73] Sheriff Dever said he was literally "flooded with calls and emails from local and federal agents who backed up his claims that the U.S. Border Patrol [had] effectively ordered them to stop apprehending illegal immigrants crossing the U.S.-Mexican border."

The next day, April 20, 2011, in a the top story in *The Washington Times,*[74] readers saw the results of that policy: Veteran journalist Jerry Seper exposed how violent drug gangs not only are expanding into the U.S., but doing so with a "disparate band of criminals known as Los Zetas." Their signature style, wrote Seper, is to decapitate and dismember victims—quite enough to qualify them as terrorists in most people's minds. Los Zetos' tentacles now reach to cities across our nation.

Mr. Seper explains how the group originally was "[t]rained as an elite band of Mexican anti-drug commandos, [then] evolved into mercenaries for the infamous Gulf Cartel bringing a new wave of brutality to Mexico's escalating drug wars."

Insecure borders constitute a national threat no matter who is behind it. Two factions actively hinder border control. One is environmental extremists, bent on placing their wetlands agenda game over national security. Another is left-leaning "one-worlders" who are hostile to the whole concept of national boundaries and sovereignty. If you don't believe that last one, listen carefully to the lyrics of late Beatles icon John Lennon's song, "Imagine." There's nothing wishy-washy about imagining

---

[73] http://www.foxnews.com/us/2011/04/19/arizona-sheriff-cites-flood-border-agents-confirming-feds-apprehension-policy/#ixzz1K3rZQZkH
[74] http://www.washingtontimes.com/multimedia/collection/violent-mexican-drug-gang-expands-into-us/

"no countries," "nothing to kill or die for," and "no religion, too."

Environmentalist Traitors.- The ostensible effort to "save" wetlands, marine life, water resources and even the air we breathe at the expense of the nation's defense infrastructure exemplifies the symbiotic relationship between the federal government and leftist extremists with respect to national security.

The evidence for outright collusion between the federal government and eco-activists appears in various forms. Judicial Watch, a non-partisan watchdog organization, exposed one of these forms in April 2011, when it revealed how the U.S. government is prioritizing environmental "preservation" over national security *by banning Border Patrol from wildlife refuges* that are heavily transited by Mexican drug- and human-smugglers.[75] It turned out that this was nothing new: Border Patrol agents have been prohibited for years, by the Interior Department <u>and</u> the U.S. Forest Service, from actively patrolling such areas, *because doing so threatens natural resources*:

"Motorized vehicles, road construction and the installation of surveillance structures required to adequately secure the vast areas are forbidden," according to Judicial Watch's online journal, "because it could endanger the environment and its wildlife."

Meanwhile, Mexican <u>drug cartels and human smugglers</u> (like the Los Zetos commandos) regularly use the large swaths of unmanned and federally "protected" land to enter the U.S.

The term *federally protected* means that areas are placed off-limits for their historical or scenic value, for their at-risk environmental status, and occasionally for defense-related

---

[75] http://www.judicialwatch.org/blog/2011/apr/border-patrol-banned-top-smuggler-routes

infrastructure. But to enviro-extremists, the nation's defense is the last priority.

An irate Republican House issued a press release[76] announcing a legislative effort to prohibit *any* federal agency— *especially* the Department of the Interior—from using environmental regulations to hinder the Border Patrol agents. The measure would essentially ensure that the Border Patrol, not federal land managers, have operational control of the nation's borders, inasmuch as these areas have become the paths-of-choice for illicit operations. The Republican House press release explains:

> ...federal land managers are using environmental regulations to prevent Border Patrol from accessing portions of the 20.7 million acres along the U.S. southern border and over 1,000 miles of the U.S.-Canada border. Border Patrol agents are consistently unable to use motorized vehicles to patrol these areas or place electronic surveillance structures in strategic areas. As a result, our federal lands have become a highway open to criminals, drug smugglers, human traffickers and potentially terrorists. This has led to escalated violence and also caused destruction of the environment.

Ironically, states Judicial Watch, these criminal operations not only endanger American lives but also cause severe environmental damage. In a piece exposing the latest evidence of complicity between the federal government and environmental extremist groups, Judicial Watch notes[77] that "Interior [Department] officials charge the Department of Homeland Security millions of dollars for conducting preapproved Border Patrol operations on its land. Since 2007,

---

[76] http://naturalresources.house.gov/News/DocumentSingle.aspx?DocumentID=23635
8

[77] http://www.judicialwatch.org/blog/2010/apr/interior-dept-impedes-border-patrol-securing-u-s

Homeland Security has paid the Interior Department more than $9 million to mitigate the 'environmental damage' of protecting the border."

All of which leads a person to wonder: Just how serious are the eco-activists about clean air, fresh water or any other talking point in their environmental rhetoric? Is it all just another agenda game aimed at snookering the public?

Another form of environmental collusion was revealed April 21, 2011, by Chuck Sylvester, landowner and co-founder of LawUSA, in LaSalle, Colorado. He detailed for the *Greeley Tribune* [78] what appears to be a joint effort by the federal government and eco-activists to control land and water resources, both private and public. The aim, he said, is to effectively shut down private, domestic enterprises "such as timber harvest, energy exploration and…cattle grazing." Mr. Sylvester explains the sleight-of-hand used by the government to wrest control from private landowners in the Midwest and South: the Equal Access to Justice Act.

"Here's how it works," stated Mr. Sylvester:

> The federal government gives eco-activists money to…file a lawsuit against the federal government [to force a stoppage of resource production]. The feds [then] respond to the eco-activist suit by asking, 'How much do you want?' and quickly write a check for [that] amount, which oftentimes includes attorney fees at $650 an hour. In contrast, the resource provider (i.e., landowner) is forced to respond [or lose everything] on their own dime.

Just six days before Mr. Sylvester's comments in the *Greeley Tribune*, on April 15, the Subcommittee on National Parks, Forests and Public Lands and the Security, Homeland Defense, and Foreign Operations Subcommittee held a joint

---

[78] http://www.greeleytribune.com/SECTION/&Profile=1028&ParentProfile=1025

oversight hearing[79] titled *"The Border: Are Environmental Laws and Regulation Impeding Security and Harming the Environment?"* to examine (for the umpteenth time!) this very issue.

One of the least understood, environmentally based incursions upon our national sovereignty is the Law of the Sea Treaty (LOST). The National Center for Public Policy Research's website provides educational resources on LOST (a.k.a. UNCLOS).

LOST would "help radical environmentalists achieve what they haven't been able to achieve through legislation," said National Center Vice President David Ridenour. He noted that the treaty would "...place a significant portion of the world's resources under the control of a U.N.-style body, and complicate our efforts to apprehend terrorists on the high seas by subjecting our actions to review by an international court unlikely to render decisions favorable to the U.S." Even Greenpeace has noted that "the benefits of the U.N. Convention on the Law of the Sea are substantial...." The U.S. Navy's use of sonar has already been challenged.

The aforementioned Government Accountability Office (GAO)—the investigative arm of Congress—is one of the few still highly respected agencies of government. It surveyed federal officers who said they continually encountered "delays and restrictions in their patrolling and monitoring operations" on federally protected (off-limits) lands. In one case, land managers took more than four months to conduct a "historic property assessment" before granting our Border Patrol permission to move in surveillance equipment.

Another GAO report, also dated April 15, 2011, "Border Patrol Operations on Federal Lands,"[80] laid out the familiar scenario, in which rabid environmentalists again trumped public safety: "...a popular smugglers' corridor, ...a 2,300-acre San

---

[79] http://naturalresources.house.gov/Calendar/EventSingle.aspx?EventID=234828
[80] http://www.gao.gov/new.items/d11573t.pdf

Bernardino National Wildlife Refuge, used by an illegal immigrant who murdered an Arizona rancher last spring."

And on it goes: Congressional investigations, reports, predictable outrage, and legislative proposals—all re-visiting the same questions, over and over, while the nation slides further into harm's way.

Sovereignty Traitors.- On February 24, 2012, Rep. Lamar Smith (R-TX), wrote a scathing piece for the *Washington Times* ("Obama budget's backdoor amnesty") detailing exactly how ineffective border security has been, and how Barack Obama was providing not only "backdoor amnesty" for illegals, but compromising both national security and, inevitably, national sovereignty.

Rep. Smith should know, as he has served in Texas's 21st congressional district since 1987. Among the most significant revelations of his article is a GAO Report finding that in 2011 "just 44 percent of the Southwestern border was under the operational control of the Border Patrol." In other words, less than half the border is under protection, despite all the nonsense about high-tech fences.

Rep. Smith further revealed that in Barack Obama's version of the non-budget, there were "cuts for several worthwhile immigration-enforcement and border security programs." Furthermore, as far back as 1996, under Bill Clinton, Justice Department records show that "40 percent of all non-detained illegal immigrants in removal proceedings simply became fugitives." Being non-detained, they simply merged into the fabric of our society—but with no intention of actually assimilating, just cashing in on America's social services. And that doesn't count all the illegals that joined gangs and other criminal enterprises. One would like to think that a few of them, at least, took pains to assimilate and contribute to this society as upstanding citizens.

More than Mere Incompetence

Is all this really just incompetence? If the Department of Homeland Security (DHS) is aware of the problem, then it also knows that 600 miles worth of "fencing"—be it high- or low-tech—*is inadequate to cover a 1,200-mile swath*. What is the agenda here?

The first hint that something beyond incompetence was at work in our post-9/11 "new-and-improved" national security measures came in February 2005. That is when it was first reported that Texas Border Patrol Agents Ignacio Ramos and Jose Alonso Compean had been sentenced to 20 years in prison for doing their job. A ditsy Assistant U.S. Attorney came up with the now-infamous charge that "it is a violation of Border Patrol regulations to go after someone who is fleeing."

The fellow they were chasing in a small town close to El Paso—Osbaldo Aldrete-Davila, a Mexican citizen—had smuggled drugs into the U.S. more than once. Even so, Davila, having been shot in the buttocks by the agents, was given full immunity to testify against the agents as well as free medical care for non-life-threatening injuries at William Beaumont Army Medical Center in El Paso.

The news reports were odd, not least because they stated that Agent Ramos had been instrumental in the capture of nearly 100 drug smugglers and the seizure of untold thousands of pounds of narcotics[81] and was even nominated as Agent of the Year, a nomination that was withdrawn following the shooting incident. Prosecutors nevertheless treated the drug smuggler as a martyr, refusing to allow testimony that would have helped the border guards.

Andrew "Andy" Ramirez, founder and president of the Law Enforcement Officers Advocates Council (LEOAC), a nonprofit law enforcement advocacy corporation, and a regular

---

[81] http://www.campominutemen.com/news/Convicted-border-agent-tells-his-story.aspx

correspondent on immigration and border security for Liberty News Network, has sorted out subsequent schizophrenic responses of our government toward Border Patrol agents. These run the gamut from strangely over-aggressive prosecutions of border agents for defending our nation from smugglers and illegals, to multiple cover-ups to hide the aiding and abetting of illegal activities on the part of officials, such as the gunrunning operation from the U.S. to Mexican cartels—especially the now-open case known as "Operation Fast and Furious." A newer legal case, in which LEOAC is representing border Agent Jesus Diaz, is pending at this writing.

In a June 6, 2011, article,[82] published in several publications, including *The New American*, Ramirez described the events of December 14, 2010—an incident along "the Rio Rico area of Southern Arizona about 15 miles north of the U.S.-Mexico border." This was a coup of investigative reporting. It led the way for other federal whistleblowers facing a veil of secrecy surrounding Operation Fast and Furious as well as an alleged, generalized war on border control agents by the U.S. justice Department.

"In a nutshell," writes Ramirez, "the federal Bureau of Alcohol, Tobacco and Firearms purposely allowed over a thousand guns—likely many thousands—to be sold to Mexican drug cartels." Ramirez's report details what happened when four members of what can best be described as the Special Forces of Border Control, the elite BORTAC (Border Tactical Unit):

> were summoned to Peck Canyon, one of the many rural pathways alongside Interstate 19 that are notorious as transport routes for smugglers of drugs, humans, and other contraband. Peck Canyon is also notorious as an area plagued by Mexican bandits known as "rip crews" who prey not only on the smugglers and illegal aliens, but also on hikers, ranchers, local

---

[82]   http://www.andyramirez.com/LNN/TNA-Project-Gunrunner-AR.pdf

police, and Border Patrol agents. Robbery, rape, and murder have become the bandits' stock in trade.

Most people know nothing about "rip crews," or for that matter, anything more than the existence of a few illegal border crossers, supposedly braving the elements and the odds in an earnest attempt to live and work in this country, given the economic disadvantages pervasive throughout South America. They know that there is the occasional drug smuggler and human trafficker, but most northeasterners, for example, think this is the extent of the problem. This notion couldn't be farther from the truth:

> Agent Brian Terry's BORTAC Unit reportedly confronted at least five bandits in the darkened ravine. Agent Terry was shot…. He shouted he couldn't feel his legs, and later…was pronounced dead. One of the bandits was wounded and captured, along with three other members of the gang. A fifth suspect was apprehended later by Santa Cruz County Deputy Sheriffs.

In the aftermath of Agent Brian Terry's death several terrible irregularities began surfacing, details of which are now legend in nearly every news outlet. In May 2012, they led all the way to Attorney General Eric H. Holder, Jr., who at this writing, is facing a contempt of Congress resolution for refusing to cooperate in an investigation. Among the troubling specifics cited by Ramirez:

- Agent Terry's BORTAC Unit was under orders to use non-lethal "beanbag" loads; [while] the bandits responded with WASR-10s, a variant of the Russian AK-47 assault rifles.
- Firearms confiscated from the bandits [that] turned out to be guns [which] had been delivered to the drug cartels via an operation of the federal Bureau

of Alcohol, Tobacco and Firearms (ATF) named Project Gunrunner.

- ATF agents, as well as the private firearms dealer who sold the guns to the Mexican cartel's buyer at the ATF's direction, had warned ATF higher-ups against continuing the program and had warned that the guns would be used for criminal purposes.
- Hundreds of guns (possibly thousands) sold to the Mexican cartel operatives under the ATF's supervision remain unaccounted for and are presumed to be still in criminal hands.

And that's just for openers. Questionable intelligence-gathering and other irregularities had tentacles reaching all the way to U.S. Immigration and Customs Enforcement (ICE), the DHS, and the Justice Department.

So exactly why, again, are Americans standing in line for invasive pat-downs and other insults in airport "security" lines?

Preparing the Groundwork for Martial Law

Any student of history knows that no good can come from a combination of extremism, fraud, graft, and national security failure. The present campaign of institutionalized harassment of law-abiding citizens is spreading a fertilizer of chaos, anarchy, fear, resentment and suspicion that eventually will culminate in a backlash. At that point, only a declaration of martial law and imposition of a police state will rein in wholesale disrespect for the law, contempt for government, and cynicism toward once-cherished institutions.

And as a matter of fact, a declaration of martial law is no longer an off-the-wall idea. Columnist and president of the Edmund Burke Institute, Jeffrey T. Kuhner reported on a March 16, 2012, Executive Order by Barack Obama—National Defense Resources Preparedness. The order gives Mr. Obama across-the-board power to do just that. Executive Orders are pretty much ignored by the American public, and often get short shrift in the media. But Mr. Kuhner's piece that appeared March 23, 2012, in the *Washington Times* revealed what's in this one:

> ...that, in case of war or national emergency, the federal government has the authority to take over almost every aspect of American society. Food, livestock, farming equipment, manufacturing, industry, energy, transportation, hospitals, health care, water resources, defense and construction.... The order empowers the president to dispense these vast resources as he sees fit during a national crisis.

Even President Franklin D. Roosevelt didn't go that far— and he was fighting a war on two fronts in World War II!

By now, every reader probably recognizes the operative words in this description: "national crisis" and "emergency"— both redefined at every opportunity. And it isn't as if the United States doesn't already have enough bills already on the books relating to national security—for example, the National Defense Authorization Act (NDAA). It has been reauthorized many times over the years, including Fiscal Year 2012. NDAA dates back to the 1960s, but has undergone so many sweeping revisions and enhancements that the Act's title barely reflects the original.

Jihadists Steal a Page from Old Soviet Handbook

In a nod to political correctness—and a thumb to the eye of Christians—our government is falling all over itself to appease ("reach out to") Islamic totalitarian ideologues. Perhaps appeasement isn't so surprising in light of the fact that Islamic jihadists learned some of their strategies from their old Soviet adversaries in Afghanistan. Infiltration, propaganda and sleeper agents are very much part of the Soviet playbook. Today, Islamic jihadists are following the same model. Meanwhile,

Americans—and, worse, our intelligence services—bury their heads in the sand.

It isn't as though we haven't been warned—by some Islamists who are not happy with the turn their former compatriots-turned-fanatics have taken, as well as by foreign allies in governments that have borne experienced terrorist attacks of their own since 9/11.

One man, in particular, has dared to single out one of the greatest threats to our nation: the Muslim Brotherhood. Frank J. Gaffney, Jr., president of the Center for Security Policy and *Washington Times* columnist, makes a strong case.[83] In a June 25, 2012 piece, he detailed how Barack Obama not only facilitated, but had "underwritten the Muslim Brotherhood's takeover in Egypt and an increasing number of states elsewhere in the Middle East."

Why should we care about that, especially if the Brotherhood maintains some semblance of order within that volatile part of the world? Just this, says Gaffney: "The Muslim Brotherhood is the prime mover behind [a] seditious campaign, which it calls 'civilized jihad'."

So-called "civilized jihad" means subversion, Soviet-style. Gaffney describes it as penetration and influence to shape policy at the highest level of government, both in the U.S. and throughout the free world, whether that government calls itself socialist or free-market. In America, says Gaffney, the Brotherhood uses a variety of front organizations, echoing the Soviet model, "as liaisons...[to] provide support to and participation in Shariah-compliant finance."

Shariah is the Islamic version of "law"—enormously intolerant in its original form, and unfriendly toward the ideals contained in the U.S. Constitution, the Bill of Rights and the

---

[83] http://www.pointofview.net/site/News2?&page=NewsArticle&id=20425&printer_friendly=1&news_iv_ctrl=-1 and
http://www.washingtontimes.com/news/2012/jun/25/muslim-brotherhoods-bait-and-switch/

Declaration of Independence. Giving the Brotherhood free reign, wrote Gaffney, is like trying to win the Cold War by giving a lead role to the KGB, or depending upon the German-American Bund organization to win World War II.

Islamic, or Shariah, law as explained by Robert D. Crane, co-founder of the Muslim American Bar Association, is based entirely on the Koran (or Quran), as purportedly revealed *verbatim* to the Islamic prophet, Muhammad, and, as such, is the "ultimate criteria for judgment on every aspect of one's individual and social life."[84] There are basically two sects, Sunni (the majority) and Shia (roughly 20 percent of Muslims).

Unelected imams, or clerics, wield complete power. Punishment for infractions—including those Americans would view as petty—include whippings, amputations, beatings, stonings, executions, beheadings, torture, body mutilation, and violent jihad (world domination) against even a *perceived* critic of Muhammad or Islam's version of God, Allah. Under Shariah, women are even less than second-class citizens and must be entirely submissive to men. (Where are Eleanor Clift and Gloria Steinem when you need them?)

Many earnest (largely Westernized) asylum-seekers fled Iran, Iraq, Syria and other Middle Eastern countries for the U.S. and other free nations in the 1970s and 80s, just ahead of the fanatical turn the region was taking. Most assimilated well into our culture without sacrificing their cultural heritage or religious beliefs.

These immigrants anticipated the emergence of totalitarian regimes that favored the most extreme aspects of what they thought were antiquated Shariah mandates that had been abandoned—for example, the mandate that non-believers ("infidels") convert to Islam or face one of the punishments listed above, along with confiscation of a citizen's property; kidnapping and ransoming foreigners for money; and genital mutilation of female children.

---

[84] http://www.islamicity.com/politics/sharia.htm

But the new crop of autocratic leaders rejected anything resembling "pursuit of happiness." That is why America is considered by Islamic totalitarians to be the Number One threat to their objectives.

Mr. Gaffney's most shocking revelation in the *Times* piece was that Barack Obama "transferred $1.5 billion of our tax dollars in a lump-sum payment" to the Muslim Brotherhood. "For him to do so," wrote Gaffney, "Secretary of State Hillary Rodham Clinton had to waive congressionally imposed restrictions" because of "justified concerns about the nature and direction of the Shariah-adherent government [that] the Brotherhood is birthing in Egypt."

Egyptians participated in their first free vote on May 24, 2012. Among the contenders were the Muslim Brotherhood's Mohamed Morsi and other, more popular choices, or so it seemed at first. Suddenly, it was reported on May 25 that Morsi of the Muslim Brotherhood was forging ahead, whereas not long before, that seemed unlikely, as he was not particularly charismatic.

Could Mr. Obama's shocking transfer of $1.5 billion, directly into the coffers of the Brotherhood have helped bankroll Morsi's candidacy?

Apparently so. On June 24, the final results were in, along with dancing in Egypt's streets. Mohammed Morsi, Egypt's first Islamic president, had narrowly defeated all the earlier-on, more popular, candidates, and finally the former prime minister, too.

What kind of message did Mr. Obama's outrageous sum send to the Middle East—or to Americans? What was Mr. Obama playing at? And why the waiver by the State Department?

Meanwhile, the United States is being forewarned by a variety of Shariah-targeted individuals around the world, many of whom once traveled freely—for example, Geert Wilders, a Dutch author, leader of the Party for Freedom, and Member of

Parliament. He states in his 2011 book that ever since he asked the Dutch government to investigate a radical mosque in 2003, he has been a marked man. Then, with the murder of Dutch filmmaker Theo van Gogh in 2004 for exposing abuses of women under Islamic law, Mr. Geert started being physically accosted and threatened. Today, he travels with bodyguards, wears a bullet-proof vest and lives in a "safe house" instead of his home.

Thus the reason, no doubt, for a growing reluctance among Americans to express concerns about such things as the precipitous rise of madrassas (Islamic schools) in the U.S.; or an Islamic "cultural center" built adjacent to the World Trade Center memorial; or Islamic charities that may, or may not, be front organizations for jihad. Even the Defense Department is purportedly tiptoeing around any mention of Islam and radicalism in the same breath.

It is understandable that Americans would try to avoid confrontation or more terror attacks via "diplomatic" solutions and various accommodations. But when Americans cannot see the difference between religious expression and a fanatical, no-holds-barred totalitarian movement; when our nation's leaders cannot differentiate between altruism and mollification, or understand evangelism versus provocation, then the nation is in trouble.

Worse, left-leaning groups are doing their best to eliminate Christian symbols altogether, including overt mentions of Christian-themed holidays and values—perhaps, to some minds, in the belief that the best defense is no religious mention whatsoever. If that is their thought, it won't work—mainly because Islamic schools and culture centers are free to teach the Koran, but U.S. schools and public exhibits cannot display an open Bible or a cross.

Which sends what kind of message about our Founding ideals to the young?

Military Response and Counteraction

Military action, or the lack thereof, is based primarily on a nation's foreign policy. The same goes for counteraction, which includes economic sanctions and humanitarian/economic aid. Therefore, the three must necessarily be considered together.

Intervention Versus War

Ever since the Vietnam War (which, contrary to Red China's successful propaganda campaign and penetration of American media, was both necessary and winnable), any attempt at military action has been viewed through the lens of radicalized anti-war protesters, both when such action is warranted and when it is not.

In the case of Vietnam, Congress never declared formal declaration of war, unnecessarily prolonged the "police action," then caved in to professional agitators and campus radicals. Marxist penetration resulted in mistaken notions about the objectives of the war, and planted an anti-war fervor in 1960s and 70s that never died out. The draft was discontinued—by, of all people, President Richard M. Nixon, who turned our military into an all-volunteer force in 1973, just the way leftist radicals wanted it.

Now comes the pundits arguing in May 2012 that the idea of a volunteer military force has been *too successful* and, therefore, we should get rid of it! Why? Because, writes Thomas E. Ricks in the *Washington Post*, going to war has been made too easy!

Richard Nixon gets no rest....

Of course, there are times when military intervention *is* ill-conceived, especially when America lacks any interest in a target country's affairs, offensive though some of its actions may be to human rights advocates and American sensibilities.

Add to that, the long-drawn out congressional process associated with any declaration of war, which means that any real adversaries get a heads-up through the media "leaks," among other things. So, the element of surprise and the capability to create a workable strategy are necessarily compromised. The enemy is always able to gear up and anticipate our moves.

Worst of all, though, is that recent administrations have felt bound to get the United Nation's permission—or concurrence, if you prefer—to launch a military strike, which is a huge blow to our national sovereignty. Indeed, Defense Secretary Leon E. Panetta argued recently that the United States only needs "international permission" to go war, not Congress's. Obviously, the U.N. isn't going to be overly sympathetic to American interests—not when its agenda game includes placing some of the world's worst human-rights abusers as High Commissioners on its Human Rights Council, in the misplaced hope that a respect for human dignity might rub off.

So, militarily speaking, what the United States generally ends up with is a never-ending series of "military interventions" and "peacekeeping operations"—many of which turn violent. President George W. Bush tried to break that trend with the invasion of Iraq—by appealing to the U.N. and NATO. We all know what he got for his trouble. Thus have "interventions" been the name of the game everywhere there is a "hot spot," putting American lives and treasure at risk.

This strategy also leaves average citizens ambivalent about the objectives of our government's various missions, since most have no idea which pundits, columnists and news reports to believe. Consequently, they leave it to the "experts," complaining only when a campaign seems to take an inordinate amount of time, as in Iraq and Afghanistan. If Iran blew up a major American city tomorrow, it is difficult to say with certainty that Americans would support a retaliatory strike.

These police actions, peacekeeping ops, interventions, or whatever one wishes to call them, are generally ineffective in the long run, however successful they may appear at the beginning. This is due to the fact that the U.S. feels a moral obligation to stay in these target regions to rebuild infrastructures and inaugurate democracies, despite often profound cultural disinclinations on the part of the country in question. Unlike in Japan in 1945, we are not insisting on unconditional surrender. And if, technically, we're tot "at war," then that option is off the table anyway.

At the same time we are busy intervening and nation-building, the U.S. conducts business with hostile countries. Countries like China share America's interests only so long as it serves their own agenda. Yes, China has developed some elements of market economics, but, on an individual level, it is hardly a "free" market. In addition, its human rights record rivals that of the Middle East, so Americans wind up subsidizing severe abuses.

Unfortunately, taxpayers are conditioned to ignore these inconvenient truths, in the hope that a permanent friendship will result, thereby avoiding any need to "intervene" at all—say, in Taiwan, should China choose to lob a few missiles in that direction.

Should Taxpayers Subsidize Humanitarian Aid?

Many Americans already contribute to various humanitarian projects through their houses of worship and charities. But the strings attached to government-subsidized aid tend to be ineffective or consistent. One has to ask, then, whether Americans should be *forced* to bankroll, through taxes, what should be a voluntary commitment to help countries in need.

In a *Washington Times* article (one of several on the subject in other newspapers), "Bush speech jumpstarts initiative to combat cancer," Paige Winfield Cunningham described September 13, 2011, how a compassionate George W. Bush was using his own namesake institution to jumpstart an initiative combating women's cancers (cervical and breast) in developing countries—primarily Africa, Vietnam, and Haiti, where such diseases are more rampant due to the high levels of AIDS/HIV. The project was part of the "Pink Ribbon, Red Ribbon," program, the goal of which was to "expand the services of clinics created under the President's Emergency Plan for AIDS Relief (PEPFAR)."

So, here was a private source, in the form of the George W. Bush Institute, providing a worthy service to the least fortunate beings on the planet, soliciting private donations from philanthropists and charities in a benevolent expression of selflessness.

But wait! In the middle of the *Times* article we discover that: "PEPFAR was initially funded in 2003 with *$15 billion* to be used primary in 15 countries with the highest rates of HIV/AIDS.... In 2008, *Congress more than tripled the initiative's funds, to $48 billion through 2013*." [Emphasis mine.]

Far be it from most Americans to wish anyone, anywhere, a gruesome death, preventable or not. But right here in the U.S., according to the American Cancer Society, were approximately 1,529,560 new cancer victims in 2010, many unable to pay the cost of chemotherapy regimens, which can run as high as $30,000, or radiation therapies, which cost upwards of $10,000, much less $40,000 for the newer photon treatments. Other expenditures typically include surgery to repair collateral body damage caused by chemotherapy or radiation.

"Insured," middle-class families are going broke to accommodate these enormous sums. Yet, our "compassionate" government steals from these taxpayers to pay for cancer screenings and treatments halfway around the world.

What kind of agenda is this? Asking Americans to donate to charities for cancer is one thing. Transferring their money to whatever nations government pleases is another.

It turns out that this scheme is a a corporate partnership between the Joint United Nations Programme on HIV/AIDS (UNAIDS), the U.S. State Department, PEPFAR, the George W. Bush Institute, and the controversial Susan G. Komen[85] for The Cure®.

With America in "corporate partner" with the U.N., this lends further legitimacy to an international body that routinely thumbs its nose at our nation's ideals of morality and justice, and makes it harder to extricate ourselves from that global body if push comes to shove.

For some reason, our legislators believe such policy makes sense: "I hope the American people understand that 6.6 million people receive life-saving medicine...[that] 6.6 million people who would be dead today now live, thanks to an effort by the American people," former President Bush was quoted as saying.

But does Mr. Bush understand that such expenditures are not specifically sanctioned by American taxpayers?

A Foreign Policy Worth Dying For: "Don't Make Us Fight You!"

Obviously, many of these problems could be avoided if the United States had a concise, viable foreign policy statement. Most candidates for public office are reluctant to come up with a firm foreign policy—possibly for fear of provoking the media, and even their assortment of sometime-allies. But failing to articulate a firm foreign policy compromises our military, renders our economic sanctions laughable (especially in Iran), confuses our allies, and does nothing to portray Americans as bold action figures—a superpower with innovative ideas.

The following might serve as a model for an unambiguous U.S. foreign policy message—penned by this author on the 10th anniversary of the 9/11 attacks and published by NewsWithViews. It reflects 21st century fiscal and domestic

[85]   http://www.mrc.org/node/39058

realities and is built around an American definition for "an Act of War":

The United States has exactly zero interest in appending foreign territory or people. We have quite enough individuals flocking to our shores as it is—from asylum-seekers to opportunity-seekers to entitlement-seekers. We are, however, committed to defending our nation and our citizens from harm, including those employed overseas. The United States therefore sends this message to the world: **Do not make us fight you!**

If you attack our country, its properties, its Territories or its private citizens going about their business in foreign lands, we will consider that an **Act of War** *and respond forcefully. You will not win. We are light-years ahead of you technologically; we have the best-prepared armed forces on the planet. Attack us, and your country will be leveled. We can, and will, demand* **unconditional surrender** *so that your people, formally sanctioned by your government or not, will not attack us again.*

This means no more nation-building. No more attempts to buy good will by providing America's enemies state-of-the-art infrastructures that we cannot afford for ourselves. If you, or your proxies, commit what we have defined as an Act of War upon the United States, then you will sit in your own rubble—assuming you survive. There will be no more pre-emptive "police actions," no undeclared wars to serve as a warning.

Regarding humanitarian aid: Our nation's many charitable organizations are free to offer services, accepting the risks and expenses of such endeavors from private donations. The U.S. Government will **neither hinder nor help** *such efforts. Humanitarian projects are, by definition, philanthropic. Therefore, the U.S. Government will no longer confiscate (steal) money from citizens, who may not wish to donate to specialized philanthropic causes. Such effort must be entirely voluntary—with just one caveat, for which a tax break will be provided to any requesting charity (lest this stipulation be seen* as an "unfunded mandate"): Any materiel used in a humanitarian effort, whether from natural disasters (e.g., famines, earthquakes) or war-caused displacement, sickness and ruin, will dispatch no supplies or literature that are not embossed with the **donating organization's logo**, clearly visible, as well as a **U.S. flag**. This action serves to curtail the practice of foreign outlaws appropriating American-made goods for re-transmittal under their own name.

As for propping up regimes deemed "friendly" to the U.S. or its interests, including the legions of staff we send to fragile and unstable nations to help construct Constitutions, safeguard voting rights and implement democracy: **The United States is no longer in the business of imposing a specific type of government on inhabitants of other nations.** After nearly 70 years, we now recognize that each country must be "ready" to move to representative government and/or pure democracy; it cannot be forced from without. Nor can the United States "police" the entire world—even in the face of what we view as grave tragedies—in the misplaced hope that U.S. interference can stabilize, over the long term, a particular region or make the world safer. Too often "friendly" regimes have taken advantage of U.S. largesse and proved hostile—to our economic interests, our physical safety and our interests abroad.

Any country seriously seeking American assistance in moving toward representative government and increased freedom is free to seek out individuals with a proven track record of expertise from among our nation's vast network of "think tanks." Any nation so inclined may solicit for-hire services from these American individuals and groups, paying the costs of any housing, travel and or other expenses that may be required. Americans thus contacted have the right to accept or decline the offer.

But be forewarned, if U.S. citizens (or family members) are deliberately harmed, such employment having been accepted in *good faith, this, too, will be considered an **Act of War**, in keeping with the aforementioned definition. The nations of the world are on notice: The United States says what it means and means what it says; it will not tolerate any form of attack upon the U.S., either as a nation, its properties or its citizens—either here within the boundaries of the United States or abroad.*

*This rationale extends to border-crossing—by foot, by air, or by vehicle—without specific, verifiable permission to do so, especially when violent acts are then committed against persons or property within the United States. Foreign nationals doing so will be vigorously pursued as outlaws, punished in our courts, then deported to their home lands. In the event their actions are sanctioned by a foreign government—i.e., via repeated attempts to cross illegally, with or without literature on evasive tactics from that foreign government—that, too, will be considered an **Act of War**.*

The United States understands that many nations have depended upon this country's largesse for years, including those with struggling economies, and countries comprising the NATO alliance and the United Nations. Understand that such generosity on our part has, in the 21st century, become an enormous burden on U.S. taxpayers, with little to show for it. We can no longer afford to subsidize foreign countries in the style to which many in those nations have become accustomed.

It is the firm belief of the United States government that the nations of the world, including emerging societies, need to learn to stand on their own feet. Their citizens must commit to raising their standards of living, just as America did some 200 years ago. It was a slow process, not without setbacks, to fully realize rights such as freedom of speech, press, assembly, religion and so forth. The U.S. had to learn as it went, including when, and how, to "draw the line." It remains an unfinished task—even for us. Other countries will discover this as well. Liberty can neither be forced nor imposed.

The United States wishes all countries and emerging nations well. We are a peace-loving people. **Don't make us fight you**.

~

CHAPTER 5
THE JUSTICE GAME

The Constitution is not an instrument for the government to restrain the people, it is an instrument for the people to restrain the government—lest it come to dominate our lives and interests." – *Patrick Henry, 1776*

The Framers of the U.S. Constitution—George Washington, Thomas Jefferson, Alexander Hamilton, James Madison, and all the others—were men who knew their subject thoroughly because they had taken the trouble to study it. They were not just a group of politicians out to make name for themselves and came up with something they thought might make them popular. They had studied the medieval systems and all the various governing documents of their day. Unlike most of the political science graduates of today's premier colleges, such as the renowned John F. Kennedy School of Government at Harvard University, they were acquainted with the great classical writings on the topic of government— Aristotle, Plato, Machiavelli, Sir Thomas More, Montesquieu, Thomas Hobbes, John Locke, etc. So they were up to their task.

They knew the results of most of the governing structures that had already been tried, and above all, they wanted to avoid a repetition in America of the tyranny that had occurred in Europe and Asia over some 3,000 years, wrote the eminent philosopher, lecturer and theologian, Emmet Fox in 1939.[86]

"If they were to read a newspaper today on events in Europe, Asia, the Middle East and Africa, other than the technology, they would find little they had not read many times concerning other civilizations," he said. They were determined

---

[86] Emmet Fox, "The American Spirit," from a lecture in 1930, later compiled into a collection, *Alter Your Life*, p. 126, Harper & Row, New York, NY 1931.

to draw up a document that would make individual or group tyranny impossible—a system of checks and balances, specific duties that belong alone to one of the three branches of government, enumerated protections for the individual from government overreach, and a method for amending the document as the years brought new challenges.

The only practical alternatives to the principles of the Constitution and the Bill of Rights are either military despotism or bureaucratic despotism—the latter being a permanent or semi-permanent elite of civil servants, whether one calls it socialism or communism.[87] Both options try to supply the masses with basic physical necessities, and both deny men and women the chance to manage their own lives, take their own risks and, in short, to "give something a try."

A "pure" democracy (i.e., no representation) is not an option for three reasons: (1) every citizens would do nothing all day long except wrangle over policies and issues; (2) in a country as vast and geographically diverse as ours, issues occur that do not affect everyone; and (3) a pure democracy always winds up a "mobocracy," and rights are easily trampled underfoot.

Of course, the concept of personal independence—very revolutionary in the Framers' day—entails a certain degree of risk and suffering, as people might make a mistake. The prisoner who is told when to get up, when to go to bed, when and where to exercise, and handed a bowl of food can hardly go wrong, but nobody wants to live like that. "Free will," a concept which underlies the entire Constitution, means sometimes making a mistake—and hopefully learning something from it and moving on.

The Constitution does not guarantee equality of outcomes, any more than it promises equality of talent, equality of personality, or equality of physical prowess. What it does promise is equality of opportunity and equality before the law.

---

[87] Ibid, p. 126.

Unfortunately, that has not been enough for the political elites and social engineers who have worked their way into positions of power and influence over the past 40 years. They have retreated from the assumptions about human beings that the Framers made in hammering out the Constitution: that the average person is basically good-natured, honest, conscientious and trustworthy. The Framers viewed the human "default" setting, so to speak, as wishing to help rather than harm.

The policymakers of the past 40 years have reverted to positions held by previous civilizations: that the average person is selfish and foolish and needs to be continually threatened and intimidated to be kept in line. Of course, nothing like that is put into a governing document, as such attitudes do not look well in writing. But in the language of legalese it means exactly that.

Consequently, the Framers' constitutional ideals about justice, enshrined in the Constitution in 1787 and the Bill of Rights in 1791 are being whittled away.

- the accused citizen's right to a "speedy and public trial";
- "the right of the people to keep and bear arms" (such "being necessary to the security of a free State");
- "the right of the people to be secure ... against any unreasonable searches and seizures..." with any search or seizure, according to the Amendment IV, being contingent on having obtained a warrant based "upon probable cause"; and so on.

These three protections alone were among first-of-its-kind guidelines for justice in a free and open society. Today, they have been twisted beyond recognition.

Instead of the constitutional requirement for a "speedy and public trial," for example, we have innocent Americans languishing in jails and detention centers with hardened convicts over a supposedly unpaid fine (see chapter 4).

Meanwhile, vicious convicted killers sit on death row, all-expenses paid by law-abiding citizens, for a decade or more after sentencing.

Basically, the United States has moved toward just three kinds of justice: the "**Justice of Pretension**," the "**Justice of Harassment**," and the "**Justice of Accommodation**." All are infused with political correctness and the misguided fixations of "the caring professions"—the latter expression being a favorite pejorative of British author/playwright John Mortimer's most beloved character, Horace Rumpole.

The Justice of Pretension

"The Justice of Pretension," (or "pretentiousness," if you prefer) means the same thing as it does in other contexts—ostensible actions which are either perfunctory, fraudulent or, as in the case of justice, have long been proved ineffective. Many good-hearted and well-meaning individuals unconsciously bolster and maintain the ruse because they have been conditioned over 40 years to uphold the new view about "justice," explained at the top of this chapter.

The Justice of Pretension is characterized by expressions like "empathy," "rehabilitation," "restitution," "psychological therapy," and "catharsis" (emotionally cleansing). The constitutional view of justice came under fire in the 1960s, with the leftist incursion of pundits, psychologists and perception-managers alluded to in chapter 4. From that time on, long-held concepts about stigmatizing certain actions, or "shame," as it was called, had no place. "Shame" was part of the old morality psychologists like Chisholm, Rees and Cameron were trying to sweep away. Thus, anybody still using the expression was portrayed as vengeful, spiteful and hateful.

Similarly, prisons and jails were viewed as "correctional," rehabilitative," and "supportive," as opposed to being a form of "reprisal" or "punishment." Punishment was now deemed "vindictive," both in prison and in childrearing.

Moreover, "breaking down taboos" came to supersede "safeguarding the public." The X and Y generations cannot possibly appreciate how this changed America.

Today's touchy-feely list of "humane" (humanistic) programs and policies were unknown to the GIs who returned home from World War II—"early release" programs for offenders, "awareness" programs for everything from homelessness to HIV, "zero tolerance" policies for carrying cold remedies, and penalties for defending one's home and family. All these, and more, were suddenly "in the interests of society."

These well-planted perceptions characterized the new relationship between crime and justice. Some sounded good initially, but played out as twisted takes on "compassion." What we actually did was subsidize, at great expense, unrepentant thugs who had no moral compass.

The late Charles Colson's Prison Fellowship and the older "12-Step Program," co-founded in 1935 by Bill Wilson and Dr. Bob Smith, for alcohol- and drug-driven crime, enjoyed the most successes under the new mantra. But as the Christian moral values came increasingly under attack, great care had to be taken to prove that inmates signed up voluntarily for these programs, lest a lawsuit drop out of nowhere, redirecting thousands of dollars from the programs just to pay lawyers.

But, even with the relatively positive outcomes of a few rehabilitation programs, the rates of new crime and recidivism (repeat criminality) soared out of control.

The recidivism rate became so bad that, in 1984, a Truth in Sentencing (TIS) law was passed to ensure that vicious predators served at least 85 percent of their sentence (with most states formulating their own versions of TIS by 1994). But by 2009, as revelations surfaced in the horrific Jaycee Lee Dugard abduction (discussed more fully later) public cynicism burgeoned.

The "Three Strikes" Law was enacted by many state governments in the 1990s. The slogan-ish label emanated from baseball, where a batter is permitted two strikes, or misses, the third strike being "out." "Three Strikes" required the state courts to impose a *life* sentence to offenders who had been convicted of three or more serious crimes; but, unsurprisingly, this "life" sentence usually came with the probability of parole.

The "correctional" system was already too broken; neither TIS nor "Three Strikes" had much effect. By the 1990s, jail time was seen as a rite of passage among many youths. The enormous population of "career criminals" viewed prison as a free meal, free housing, medical care, a chance to meet other "enterprising" offenders, and even get free education as part of a "rehabilitation" program if one really wanted to.

Not a bad deal for the "gainfully *un*employed!"

"In summary, both Three Strikes and Truth in Sentencing have had few observable short-term impacts on the volume or composition of correctional populations," wrote Elsa Chen in a 2001 document for the Justice Department.

As for the danger, lack of privacy, regimentation (such as it was), the occasional sadistic "correctional" officers, it wasn't so different from the unstable life many thugs and gangsters had already been living.

Older inmates—offenders who had committed crimes in another era, when justice was less about politics and "rehabilitation," and more about safety—were scared to death of the new arrivals. Today, fear of rape has become a "central defining characteristic" of the prison experience.

In 2007, the Bureau of Justice Statistics (BJS) reported that out of a national prison population of 1,570,861, more than 70,000 prisoners were sexually abused—which translated to about one in 20 inmates, according to the Human Rights Watch organization—conversely, a 1978 study federal of inmates reported 0.6 percent of inmates were victimized in that way.

Random Acts of Savagery

The sheer audacity and viciousness of broad-daylight attacks began surging between 1966 and 1986: carjackings in grocery parking lots; knifings and other physical assaults at subway stations as well as on the underground trains; and abductions of children on playgrounds, in busy shopping centers and at bus stops. In New York City alone, violent crime rates more than tripled between those years. By 1984, the subway had become a symbol of law enforcement's ineffectiveness, according to the Metropolitan Transit Authority.

The Justice Department estimated that, between 1987 and 1992, about 35,000 carjacking attempts took place each year; between 1992 and 1996, about 49,000 annually. Among the most notorious was the September 1992 carjacking by two men of 34-year-old Pam Basu, a research chemist, in Savage, Maryland, and mother of a little girl strapped to a car seat going to her first day of preschool.

Mrs. Basu was carjacked at a stop sign, a mere 100 yards from her house—a crime unexpectedly caught on video by her husband, who had intended to record his daughter's inaugural trip to pre-school. To Mr. Basu's horror, he recorded instead two thugs who emerged suddenly from the bushes, pushing their way into his wife's car. Mrs. Basu subsequently became entangled in her seatbelt while trying to rescue her toddler. She was dragged over a mile to her death. The criminals finally threw the seat containing the little girl from the car. Thankfully, she was left unharmed on the roadside.

Congress declared carjacking a federal crime that same year. Although Basu's killers were sentenced to life in prison, the younger of the two, Bernard Miller, then 17, became eligible for parole in 2010. Since a book on the crime came out in February 2012, *Fatal Destiny: The Carjacking Murder of Dr. Pam Basu*, by retired police sergeant and author James H. Lilley, the notoriety of the deed hopefully will keep both perpetrators off the streets permanently. So far, one of the convicts' attempts to be paroled on the basis of "ineffective counsel" has failed.

The pervasiveness of sophisticated devices and computer systems has prevented and discouraged theft of *unattended* cars, but the general rise continues—often with deadlier results. Perpetrators now hang around parking lots and underground garages, looking for individuals leaving or returning to their vehicles, then pounce. Or they wait at stop lights and stop signs, looking for someone who seems vulnerable.

Case Study I: "Justice Journalists" Vilify Self-Defense

In 1981, a then-34-year-old, bespectacled electronics entrepreneur, Bernhard Goetz, suffered permanent damage to one knee and his chest at the hands of three youths at a subway station. They attempted to rob him as he carried equipment. They were later charged only with "criminal mischief."

Goetz, though injured, helped a nearby off-duty police officer arrest the youths. But he was put off by the fact that he himself spent more time at the police station than the thugs who attacked him. He decided then and there that he'd better purchase a gun for self-protection, as clearly no one else was going to protect him in a city where the crime rate was out of control according to every opinion poll. Goetz was turned down for a gun permit on the grounds of "insufficient need," even though he routinely carried expensive electronics and substantial amounts of money for legitimate business transactions. So, on a trip to Florida to visit family members, he purchased a handgun.

The incident in New York had both scared and scarred him. Even though he thought, like most victims, it had probably been a one-time thing and would never happen again, he was later reported to have commented: "Prior to being mugged I did not feel I had to carry a gun," Goetz said. "[But] you can't let yourself be pushed around. You can't live in fear. That's no way to live your life."[88]

Then, three years later he was accosted again, this time inside a subway car by four youths, each of whom had already been arrested and/or convicted on criminal charges, but who, nevertheless, were roaming the streets. In fact, several reports from 1984 stated the foursome seemed to be on their way to rob some video arcade machines. One youth demanded Goetz's money; another cut off the passageway out of the car; and a third attacker, James Ramseur, according to witnesses, hovered menacingly while holding a screwdriver. Goetz figured he was really in for it this time; so he pulled out his gun and shot them, injuring all four, one critically.

Because of the public backlash against openly vicious and uncontrolled crime, Goetz became a hero to some, but a villain to leftists in the media. He was dubbed "the Subway Vigilante" by mostly unsupportive journalists and wound up serving six months for carrying the unlicensed firearm.

But there's a clincher in this story—and you rather have to dig to find it, not because it wasn't reported, but because of the *way* it was reported:

In December 2011, the screwdriver-holder in the attempted mugging, James Ramseur, committed suicide 27 years to the day after the Goetz attack. The media fixated on the obvious link—the date of the suicide—even getting a quote from Goetz, who made a similarly natural assumption: "Sounds like he was depressed."

---

[88]http://www.brainyquote.com/quotes/authors/b/bernhard_goetz.html#wGX1CVSeM 93v6S4K.99

Most of the news reports went on to imply that Ramseur probably held a fierce grudge against Goetz's public-hero status, while the four attackers were simply seen as criminals, even though one had been paralyzed by Goetz in the shooting.

Was that paralytic James Ramseur? You have to go back to the original incident to find out—but no, he wasn't. In fact, what only a few reports mentioned, and then only in passing, is that Ramseur subsequently served 25 years *for raping and sodomizing a pregnant woman in 1986.*

Look at that year again: 1986.

Goetz was accosted by Ramseur and the others in the subway car in 1984. For saving his own life, Goetz served six months for (horrors!) carrying a weapon for self-defense purposes. The press, meanwhile, created a public perception of Goetz as a "vigilante"—so much so that a few people actually started believing it.

Meanwhile, Mr. Screwdriver-holder was *where*? Out on the streets, raping and sodomizing someone who was definitely in no position to fight back! Much later, it was revealed that Ramseur had had major run-ins with the law even *before* the 1984 Goetz incident.

So why *did* Ramseur kill himself on 27th anniversary of the Goetz incident?

It doesn't take a rocket scientist to figure it out: More than likely, the nerdy Mr. Goetz looked like just another easy mark, whereas he was the only one who'd ever fought back and lived to tell about it! He had surprised the thugs by taking on four big, strong, menacing attackers. Ramseur, no doubt, had relived that moment over and over during his 25 years in prison on the rape-and-sodomy charge, and he seethed at the thought that an unimposing figure like Goetz could have been the only one to foil him.

While most people probably didn't put this information into the context of a timeframe, it was hiding in plain sight. This is how perception management is propagated in the media. Reporters do it because (a) they are trained that way in modern schools of journalism, and (b) the editors of liberal-leftist publications *want* the facts spun that way.

Thus, most of the reports on Ramseur's suicide made it appear that, because of the timing, he killed himself over *Goetz's actions* that day in 1984. Well, yes, sort of. Goetz refused to be a doormat for a crime in-the-making—perhaps, in Ramseur's case, one not so unlike the one he perpetrated on the pregnant woman two years later! Only as an *aside* do we learn that Ramseur went free to commit that savage crime.

Oh, and not a single story speculated on the mental state of the poor woman Ramseur brutally assaulted in 1986, or the fate of the child she was carrying—or for that matter whether either of them was alive or dead.

So, what lessons are we to take away from such reporting? Even if one puts the best face on it and assumes that Goetz overreacted to a demand for money from four scary-looking young hoodlums, the public will take away five subliminal messages:

1. Political correctness trumps everything else: the   four youths were black and Mr. Goetz was white —not   mentioned overtly in the reports—so both   "justice" and the media must err on the side of political underdogs.

2. People   are   supposed   to   negotiate   with intimidators for their safety, not defend   themselves or carry a weapon in case   "negotiation" doesn't work out.

3. Law   enforcement   does   not   exist   to   protect   the weak.

4. No one has a stake in your personal safety but   you.

5. If   you   dare   to   defend   yourself   or   your   property, your   actions   will   be   taken   out   of   context   by   a lapdog-liberal press until public opinion is   swayed against you.

Case Study II: Double Standards for Public Figures

Of course, if you are a larger-than-life public figure, with politically correct credentials, the game and the agenda are a bit different. To wit:

Syndicated columnist and television commentator, Carl Rowan, was an outspoken advocate of strict handgun control, going so far as to call for the mandatory, complete disarmament of civilians. Dubbed "the most visible black journalist in the country" by the *Washington Post*, Rowan argued in a 1981 essay that "[a]nyone found in possession of a handgun except a legitimate officer of the law goes to jail—period."

Then, in June 1988, Rowan was arrested and charged with using an unregistered weapon to wound a teen-ager who intruded into his backyard to take a dip in Rowan's pool at his upscale Washington, D.C., home. Unbelievably, Rowan argued *that he had the right to use whatever means necessary to protect himself and his family.*

When suddenly apprised of his own duplicitous argument, Rowan offered up a variety of contradicting excuses, saying there had been threats on his life, including by the Ku Klux Klan. Then he alleged he had fired because the youth was trying to break into his house (or, was it the backyard?) and refused to stop when ordered (or, were any words exchanged at all?). He also said the pistol he used was exempt from the District's strict gun-control laws because it belonged to his older son, a former FBI agent.

Predictably, District officials became suspicious of Rowan's various justifications and charged the columnist with violating the same laws he had spent years advocating. The highly publicized trial ended with a hung jury (surprise!), and the judge hearing the case declared a mistrial.[89]

---

[89] When Mr. Rowan passed away at age 75 in September 2000, several sources resurrected the details of this case, including the *Washington Post*, CNN and the *Wall Street Journal*.

Case Study III: Stupid Criminals, Clueless Victims

Today, victims of crime typically are told that police officers rarely investigate "run-of-the-mill" incidents of burglary or vandalism—that is, unless the complainant is well-known. Interestingly, those well-connected don't seem aware that they received preferential treatment when investigations are made on their behalf.

A case in point occurred in 2011, when a prominent liberal columnist, Marc Fisher of the *Washington Post*, detailed his own home invasion/burglary case[90] in a May 13 piece.

The facts of the case in Fisher's column are worthy of late-night comedian Jay Leno's favorite routine entitled "**Stupid Criminals**"—although, in light of Marc Fisher's column regarding the break-in at his home, Mr. Leno might want to add a new segment to his repertoire and call it "**Clueless Victims**."

In what can only be described as a bizarre twist of fate, burglar Rodney Knight chose the wrong house in December 2010, when he broke into, and ransacked, Fisher's place in the District of Columbia while carrying a loaded gun. Later, exhibiting defiant audacity, he posted photos of himself gloating over his grab-bag of plundered goods *using Fisher's son's laptop and Facebook account*, even going so far as to show himself wearing Mr. Fisher's new winter coat.

Fisher's first surprise, he wrote, was the speed with which the police responded to his 911 call. Even so, the police told him: "We do not have the resources to take this kind of crime seriously. ...The system [is] too overwhelmed by more serious offenses. Sure, [we'll] dust for fingerprints, but...no one [will] ever look at them."

Thanks to the burglar's stupidity in posting his crime on Facebook, identifying him was a shoo-in. Nevertheless, wrote

---

[90]   http://www.washingtonpost.com/opinions/the-facebook-burglar-robbed-me-why-wasnt-it-taken-seriously/2011/05/11/AFrIyp2G_story.html

Mr. Fisher, the prosecutor offered to dismiss half the charges against the burglar in exchange for a guilty plea—anything, apparently, to avoid a trial. Knight's defense counsel even tried to get the judge to "go easy on" his 19-year-old client—because he had "a fairly minimal criminal history."

Fairly minimal? Seven arrests in two states plus the District of Columbia, two for which he never bothered to show up in court, and a lengthy juvenile record, too. If Knight was 19 when he broke into Fisher's home, then the seven arrests occurred over less than a two-year period, because before that he was still a minor.

So, in D.C. Superior Court in the spring of 2011, at his sentencing, a new-and-improved Robert Knight, decked out in a presentable wardrobe he probably would never have selected on his own, ate humble pie and asked for Fisher's forgiveness. Fisher correctly noted that it "hardly mattered. The criminal justice system—from the cops to the prosecutors to the judge— had already given [the offender] plenty of breaks." This time, instead of the 15-year-sentence he would have received had he gone to trial and been convicted by a jury, Knight got only "27 months for the burglary and 17 months for the weapons offense." Fisher was surprised again when he was assured that this pittance represented "an unusually stiff sentence 'for a burglary'; [and that] even a relatively modest prison term is unusual for a property crime."

Fisher never seemed to recognize that both the speedy response by police to his call and the sentence handed down to the burglar, resulted from the fact Fisher was a prominent journalist for the *Post*.

Fisher was so naïve that he wondered aloud in his May 2011 column why apprehensions and convictions were so rare! And why *weren't* property crimes taken seriously? And why *did* Knight's defense counsel ask the judge to "go easy" on Knight—arguing, apparently with a straight face, that his client's criminal history was "fairly minimal"? Why did the

Assistant District Attorney heap praise on the burglar's so-called "cooperation" when, in fact, he had lied about his reason for being in Fisher's house (being "hungry")?

Fisher did allow that: "Eventually, a crackerjack detective with a strong interest in social-media-related crime [e.g., Facebook]…took over and gave the case far more attention than most burglaries get."

Well, duh… Everyone on the force was no doubt told that Fisher was a columnist for the *Post*, and the last thing local law enforcement needed was a black eye in the *Post*.

Everyone but the columnist—and maybe some of his liberal colleagues at the newspaper—probably recognize the scenario Fisher describes as "coddling of criminals" and "promoting a culture of criminality." Most people know that the entire scenario—from police response, to investigation, to plea deals, to sentencing—has little to do with the "justice."

As for Rodney Knight, the burglar—should he ever decide to 'go straight'—he will find that his jail time, and even the Facebook frolic, probably won't hurt him. His choice of victims, however, and the resulting columns and blogs about him will probably follow him longer than his rap sheet.

Case Study IV- Child Torture-Murders

Over and over, we read and hear about how government works to protect children, while actual policy reflects "catch-and-release." Obviously, the idea that a child can "negotiate" his or her way out of a bind is pretty much a non-starter for a 7- or 10-year-old, and a gun—or any other weapon, for that matter—is going to be of little use to a youngster that age under attack.

The enormous uptick since 1966 in incidences of child abduction/torture-murders by persons unknown to the victim shows more than just a rise in predators. It reflects serious flaws in the criminal justice and parole systems. The avalanche of TV crime-dramas built around vicious child assaults isn't helpful. Neither are gore-filled video games seductively labeled "Mature Audiences." Some neurologists, like Dr. David Hilton, say there is now proof, for example, that pornography is addicting.[91] Graphic sexual images have been known to shock some youngsters so completely that they never exhibit *any* interest in sex. Yet, except for actual use of children in sex acts, pornography is no longer stigmatized.

While the flurry of government programs aimed at recovering missing and abducted children, along with the various "alerts," registries, and "awareness programs," have met with some success, they have had little or no effect on *the rise in incident **rates***, which is all that matters.

For every child found, there are untold numbers of lives ruined. A child, in particular, cannot just "get over" a sexual assault or abduction. It remains seared into the consciousness forever. Only the mentally and emotionally tough manage to "put it in perspective," and "move on."

Like every other category of crime, the mid-1960s saw the greatest number of convicted violent predators released from prison, under a ridiculous system of sentencing and laissez-faire guidelines for parole. A July 8, 2009, opinion piece in the *Washington Times*[92] by Lovisa Stannow, executive director of Just Detention International, revealed a new national disgrace— the rate of release of prison inmates, a shocking 95 percent of all convicts. If this statistic is even close to accurate, it is no wonder that our nation is awash in violent crime by repeat offenders with long "rap sheets."

The result is a society that suspects everyone, feels unsafe, and holds law enforcement in contempt. What follows is a chronological sampling of high-profile cases between 1972 and

---

[91] http://www.washingtontimes.com/news/2010/jun/20/hagelin-addiction-to-porn-is-real-destructive/

[92] http://www.washingtontimes.com/news/2009/jul/08/responsible-for-those-in-custody/

2011, with the FBI caveat that most such crimes go unreported (this, no doubt, will make everybody feel better):

Steven Gregory Stayner.- Lured and abducted in 1972 at age 7. He was molested and held until age 14 when he escaped and helped rescue another even younger victim, Timothy White. The perpetrator already was a convicted child rapist named Kenneth Parnell, who had only served three years for the 1951 sodomizing of an 8-year-old boy in Bakersfield, California. He was sent to state prison for the Stayner-White abductions, and paroled again in 1985. In April 2004, Parnell was finally returned to prison for trying to buy a 4-year-old boy. A woman who made home deliveries turned him in—after Parnell attempted to get her help in obtaining an African-American boy, along with a birth certificate! Gratefully, Parnell died of natural causes in prison January 21, 2008, before he could get released again to seize another child.

Etan Patz.- The first major public recognition of child abduction-murders. In 1979, Etan became the first child to appear on a milk carton in law enforcement's weak attempt to gain information from the public concerning missing children. Then six-year-old Etan had movie-star looks going for him, so the Center for Missing and Exploited Children[93] inaugurated the now-defunct milk carton campaign using his picture. Thirty-three years too late, in May 2012, a tip resulted in what some believe might turn out to be a break in this "cold case." The suspect, who allegedly confessed, is being held at this writing in a jail's psychiatric hospital ward.

Adam John Walsh.- A 7-year-old boy who was abducted from a Sears Department Store at a mall in Hollywood, Florida, on July 27, 1981. His head was later found severed from his body, about 120 miles away. His story was made into the 1983 television film *Adam*, seen by some 38 million people at its

---

[93] The Center is largely funded by the Justice Department, with the idea of not only of getting help from the public, but also of raising awareness that might prevent child abduction, child sexual abuse and child pornography.

original airing. Convicted serial killer Ottis Toole confessed to the boy's murder but was never tried for the crime due to loss of evidence. He died of natural causes in 1996, and authorities felt certain that he was, in fact, the perpetrator, and closed the case. **Adam's Legacy:** John Walsh, Adam's father, helped create the Center for Missing and Exploited Children. He hosted the television show, "America's Most Wanted," and created the national sex-offender registry.

Jaycee Lee Dugard.- Probably the best-documented and most long-term case on record, where the victim (then age 11 in 1991) actually survived 18 years of hell to reveal details of her torture-abduction at the hands of Phillip and Nancy Garrido—and to sue federal and state officials for "gross neglect." We will return to this case further on, as it exemplifies everything that is wrong with American criminal justice. **Jaycee's Legacy:** The JAYC Foundation, Inc., founded by Ms. Dugard to help both the victims of abductions and their families in the aftermath of similar traumatic experiences.

Polly H. Klaas.- The 12-year-old was snatched from her home in Petaluma, California, during a slumber party in October 1993. Almost two months later, Richard Davis, who was already being hunted for violating his parole, led authorities to her body and confessed. He was sentenced to death, but remains on death row (what else is new?). In fact, he had a history of sexual assault dating from 1976. He even faked a suicide attempt and escaped from a Napa State Hospital and went on a four-day crime spree, mainly assaulting women—one beaten with a fire poker. Paroled again following vicious sexual attacks and other assaults on women, the high-profile killing of Polly Klass ended his career (one would hope!). **Polly's Legacy:** Her murder prompted the aforementioned "Three Strikes" law.

Amber Hagerman.- The 9-year-old girl was abducted in January 1996 in Arlington, Texas, while riding her bike near her grandparents' home. Her body was found four days later with her throat cut in a drainage ditch. No arrests were ever made. According to witnesses, a man yanked her off the bike and threw her into the front seat of his pickup truck, then sped off. **Amber's Legacy:** The Amber Alert system, now adopted in all 50 states, to help find abducted youngsters. The national program has helped rescue of hundreds of children, but the *rate* of child abductions and sexual assaults nevertheless keeps rising.

Xiana Fairchild.- This 7-year old girl from San Jose, California, was snatched in 1999 by Curtis Dean Anderson on her way home from school. He was also responsible for an earlier sexual assault of two young girls. Xiana Fairchild's skull was found nearly a year afterward, and Anderson apparently filmed the entire strangling and molestation. He later confessed to having kidnapped and molested an 8-year-old girl from Vallejo, California, the following year. The child (name withheld) managed to escape after two days of being shackled to the front seat of Anderson's car by diving through an open window and flagging down a passing truck, and Anderson was then finally apprehended. It took another five years for the Fairchild case to come to trial. Anderson eventually claimed to have murdered 15 other children. He died in a prison hospital in 2007, so he was unable (gratefully) to obtain early release.

Elizabeth Smart.- A now-renowned 14-year-old girl, Elizabeth Smart, was kidnapped in 2002 from her bedroom, then raped and held for nine months. But even though perpetrator Brian David Mitchell was picked up immediately after he was spotted with Elizabeth, and was tried, along with accomplice, Wanda Eileen Barzee, his conviction was far from "speedy." It took almost 10 years before he went to trial. Elizabeth is one of the few who were able, eventually, to move on with her life. She recently married.

Siblings Dylan and Shasta Groene.- Kidnapped in 2005 by Joseph E. Duncan, III, a convicted serial killer and a sex offender at least as far back as 1997, maybe farther. Many of the crimes occurred during Duncan's parole from 1994–1997. Shasta Groene was found alive at a restaurant with Duncan, but two adult family members had been abducted and murdered. Dylan's remains were found in a remote area in Montana. Duncan was sentenced to die for the kidnapping, torture and murder of 9-year-old Dylan Groene, after murdering his mother, brother and mother's boyfriend in their home. It was reported in March 2012 that the U.S. Supreme Court has refused to overturn an appeal. Duncan has since confessed to other child murders.

Taylor Behl.- A 17-year-old college freshman from Vienna, Virginia, who had moved to Richmond in August 2005 to attend Virginia Commonwealth University. Two weeks later, her body was found in a ravine. Benjamin Fawley, a man who, according to Taylor's mother, she had "only" had sex with "once out of curiosity" (as if that were perfectly okay for a 17-year-old), claimed that the girl died accidentally while they were performing a consensual, kinky-sex act. Fawley said he panicked and dumped her body. Behl and Fawley were captured on surveillance footage leaving Taylor's dorm together, apparently amicably, after she went to her room earlier that night. But amicable or not, Fawley was 38 years old with a rap sheet that included 16 counts of child pornography, attempting "indecent liberties with children," and "contributing to the delinquency of a minor."

Elizabeth Olten.- The 9-year-old girl was murdered out-of-the-blue by a 15-year-old neighbor, Alyssa Bustamante, in a small town west of Jefferson City, Missouri. It took three years before Bustamante went to trial, but maybe this time the wait was worth it. Her journal diary was found, and forensic experts had to use special techniques to see through the blue-ink used to cover up her original journal entry. They read the relevant portions aloud. She wrote: *"I just f- - - - - g killed someone. I strangled them and slit their throat and stabbed them and now they're dead. I don't know how to feel..... It was ah-mazing. As* *soon as you get over the 'ohmygawd I can't do this' feeling, it's pretty enjoyable. I'm kinda nervous and shaky though right now. Kay, I gotta go to church now…lol."* The most Bustamante (now 18) can get for her crime, apparently, is life <u>with</u> a chance of parole. She could be out in as little as 10 years. (The Justice of Pretension demands at least that.) But Bustamante's journal entry speaks volumes to how desensitized children have become to the grisly acts they see played out in video games and on television.

Sarah Haley Foxwell.- An 11-year-old from Salisbury, Maryland, taken from her bedroom the week before Christmas in 2009, and found dead on Christmas Day. Thomas J. Leggs Jr., 30, the indicted suspect, was listed on both Maryland and Delaware's sex offender registries, with other convictions for burglary and destruction of property. He had convictions for a sex offense, and also the rape of a minor, along with multiple parole violations. Yet, he eluded any substantial jail time.

Leiby Kletzky.- An 8-year-old boy from Brooklyn, New York, disappeared on July 12, 2011. His dismembered remains were found two days later. The confessed killer, Levi Aron, age 35, used a lethal drug cocktail to smother the boy. He was located via surveillance cameras along the boy's route from his day camp toward home. (This, of course, will serve to validate the need for more surveillance cameras.)

Moreover, we have an America filled with gee-whiz technologies that allow investigators to track and monitor nearly every aspect of our lives, opinions and whereabouts, along with financial transactions. Experts can cross-match anything from credit cards, to phone calls, to passports and vaccination records.

Yet, we cannot find (or keep locked up) obvious threats to public safety that are under our noses.

Less Than 20 Years to Disable Law Enforcement

Let's look at some timeframes for a moment. Parents who have children in K-12 institutions today likely do not recall what law enforcement was like in America before the crime spike that began in 1966 and was out of control in the big cities by 1976—coincidentally, the 200th anniversary of the U.S. Constitution.

So, let's subtract another ten years, and go back to 1956, before the crime "spike," and put this into the context of a single community: a then-middle-class suburb of Washington, D.C.—Chevy-Chase, Maryland—which this author described for the *Washington Post* in 2005.

The District of Columbia in 1956 was not known then as a murder capital, and Chevy Chase was a bedroom suburb filled with everything from plain, uninspired two-story colonial, brick homes that are now over a million dollars, to larger houses for big families that have been retrofitted and re-retrofitted to accommodate the $3- or $4-million-dollar price tag.

Porches, where any existed, were screened-in. Basements were mostly "unfinished." Dogs ran loose. Everybody set off fireworks and sparklers bought from local vendors on the Fourth of July. Most kids walked to school or used public transportation from about age 8. Only a few took the school bus.

A fellow whom neighborhood kids knew only as Sgt. Bradshaw was a frequent visitor in his patrol car at odd times during the day and evening. Homeowners could call the police department if they were going to be away, and ask them to take an extra look during their rounds. They could rest assured that somebody from the force would double-check the premises. Police were respected, and officers went out of their way to make friends with the neighborhood children.

Sgt. Bradshaw always had a smile for the youngsters on his beat. He'd stop and toss a few balls to the boys, ask about the folks or the new baby, and patiently explain why something kids might be doing was dangerous—like standing on their sleds and zooming down an ice- and snow-covered street (made even icier by pouring buckets of cold water on it).

One summer afternoon, Sgt. Bradshaw was making his rounds along Kirkside Drive in the suburb, when he came upon a group of girls, huddled together, whispering and looking ominously down the street.

"What's going on, ladies?" he joked, poking his head out the car window.

The girls looked at each other with embarrassed giggles, at a loss for words. Sgt. Bradshaw took in the scene of eight-to-10-year-olds. He knew intuitively something was up. Sgt. Bradshaw also knew most the kids' names. A girl named Patty looked like his best bet for a straight answer.

"Patty," he asked, "is there something I should know here?"

"Um, well," Patty stammered, "this man in a green car asked us if we wanted to see something cute."

"Uh-huh…" said Sgt. Bradshaw, waiting.

"We thought it was a puppy," another girl said, "because he reached down in the car."

"I *think* he said 'puppy'," offered a third child, although the rest weren't sure.

"Well, what did the puppy look like?" asked Sgt. Bradshaw, choosing his words carefully.

"Um, it wasn't. It was his …."

"His pants were undone," interrupted a 10-year-old.

"I see," said the officer, evenly. "A green car, you say?"

None of the girls would have known, or cared, about a model number, make or license plate, so he didn't ask; but they all agreed the car was dark green, pointing to the ivy in a nearby flower bed.

"Did any of you notice which way the car was going, or whether there was anyone else inside?"

"No, no one else. He went down the street."

"It turned that way," two girls said at once, gesturing to the right.

"Thanks, girls," said Sgt. Bradshaw. "You did the right thing telling me. Well, I'll be off now."

Sgt. Bradshaw drove away at his usual meandering pace, but they heard the siren blare and engine race as he turned the corner at Kirkside Drive.

The next day, one of the group overheard their parents saying that Sgt. Bradshaw had caught the man in the green car that same day, just as the fellow was leaving the scene of yet another "indecent exposure" incident. He didn't need to read the man his "rights." The guy was locked away for a very long time.

With the assaults and murders of countless children since those days, there is cause to reflect upon Sgt. Bradshaw and the lazy summer days of an era when whole families sometimes slept in the famous Rock Creek Park that runs from Maryland through parts of the Nation's Capital on hot nights; when little kids played in the street, expecting the best of people, not fearing the worst. But even in that age of innocence, most children had a sixth sense when something was "off," as with the man in the green car. They didn't need explicit lessons in "good touch-bad touch" to activate their alert systems.

Nobody called it "community policing" back then, because officers like Sgt. Bradshaw already operated that on that principle. Police were encouraged to know their neighborhoods and have a regular beat instead of rotating among vicinities and distancing themselves from the public they served. They didn't wait until youngsters were traumatized or killed to catch miscreants—which is probably one reason why hardly anyone ever heard of child snatchings, rapes and torture-murders until much later. Detectives didn't expect 8-year-olds to repeat grisly details, or for citizens to have to hire private security or appoint one of their own to do patrol duty in gated communities. The police did the jobs citizens paid them to do—that is, gathering information discretely and protecting communities with wisdom and common sense.

No, 1956 wasn't perfect—and inflation has now made once-unremarkable communities like Chevy Chase into domains of the very wealthy, or nearly so. But, posh or not, the Sgt. Bradshaws are gone with the wind. The fact that it took less than 20 years to happen should give us pause, because changes of that magnitude over such a short timeframe are not a reflection of naturally evolving "community standards."

The liberal-left response to the question "why" is typically *poverty*. Yet, unlike in 1956, the poor have access to subsidized soup kitchens, heated and air-conditioned shelters, all manner of social services, job training programs. Minorities do not have to run the Jim Crow obstacle course to get an education or a job.

The Morphing Definition of American "Poverty"

The media vastly exaggerates grinding poverty in America, which, compared to other nations, is virtually nonexistent.

The recession and housing debacles notwithstanding, many people misunderstand poverty. The rationale of increased spending for "poor children" never ceases to resonate, thus education agencies, among others, can usually secure more funding on that basis.

But, recent research into what constitutes "poverty" in America is a mind-bender. A study based on the government's own statistics by The Heritage Foundation's Robert Rector was detailed in the *Washington Times*[94] on July 25, 2011:

The average household defined as poor … has a microwave, a washer and dryer, a dishwasher, a coffee maker, and a cordless phone. Half of poor households have a computer…, two color televisions and a DVD player, along with a video-game system such as an Xbox or a PlayStation for those households with children…. [W]elfare expert Robert Rector [reveals] in a new study [that] "…the houses and

---

94   (http://www.washingtontimes.com/news/2011/jul/25/what-really-is-poverty/)

apartments of America's poor are quite spacious by international standards. The typical poor American has considerably more living space than does the average European.

Fast-Forward to Generations X and Y

Generations of parents and grandparents had walked or taken public transportation to school when they were youngsters. But, by the year 2007, even before the Jaycee Lee Dugard rescue, most mothers and fathers had decided they could no longer allow their little ones to make their way even to the designated pickup spots for school buses four blocks away.

Today, parents not only physically drive the few blocks to deposit their children at the appropriate intersection, *but then hang around until the school bus actually appears*. For all that, parents could have driven their youngsters to school themselves (if they didn't mind paying for the extra gas)! A May 16, 2012, *New York Post* article, "Bronx School Janitor Foils Kidnaper," by Kevin Sheehan and Beth Defalco,[95] captures the ubiquitous sense of helplessness.

These parents have reason to worry: According to the U.S. Department of Justice at the time of ABC's Dugard-Sawyer broadcast in 2011, some 20,000 youngsters are abducted by strangers every year. Most are returned fairly soon, some assaulted, some not. But many of these children are held long-term, and only about half return alive, most of those severely abused.

Lawsuit Shows Zero Accountability for Officials.- Two years after Jaycee Lee Dugard's serendipitous rescue (due to uncharacteristic carelessness on the part of her abductor, Phillip Garrido), the true facts surrounding her harrowing ordeal came to light. The agonizing story was revealed in a television

---

[95]http://www.nypost.com/p/news/local/bronx/don_mess_with_mr_clean_0xiW7ZNda kVOTLk48luxcK

interview between Ms. Dugard and ABC's Diane Sawyer. Jaycee was "tasered" at age 11 by convicted rapist Garrido and his girlfriend-accomplice (a fellow inmate, also paroled) as Jaycee walked along her regular route to school. She was handcuffed and held in a backyard shed, repeatedly raped and otherwise abused for 18 years. She gave birth (the first time at age 14) in Garrido's backyard prison, surrounded by attack dogs to prevent her escape. Both parolees abused her emotionally with ongoing good guy/bad guy theatrics and threats.

Ms. Dugard showed a strength of character unmatched by any a prisoner-of-war survival story: nearly two decades of sexual torture and confinement in a paroled convict's makeshift, backyard tent, where she was impregnated twice and forced to give birth in the filthy environment of her surroundings—babies she nevertheless nurtured and even schooled during the ordeal, using makeshift equipment. She continues to care for them to this day. The harrowing details are detailed in her book, *A Stolen Life*.

Parole officers time and again overlooked Phillip Garrido's failed drug tests, as well as what should have been obvious signs of foul play around the pair's home during some 60 visits. Like so many other things in the modern, bureaucratic world, process superseded substance—a phenomenon that had come to characterize government employment. Officials apparently were too busy focusing on their clipboards' check-off sheets to actually bother looking around for suspicious activities.

Prison psychiatrists knew Phillip Garrido well. He had been given psychiatric drugs to "control" his erratic thoughts and fantasies. ABC's Diane Sawyer says everything Garrido did was supposed to have been monitored once he was released. Clearly, that hadn't happened.

Garrido's rap sheet was a long one: A first arrest was in 1972 for raping a 14-year-old girl, who was so terrified she couldn't testify. Without the capability for DNA analysis back then, the case collapsed. But three years later he abducted a woman and took her to a storage container, where he raped her over and over for eight hours. She finally escaped, and he was convicted. He was sentenced to 50 years for that crime, but despite the viciousness of the assault, Garrido served only one quarter of that time. Then, he met Nancy, another inmate, and married her in prison. Once paroled, the duo set about scouting for female children to abduct.

After Dugard's rescue and the Garridos' trial, it was revealed that the couple had shot numerous videos of children—including one showing a young girl who looked a lot like Jaycee, being lured toward their van. For the crime against Ms. Dugard, Phillip Garrido was sentenced to 431 years behind bars, and Nancy got 36 years to life for her role. Due to the extremely high-profile nature of the case—like the infamous Charles Manson clan involved in the 1969 Sharon Tate-Leno/Rosemary LaBianca murders—the Garridos will probably stay in prison, but one never knows.

That officials had bungled their appointed rounds at the Garrido home was a "no-brainer." Ms. Dugard received a hefty compensation from the State of California in the aftermath, probably hoping to minimize public outrage. But Jaycee Dugard decided she needed to "send a message" to the entire judicial system, which she recognized was deeply flawed, since both federal and state officials were at fault. She didn't need more money, so she decided she would donate whatever she received from the lawsuit to other victims of abuse. Thus, the JAYC Foundation. Her lawsuit justifiably cited "gross neglect" by federal and state officials.

But a new shock surfaced. Over the years, the government at all levels had *insulated itself from prosecution*! The Dugard lawsuit revealed that government had surreptitiously implemented strong immunities that shielded officials—at the federal, state and local (county) levels. Weighing in on Dugard's lawsuit prospects in 2011, author and attorney Norm

Pattis explained that "sovereign immunity typically bars suit against the federal government."

With a sickening thud, parents were disabused of all remaining notions about police officers riding to the rescue. Parents of all political persuasions suddenly realized they could not count on the U.S. justice system at *any* level to protect them or their children from perverts. Indeed, with the advent of political correctness, even the word "pervert" had been banished.

The Justice of Harassment

At a conference in Michigan where this author served as a speaker, a woman approached during a book signing. The speech apparently touched a chord, and she wanted to recount what had happened to her the year before. Book signings tend to bring out such people, who want person-to-person contact with the author; but, what this mother of four homeschooled children had to say was a conversation-stopper. It epitomizes the Justice of Harassment.

It all started when Lucy Smith (not her real name) thought one of her youngsters might have a fever. She took the plain, old-fashioned thermometer from the shelf (i.e., the non-digital kind) and placed it in the little girl's mouth as usual. After reading it—the temperature was just slightly high—she used alcohol to sanitize it and started "shaking it down" like most people do, before putting it away. At that moment, another of her children boisterously entered the bathroom to ask a question, and in the process jostled Lucy so that she dropped, and broke, the thermometer on the hard floor tiles. She saw exactly where it landed.

She told the two youngsters to leave immediately—they, like Lucy, had been a fair distance behind where the thermometer lay in pieces—and she shut the door. Lucy donned rubber gloves, grabbed a cleaning towel and proceeded to first get all the pieces up and then scrub down the entire floor with a disinfecting cleaner, which was gratefully under the sink, to ensure no mercury had escaped. She did this twice, with two cleaning towels, and then used another to dry it down. She took off her sandals, and cleaned them thoroughly, too, and the sink and tub. She stepped out of the bathroom, closed the door, and told the children to use another bathroom. She bagged the used cleaning towels and threw them away, thinking she had done all she knew to do.

But then, being the responsible and thorough person that she was, she went to the refrigerator door and grabbed off the number of the Poison Control Center she kept there. She told the person on the line what had happened and what she had done about it and asked if there were any additional precautions she should take. They said not to worry; someone knowledgeable on such matters would get back to her. Lucy went about her business, and soon heard the doorbell. A no-nonsense lady asked if she was Lucy Smith and demanded to see the room where the accident had occurred. The bathroom in question sparkled, having just been scrubbed down, but that didn't matter to the lady from Social Services (one of the "caring professions"). She demanded that Lucy call in a professional to remove and replace every single tile in the bathroom, as well as the carpet in the adjoining bedroom, and then clean or toss out any shoes the two children might have been wearing.

Now, Lucy is a very quiet, unassuming woman, the kind who never raises her voice. If anything, one might have described her as "mousy." But the expense and time involved in hiring someone to virtually renovate the bathroom and re-carpet the bedroom seemed like gross overkill. She would have said so, but the shock on her face must have said it all. That was all the woman from Social Services needed to see. She told Lucy that if she refused, she would have to report her and all the children would have to be placed in foster care until Lucy complied.

"What school do your kids go to?" she demanded.

Lucy explained that she homeschooled them. The woman from Social Services harrumphed.

Lucy wanted to talk to her husband first, but the woman said, "Well?" Then as an afterthought, she added, "If you don't have someone in mind to do the job, I can see that you get a list. But it needs to be done right away. Nobody can use these two rooms until the work is finished. You're just lucky I'm not including the whole second floor of this house. But since you apparently did a good job, this should be enough."

Afraid and shocked, Lucy agreed, signed a piece of paper, and called as soon as the dates and times had been set up to do the work. Social Services checked back one more time later, and apparently were satisfied.

Wouldn't it have been nice if that much thought had gone into checking the premises of Jaycee Dugard's captor, Phillip Garrido?

Criminalizing Normalcy

The only people, it seems, who can any longer be safely harassed are parents! Examples of parents being criminalized for "neglect" and "child endangerment" abound—often for trying to protect their own children. For example, a parent might reject chemotherapy for a child's cancer, particularly if the youngster has already undergone painful, unsuccessful treatment and is too frail or exhausted to continue treatment.[96]

Many parents also refuse to administer psychiatric drugs for typical childhood misbehavior. Then, there's the legitimate concern over all-in-one vaccination cocktails, given the sudden huge spike in autism since these started being routinely administered. Experts have denied any of the vaccines are at

---

[96] http://ir.lawnet.fordham.edu/cgi/viewcontent.cgi?article=3264&context=flr

fault, but have tiptoed around the issue of combination vaccinations.

There is no respect at all for legitimate parental concerns. Here's an example of government's over-the-top, harassment approach that occurred in the State of Maryland in 2007:

A group of parents voiced objections to their small children getting too many vaccines at one sitting. After getting the brush-off, they simply declined the vaccination mandate. So, in November 2007, Maryland officials herded their youngsters into a Prince George's County courthouse, guarded by armed personnel with attack dogs.[97] Inside, the children were forcibly vaccinated, under orders from the State Attorney General, thereby stripping parents of any legal right to decide how they wished to protect their offspring from infectious diseases. Health authorities even threatened, by innuendo, to jail parents for up to 30 days if they continued to resist—thereby suppressing both public discussion and parental prerogatives.

"Medicalizing" Political Dissent

A study which drew gasps of outrage from the conservative, or simply the politically incorrect, community in August 2005 was a $1.2 million, taxpayer-supported product of National Institute of Mental Health and the National Science Foundation. It alleged that adherence to conventional moral principles and to limited government are signs of mental illness. NIMH-NSF scholars from the Universities of Maryland, California at Berkeley, and Stanford University attributed notions about morality and individualism to "dogmatism" and "uncertainty avoidance." Social conservatives, in particular, were said to suffer from "mental rigidity," a condition which, researchers said, is probably hard-wired, condemning traditionalists to a lifelong, cognitive hell, with all the associated markers of mental illness: "decreased cognitive

---

[97] http://www.npoa.us/?p=19

function, lowered self-esteem, fear, anger, pessimism, disgust, and contempt."[98]

There have been several such "studies" to medicalize, and in the process, stigmatize, the politically incorrect. Take the work of University of Manitoba associate professor of psychology Robert Altemeyer: He has developed a Right Wing Authoritarian (RWA) Scale, to identify those harboring "authoritarian tendencies." Even ordinary traditionalists—those who don't specifically endorse liberal-leftist dogma—are characterized as "cognitively rigid, aggressive, and intolerant."

In December 2010, scientists at the University of London said that conservatives have an enlarged "fear" area in their brains, and smaller areas associated with courage and optimism. The London Telegraph reported:

> Scientists have found that people with conservative views have brains with larger amygdalas, almond shaped areas in the centre of the brain often associated with anxiety and emotions.
>
> On the other hand, they have a smaller anterior cingulate, an area at the front of the brain associated with courage and looking on the bright side of life.
>
> The researchers say there is a direct correlation between the sizes of those areas and one's political views.

There are many more "studies" of this sort cropping up. They are reminiscent of the approach to political dissidents taken by the Nazis in the 1930s and 40s, then again under Stalin and his successors in the Soviet Union and its satellite countries. In fact, Russian officials appear to be still at it. Just ask Larisa Arap, detained in 2007 by Russian military police during a routine medical exam, as punishment for having collaborated on an article describing police abuses of peaceful

---

[98] "Political Conservatism as Motivated Social Cognition." Psychological Bulletin 129(3): 339-375, also online at http://www.apa.org/journals/bul/503ab.html.

political dissenters under the cover of "punitive psychiatry." She was finally released from the Murmansk psychiatric ward, complete with threats to her entire family if she spoke out. She has since been rescued.[99]

As lately as 2009, the Chinese Communists were doing more of the same, as per a report by PBS News Hour showing political dissidents in China being forced into to psychiatric hospitals.[100]

So, if you have one of those "DON'T BELIEVE THE LIBERAL MEDIA" stickers on your car, beware. Your number may come up in the next edition of the Diagnostic and Statistical Manual of Mental Illnesses (DSM), considered the bible of psychiatry and taken very seriously by the nation's courts.

Anybody can see where this is going. And here's the thing: If one side can do it, so can the other, as soon as the political winds change.

Digital Tricks

In the light of the uptick in violent crime, the concept of security cameras seemed to make sense in 2007—in stairwells, at entrances to office buildings and subway stations, etc. An ABC News/*Washington Post* poll found in July of that year that 71 percent of Americans favored increased video surveillance.

But by 2009, advanced monitoring systems of one kind or another were proliferating around the country for dual purposes—"traffic" cameras, tolling cards attached to vehicle windshields, subway SmartCards, key cards for entry into restrooms and parking lots, offices, hotels, and more. D.C. Mayor Vincent C. Gray joyfully announced on March 27, 2012,

---

[99] "Activist tells about torture and captivity," by David R. Sands, the Washington Times, Oct. 16, 2007

[100] See Video: Chinese Dissidents Committed to Mental Hospitals) http://chinadigitaltimes.net/2009/09/video-chinese-dissidents-committed-to-mental-hospitals/

a plan to blanket "the entire city" of Washington with cameras as part of a "traffic calming initiative," prompting jeers from many D.C. Council members. They decried the vast expansion of "gotcha situations" to allow the city to close a $172 million gap in the District's budget for 2013. The Nation's Capital, meanwhile, remains among the highest for city violence and crime—even with its existing cameras.

Average citizens initially believed that with the new technologies, law enforcement officers would be freed up to spend more time in unmarked cars—as in, patrolling their beat—preventing crimes and catching those in progress. Still others took the optimistic view that the fines collected from red-light cameras and speed traps would be used to pave roads, repair street signs and provide more trucks to sand snowy highways in winter.

None of these "good purposes" materialized.

No sooner had the public accepted the new whiz-bang technologies, than government began integrating the various digitized tools and using them in schemes aimed at ripping off upstanding citizens.

Here's how the whole camera-revenue agenda game works: A company approaches state or county officials with an offer to bear the entire cost of installing so-called "traffic" cameras on "x" number of streets in return for approximately one-half of the revenues generated from fines.

Alternatively, officials from the county or state solicit competitive bids for installing revenue cameras, hoping for the best deal. The winner will be the company submitting a proposal that would jam up roads for the least amount of time, put in cameras the most cheaply (configured, of course, to serve multiple purposes) and request a lesser "cut" of the resulting revenues.

For example, according to a *Washington Times* editorial[101] on June 8, 2012, Montgomery County, Maryland, including nearby incorporated cities were:

> ...paying Affiliated Computer Services (ACS), a Xerox subsidiary, $16 for each ticket the company issues. ...These jurisdictions re-wrote their contracts in 2009 to affirm that ACS does not "operate" the speed cameras, since the law only bans "operators" from receiving per-ticket compensation. ACS and other similar firms install, own, maintain and calibrate the cameras. They take the photographs, determine who's guilty, prepare evidence for court trial, mail out tickets, collect the fines, pursue those who don't pay and run public-relations campaigns to defend the program.

Look again at the last line of the quotation above. It says ACS runs "a public-relations campaign to defend the program." That is perception management—in this case, a ruse aimed at making average citizens believe the speed-camera agenda is about government looking out for public safety, rather than a you-scratch-my-back-and-I'll scratch-yours revenue-sharing scheme.

Maryland's Prince George's County Revenue Authority sees big dollar signs, too. The *Washington Times* reported[102] the previous month that the Authority expected to double its haul in the 2012 fiscal year, to about $55,700,000.

Readers of this section are urged to go online and read the full editorials alluded to here, because they exemplify how individuals are being criminalized for harmless, ordinary conduct in the absence of real investigative police work—the kind that might have saved Jaycee Lee Dugard from 18 years of horror.

---

[101] http://www.washingtontimes.com/news/2012/jun/8/enough-schoolboy-excuses/
[102] http://www.washingtontimes.com/news/2012/may/28/speed-camera-explosion/

Proactive Waste in the Service of Harassment

Policing has moved from a proactive approach to safeguarding citizens to a harassment-driven mandate to fleece the public. Much of the resultant spending, under the guise of "safety," could be described as *proactive waste*. Among the most obvious are flashing digital billboards; speed bumps; so-called "safe speed" cameras; and red-light cameras, with *deliberately shortened* times for yellow-amber lights. Entrapment and over-reach are pervasive.

Flashing Billboards.- Millions of tax dollars better spent on criminal investigations—or even road signs announcing upcoming streets and freeway junctions—have been dumped into electronic billboards that tell one virtually nothing they don't already know, or give information such as toll-free numbers for hot-tips that the driver won't remember and can't write down.

Do we really want Uncle Sam reminding us to "go green" and "recycle" every few miles? If you think flashing digital signs in the name of "intelligent transportation" are a taxpayer rip-off, just wait!

Speed Bumps.- There's never enough money to repair potholes, clear debris or monitor parking lots for thieves and rapists, but plenty of dough is somehow available for hard-to-gauge, variable height speed bumps that cost taxpayers between $1,200 and $2,000 a pop. Installed, as they are, using different heights, colors and materials makes it a sure bet that, sooner or later, nearly every driver will suffer damage to a vehicle, especially when "bumps" are covered by snow or wet leaves. These bumps, especially the hard-to-see, decorative brick ones that are higher than expected, are hard on many people's back, difficult for ambulances and other emergency vehicles to negotiate, and can cause toddlers and pets to throw up in the vehicle.

Speed Cameras.- With the advent of so-called "safe-speed" cameras, the term "gotcha justice" came into vogue. A prime example was the bicycle supposedly caught on camera going an impossible 57-miles-per-hour that came to light in Prince George's County, Maryland, in 2011. Less cynical and more naïve folks put the bicycle incident down to mis-calibrated machines, but investigative reporters have found hard evidence that the arbitrary speed-limit postings are often dangerously low to entrap tourists and those who don't use a particular road often.

"Speed" cameras take pettiness to new heights as a creative form of taxation, while masking an underlying purpose of interconnecting surveillance.

A February 10, 2012, *Washington Times* editorial[103] noted: "The District of Columbia ignores decades of traffic engineering research that have concluded [that] the safest speed is determined by measuring how fast 85 percent of traffic is moving in safety. Ignoring the science and arbitrarily setting an ultra-low limit on a freeway creates a cash cow."

In the real world, the dangerous drivers are the ones weaving in and out of traffic, tailgating, honking at drivers to get out of the way, driving in two lanes at once, and making hairpin left-turns in front of oncoming traffic. Ever see one of these get ticketed under "Aggressive Driver Imaging"?

Red-Light Cameras.- With the roaring success of ubiquitous "safe speed" cameras, it is unsurprising that governments would make driving more dangerous for average citizens in the interest of raising revenue. The National Motorists Association revealed, for example, that six cities this year alone were caught deliberately shortening the timeframes for yellow/amber lights in an attempt to increase revenue when, in fact, it has been

---

[103] http://www.washingtontimes.com/news/2012/feb/9/speed-camera-unrest/

proved that *extending the seconds of these same lights actually reduces accidents.*[104]

Once drivers realize that traffic has inexplicably stopped, they often slam on the brakes, causing their own vehicle to be rear-ended, along with possibly a chain reaction going back several car-lengths. This results in great expenses to drivers, including raised insurance rates, not to mention the shock of either being hit, or hitting someone else's vehicle.

Somehow, the question of entrapment has failed as a legal constraint on government or camera contractors.

Stripping for Justice

Other patterns of harassment are showing up in unlikely disguises. Here's how the April 2012 U.S. Supreme Court handed down a 5-4 decision relating to strip-searches strip-searches for petty offenses (alluded to briefly in Chapter 4) played out in New Jersey:

Albert Florence was probably the first beneficiary of the new strip-search policy. Arrested on a warrant for an "unpaid" fine—which he had actually paid!—Mr. Florence was shuttled between two jails. Thus, two strip searches. Officers were waiting to find out if the man was telling the truth.

The justification? Security trumps privacy in dangerous environments.

What dangerous environment, you ask?

The jails! The ones Mr. Florence never should have been taken to...

Military-Grade Crowd Control

A front page headline in an October 2009 report in the *Washington Times* read: "Police buy military-style sonic

---

[104] http://www.motorists.org/red-light-cameras/effect-yellow-timing

device."[105]

If you're an *aficionado* of spy thrillers, you may already be aware that Long-Range Acoustical Device (or LRADs) are used to disperse troublesome crowds and angry protesters by emitting a piercing sound dangerous (and painful) enough to permanently damage hearing and temporarily distort vision.

People might be excused for assuming these devices would be used solely on violent, out-of-control mobs, looters and vandals.

Most people think of crowd control in terms of barriers, barricades and belt-like stanchions to keep huge throngs from stampeding. For riot situations incited by professional agitators, where rocks, bottles and Molotov cocktails are hurled at innocent bystanders and at security teams guarding official conferences—police typically have used smoke grenades, tear gas, batons and foam bullets to keep order.

Not anymore.

Thanks to Department of Homeland Security (DHS) grants, local police departments around the country are ordering these devices, and they have already been used at some of the country's more spirited town-hall meetings on health care. According to the manufacturer, American Technology Corporation (ATC), based in San Diego, they exist solely to "influence [people's] behavior and gain compliance."

Well, that's comforting.

Using a military-grade weapon that permanently damages hearing to "influence behavior" and "gain compliance" is a far cry from traditional crowd control.

Government Fed Up With Freedom of Information

With the U.S. Justice Department and Attorney General Eric Holder continually under fire, it came as something of a

---

[105] http://www.washingtontimes.com/news/2009/oct/01/police-buy-sonic-device-to-subdue-unruly-crowds/

surprise, even to Capitol Hill insiders, when the Freedom of Information Act, or FOIA, was suddenly in the crosshairs in 2011.[106]

On October 30, 2011, new rules were advanced by the Department that would have not only denied the public access to documents, but encouraged bureaucrats to lie outright, telling requesters that either the documents they were seeking never existed or that they don't exist now.

Turns out, that the practice had been going on for decades, something many suspected but couldn't prove, until it was revealed in a FOIA lawsuit filed by the American Civil Liberties Union (ACLU) of Southern California. Thus, the ACLU had to swallow hard and agree that the proposed rule change would mean that Obama was "authorizing agencies to lie."

The announcement was promptly picked up by major news outlets. Legal Counsel for the Sunlight Foundation, John Wonderlich, wrote a stinging letter to the Department, decrying the blatant retreat from open-government policies. Seth Mendel blasted the proposal in *Commentary Magazine.*[107]

Yet, strangely, just the month before the rule-change announcement, the White House had approved a new post to FOIA's website, officially releasing its Status Report on Open Government.[108]

Talk about "*chutzpah!*" The website actually boasted of "substantial steps to increase participation and collaboration in government, and to make government more transparent." It cited "the Administration's unprecedented efforts to promote greater disclosure..., [with] a focus on improving the FOIA process through the use of technology."[109]

[106] http://www.washingtontimes.com/news/2011/oct/30/justice-seeks-reduction-of-foia-access-on-operatio/
[107] http://www.commentarymagazine.com/2011/10/31/foia-aclu-obama/
[108] http://www.whitehouse.gov/blog/2011/09/16/status-report-administration-s-commitment-open-government
[109] http://www.justice.gov/oip/foiapost/2011foiapost31.html

With the uproar over its duplicity, the Justice Department withdrew the proposed rule change—for the time being. If the administration was "testing the waters" of public reaction, they managed to get even the ACLU to balk.

FOIA was initially signed into law[110] by President Lyndon B. Johnson on July 4, 1966, and was amended so as to cover electronic records[111] in 1996. Congress actually sought to strengthen FOIA in the wake of the Watergate scandal in 1974. After negotiations between Congress and the Ford Administration broke down, Congress passed the strengthening amendments to FOIA, which the President then vetoed. But the majority-Democrat Congress swiftly voted to override the veto. Clearly, it was in their interest, following Watergate and the unpopular Vietnam War, to at least make a pretense of openness.

But, the political winds changed. Conservative watchdog organizations, such as Judicial Watch, and Accuracy in Media soon discovered how to make the new openness policy (a.k.a. "transparency") work for them. Traditionalists, values-voters, constitutionalists and the conservative print media had made it abundantly clear during the scandal-ridden Clinton era that they intended to capitalize on FOIA.

Should the FOIA office eventually get the exemptions it wanted—especially the part about giving staff *carte blanche* to lie to requesters about the existence of records, as opposed to merely declining to provide them—petitioners would be prevented even from appealing the decision. In legalese, that's called "challenging the application of the exemption." Due process and other protections would be undermined.

The attempt to transform FOIA would also have made it more difficult to obtain "fee waivers," something typically provided to the media, part-time reporters and online journalists, to circumvent often prohibitively exorbitant fees

---

[110] http://www.gwu.edu/~nsarchiv/nsa/foia/special.html
[111] http://www.gwu.edu/~nsarchiv/nsa/foialeghistory/legistfoia.htm

associated with FOIA requests. This is probably the main reason the ACLU stepped up to the plate.

All this presents a dilemma for Big Government liberals and leftists, who never were keen on being held accountable to the "unwashed masses" anyway, and are even less so now. Their rationale is that average citizens ("nonprofessionals") don't understand the issues. But saying so, of course, is still political suicide.

The Justice of Accommodation

The Justice of Accommodation is closely aligned with political correctness, and employs some of the same double-standards and hypocrisy we have seen, but with a different motive, or agenda. This time, it's only that the press, or a particular socio-demographic bloc, needs to be mollified, but political factions *within the governmental hierarchy* and "tight" with the sitting administration must be accommodated— especially if appropriations, career promotions, entitlements or agenda items are at stake.

One such proposed accommodation was the Dream Act. It didn't pass in 2012, along with the various iterations of amnesty before it, submitted by various administrations. Most people, however, seem to believe Mr. Obama's Dream Act *did* pass. That is because five months before the presidential election, the Obama administration saw fit to unilaterally rewrite a portion of the immigration law, and implement it by use of executive power![112] This, of course, served to bypass Congress—the only branch constitutionally tasked with writing law—and now threatens to unravel the entire constitutional framework unless the people respond with an enormous backlash. That isn't likely, given that most Americans are unclear as to how, and whether, the Dream Act passed at all.

---

[112] http://www.fairus.org/news/obama-bypasses-congress-declares-dream-act-now-in-effect

If we are going to herd respectable citizens around like cattle at airports—ordering them to present for inspection, as it were—then people have reason to expect a serious approach to immigration.

Immigration Games

The immigration conundrum is a messy thing. On the one hand, nearly everyone in America is an immigrant, if you go back far enough. On the other hand, we have infiltrators, criminal drug gangs and terrorists in an age of easy travel options that take mere hours, not weeks or months. No politician wants to be responsible for the results that could ensue from that.

Yet, a third consideration is left unstated, although it is well-known: Illiterate or non-English-speaking immigrants, unfamiliar with our form of government and the nuances of campaign rhetoric, are easy marks for vote-getting at election time. As a result, immigrants have become pawns.

Obama Tries to Rewrite Immigration Law.- If we had stuck to the rules in place when Ellis Island was the main gateway to America, we might have had a set of guidelines instead of mass chaos.

Barack Obama's misguided rewrite, supposedly in the interest of innocent children who were brought to America by their parents illegally (Mr. Obama claims the Dream Act would "only benefit 800,000 people")—is just one more amnesty-style accommodation. Mr. Obama claimed that the only illegals eligible under his rewrite would be those with no criminal record and who had jobs. But, according to Jon Feere, the legal policy analyst at the Center for Immigration Studies, it is well-established that many "illegal aliens hold[ing] jobs have acquired their positions through deception and are often engaged in ID theft, Social Security fraud, and I-9 form fraud...." Furthermore, he wrote in the *Washington Times* June

20, 2012,[113] "the Obama administration [has a] policy of giving 'low-level offenders' a pass."

Mr. Obama also claims that his small fix to existing law would benefit only children having no culpability in their status as illegals. Compassionate though that may sound, said Feere, Mr. Obama's plan "does not include any language requiring applicants to prove they were 'brought' into the United States by their parents."

Andrew P. Napolitano, author, former judge, and current senior analyst for Fox News Channel, pointed out that it is not the President's job to rewrite law and that attempting to do so was to bypass Congress and disregard the Constitution.

But the larger issue here is American assimilation. That used to be expected, and now it's discouraged. Here's what President Theodore Roosevelt wrote in 1907, and it pretty well sums up the expectations of the Framers of the Constitution and many generations of American citizens, including earlier immigrants:

> We should insist that if the immigrant who comes here does in good faith become an American and assimilates himself to us he shall be treated on an exact equality with everyone else, for it is an outrage to discriminate against any such man because of creed or birth-place or origin. But this is predicated upon the man's becoming in very fact an American and nothing but an American. If he tries to keep segregated with men of his own origin and separated from the rest of America, then he isn't doing his part as an American. There can be no divided allegiance here.... We have room for but one language here, and that is the English language, for we intend to see that the crucible turns our people out as Americans, of American nationality, and not as dwellers in a polyglot boarding-house; and we have room for but one soul loyalty, and that is loyalty to the American people.

---

[113] http://www.washingtontimes.com/news/2012/jun/19/obamas-amnesty-dream-presidents-measure-is-much-mo/print/

The great historian, Henry Steele Commager, put it another way in 1950 in a piece for Time, Magazine: that the goal of American schooling should center on passing along a "common body of knowledge," which children could then take into whatever profession or avocation they wished.

> *Poets like Bryant, Longfellow and Whittier; painters like Trumball, Stuart and Peale; historians like Jared Sparks and George Bancroft; schoolmen like Noah Webster with his Spellers, William H. McGuffey with his Readers—these and scores of others popularized that common group of heroes and villains, ... images and values, of which national spirit is born.*

How many immigrants—or even natural-born citizens—recognize even half of these famous Americans today?

Whatever Happened to Sponsorship?

In 2005, the Center for American Progress released one of the best assessments on record of the costs of illegal immigration. Today, some 11 million undocumented persons currently in the U.S., to say nothing of the 500,000 or more that cross the border each year. CAP's statistics were of the associated costs were based on 10 million illegals.

CAP's data analysis estimated the cost to taxpayers being at least $206 billion over 5 years (or $41.2 billion annually), and possibly as high as $230 billion, even in 2005. Apparently, the Center arrived at this figure after assuming that 2 million would leave the U.S. of their own accord—which seems something of a stretch. But, to put the $41 billion in perspective, CAP indicated that the figures would exceed the then-annual budget of the entire Department of Homeland Security.

In researching "sponsorship," it appears laws are still on the books. "If you do not have a college degree or skills that are in demand…you must have a job offer with a U.S. company that is willing to sponsor you for a labor certification. This process takes many years to complete but leaves you with a green card," states a government website. Most agencies offer similar advice to prospective immigrants.

Also, immigration laws state that in order to protect U.S. citizens, a visa is denied to certain applicants, among them, those who:

- have a communicable disease, or a dangerous physical or mental disorder.
- have committed serious criminal act(s).
- are known terrorists, subversives, members of a totalitarian party, or former war criminals.
- have used illegal means to enter the U.S.

There is a purpose for these laws. For example, it was reported in several news outlets that a homosexual Mexican man with AIDS, living in San Francisco, was granted asylum in August 2005 by the 9th U.S. Circuit Court of Appeals, reversing an earlier ruling of deportation for overstaying his visa. Why? Because the man would face persecution for his condition and orientation in Mexico.

Okay, but get this: The man was working as a *waiter*—as in food service—at a local hotel.

How does a fellow with a compromised immune system get a job working around food, and what happened to the prohibition against "applicants with communicable diseases"? Have this nation's leaders lost their collective marbles?

Time and again, we read stories describing the travails of dispossessed immigrant families who were brought to the U.S. as refugees or asylum-seekers, but aren't making it, even with a lot of help from social service agencies: migrant workers from Mexico, Haiti, and the Dominican Republic; a Somali family.

We can sympathize with these individuals. But American citizens living here lead harrowing lives, too. This isn't the right time to be straining our resources and accommodating illegal immigrants, *especially those who have no intention of assimilating or becoming "Americanized."*

New immigrants have been a good thing for America. They keep us "fresh," and remind us of the blessings we have that downtrodden and totalitarian other countries do not. They remind us what a "work ethic" is about. However, no new citizen should be over here right now without a sponsor—that is, a *full* citizen with a spotless record who will take responsibility for the applicant. It's dangerous for us, and for the immigrant in a world of random terrorism.

Former Rep. Tom Tancredo (R-CO) and former House Speaker Rep. Newt Gingrich (R-GA), are right when they insist we need to get a handle on America's out-of-control immigration problem. As of August 2012, the Obama administration was still sticking to its no-deport policy.

But if government expects the public to get behind the Patriot Act and be inconvenienced by anti-terrorism programs, then it has to see seriousness elsewhere. The 2012 passage of H.R. 1388, giving Hamas, the terror organization, $20 million to immigrate to the U.S. as part of Hamas Refugees—to pay for housing, food and transportation—is not viewed by most taxpayers as indicative of seriousness.[114] This bill was barely mentioned by most of the press (e.g., as a moving ticker on the bottom of the CNN screen).

The Department of Homeland Security (DHS) should be immediately be made to *decide on a cut-off date* for categorizing persons as "illegal." Those so categorized should be located and identified. A list of key points should be applied in questioning those classified as *illegal*—among them: "Where are you taking English classes, and classes in American history and the U.S. Constitution?" Not "are you," but "where are you?" This is an indicator of commitment to assimilation;

---

[114] www.thefederalregister.com/d.p/2009-02-04-E9-2488 or
http://www.thefederalregister.com/d.p/2009-02-04-E9-2488%3e

classes in American history and the Constitution are two other requirements. They must supply proof. Then apply the simple four-point sponsorship-test-items listed above. If all but, say, one item is satisfied, DHS or U.S. Immigration Control Enforcement (ICE) might use its discretion to direct the illegal immigrant to help for the one unsatisfied point—with a requirement for follow-up within days, not weeks. If the immigrant fails to show up, then he is *off the list* for remaining in the U.S. We simply can't take the risk. Illegals who have arrived in the U.S. illegally, cannot be allowed to treat their status like a parking ticket—not in an age of terrorism. Their alternate option is deportation. This is the job DHS and ICE *should* be doing. They should not be accommodating leftist opportunists looking to remake the political landscape use hapless immigrants as pawns in their scheme.

On August 23, 2012, 10 ICE agents and deportation officers filed a lawsuit in a Texas federal court over the administration's non-deportation policy, alleging that they were, in effect, being forced to violate their own oaths of office under threat of reprimand.[115] This serves as a warning to us all concerning the slapdash, misguided path America's leaders have taken with respect to immigration.

Accommodating America's Enemies

It was briefly discussed in chapter 4 how the nation's leaders are increasingly tolerating—in actuality, accommodating—Middle Eastern jihadists.

Now there's another twist that affects the criminal justice system. The Associated Press reported, for example, that Ohio has removed pork from the menu of state prisons in response to a lawsuit brought by Muslim inmates. The move was, said state Corrections Department spokesman Carlo LoParo, "a way to

---

[115] http://www.cnn.com/2012/08/23/us/ice-agents-lawsuit/index.html

accommodate religious preferences without jeopardizing prison security."

This author was detailed for a time to the Office for Civil Rights in the U.S. Justice Department. Among the duties was that of responding to inmate mail—usually complaints about prison conditions or a demand for special accommodations. Hundreds of letters were from inmates who had changed their name from their given, American name, to an Islamic one, followed by their prison inmate number. Could there be a jihadist recruitment program going on there. If Christians couldn't proselytize, then neither could Muslims or Wiccans (yes, that means "witches") or anybody else.

The issue fell pretty much on deaf ears, although a couple of years afterward, several newspapers did, in fact, report that there was recruitment by prison clerics, among others.

As for demands, the Muslims wanted, among other things, prayer rugs. The Rastafarians said it was part of their religion to wear their hair *very* long, preferably in "dreadlocks," and they were offended by prison officials who demanded that Rastafarians get a haircut. The Wiccans wanted feathers and candles. And so on.

It was not as if officials were burning Korans or denying religious materials to inmates who wanted them. These were not complaints about religious intolerance. They *were* about "endorsement," which translates to "accommodation."

Of course, there was no "accommodation" when it came to programs that might be loosely connected to Christianity (say, by alluding to a Higher Power, not even to Jesus per se), such as the familiar "12-Step Program" for substance-abuse.

In pursuing this duplicitous policy, our government is compromising national security, because many of the "turned" inmates will get early release.

The Amazing Race (Card)

Today, nothing plays as big a role in agenda-ridden setting of accommodation politics as the issue of race.

The major mission of the 1960s counterculture movement was an anti-Establishment message of tearing down barriers of acceptability (the usual route to destabilization). From that perspective, the civil rights movement constituted convenient add-on. From the civil rights' leaders perspective, the counterculture movement was a convenient ally. Neither faction at the time recognized the lengths to which professional agitators for the U.S.S.R. and Maoist China were playing in their respective agendas—and those who did know didn't particularly care. Blacks served as the Communists' "proletariat"; Anglos served as their "bourgeoisie." It was perfect. America was clueless.

Moreover, all three sides had their own agenda. Between anti-war activism, shattering moral taboos, pitting parents against children and children against parents, and inciting violence on "behalf" of civil rights, America would be forced into hostile camps. In the process, the real enemies of America, the Marxists and culture radicals, believed they could inflict a knockout blow to Americanization, or "assimilation"—not only as that term applied to blacks, but to Hispanics and any other blocs of newcomers to our shores.

The last thing professional agitators wanted was a united America. The Weather Underground (cofounded by Mr. Obama's early mentor, Bill Ayers) actually talked about killing some 25 million American citizens to send a message to the rest! Louis Farrakhan's Nation of Islam (predominantly black) sought to aggressively and violently pit blacks against white, as the original Black Panther Party. The New Black Panther Party is still calling for militancy against whites, yet receives no reprimands from the Department of Homeland security concerning "making terrorist threats"—clearly in accommodation to Mr. Obama's past ties with certain members of the group.

But the larger reason behind government's disinclination to rebuke such high-profile activists is psychological. In their heyday, the groups employed psychological tactics never before seen in the U.S. It is a testament to the strength of the Framers of our Constitution that this nation *didn't* dissolve into another civil war there and then, as have other countries—and with much less provocation.

Brown v. Board of Education Fails to Foil Segregation.- African-Americans had fought hard for this country, and many died for it in World War II. It was past time for reconciliation. From 1951, when fourteen black parents tried to enroll their children in white schools, Anglo-Americans of every extraction (but mostly Western European) already knew, deep down, that racial segregation was not a winner—not for the country, not for the workforce, and not for communities.

Granted, there were pockets of die-hard discrimination, especially in rural areas. But, the fact was, many black families could trace their lineage in America farther back than their white counterparts. Many blacks had already proved their intellectual capacity and were tired of being relegated to second-class status. They wanted to take a place alongside other groups that had immigrated to our shores. All they needed was an equal chance to do so, regardless of how they got here— beginning with the schools.

Unfortunately, the schools were already under attack by leftists, several years before the 1954 *Brown v. Board of Education,* thanks to those who had laid the groundwork in 1946-47—entities like Drs. Brock Chisholm, J.R Rees, and the NEA (see chapter 4).

But, decades of essentially forced illiteracy, menial jobs and broken-up families had created a no-win situation for blacks and contributed to a perception of inferiority. This had the effect of producing an unusually strong bond among people of color nationwide—as well as a culture of dependency and victimization. Simply waving a piece of paper in 1954 banning segregation in schools in *Brown v. Board of Education* didn't affect restaurants, theaters or realty companies, and it was not going to solve the larger problem of acceptance and assimilation. This reality made the nationwide bond among blacks even tighter.

Lincoln Assassination's Unforeseen Impact.- Had Abraham Lincoln not been assassinated after his Emancipation Proclamation ended slavery, the steps toward full citizenship and assimilation might have been addressed quite differently— and much sooner, with greater compassion. President Lincoln had made his case eloquently in a series of seven famous debates in 1858 when he ran against Franklin Douglas.

Unfortunately, Lincoln never got the chance to follow through, so blacks were left to wander about on their own, suddenly free but with no place to go, no means of financial support and no action plan. The abolitionist movements and Underground Railroad of years past foundered—a few charities here, a business operation there, a friendly abolitionist somewhere else—but no brainstorm vivid enough to capture popular backing. Many blacks tried to go back and work for the same people they had been freed from—this time for money. Sometimes that worked, but usually it didn't.

The choices ended up boiling down to two options: recoil in isolation, or become aggressively audacious.

Actually, there was a third option, but most either didn't think of it or didn't know how to go about it: patronage. Find a benefactor and use that as a springboard to a career or trade and independence. That's what smart, talented young men without means had done in the Old World to support themselves. For example, Leonardo di Vinci. It's what many new, and initially unpopular, immigrants in America did, too.

But there was a difference between "other immigrant groups" and American blacks:

- Most American blacks didn't come to this country willingly, and they couldn't "go home."
- Western European immigrants typically had been exposed to some education, handed down by their families, if nothing else, and literacy was encouraged, not the other way around.
- Except for the Asians, most of America's "willing immigrants" didn't look all that different from other Americans.
- Non-African immigrants hailed from patriarchal backgrounds with their own culture more-or-less intact.

Moreover, black Americans were at a huge disadvantage if they hoped to make it in America. And because literacy for blacks had been roundly discouraged to sustain slavery, education was not always understood by young blacks as the "ticket" to prosperity that had benefited other immigrant groups.

Frederick Douglass Lights the Way.- The eminent black orator and writer, Frederick Douglass certainly had education figured out. Having experienced both the best and the worst conditions under slavery, his fortunate exposure to reading and writing (when it was actually against the law for blacks), led him to declare that "knowledge is the pathway from slavery to freedom."

Those pioneering parents who tried to enroll their kids in white schools in 1951 saw the benefits of education, too, of course. But, unfortunately, that message didn't get through to some of their youngsters. Possibly because they were, after all, just children, trying to make their way during a period of upheaval, they understood school mainly in the context of breaking down "white" barriers. Once they were there, some didn't know quite what to do. Technically, they were "in," but the races weren't mingling. This resulted in two things: a black community knitted even more tightly together—tighter than the Irish, the Jews, the Italians or the Dutch—and a massive effort at social engineering based in psychology and politics. It wasn't a good mix.

Second, and most obviously, blacks looked very different. They could not just melt into a crowd and sprout intellectual, musical or athletic genius—unless, of course, like Frederick Douglass, they had very strong personalities, an optimistic spirit and unwavering motive. Upon reaching freedom in New York in a madcap 24-hour escape from a cruel "slave-breaker," Douglass wrote: "Anguish and grief, like darkness and rain, may be depicted; but gladness and joy, like the rainbow, defy the skill of pen or pencil."

Not exactly the musings of a moron…

Third, their society and cultural background was matriarchal from the beginning. Even Frederick Douglass wasn't sure who his father was. Worse, their native African culture was deemed too "primitive" for Western tastes and subsequently discarded. So, this was not just an American-Anglo phenomenon, but extended to many countries to which blacks had been taken during the height of the horrendous slave trade. Indeed, some of the chieftains back in Africa had sold them out to slave traders for trinkets—a fact not lost on the earliest generation of slaves and passed along by word of mouth to their offspring, who predictably responded by rejecting their "native" culture.

Slavery's Negative Legacy to Black Families.- As if all these things were not enough to keep blacks from becoming "fully Americanized," encouragement by white overseers to reproduce without benefit of marriage and dividing up families for resale, helped to de-stigmatize illegitimacy among crucial generations of blacks. Many blacks coped by detaching their feelings from family, never knowing when they might be broken up. Who could blame them?

The matriarchal nature of the old culture sustained parental bonds between *mother*-and-child, but not so strongly between *father*-and-child. Even so, by the 1930s, most blacks had adopted Christian dogma, in which marriage and fidelity played a large role, so Americanization progressed, if slowly.

Again, we can refer back to Frederick Douglass. As soon as he arrived in New York, he sent for the woman he loved, Anna Murray. They married—and stayed married until Anna's death 44 years later—raising five children within marital bonds. Thanks to people like Douglass, and of course the simple passage of time, Americanization, Christianization and literacy slowly began to take hold. But until blacks had a good reason to look out for America as much as to look out for themselves, real assimilation couldn't take root.

So, after the *Brown* decision, there came Jim Crow—better described, perhaps, as "the way things were." No reason. It simply was what it was.

Blacks Surmount the Odds and a Leader Emerges.- Martin Luther King, Jr., and many of his fellow civil rights advocates helped change all that—although the truth was, it was starting to change by itself. The eminent writer-researcher-educator, Thomas Sowell, found that the rise of blacks in professional and other high-level occupations was greater during the five years *preceding* the Civil Rights Act of 1964 than the five years afterward. Peculiar, to say the least.

Walter Williams, columnist, professor and holder of doctorates in economics and law, points out that poverty among black families fell from 87 percent in 1940 to 47 percent in 1960—*before* anti-poverty legislation took effect. Black poverty fell again by about 17 percent between 1960 and 1980, but of that, only 1 percent of the decline occurred in the 1970s, *when civil rights for African-Americans was supposedly at its peak.*

These statistics suggest that had something not gone terribly wrong, by the 2000s African-Americans would have assimilated more or less across the board, with roughly the same percentage of professionals and menial laborers as other immigrant groups. Along with that would have come social inclusion.

By way of comparison, take the waves of Japanese immigrants. Despite the short period of detainment following the scare of Pearl Harbor, Japanese have not generally suffered the same discrimination in America as whites. If any group was ripe for ostracism, it would have been the Japanese, given the well-publicized horrors of the Bataan Death March and other atrocities during the Second World War. But most of the residual ill-will petered out by the 1960s, and Japanese immigrants took their place beside other immigrant groups and assimilated—with elements of their native culture remaining intact. The reasons for this are not easy to pin down.

The War aside, blacks unconnected to the civil rights movement in the 50s or 60s *were* making it. The famous contralto Marian Anderson may have gotten the cold should from leaders of the Daughters of the American Revolution (DAR) when her agent tried to book her at Constitution Hall, but she had already performed all over the world, including in New York at Carnegie Hall. Whites were coming to the conclusion on their own that incidents like the DAR snub were over-the-top. By 1962, the tide of black ostracism had started to turn on its own.

The World Sees Blacks Through New Eyes.- Black entertainers—from the Ink Spots from the 1930s and 40s to the Coasters in the 50s and the early "Motown" (Record Corporation) greats of 60s—dressed in the sort of attire that, even when flamboyant for the stage, was also pristine; they displayed a combination of class and humility for the applause from majority-white audiences. Martin Luther King, Jr., always appeared in a coat and tie. Posters and photos from the 60s era almost invariably showed marchers in what we would now describe as "business attire" or "good casual." For the most part, demonstrators comported themselves respectfully, save for a few individuals who traipsed through the Tidal Basin in Washington, D.C. Today, white teens in blue jeans do that routinely.

Interestingly, because radio had the greater audience of that period, white teenagers couldn't tell, for the most part, whether singers were white or black. In looking at old clips on PBS' popular "Doo-Wop" series, many of the now-grown kids from this author's generation are surprised to learn that their favorite singers were black.

The "Doo-Wop" series is built around reunions of original rock-'n-roll groups, both white and black. But, while their individual voices are unique—thus their fame—one often cannot tell, without the benefit of an album cover, or old TV clip, what race anybody is.

The ubiquity of radio may have had some bearing on this phenomenon, as listeners were accustomed to being able to understand the words to a song—whether the lyrics were silly, romantic or dramatic. If audiences of the day couldn't comprehend the lyrics, entertainers were toast, regardless of their ethnicity.

Enunciation aside, songs of the era expressed an amorous sentimentality, incorporated complex harmonies, were hold-your-sides funny, or evoked an entreating innocence that connected sex with affection—Sam Cooke, Chubby Checker, Brook Benton, Ray Charles, Dinah Washington, the Supremes, Diana Ross, Nat King Cole, Louis Armstrong, even the later Pointer Sisters... If any of them had an axe to grind, they kept it to themselves.

Jazz pianists were making a splash, too. Most hadn't had any actual lessons, but somehow they had learned to play by ear and by watching others. Not only that, the music itself was unique in its complexity. The tunes were upbeat, contagious, sensuous in a pleasant sort of way, and highly emotive. Sammy Davis, Jr., and Ben Vereen mesmerized audiences with their feet. Vereen came to the attention of the all-time great choreographer Bob Fosse, who nurtured his talent. The two became fast friends.

The world was taking notice.

Snatching Defeat from the Jaws of Victory.- Then something happened; the movement got derailed, and with it the gains many blacks had made on their own.

The illegitimacy rate among blacks in 1940 was down to approximately 15 percent. By 1965 it had climbed to about 24 percent, compared to 4 percent among whites. Today, black illegitimacy stands at over 70 percent (2010 government statistics), about three times the national average, even in these liberal times. Among the reasons theorized is that welfare laws, over time, created a financial incentive for poor mothers to stay single. But that doesn't explain why many black schoolgirls actually competed to see who could get pregnant first, even with all the school programs that work to counter it.

The Spoilers

Unknown to many earnest people in the civil rights movement, the same Marxist infiltrators who took to college campuses to rabble-rouse against the Vietnam War, preach "free love," and bomb police cars, were also busy inflaming blacks. While leaders like Martin Luther King, Jr., never once advocated rioting and pillaging, as soon as he would leave a place where he had been speaking or leading a march, in would come the leftist spoilers inciting violence and looting, *exactly the way a young Josef Stalin had done in his home town of Tiflis, Georgia* (part of the former Soviet Union).

It is fascinating to read Simon Sebag Montefiore's meticulously documented historical account of *Young Stalin*. His scheme in Tiflis (modern-day Tbilisi) to increase his name-recognition was intended as a way into Vladimir Lenin's inner circle. But tactics-wise, the parallel between Stalin's organizing of a group called "the Outfit" to incite bank robberies in Tiflis, and those of behind-the-scenes tacticians during the 1960s civil rights movement is simply unmistakable.

American "revolutionary" leaders were culled by trained "handlers" from college campuses, labor unions, entertainment, and youth groups. Their foot-soldiers, in turn, were a mixed brew. Some were just unhappy misfits—angry at their parents and life in general. Others were extremists hawking a variety of silly issues—from the "right" to wear long hair and torn jeans, to "save-the-whale" campaigns. Then, there were hangers-on, who just wanted to be a part of something, and idealistic grassroots activists who wanted "to make a difference." Along the way was the usual assortment of nitwits with too much time on their hands.

Race to the 2000s.- According to Justice Department figures, blacks are six times more likely than whites to be homicide victims, and a whopping 94 percent of black victims are murdered by blacks. Like many recent writings by black columnists and authors, Robert L. Woodson, Sr., founder and president of the Center for Neighborhood Enterprise, decries the crisis of "rising gang violence and black-on-black warfare in the nation's cities...in the course of just one weekend." He was alluding to the year 2012 in Chicago, "the site of 40 black-on-black shootings, even of which were fatal."

Dr. Walter Williams found that the high-crime rate of many majority-black communities has turned what were once nice neighborhoods into economic basket-cases. Worse, the violence has caused upstanding individuals, black and otherwise, to move away, thereby leaving a slum.

African-Americans who worked, and succeeded, in escaping such tawdry environments are called "Oreos" and "Uncle Toms" by their own race. Those who yearned to be a part of the system, not at odds with it, had to work harder than ever to prove they were successful in their own right, not on account of some government program. The once tight-knit black community was turning against itself.

African-American Icons Try to Save the Movement.- People like legendary comedian Bill Cosby, who left the "projects," got a Ph.D., and his own TV show, were embarrassed. He, and many others who had advocated for civil rights in the 1960s and 70s—escaping poverty and rising above racial discrimination to the point where they had thoroughly assimilated—could hardly believe what was happening. Professional African-Americans who had pulled themselves up by the proverbial bootstraps didn't want to turn their backs on their race; on the other hand, they could not just sit back and watch the seeming lurch backward so many of their brethren had taken.

So, Cosby spoke out—to black audiences in 2004, including the National Association for the Advancement of Colored People (NAACP)—and gave them all a piece of his mind, saying "[t]his is not what I marched for." He criticized their demeanor, rap lyrics, prison-like garb and black enunciation, which was virtually unintelligible, especially among the young—quite unlike the language of the "projects" where Cosby had grown up in virtual poverty. Black songwriters of yesteryear had been brushed aside: Upbeat was exchanged for ugly. Seductive moved to sadism. Beautiful to brutal. Romantic to repulsive.

What on earth had happened?

And because Bill Cosby was who he was—a beloved, household-name actor and comic—he got away with it, more or less. But it was already too late to have the necessary impact.

On May 25, 2012, the aforementioned Robert Woodson wrote one of the most poignant columns on record[116] regarding epidemic levels of graft and corruption among household-name black professional groups and public officials, such as the congressional Black Caucus and former Louisiana Rep. William Jefferson, to name just a few. Woodson was right that many, if not most, of the instances of corruption he cited were not widely reported. With the exception of Rep. Jefferson and the extortion-bribery-fraud scandal involving former Detroit Mayor Kwame Kilpatrick, this author checked every allegation to be sure there wasn't some mistake. The amounts of money involved, and the sheer audacity of the crimes, were obscene.

Just as educational opportunity for blacks in the 1954 *Brown* decision didn't translate into automatic assimilation and high literacy, the ugly truth, reveals Woodson, is that "African-American political power didn't [even] protect civil rights...."

We now live, says Woodson, "[i]n an era where race has begun to serve as both a shield (rebuffing legitimate criticism as evidence of racism) and a sword (attacking dissenting opinions as racist)."

That had already proved to be an understatement.

Stalinesque Sequels

In 2002, the Republican U.S. House Majority Leader Trent Lott lost his speakership over a celebratory remark he made in 2002 to honor a dying Senator Strom Thurmond, then celebrating his 100th birthday. By then, every word, symbol and expression was being scrutinized for perceived racial slur.

Senator Thurmond (R-SC) had served for 48 years and was a product of a segregated South. He was also a decorated World War II veteran who had voluntarily left a prestigious job as a judge in 1942 to serve the U.S. Army, participating in one of

---

[116] http://www.washingtontimes.com/news/2012/may/24/black-on-black-crime-in-the-suites/

the deadliest battles, the Normandy Campaign of 1944. As Senator, he chaired the Senate Armed Services Committee in which he had an understandably strong interest. In the 1960s and 70s, Thurmond became very concerned about activism against the United States by leftist agitators—which infuriated the counterculture press.

So, what happened at Thurmond's centennial birthday party to Trent Lott in 2002 was payback for taking on leftist agitators. They seized upon the Senate Majority Leader's benign plaudit and turned it into a major issue. His words were: "When Strom Thurmond ran for president, we [Mississippi] voted for him. We're proud of it. And if the rest of the country had followed our lead, we wouldn't have had all these problems over the years, either." That was taken for a racial slur.

In 1948, Thurmond ran for President on a "Dixiecrat" party ticket, back when the word "Dixie" was acceptable. Thurmond also once challenged the Civil Rights Act on the grounds of Separation of Powers under the Constitution. But what Lott was referring to when he said "these problems," was States' rights, the 10th Amendment, which was what the Dixiecrat Party was primarily about in 1948. The civil rights movement wouldn't occur for another 20 years.

For that one comment, Lott was tried in the press and forced to resign as Majority Leader. As usual, conservative colleagues were of no help.

Quite a different story played out in 2008, when Democratic Senate Majority Leader Harry Reid made a far worse gaffe. Reid said he thought then-candidate Barack Obama might have a good shot at the White House because he was "light-skinned" and spoke "with no Negro dialect, unless he wanted to have one."

The insult was dismissed as "no big deal."

This kind of word-parsing should have come as no surprise. In 1999, the word "niggardly" was stupidly misconstrued as a racial epithet (it means *miserly* or *stingy*) by a black colleague in the D.C. government, just as use of the term "Dixie," which refers to the large swath of southern states, was by that time tantamount to supporting slavery.

The man who launched the 1999 controversy was David Howard, a white aide to then-Mayor Anthony A. Williams. Howard was referring to the budget. The official complaint over the use of "niggardly" said more about state of literacy in the U.S. than it did about political correctness. But so fierce was the firestorm—until somebody bothered to look the word up in the dictionary—that Howard ended up tendering his resignation over the incident, and Mayor Anthony, a black man, accepted it. Upon dissemination of the dictionary meaning, the Mayor offered Howard his job back, but Howard wisely refused.

Meanwhile, in a timely, but unrelated, incident just one week after Mr. Howard's supposed gaffe, a junior-year African-American English major (and vice-chairwoman of the Black Student Union) at the University of Wisconsin revealed she didn't know much about English when she was offended by her professor's use of the same word in a course on Chaucer, the 17th-century poet. "I was in tears, shaking," she complained to the faculty.

The upshot of both incidences was a national debate on racial sensitivity. Even Julian Bond, the renowned then-chairman of the NAACP, was aghast at what he called "hair-trigger sensibility" on race. "Seems to me," quipped Bond, "that the mayor has been niggardly in his judgment on the issue...Mayor Williams should bring Howard back—and order dictionaries issued to all staff who need them."

~

Chapter 6
THE CAMPAIGN GAME

[W]e hear the same liberal lament: 'Our political system is broken because of partisanship.' This is untrue.... The argument tries to pit politics against principle. Democrats are using their own convoluted brand of partisanship, a cynical, feel-good version of 'Can't we all just get along?' after they have already stacked the deck against reform.... [Their] political claim prevents discussion of the real problem the nation faces.... *-- Thomas N. Tripp, author and secretary, American Conservative Union Foundation, in an op-ed for* **The Washington Times***: "The myth of bipartisanship," November 25, 2011*.

Mr. Tripp got it half right in the quotation above, especially the part about "pitting politics against principle." The "Free-To-Be" generation and their progeny say they want *bipartisan politics*. Consensus. Compromise.

No, they don't... What they want is "unanimity," which is altogether different. They have been conditioned to expect leaders and a government in which everyone thinks alike.

This is part of the phenomenon Mr. Tripp, among others, refers as a "stack the deck?" But how, exactly, is that accomplished?

Them Versus *Us*

First of all, we should be clear about who *they* are, as the term "liberal" is something of a misnomer—a word not at all reminiscent of its 1770s-era usage. What Tripp calls "liberal Democrats" are in reality committed socialists and globalists (the latter meaning that U.S. national sovereignty is not a big deal to them). They adhere to, or may have subconsciously absorbed in school, a Marxist view of egalitarian economics, highly regulative governance, and an overarching international body as an ultimate arbitrator.

This, of course, was the communist view, too. The difference with American Marxists (if they know who Karl Marx was) is that they don't really expect to see tanks roll down the street, or individuals dragged from their houses to an equivalent of Lubyanka prison[117]. But, then, neither did the average Russian, Latvian or Hungarian, until people got caught up in the "machine," or, as was the case in many countries, signed on to so-called "wars of liberation." For these reasons, the term *leftist*, or *left-winger*, not "Communist," is used to describe persons who endorse, or acquiesce in, the Marxist-socialist-globalist vision.

Since the Reagan Administration, the Left has determined never again to get blind-sided by the likes of a charismatic conservative.

The Standard Operating Procedure the liberal-leftist camp today is to *pre-empt* any opposition to the socialist agenda by "stacking the deck" against its various nemeses: conservatives, constitutionalists, Christians, traditionalists and patriots. For the sake of convenience in this chapter, let's just call all five groups as CCCTPs.

Is this fair? No, it is not. So why lump the five together? Because—and this is important—***the Left paints them all with the same brush anyway***. It's about the "game"—remember?

Obviously, some conservatives are not Christians, and some constitutionalists are not ardent traditionalists, and some patriots are not social conservatives. But to the Left, it doesn't matter. All are under attack. That is what the Agenda Game known as "the stacked deck" is all about.

So this means that if, for example, a Jewish person is a defender of traditional Judeo *and Christian* values, or if an atheist decides to become an outspoken champion of Western culture—these individuals shouldn't wonder why they are targeted as "one of those wacky Christian Bible-thumpers." Yes, that will happen! This is a key example of how "stacking the deck" is actually played.

Why does the liberal-left do this? Because it can!

Therefore, defending oneself against such attempted smear attacks such *is only going to bring on more of the same*. The target

---

[117] http://www.articles.latimes.com/1991-09-07/news/mn-1571_1_lubyanka-prison

subject will be lucky to ever get the chance to debate the issue of traditional values or Western culture. He or she will spend *all* the time defending against the smear.

This is how bullies operate; this is high-stakes political combat in action. Leftists force the politically incorrect "miscreant" to argue on the terms decreed by the leftist media—which in the above case is to say, on the basis of a smear: name-calling.

As long as CCCTPs fail to understand the game, they will keep playing "defense" instead of forcing leftists to argue serious topics. They will not win—*even if they get appointed or elected to a post*.

That is why the Supreme Court has moved slowly toward decisions that favor the Left, or socialism. That is why cabinet appointees keep taking the country inexorably leftward. No prospective Justice or political appointee today is going to make it past the leftist censors in the bureaucracy, media or Congress—unless that candidate is perceived to be at last malleable.

How "Deck-Stacking" Works

With every new election cycle, it matters less and less which candidate one votes for, as each contender works to ensure that his or her campaign rhetoric "plays it safe" in the media. They float proposals that will please their base but have zero chance of passing any Congress, liberal or conservative, because of intransigent vested and/or special interests. Those who refuse to play that game are soon "out"—marginalized. The same goes for prospective appointees who require congressional approval.

The punishment for missing a beat is career-shattering—at least for any politician even slightly to the right of center.

Of course, the double standard is palpable. Leftist presidential candidate Bill Clinton could admit[118] to having tried marijuana with no repercussions, but President Ronald Reagan's conservative Supreme Court Justice nominee Douglas H. Ginsburg was forced to

---

[118]

http://www.time.com/time/specials/packages/article/0,28804,2007228_2007230_200725 8,00.html withdraw his name as a contender[119] after having admitted to the same thing.

This incident occurred shortly after Reagan's first nominee, Judge Robert H. Bork, was defeated in the Senate in a disgraceful "show trial" for his views on civil liberties and social issues. The more important focus—his stellar qualifications—barely came up. Reportedly, some members of the media even went so far as to peruse video stores to see what films he might have rented, and libraries for which books he might have checked out—to dig up dirt. They found nothing.

In recent history, only Justice Clarence Thomas[120] has demonstrated the intestinal fortitude to prevail over the "stacked deck." It is worth the reader's while to revisit those 1991 hearings[121], as they were among the most vicious of all time. Justice Thomas managed to rebuff the power players with class, resolve and dignity. Whether he could do the same today, with the leftist power machine being even stronger, is probably a question he will not have to face, although the Left continues to dissect his, and his family's, every move.

Thus is the deck "stacked" against CCCTPs. Liberals, globalists and leftists ultimately get a free pass, no matter how they behave or what they say, while every utterance of a conservative or traditionalist is scrutinized.

So, here is the situation bipartisan-minded citizens now face:

They attend town-hall-style meetings, sit on committees and focus groups, deliberate with the heads of community associations, and debate leaders in their houses of worship. Unfortunately, the CCCTP camp no longer has legitimacy in the media or in major institutions, and their liberal-leftist counterparts do. This makes it easy for professional "facilitators" to divide such forums into two hostile, opposing factions—and then make it seem as though CCCTPs

---

[119] http://www.nytimes.com/1987/11/08/us/ginsburg-withdraws-name-as-supreme-court-nominee-citing-marijuana-clamor.html?pagewanted=all&src=pm
[120] http://www.en.wikipedia.org/wiki/Clarence_Thomas
[121] http://www.annoy.com/sectionless/doc.html?DocumentID=100506

are inflexible, dogmatic and obstructionist when no "consensus" is reached.

Of course, all the "compromising" will occur on the side of CCCTPs, rarely or never on the Left's—**unless** the issue is of no real concern to liberals and leftists. In that case, the Left can afford to throw a bone to CCCTPs now and then, having accrued powerful friends in the media, the education system (including teacher-training institutions), schools of journalism, high-profile news outlets, entertainment, and even among some religious hierarchies. The Left has absolutely nothing to lose by picking and choosing its battles on its own terms.

Leftists agitators achieve their goal of pre-emption *by creating a psychological environment* so that any issue always moves on the Left's own terms. Essentially, *they decide what their quarry is going to think about and for how long,* and at this point in time the Left has stockpiled enough credibility among major institutions to pull it off.

This deck-stacking also narrows the field of potential political candidates. It is important to continually remind oneself when reading or listening to what passes for debate and editorial analysis, that what is typically being purveyed is PM masquerading as PR.

Perception Management v. Public Relations

Perception management (PM) was discussed at some length in chapter 5 in the context of "justice," but not in the context of political campaigns, or "bipartisanship." For this we need to compare it to a close cousin—public relations (PR), or marketing.

The purpose of public relations (PR), or marketing, is to sell you something that you might need and would fit into both your budget and your lifestyle—say, a new brand of coffee, or a more convenient type of frozen dinner, or maybe a better chair that allows you to use your laptop without spilling your coffee. PM, on the other hand, would be used to trick you into believing that your coffee is really hot cocoa, and that you actually *want* hot cocoa, not coffee. Not only that, your clumsiness with the, er, cocoa will be construed as "inattentiveness," which means you may want to try a drug for Attention Deficit Disorder!

So we see that both PM and PR utilize persuasion. But PR is built around "service"—with an emphasis on something you might actually need or use. PM is built around deception, pure and simple—with the emphasis being on something you would probably reject on your own. Whereas PR organizers typically *welcome* dissimilar viewpoints—because it might lead to a *product* or idea with mass-appeal, PM coordinators will place nothing on the agenda for discussion that cannot in some way be twisted or made useful to their employers on the liberal-left.

This is not to say that the PM coordinator doesn't allow occasional comments or viewpoints that run contrary to the socialist-left party-line. But doing so comes with a caveat: "Can my opponent's remark or opinion be made useful to my agenda?" If the answer is "yes," then any viewpoint, idea or rationale offered by a CCCTP will only be aired or publicized with the expectation that either the viewpoint itself, or you, the opponent, *can be discredited when the time is right* (think businessman Herman Cain's fleeting run for president in 2011).

What is called "negative campaigning," or creating "bad PR," is often another aspect of perception management—so it's no wonder that people get confused. True, sometimes a bad product, per se, creates its own "negative PR" and is pulled from the market. But in PM, if the proper *psychological climate* has been created, then *it will not matter* whether an allegation is true, or entirely twisted and/or trumped up. With enough financing and repetition in the media, the charge itself will be enough to bring down an opponent or potential candidate.

Knights of Columbus head, Carl Anderson, came out in 2012 slamming the practice of "personal vilification." He cited a July 2012 Knights of Columbus-Marist poll[122] showing that nearly 8 in 10 Americans, or 78 percent, say they are "frustrated" by the negative tone of political campaigns. They will have to continue being

---

[122] http://uspolitics.einnews.com/pr_news/106694121/ new-poll-finds-nearly-8-in-10-americans-frustrated-by-tone-of-political-campaigns

"frustrated" until such time as they understand hardball PM, or political combat.

Fabricated charges, well-publicized in advance of any evidence (perfectly doable in today's high-tech, special-effects-laden age) can even displace a well-considered piece of legislation, so that it is rejected out of hand, without so much as a congressional hearing, and its backers maligned in the mainstream press.

The opposite is also true—mostly for the benefit of leftists, as they are better financed: Recall in 2010 then-House Speaker Nancy Pelosi's infamously flippant remark to Congress about the 2,700-page ObamaCare proposal: *"We have to pass the health care bill so that you can find out what's in it."* If a CCCTP had made such a gaffe, that lawmaker would probably have been officially censured or even replaced.

These are all signals that our government is moving beyond the ability of "we, the people" to control it—that it is not flourishing in the service of Americans but, rather, is guided by the well-orchestrated tenets of PM.

Think of it as you would a real orchestra; that serves as a good analogy here: When the conductors (the leftist elite) tap their baton, all the various front groups open their "sheet music." Once the audience (average citizens) hears is the "concerto," it is played so smoothly one can barely discern its separate instruments.

The "Slumdog Billionaires" of Politics

These chapters have alluded repeatedly to second- and third-party high-financing of the leftist agenda. With an increasingly left-leaning global presence has come billion-dollar donors with enormous access to power as well as means—e.g., Open Society Institute chairman and international investor George Soros, Las Vegas casino tycoon Sheldon Adelson, Hyatt hotel billionaire Penny Pritzker, investment icons James Crown and Warren Buffett, entertainment mogul Haim Saban, "hedge-funders" Marc Lasry and Tom Steyer, and entrepreneur Johnny Chien Chuen Chung.[123] These are just a few of the better-known examples.

However, with the advent of super-PACs in 2010[124], even shadowy figures now find it feasible to thoroughly circumvent the financial disclosure process and influence election outcomes. Of course, famous left-wingers like George Soros make huge donations to ultra-left super-PACs. Soros' super-Pac was so well-endowed in 2012 that it financed operatives to "track" and "tail" (let's call lit what it is: "stalking") Republican candidates[125], with the aim of monitoring and recording any statement, misstep or flub conservative contenders might make—even something that can be taken out of context and twisted—before disseminating it widely.

But how about less-recognized super-Pac figures?

Online journalists Kathy Gill and Tom Murse help explain the difference between a PAC and a super-PAC, as well as ill-fated earlier attempts to rein in anonymous big-spenders, individual and otherwise.

According to Gill, a PAC is simply a Political Action Committee, which first emerged around 1943. PACs can contribute *fixed* amounts garnered from corporations, unions, individuals and associations. A single individual is permitted to donate as much as $5,000 a year to a candidate, or to the candidate's registered committee ($2,500 in the primary and the remainder in the election *per se*). A PAC[126] allows for pooling the contributions of these donors *and* provides a further $15,000 to any party's official national committee. Not only that, a PAC can give up to $5,000 to another PAC.

Obviously, the PAC set-up was already a coup for high-rollers against typically small-potatoes middle- and lower-class donors with only $25-$250 to spend.

---

[123] http://articles.chicagotribune.com/1997-07-30/news/9707300004_1_dnc-officials-white-house-christmas-johnny-chien-chuen-chung

[124] http://uspolitics.about.com/od/firstamendment/a/ What-Is-A-Super-Pac.htm

[125] http://weaselzippers.us/2012/08/28/george-soros-at-it-again-paying-for-trackers-to-hunt-for-dirt-on-gop-candidates/

[126] http://uspolitics.about.com/od/firstamendment/a/ What-Is-A-Super-Pac.htm

But even this was surpassed in 2010, with a landmark U.S. Supreme Court case, *Citizen United v. Federal Election Commission*, which virtually launched the super-PAC.

A super-PAC places *no* restrictions on *who* contributes or *how much* they contribute. "They can raise as much money from corporations, unions and associations as they please and spend unlimited amounts on advocating for the election or defeat of the candidates of their choice," writes online journalist Tom Murse.

Unbelievably, the U.S. Supreme Court decided that limiting corporate and union spending to influence elections was unconstitutional. The 5-4 decision tossed out the 2002 Bipartisan Campaign Reform Act (commonly known as the McCain–Feingold Act (BCRA), although BCRA was neither effective nor particularly "bipartisan." But it furthered the *pretense* of reining in "electioneering communications" to some extent.

But, with the advent of super-PACs, which came just in time to affect Election Year 2012, the very wealthy would be able to "give" to the same candidates numerous times under different venues. The decision also allowed (without saying so directly, of course) unions, corporations, associations and so forth, to channel the dues of members, including the funds of employees who are forced to join because of collective bargaining laws. A portion of the pot of dues collected is redirected into candidates, many of whom union members might not otherwise support—an action which borders on extortion.

The entire issue of campaign "donation" has become a national security and sovereignty problem, because foreign nationals—some of them unfriendly to American ideals and core policies—are funneling money into U.S. elections. For example, as far back as the Bill Clinton campaign, there were allegations of illegal campaign contributions from the Chinese government. The unspoken and unwritten understanding was that the Chinese could purchase American technology if they funneled money into a winning campaign. The down-side, of course, was that the technology they bought from us could, in turn, be used to level American cities. Thus, our two countries are entwined, economically and politically; it would be very difficult at this point for the U.S. to extricate itself.

To compete, the Republican Party has been dragged down along with the Democrats, so that, with rare exceptions, the major parties have, in effect, succumbed to the kinds of games enjoyed by the "cocktail set." This pejorative was alluded to in this book previously; in this context, "cocktail set" means wealthy political "junkies" who hobnob with the rich and famous, caring not at all about the political outcome, but, rather indulging in the game itself—rather like betting on a racehorse!

All this has had a dispiriting effect on individual and grassroots participation, knowing they cannot possibly contribute enough money to have a say on issues vital to this nation once the election is over.

The "Caring" Contributor

Many election-watchers scratch their heads in wonder at wealthy icons like Bill Gates, Warren Buffett, Stephen Spielberg, etc., who donate millions or billions to left-leaning candidates and causes around the world but invest practically none of their largesse in America—*even when a niche exists that could make them a lot of money and create jobs, too.*

Take, for example, America's 1940s electrical infrastructure in many major cities like the Washington, D.C. area—the Nation's Capital, of all places. The Potomac Electric Power Company (known as Pepco) is the dysfunctional public utility that purports to supply electric power to most of the area, including Montgomery County, Maryland—one of the nation's most highly taxed areas. The power goes out every time there is a thunderstorm or moderate snow—for days, if not a week or more—let alone a rare "derecho"[127], hurricane or ice storm. Among the costliest of week-long outages occurred on June 9, 2012, when a derecho packing 60- and 70-mile-per-hour winds moved through the area in a mere 10-15 minutes. But the outages lasted through the holiday week of Fourth of July, with 105-degree temperatures. Hundreds of millions of dollars in damage was

---

[127] http://www.erh.noaa.gov/lwx/events/svrwx_20120629/

done to the area's economy—and the sealed windows of modern buildings didn't help because they allow for no fresh air.

Between an inability to get to work, remain in a "sealed" office building, or to get any work done at home, the above-ground power-line issue again took front and center stage. Spoiled food (including in grocery stores where backup generators finally gave out) and shuttered businesses added to calls for a reconfigured power-line structure.

"People are fed up with power outages. We need a game-changer," said DC Mayor Vincent Gray.

Hello? Mr. Buffett? Mr. Gates? Are you there? Oh—you're in Bangladesh? Sorry to bother you.

Pepco has had to bring in crews from as far away as Louisiana to restore power in recent years, and it's not as if severe weather is new to the Washington metropolitan area. From as far back as the 1950s, when Hurricane Hazel roared in, and snow drifts sometimes made it impossible for people of that era to open their garage doors, this problem has existed. But that was before the Internet and cable –TV made underground infrastructures the norm for newer communities, thereby facilitating retrofits for older neighborhoods.

The D.C. area is hardly alone in this problem, but being the Capital of the United States makes it a national security issue. The time is ripe for an entrepreneur with plenty of capital to buy out companies like Pepco and undertake an extreme makeover of our country's crumbling utility systems. This would also generate literally hundreds of thousands of jobs, considering the number or cities experiencing long-term outages. Even with re-training of workers, the investment would pay off big.

So, why are these icons like the Bill and Melinda Gates Foundation and big-name entertainers dropping money down a bunch of basket-case rat-holes that have never managed to make use of what the United Nations and private donors have already given?

The reason is that investing in American infrastructure is not "showy," but throwing good money after bad half a world away is. No one would argue the merits of helping these struggling populations. If billionaires want to do that, they could actually generate more money toward that cause by investing in infrastructure projects here at home. These would pay off handsomely to those with enough capital to invest in them, and would add to their income in the long term.

This should be a top issue for political candidates. Unfortunately, the globalist-leftist camp is not interested in such logic. How much more satisfying it is to saturate the airwaves with emotionally evocative devastation and distraught victims in foreign lands! That's what they believe increases viewership and a steady stream of advertisers—for products that will be of no use during a massive, long-term power outage.

High-Stakes Candidacy Mimics "High School"

Today's political campaigns are little more than popularity contests. Beginning with the 1992 election campaign of Bill Clinton, the biggest question of the day was "boxers or briefs"[128]. Mr. Clinton's "handlers" sought to give him a "cool" persona by encouraging him to don sunglasses and play saxophone on Arsenio Hall's TV show[129]. From that time onward, it was as if our nation's presidential candidates were running for Student Council instead of the highest office in the land. Which candidate today, not being at least passably photogenic, has any chance on the public stage of electoral politics?

Where did Americans get the message that it was mandatory for a candidate to be physically attractive? In school! (We will see how this idea gets transmitted in chapter 7.) Meanwhile, has most of the developed world become imbued with the notion that popularity, position and status is defined by whatever "look" is deemed "hot" at a given time, and without that, the person's "message" to voters and constituents is inconsequential.

---

[128] http://www.time.com/time/specials/packages/article/ 0,28804,2007228_2007230_2007258,00.html

[129] http://articles.baltimoresun.com/1992-12-27/features/ 1992362178_1_clinton-arsenio- hall-hall-show

Indeed, the main task of modern campaigns is to ensure that every voter sees your face stamped on everything that stands still. Every time people open their newspaper, go online, turn on the radio or TV, see a passing bus or billboard, the candidate's smiling face and name must be staring back. In other words, the face and name carries more psychological weight than whatever policies or promises the candidate makes.

Whatever Happened to Conservative "Turf"?

The quandary, of course, is how to take back the reins of debate. This produces yet another dilemma: Getting the Left to debate issues on CCCTP turf.

Many, of course, will say there is plenty of conservative turf, and go on to cite a list of well-known (at least well-known to die-hard conservatives) think tanks and media groups: the Heritage Foundation, the *Washington Times*, the American Conservative Union, the American Enterprise Institute, Eagle Forum, Hillsdale College, the *Weekly Standard*, Concerned Women for America, the Media Research Center, the Family Research Council, and so on.

But let's just suppose, for the sake of argument, one of the organizations above decided to host a debate, inviting established speakers and experts from all political sides. The topic could be anything: climate change, female military staff on submarines, gay clubs in schools, displays of Christian crosses on tax-supported properties, Medicare reform, drugging rowdy schoolchildren, private-property rights, domestic oil drilling, cultural enhancement.

Question: What are the chances that any known entity on the liberal-leftist side would sign on to a debate at the above institutions?

If you said "slim to none," you can move to the head of the class. Conservatives, constitutionalists and traditionalists have no "turf." *Nada. Nyet.* Isn't gonna happen....

Now, suppose CBS, ABC, NBC, PBS, CNN, Brookings Institute or the Aspen Institute for Humanistic Studies hosted one of the same forums, same topics?

Why, Mitt Romney would be falling over Louisiana Gov. Bobby Jindal, who would be elbowing both former Secretary of State Condoleezza Rice and former Rep. Paul Ryan out of the way in a mad dash to secure a spot on a podium—to debate, of all people, Al Gore—even though not a single one of the five may have the credentials to debate the topics at hand. But never mind, even if politically amenable "experts" were brought in, the result would be the same. The liberal networks and policy organizations would enjoy standing-room-only attendances and 100-percent acceptances to debate.

Where did the conservative "turf" go? Their office buildings are still standing; the presses are still running; the revolving door of "fellows," "senior analysts," and policy wonks still work hard in cramped offices. Yet they receive only occasional invitations to serve as resident expert or participate in discussions on PBS.

What happened is, that anybody perceived by the media as "conservative"—regardless of the number of doctoral degrees—has no legitimacy with the "mainstream" media, so their findings either receive no mention at all, or are ridiculed by those who hold the reins of the agenda: the liberal-left.

CCCTP Republicans and "conservative Democrats" dropped the ball in the 1970s. They failed to invest heavily in media while it was still relatively cheap—"buying out" or "buying up" as many existing newspapers and local TV or radio stations as possible. By the time the Reagan Revolution came along in 1980, it was too late. The damage was done. Conservatives were playing catch-up, and have been ever since.

Less extremist, old standby newspapers like the *Washington Star* and *Dallas Times-Herald* were edged out in the 1980s and 90s, replaced by liberal-leftist empires. When our foreign allies started worrying that their own days were numbered if this nation caved to one-sided coverage, a few tried to help launch more balanced fare. What did conservatives do? They complained—about the owners, their religion, whatever—without even trying to understand why our allies were worried! And, more to the point, without putting out the capital for such ventures themselves, until it was way too late. Good

CCCTPs were too busy propping up the Republican National committee and other Party offices. What good did they imagine their largesse would do if there was nothing in America except a hostile press and hostile college professors "educating" their kids?

This strategy had the effect of emboldening the leftist war on "conservatives."

Consequently, today, most of the truly comprehensive research papers stay "in-house." They are passed around CCCTP organizations instead of being broadly publicized, including those by noted "conservative" scholars with advanced degrees in difficult subjects like biochemistry, geoscience, medicine, astrophysics and forestry.

CCCTPs may not be able to recapture lost opportunities, and giving the Left enough rope to hang itself didn't quite work out, either. But what conservatives *can* do now is to start reframing the various debates, and utilizing the lessons learned from "perception management." To that end, CCCTPs should not be looking to *level* the playing field, they should be remaking it.

How to Concede in Politics Without Really Trying

Most adults recall the iconic musical comedy, *How To Succeed In Business Without Really Trying*. It is still a mainstay of annual high-school school plays, drama schools, and replays on classic-movie channels. The title speaks for itself, and the entertainment experience remains uproarious.

Over the past few years the Republican Party, the Tea Party and various activist organizations (including even some Libertarians) have produced their own adaptation on the theme—a dark comedy that would be funny in any other era. While the tendency in politics to criticize one's own always smacks of treason, it is time for a reality check.

Joseph Curl delivered one such critique in his April 10, 2011, piece for *The Washington Times*, just ahead of Campaign 2012[130]. He

---

[130] http://www.washingtontimes.com/news/2011/apr/ 10/curl-trump-shows-lightweights-how-to-pound-obama-i/

stated, in essence, that even publicity-hound Donald Trump knew more about strategic politics than the current "sad sack" cast of characters with their hats in the ring[131].

The columnist accused the then-long list of dark-horse candidates of being full of "baggage," but without ideas. These, Mr. Curl said, in essence, were "hotshots" who could be counted on to take potshots at the Left instead of demanding the proverbial pound of flesh.

The question CCCTP candidates should always ask themselves is: *If I were a left-leaning political tactician, what action on my part would be sure to drive prospective supporters to another camp?*

The most sure-fire way to alienate grassroots conservatives and traditionalists is for candidates and even conservative officials to give the impression they are "too good" to respond to average constituents.

Simon Cowell or Ronald Reagan?- Twenty-five years ago, the late President Ronald Reagan was still penning personally handwritten notes to struggling conservative supporters, respond extensively to their exact questions, advise them on issues within his sphere of influence. This was before the ubiquity of the personal computer, which made things both easier and harder. Mr. Reagan would also helpfully annotate the writings of interns and new-hires to suggest improvements on their work, rather than passing the job to an aide.

He directed his staff to send hand-written, personalized Christmas cards to a virtual "unknown," whose only bid to fame may have been writing something nice about him in a letter-to-the-editor or opinion column that appeared in a newspaper out in the boondocks. (*This author should know, having received all of the above at one time or another, from Mr. Reagan, both when he was Governor in California and as President of the United States.*)

A then-ingénue named Peggy Noonan revealed in her first book[132], how President Reagan red-lined her early speeches for him—but without any snide remarks or putdowns. Too many conservative

---

[131] http://www.conservative.org/cpac/
[132] http://www.search.barnesandnoble.com/What-I-Saw-at-the-Revolution/Peggy-Noonan/e/9780812969894

leaders today come across more like *American Idol*'s Simon Cowell, not the classy Ronald Reagan.

All "Revved Up"—With No Place to Go.- Years ago, there was a TV commercial that showed a coach revving up his football team at halftime. He was in top for; had the full attention of his team. Soon his players were chomping at the bit, all set to go out there and do their coach's bidding. They surged toward the door—only to find it locked. Whereupon, they crashed into one another, injuring themselves, with no affect whatever on the locked door. It was very funny at the time.

Many constituents today would identify with that ad. They keep up with the issues, read piles of books and articles, listen to CCCTP commentators, and finally work up the kind of sought-after "go-get-'em" resolve that candidates crave. Then, as soon as these burgeoning activists swing into action, they are irked and dismayed to find the "door locked"—unable engage a leader or official on any issue of importance to them.

Conservatives of any stripe simply don't have the political capital to be "full of themselves." This isn't the time to play the role of an exclusive fraternity, complete with the secret handshake.

There is a place for blogs, comment boxes on websites and donor registries. Granted, in today's interconnection-overload society, one does need to weed out the occasional "nut-case," potential security threat, spam or phishing expedition, and what some refer to as "permanent pen-pals." This author has received them all, and so have most newspaper and magazine editors, organizational chiefs and legislators.

The pervasiveness of the Internet has produced both the expectation of "connectedness" and a disdain for one-on-one interaction. The advent of, first, e-mails, then texting, mass-distribution, Twitter and Facebook has made in-person confrontation unnecessary; yet people still expect *personalization*.

As a result, individualized responses to constituents have morphed into what is called the "boilerplate" letter, one for every conceivable occasion—and immediately recognizable if you know what to look for. The first paragraph (usually just one sentence) is tailored to provide space for a constituent's name and something that passes for the issue in question, and the rest offers feel-good pap and organizational drivel.

Online, the constituent gets the proverbial pop-up box for abbreviated comments, and a drop-down menu of pre-selected topics—which may, or may not, match the issue the constituent wants to address. Any phone numbers placed on the website will be answered by a receptionist and directed to an aide, never to the official—even if the constituent and the official were once friends! Anybody, after all, can say they have a personal relationship with the official. The status symbol of having "arrived," at least in political circles, seems to demand removing oneself above the *hoi polloi*—which sends this message to constituents: "I'm too important to bother with you."

This isn't to say that it's easy for officials, candidates or heads of organizations to respond to hundreds of calls, e-mails or letters without significant staff. Thanks to mass-distribution e-mails, even relatively well-known people, such as columnists, receive avalanches of daily communications via the electronic medium, more than were ever delivered by the pre-electronic-age Post Office. So, while the task can be overwhelming for those without the ability to hire large staff, the alternative is worse.

Too many conservative leaders have a skewed view of their own importance and popularity. What these egotists don't realize when they brush off knowledgeable individuals who attempt to contact them, is that these same ignored people increasingly are "finding" *each other* via Internet "conservative" groups. But they are not just "connecting"; *they are also passing along the fact that their attempt at contact with a legislator or group head was virtually ignored*!

All that said, the fact is that, mixed in with the unwanted goofballs and scoundrels, is the "gem"—that key individual who has important information, or a brilliant idea that could change the course of a campaign—and maybe the direction of a nation. Cut these folks off, or force them to air their concerns on blogs—which amounts to "venting" solely to one another—and CCCTPs lose. Perhaps this time for good.

Do We Have the Confidence to Run The Republic?

The real political question, if CCCTPs will face up to it, is whether the Republic has the self-confidence to run itself—which, of course, is the conservative Republican and Tea Party view—*versus* whether an elite should make decisions for a public which is too stupid to make wise choices on its own. The latter is the liberal Democratic view, the authoritarian view (as in monarchies), and the Marxist-totalitarian view.

Communism and socialism, at their core, are about a strong government that "knows" what is best for the masses. None have succeeded, and the attempt often turns into a totalitarian nightmare. But for some reason, many of America's citizens think we need to try it here. They apparently have little confidence in the average person—despite all the emphasis in today's schools on self-esteem.

~

CHAPTER 7
THE EDUCATION GAME

> I think we can say that the Constitution reflected an enormous blind spot in this culture that carries on until this day, and the framers had that same blind spot. ...The Supreme Court never ventured into the issues of redistribution of wealth and sort of more basic issues of political and economic justice in this society.
>
> The Constitution is a chart of negative liberties; [it] says what the states can't do to you, but it doesn't say what the federal government must do on your behalf. *--Barack Hussein Obama, in a radio interview, 2001*[133]

Education is the game-changer conservatives love to hate. But education will determine, ultimately, on which side American will fall in 2013 and beyond—Nanny State socialism or representative democracy. The above quotation tells us exactly where Barack Obama stood long before he was elected, had more of the nation's voters bothered to check out his past statements. The former "community activist" and Harvard law scholar said plainly that he had a different view of the role of government in society from the Framers of the Constitution.

It was inevitable, then, that once elected, Mr. Obama's vision would be reflected in his choice of Secretary for the U.S. Department of Education, and in all the various projects and programs that were developed and supported by that agency under his administration.

At least 90 percent[134] of children attend public (government) schools, where every new class of high school graduates since 1966 has been indoctrinated into ever-more-leftist ideologies during their K-12 years.

The most visible reason for this is that the campaign to do so was spearheaded by the National Education Association (NEA) and its co-founded brainchild, UNESCO (the United Nations Educational, Scientific and Cultural Organization).

---

[133] Thanks to Robert Knight, senior fellow for the American Civil Rights Union, for locating this quotation.

[134] http://www.educationbug.org/a/public-schools-vs--private-schools.html

Over the years since 1947, the NEA and UNESCO have conspired with other left-leaning organizations, including a vocal cadre of leftist psychologists (see chapter 5) to ply schools with extremist propaganda, phony standards and invasive questionnaires masquerading as academic tests.

Then, there's incoherent, skewed and ill-defined instruction in critical subjects like history, math, literature, economics—and now even science—until the sheer capability to sustain a *republic* (assuming pupils know what the term means in a post-Obama world) is in jeopardy. The opening quotation from Mr. Obama is symbolic of the nature of today's academic instruction.

Many private (and even some religious schools) contain similar leftist offerings, thanks to compromised departments of teacher preparation in the universities, which obtain grant monies from government, as well as influential foundations, associations and institutes of the-and-that—all with predominantly leftist staffs. The old Soviet Union may be technically defunct, but the cultural Marxism brought here by Cold War agents between the 1950s and 1980s did incalculable damage.

Every new crop of high school and college graduates, regardless of career path, has been more left-leaning than the last. Classroom debate has long since veered away from "academic freedom" toward manipulated, if not mandated, "political correctness." Infractions are characterized as "hate speech"—with punishments ranging from ridicule and ostracism to suspension, expulsion and "psychological counseling."

Most conservatives simply do not "get" the strength of their opponents. Like the late, well-connected columnist, Tony Blankley, they think that "three presidential administrations and six Congresses from now"—when the U.S. Treasury is expected to have run out of money (in 2024)—the masses will demand conservative-traditionalist-constitutionalist government. They don't want to face the reality of 45 years of educational mayhem.

Now-grown children of the 1960s, 70s, and 80s constitute most of today's "voting public." Statistically speaking, most can be found watching reruns of *Friends* and *American Idol*. The few who avail themselves of more serious fare like PBS' *Frontline* and who read *The Economist* do not realize they may still be getting a highly condensed, skewed view of the events, often without context. Most people feel they don't have the time (or the incentive, even with the Internet) to do the kinds of in-depth research it takes to correct any misperceptions.

While certainly there are balanced programs and publications out there that generate hundreds of thousands of subscriptions and Internet "hits," these reports and op-ed pieces, no matter how worthy, still require the reader or viewer, in today's era of information overload, to compare them with their equivalents in various opposing forums—i.e., publications and presentations having a different slant.

Although, subconsciously, people realize the need to know what "the other side" is saying, those who do not make their living from this sort of activity simply are not moved to dissect every report or analysis and compare it with five or more other versions. This is especially true of topics which, at first blush, do not appear controversial—such as "traffic" cameras, which arguably have ramifications beyond the obvious. Thus, a troubling pattern of government incursion into everybody's daily life has been allowed to establish itself—which, of course, is the essence of "statism."

Some conservative icons and pundits make it sound as though there is plenty of time in which to turn the country around—at least until the country goes broke in a dozen years or so. Like the late columnist, Tony Blankley, they overlook that crucial connecting dot—education—the link that busts their "optimistic" visions to Kingdom Come.

Education Dept. Throws U.S. Kids Under the Bus

One had to give Education Secretary Arne Duncan credit for *chutzpah*. He handed pundits a perfect line when he told Congress (again!) in July 2011 that the Education Department needed a 13.3-percent increase because "you can't sacrifice the future to pay for the present." Never mind that the 4,200-person agency, and its ever-morphing alliance with leftist groups, has *already* comprised the future—not only in terms of children's immediate well-being, but in terms of the debt they will inherit.

The education budget has swelled along with the rest of the nation's debt. In 2011, the education budget stood at $68.3 billion. In Barack Obama's FY 2013 budget proposal, which didn't pass, education funding was set to increase by another $1.7 billion (a 2.5 percent increase over FY 2012). These increases would have come on top of the $98 billion provided to the Department of Education in 2009, as part of the so-called "stimulus" package—not to mention the $10 billion "EduJobs" bill passed in the summer of 2010.

Like the "EduJobs" bill, which most of the public has already forgotten, if they heard about it at all, the Obama administration was looking to sneak in a further $60 billion for *new* programs—spending that would be supplemental to the FY 2012 enacted budget and the FY 2013 requested budget. As for results emanating from such expenditures over the years, the only applicable description is "flat."

The number of add-ons and "new" programs that rarely make the news is astounding:

- $5 billion: RESPECT Project (Recognizing Educational Success, Professional Excellence, and Collaborative Teaching), aimed at attracting good teachers;
- $25 billion: Keeping Educators in the Classroom proposal), intended for hiring (or re-hiring) more teachers;
- $3 billion (annually): the STEM (Science, Technology, Engineering, and Mathematics) initiative, targeted mostly to girls and minorities since FY 2010. Some 13 federal agencies invested in 209 programs, 90 percent of which duplicated at least one other education program, with no tangible evidence that STEM works;[135]
- $22 million in investments from the private sector to compound the government "commitment" to improving math and science;

---

[135] http://edworkforce.house.gov/news/documentsingle.aspx?DocumentID=276133

- $80 million: another new (and improved?) "competition" aimed at teachers preparation in math and science
- $1 billion+ for at least 10 new multiyear programs since FY 2008, a few now defunded, aimed at educating the poor.

Ever-Earlier Childhood Education Programs

As indicated in chapter 3, Head Start began in 1965 as an 8-week, pre-K summer program for low-income youngsters thought to be at risk. Head Start and its sequel, Project Follow-Through in 1967, merged to become the opening salvo in an intensive effort to get children enrolled in school (and away from parents) at ever-younger ages. Preferably, children would hop out of subsidized day care on into government schools.

Head Start morphed into one of the longest-running anti-poverty programs in U.S. history, with its own federal office run out of the U.S. Department of Health and Human Services (HHS). Thus, did schools get into the business of feeding children, which morphed into a demand that all school districts, poor or not, provide meals—and, in 2012, for the first time, specific *kinds* of meals, at that.

HHS' involvement had the side-effect of moving schools further away from academics—for pitifully little result considering Head Start's discouraging track record[136]. Even HHS' own Longitudinal Study has admitted to "only a few statistically significant differences in outcomes at the end of first grade...," and in some cases even "negative impacts."

Obama's Early Learning Challenge

The latest variant in a long series of early-childhood education efforts is Mr. Obama's Early Learning Challenge (ELC), a joint venture between the Departments of Education and Health and Human Services. The Obama administration announced on April 9,

---

[136] http://www.acf.hhs.gov/programs/opre/hs/impact_study/reports/impact_study/executive_summary_final.pdf

2012, a $133 million program for which states could apply for an ELC grant. This sum was set aside from the administration's primary program, Race to the Top (RTTT), which we shall examine further on. From the government website[137], it appears that some 35 states plus the District of Columbia and Puerto Rico have applications pending at this writing.

"Successful" applications means parents releasing their children into government hands much sooner.

ELC serves a dual function in that pupils and their parents can be scrutinized ever more closely in a final push to assure that the upcoming generation is populated with left-leaning liberals. One link for an "approved" early childhood program during the Bush administration, accessed through the National Center for Education Statistics, suggests that children were being assessed on how well they interacted with parents in a playroom (via one-way "windows"?). This, and other "oversight" measures by government, fulfills the prophetic vision of John Dewey's contemporary, Paul Popenoe, who wrote this telling comment in the *Journal of Heredity* (of which he was editor) in 1926:

The education system should be a sieve, through which all the children of a country are passed.... It is very desirable that no child escape inspection....

In the case of ELC, agents from the Education Department's Implementation and Support Unit carry out their on-site inspections of each state receiving federal dollars. The recipient states, in turn, must oversee each local district and its schools, and keep records that can be turned over to the federal agency.

One cannot help but wonder why state officials holler about State and local rights when they sign on, in effect, to grant "competitions" like this. What part of "federal" do state officials not understand?

---

[137] http://www2.ed.gov/programs/racetothetop-earlylearningchallenge/awards.html

Which leads to a key issue that requires the voter's comprehension: What Big Government means when it offers the "carrot" of federal dollars to states via a "competition."

How "Competition" for Education Dollars Works

State Departments of Education are virtual clones of their federal parent, the U.S. Department of Education (DoEd). The state versions are referred to generically as State Education Agencies (or SEAs). The SEAs receive what is called "pass-through" money from the DoEd, plus additional revenues from *state* taxes. Every time an SEA takes federal bait, it loses some of its autonomy because of federal oversight. That's the "stick": oversight. The same goes for local education agencies (LEAs) where the individual school districts reside. The LEAs receive pass-through dollars from the states, and kick in their own revenues through means like property taxes.

Thus each individual school is getting a mixed "pot" of money— federal, state and local agencies. You pay your taxes into all of them, but as a mere citizen, you have no clout, because you have no "stick." Local and state agencies must, inevitably, report to, and do the bidding of, the U.S. Department of Education, because its "pot" of tax money is larger and takes precedence ("carrot" and "stick," remember?).

At this juncture it is difficult to imagine how much more "autonomy" state and local agencies have left to lose!

Mr. Obama's early childhood program, the ELC solicitation, follows a textbook competition-and-oversight scenario, a game typical of all federal agencies providing grant monies to states for various purposes.

The federal Department, in this case the DoEd, grades each state's application according to a rating scale. The "winners" of competitive programs are supposed to provide the federal entity with a "proposal," similar to that of private companies responding to a solicitation (or "bid") from any other agency, public or private. The responses that will get the largest share of federal tax dollars will not necessarily be those who say they will do the job cheaper, as with the private-sector proposals. The most successful state responses will be those who satisfy not only the federal criteria, but also the "between the lines" expectations of the sitting administration.

Other states may be "successful" in obtaining greenbacks as well, but it will be a somewhat lesser amount of the "pot" allocated for the program ($133 million for ELC). The "competing" states must also kick in investments out of state revenues (taxes). Of course, the allocated federal monies, with or without state revenues, never ends up being enough.

The government takes pains to ensure that the parameters of these "competitions" are not out of reach for any state—after all, the feds *want* as many as possible onboard! And they want the states to "sell" the program to local school districts and parents because doing so will place more pressure on Congress to appropriate money for similar programs.

The federal government purports to allow each state to implement its "own" version of a plan—within the guidelines specified by the feds in the grant solicitation. Left unstated, but understood, is that the state's *actual* program must reflect the administration's political agenda. The federal government reserves the right to determine *how well* each grantee is "complying," by sending its own inspection agents to each site where an ELC exists.

This was how the U.S. Department of Justice, for example, conducted its grant-oversight inspections for its Community-Oriented Policing Services (COPS) program[138] in the 1990s, and how its Office of Juvenile Justice and Delinquency Prevention's[139] determined who would continue receiving anti-gang grants.

So, when the Obama administration calls its solicitations a "contest" for a "share" of the $133 million "pot" committed solely to ELC—carved from the overarching stimulus package of $4.35 billion (see chapter 3)—it's the same game that has been applied to state (and, for that matter, local) agencies since the days of Lyndon Johnson's Great Society Programs.

---

[138] https://www.ncjrs.gov/pdffiles1/nij/183644.pdf
[139] http://en.wikipedia.org/wiki/Office_of_Juvenile_Justice_and_Delinquency_Prevention

The overriding goal of these "competitive" solicitations is to make state and local agencies increasingly dependent on the federal government so that they have *no choice* but to buy into phony reform programs like Race to the Top (RTTT) and early childhood component, ELC.

Unlike private companies, which typically pick and choose which grant solicitations they want to respond to, state and local agencies that depend on tax revenues from their own end as well as from federal largesse find it increasingly unwise to decline the invitation, as doing so could be interpreted as disapproval of an administration initiative—never a good "career move."

Moreover, nationalization of education is a *fait accompli*. Even some private schools find themselves entrapped because they accepted federal dollars for some small thing—like "enrichment services" to eligible children, or wheelchair-accessibility to their bathrooms, things they could probably have afforded themselves way back when, had they been so inclined. Even the voucher program allows private and religious schools to take federal funds. Pretty soon, one thing leads to another, and schools find themselves dependent upon federal tax dollars! They discover they can't say "no" to anything.

How Parents Lost Their Prerogatives

For concerned citizens seeking a turnabout in American politics overall, it is important to recognize that today's schools are the single most influential factor in that process. As government alternately encourages, bribes and deceives parents into handing over their youngsters to be schooled at ever-younger ages, usually prior to the age of reason, which is thought to be around seven years of age,[140] parental values have less chance of taking hold.

---

[140] http://www.uic.edu/classes/psych/psych270/moral.htm

The rationale behind these toddler programs is that most parents are ill-equipped to do the job—that is, they lack the required skills, psychiatric knowledge, time and resources[141].

Once a parent enters the child "into the system"—be it a public or private entity (exception: non-accredited neighborhood co-ops)—one or more levels of government oversight kick in, monitoring the child *and evaluating parents* to a greater or lesser extent. If you don't believe it, try keeping your child home from school for a week without some exceptionally good reason and see what happens. In most states, homeschoolers already have to submit lesson plans and curricular outlines to the state for approval; so, with states signing onto programs like ELC, homeschoolers may soon be submitting plans for their 3-year-olds, not just for the typical K-12 grades.

Obama's Race to the Trough

American education has seen one "reform" movement after another. A list is found in the next section. The most recent incarnation, however, is "Race to the Top"[142]. It was initiated by the Obama Administration in 2009. RTTT, as it is known, is structured around a serious-sounding centerpiece called the "Common Core of State Standards Initiative Project,"[143], or CCS for short. CCS was set for implementation in at least 46 states in 2012.

Unlike Early Learning Challenge, CCS is a mandate, not a grant. No states "compete" for this money because the "standards" are set by the federal government. SEAs receiving DoEd dollars for any purpose are obliged to accept them. But like Early Learning Challenge, CCS is supposed to pass itself off as a "state-led" initiative, even though it is part of a federal initiative.

The difference is the "middleman" who coordinates the effort. As with most mandates from On High to the states, the coordinating entity is the National Governor's Association (NGA), through its Center for Best Practices ("NGA Center," for short). The "Best

---

[141] http://www.associazionegiovannadarco.org/importance-of-early-childhood-education/

[142] http://www2.ed.gov/programs/racetothetop-earlylearningchallenge/index.html

[143] http://www.corestandards.org/

Practices" moniker hails back to the Effective Schools (reform) Movement in the 1970s.

Like its "reform" predecessors, the Common Core of Standards can neither be described as academic nor substantive. CCS is rife with the usual misrepresentations. For example, the "Common Core" Math Standards do not focus on attainment of chronological steps along the path to competency at incremental levels, such as Algebra I, Geometry and Algebra II, Trigonometry, etc., but, rather, all of these are treated, essentially, as one. This makes it virtually impossible to tell which skills have been mastered by students and which have not. One cannot improve instruction this way—but, then, "academic instruction" is not the purpose of today's schools.

Similarly, in English, the high-school-level standards do not set grade-level-specific achievements. Spelling and grammar are fused with literature and vocabulary, which, of course, they *eventually* are once a child has mastered the fundamentals. But that's the point: The student *hasn't* mastered the fundamentals.

Additionally, the emphasis in Literature is on modern works, not on appreciating the contributions of the classical masters in various disciplines. One is free to enjoy the great classicists, or not, but *only if one knows about them*. Today's high school seniors, and even many college graduates, have little idea what the philosophers, scholars and artists prior to 1945 said or believed, even though their works greatly affected the evolution of governance in Europe and, in turn, America—underscoring the reasons why the U.S. took such a different route.

Can states decline the "standards"? Sure they can—if they want to lose their federal funding.

Dependency Leads to Federal Takeover

Given that every state in America is dependent at this point upon federal education dollars for its public schools (and some private ones, too), the so-called "standards" are, in effect, nationally imposed. On May 22, 2012, an irate-sounding Rep. Duncan Hunter (R-CA), chairman of the U.S. House Subcommittee on Early Childhood,

Elementary and Secondary Education, dismissed the RTTT reform plan—CCS, ELC, and all—calling the whole shebang "an unprecedented expansion of federal intrusion into local education decisions, adding to the boondoggle of bureaucracy already challenging teachers, principals and superintendents."

"I urge the president," Rep. Hunter said, "to stop dedicating more taxpayer dollars to new programs with questionable impact."

To be entirely fair to the Obama administration, one needs to understand that Rep. Hunter has been a fixture on Capitol Hill since 1981, a product of the "Reagan revolution." So, he knows quite well the history of federal interference into state and local education, under both Republican and Democratic presidents. Why he would wait until 2012 in the Obama administration to stand up on his hind legs and bark probably has more to do with partisanship than principle.

"Reform" Measures: Same Old Song, New Lyrics

Most people alive today only remember "reform" measures that date from around 1970, even though many of those originated much earlier, sometimes reappearing under new names whenever they finally got a black eye with the public. (All the following can be found by typing the titles into a browser):

- The **Effective Schools Movement** (Carter and Reagan administrations);
- **Mastery Learning**, an older program revived around 1980 under then-Education Secretary William J. Bennett;
- **America 2000** (George H. W. Bush administration);
- **Goals 2000: Educate America Act** (Clinton administration), the centerpiece of which was a program called **Outcome-Based Edu**cation [144] in 1993; and
- **No Child Left Behind** (**NCLB**) in 2002 (George W. Bush administration). A centerpiece of NCLB was, and remains, the **International Baccalaureate** (**IB**), which most people

144 (http://en.wikipedia.org/wiki/Outcome-based_education)

mistook for its pre-World War II European counterpart, called simply "the Baccalaureate." The Baccalaureate was rigorous. Its IB successor is politicized.

None of these programs truly expired; they just got reorganized and reshuffled. All are tied in some way to the ever-expanding 1965 Elementary and Secondary Education Act (ESEA). One administration after another added on Titles and Sections to the Act, which is why the ESEA is rightly called "the enabling legislation of education."

ESEA came out of Lyndon B. Johnson's Great Society Program, and never produced an iota of improvement in academic achievement. Titles I, III and IV proved particularly onerous—making the Act's continued reauthorization every few years absolutely essential to government. It was also essential to get every state onboard with a series of "reforms" so that all state and local education agencies would in some way be at the mercy of federal dollars.

Perversely, Section 103b of the Act[145], specifically prohibits the federal government from involving itself in state or local curriculum. But then, further down, Section 209 provides a loophole. It allows the DoEd to split hairs and claim it merely funds *development* of curricular *frameworks* and instructional *materials*, not the forbidden "direction, supervision or control of curriculum."

Such obfuscation sails right past most journalists. Their reports drop what editors might interpret as "wordiness." As a result, people misunderstand how tax dollars are spent.

Moreover, education "reform" and "remediation" agendas are played out, over and over, utilizing the aforementioned National Governors Association (and its Center for "Best Practices") in concert with the Council of Chief State School Officers, the Education Commission of the States, the U.S. Commission on Uniform State Laws and other, less well-known, federally funded agencies and private foundations –all ensuring that the agenda stays afloat.

---

[145] http://www.eric.ed.gov/PDFS/ED180121.pdf

Don't Know Much About…Anything

In 2011, just as young people were headed to universities across the nation and the K-12 back-to-school season was in full throttle, a front-page *Washington Times'* headline disclosed on August 17: "Scores show students aren't ready for college—75 percent may need remedial classes." A May 25, 2012, report in the Associated Press (AP) seconded that finding: "SAT reading scores for the high school class of 2011 were the lowest on record, and combined reading and math scores fell to their lowest point since 1955."

Then, a Spring 2012 study (Remediation: Higher Education's Bridge to Nowhere)[146] by the Washington-based nonprofit group, Complete College America (CCA), pointed to research showing that college-level remedial courses had come way too little too late for most students, delaying job opportunities and exacerbating student-loan debt.

CCA works to increase college graduation rates in the United States. Its president Stan Jones, stated in an AP interview that the remedial approach isn't cutting it: "Simply putting [pupils] in three levels of remedial math is really taking their money and time with no hope of success."

A number like 75 percent (or 1.7 million young people) gets people's attention. Tthe *Times* article quoted another education advocacy group's finding that "80 percent of college students taking remedial classes [in 2008] had a high school GPA of 3.0 or better."

What? *Even when students score well, they don't know much.* How is that even possible?

We could ask Darryl Robinson, a hard-working graduate of a D.C. public charter school, who wrote a sobering article[147] for the *Washington Post* on April 13, 2012, about his experience as an incoming freshman at Georgetown University: "The gap between what I can do and what my classmates are capable of is enormous." Despite an early, severe speech impediment, which isolated him for a

---

[146] http://www.completecollege.org/docs/CCA-Remediation-final.pdf
[147] http://www.washingtonpost.com/opinions/i-went-to-one-of-dcs-best-high-schools-i-was-still-unprepared-for-college/2012/04/13/gIQAqQQAFT_story.html

long period, he overcame it and "aced" all his classes at the charter school. Even with put-downs by teachers, which included condescending remarks when he did well, he continued to excel! "In high school," he wrote, "I maintained good grades simply by listening and giving them what they wanted to hear: themselves. ...[A]s long as I was respectful, I was a great student."

Robinson says it wasn't until his junior year at the school that he actually opened a textbook "to learn material that a teacher had not given to me verbally. It was for Advanced Placement (AP) Human Geography, my first AP course."

Human Geography? It sounds like a take-off on "demographics" or maybe "cultural diversity." What happened to physical geography? But...we digress...

Robinson says Human Geography was the hardest AP course, along with his AP English thesis, he ever had in his high school experience.

Robinson says he stays in contact with his old friends, many of whom are attending other East Coast colleges. All apparently agree that their high schools, charter and otherwise, did not prepare them adequately for university-level studies—"even when they [the schools] tried."

One of Mr. Robinson's greatest surprises is the degree of academic independence and self-motivation he had to muster in order to succeed at Georgetown University. No serious student can "sit back and merely listen to a teacher," but rather, he or she must go "out and get the material, read more than what is required, and [do] exercises" that the student constructs for himself." This level of dedication, says Mr. Robinson, left little free time for socializing—but, it has finally paid off. He is no longer "floundering" at Georgetown University.

We can only stand up and cheer for Mr. Robinson. He will make a terrific employee, and has all the characteristics of an outstanding American.

However, in reading the whole of his story (strongly recommended, see footnote), he reveals the hideousness of K-12 education that leaves potentially high-achieving pupils like Mr. Robinson dispirited, and with gross misconceptions about what true scholarship and a "well-rounded education" really are. If students truly decide to break outside the mold of mediocrity and excel, they won't have time to party or protest.

The Plain Truth from the Horse's Mouth

At least one luminary in an otherwise sorry lot at the U.S. Department of Education (DoEd) decided not to sugar-coat it: Long-time former U.S. Commissioner of Education Statistics Pascal D. Forgione, Jr., Ph.D., has been *persona non grata* within the Department's hierarchy ever since he issued a scathing indictment of America's K-12 schools in 1999. As reported by this author in a 2011 article,[148] Dr. Forgione's speech eventually surfaced on the Internet, despite mighty efforts by component agencies like the National Center for Education Statistics (NCES) and the Institute of Education Sciences (IES) to scuttle it.

Dr. Forgione is highly credible. An Internet search of his various appointments, reports and testimonies over the years reveals an intimate familiarity with all aspects of DoEd's data-collection, assessment and computer systems, as well as international, cooperating agencies working directly or indirectly with the U.S. education establishment. So, when Dr. Forgione says that pupils' ongoing poor showing in science, math and reading are tied to weak curriculum, he ought to know!

"Our idea of 'advanced' is clearly below international standards," he admonished in his now-infamous speech. He quoted Distinguished Professor Dr. William Schmidt, executive director of the National Research Center and its Third International Mathematics and Science Study (TIMSS)—the one test that has proved a real measure of what K-12 pupils actually know. Dr. Schmidt describes U.S. textbooks as "treat[ing] topics with a 'mile-wide, inch-deep' approach." He points to a "typical U.S. eighth-grade math textbook [that] deals with about

---

[148] http://www.thenewamerican.com/culture/education/item/362-education's-armageddon

35 topics. By comparison, a Japanese or German math textbook for that age would have only five or six topics."

Dr. Forgione quotes other worthies such as Jean McLaughlin, president of Barry University, who has long criticized the public schools' foray into "social re-engineering" at the expense of proficiency in subject matter. This view was seconded by the superintendent of the nation's fourth largest school district in Miami-Dade, Florida, who complained: "Half our job is education, and the other half is social work."

It's more like 61 percent—a combination of attitudinal propagandizing, personality profiling and mental-"health" screening[149].

Dr. Forgione exposed how schools systematically let kids down. "By grade 4, American students only score in the middle of 26 countries reported. By grade 8 they are in the bottom third, and at the finish line, where it really counts, we're near dead last. It's even worse when you notice that some of the superior countries in grade 8 (especially the Asians) were not included in published 12th grade results. They do not [even] need 12 grades." (It is worthy of note here that, in quiet defiance of political correctness at many elite universities, Asians are required to score 140 points higher on the SATs than whites, 270 points higher than Hispanics, and 450 points higher than African-Americans.)

However, the DoEd soon devised a remedy. Given Dr. Forgione's stinging reproach, department heads at NCES talked European educators into integrating the TIMSS with the National Assessment of Educational Progress (NAEP), then watering both down to reflect the United Nations' psycho-political and social engineering goals rather than intellectual ones. Beginning with the 2011-2012 school year, the TIMSS was merged with the U.S.'s NAEP. Academic testing has quietly been renamed an "assessment" for a reason—because it is not a test!

A "Test" or "Not a Test": That is the Question

The DoEd's National Center for Education Statistics (NCES) is probably the most crucial and influential component of the Education Department. It defines the difference between an assessment and a test: "An *assessment* is any systematic procedure for obtaining information from tests and other sources that can be used to draw inferences about characteristics of people, objects, or programs." Another major source, *Constructing Curriculum for the Primary Grades* by D.T. Dodge, et al., states (emphasis mine): "Assessment is the process of **gathering information about children** in order to make decisions about their education. Teachers obtain useful information about children's knowledge, skills, and progress by observing, documenting, and reviewing children's work **over time** [a.k.a. longitudinal study]. **Ongoing** assessment [also] occurs **in the context of classroom activities**."

What they are talking about here is "noncognitive feedback," intended to determine opinions on issues, ranging from the importance of the United Nations, to sexual orientation and climate change. Anyone schooled in marketing, public relations or perception management would recognize the formula: what-would-you-do-if queries; confession-style probes; and psychological "fishing" expeditions. There is never a "right" or "wrong" answer, only "preferred" ones, as explained in tightly held guides for analysts known as "Interpretive Literature."

Such surreptitious methods of data-collection allow attitudes and worldviews to be tallied and followed over the child's school years, then on into college—and even the workplace. Former students have been surprised to discover that an assessment question they answered at age 16 affected not only their college acceptance but also their career path.   They are even more dismayed when they receive "follow-up surveys" well into their adult years.

Take, for example, the March 23, 2010, commentary by *Washington Post* staff writer Justin Moyer entitled "Government surveys high school seniors, and then tracks them for decades"[150]. In this first-person narrative, Moyer described how, in his not-terribly-distant younger days, he was given a survey in high school that "looked like the SAT [Scholastic Achievement Test]," as it was printed on a type of paper that resembled that of standardized tests. He didn't think too much about it at the time and was told "[p]articipation was voluntary" and that "[a]nswers...would remain anonymous."

He answered questions about drugs ("Had I used tobacco, alcohol, marijuana, heroin, cocaine, methamphetamines? How often?"), sex (what kind, specifically, and how often?"), and driving habits ("From where?" "To where?" "How often?")

He was only 16: "There wasn't much to hide."

Then, that all-important "but," in hindsight: "But there was no taking it back," Moyer wrote. "Apparently I'd signed up for a long-term project: No matter where I went or what I did, follow-up surveys dogged me.... I moved to Connecticut...to Cape Cod...to Washington... [all] around Washington. But about once a year, I'd open the mail and see...another survey, embossed with the logo...'**Monitoring the Future: A Continuing Study of American Youth**.' Return address: the University of Michigan."

Unbeknownst to Mr. Moyer, he was describing a "longitudinal study." And today, kids a lot younger than 16 are getting them. The aim is to assess psychological and political attitudes, to see who is swallowing the propaganda that passes for academics, and, more importantly, who is either waffling or "not buying." If too many don't "buy," then curriculum is altered using a more heavy-handed approach.

That's precisely what we're seeing today. The curricular propaganda is morphing right along with the technology to collect, store and "share" information that reveals whether youngsters are "internalizing" (absorbing) politically correct biases. If they are not, then "remediating" (nor to be confused with *remedial*) curricula are

---

[150]   http://www.washingtonpost.com/wp-dyn/content/article/2010/03/22/AR2010032202847.html?hpid=sec-health

brought to the classroom then and there. "Remediating" curricula are *re-education* programs.

As for whether or not students are "internalizing" any actual academic information, the answer is: "apparently not." Even with little of an academic nature on assessments (or tests), teachers have to help students cheat[151] to make themselves and their school districts look good!

On June 22, 2012 it was reported in most major news outlets that teachers at three Washington, D.C., schools were being fired for "help[ing] students choose the right answers on the Comprehensive Assessment exams." Other schools had been "flagged for irregularities" and "security violations," such as allowing students to use a cell phone, during which they could coordinate a "bathroom break" with other pupils. This follows on the heels of a similar cheating scandal in Atlanta, Georgia, and Houston, Texas, both in 2011.

In the past, many states have not allowed teachers to see or proctor assessment tests. Proctors were (and in many cases, still are) brought in from outside the school system. Questions are kept from teachers and curious parents alike—mostly to avoid controversy over items that might call for a personal opinion, or be perceived as political, not over fear of cheating. A 1991 book exposing[152] the scope of attitudinal testing under the cover of academics, discusses the case of a young boy in Allegheny County, Pennsylvania, who, realizing that something was amiss, told his mother afterward: "There's no way anyone could cheat on a test like this!" He was referring to the fact that the responses mostly called for opinions.

But bringing in proctors is expensive—thus the change in policy in some districts. The flip side is that any allegations of teacher cheating[153] can cost as much as a million dollars in investigation fees, especially if legal cases are outsourced to law firms by school districts

---

[151]   http://www.wtop.com/41/2915280/Teachers-to-be-fired-for-helping-students-cheat-
[152]   http://www.halcyon.org/obe.html
[153] Threat of lawsuits by parents over psychological-style questions are rarely taken seriously by the media or the courts, and are, in any case tremendously expensive, even when parents win. The 1995 case, "Allegheny County Pennsylvania Parents Coalition vs. Western Psychiatric Institute & Clinic," is among the more interesting.

in order to avoid accusations of bias. Catch-22 again—and pupils are no better off for the expenditure.

Propagandizing: The School's Primary Job

One would think a 2009 study by the Program for International Student Assessment, among others, showing U.S. students ranking internationally 25th in math, 17th in science and 14th in reading would have put a damper on the political adventurism in the classroom. This study compared 15-year-old students among member nations of the Organization for Economic Cooperation and Development.

Instead, propagandizing is more pervasive than ever, with the help of far-left extremist groups.

For example, beginning in the 2011-2012 school year, Maryland launched an "environmental literacy" graduation requirement. It was subsidized by at least one advocacy group most folks had never heard of, No Child Left Inside Coalition (NCLI)[154]. According to the Competitive Enterprise Institute's Matthew Melchiorre, who reported on August 31, 2011, for the *Washington Times,*[155] the Maryland State Board of Education approved the requirement "at the behest of organizations that promote a far-left political agenda based on misinformation and anti-capitalist fervor." NCLI pushes "major societal change…in response to global warming"—that is, "central planning, sustainable development, and de-industrialization based on climate-alarmism…." As we will see in Chapter 8, global-warming theory has been thoroughly discredited by experts, who have discovered weather changes to be cyclical phenomena related to sunspot activity.

The Maryland curriculum is the kind Drs. Forgione and Schmidt condemned when they alleged that weak curricula and poor texts were letting kids down. The Maryland environmental curriculum's stated intent is to convince students that "human impacts threaten current global stability…," writes Melchiorre, as well as "the long-debunked

---

[154] http://www.washingtontimes.com/topics/no-child-left-inside-coalition/
[155] http://www.washingtontimes.com/news/2011/aug/30/propaganda-posing-as-environmental-literacy/

notion that population growth has made resources scarcer." Assignments for this type of fare frequently involve door-to-door petition drives—homeowners are probably familiar with these—and take time away from the hard sciences.

Case Study I: Real-World Results of "Junk Science".- In visiting an ailing, 88-year-old relative at a nursing home in 2011, this author got an unexpected opportunity to see, up-close-and-personal, what happens when schools skip over basic science.

It was a small problem, but one with big results for the patient, who was unable to make use of a "call cord," hooked up to a switch, which, in turn, alerted the nursing station down the hall that a bedridden resident needed help. In this case, the patient was an elderly stroke victim whose speech had been impaired, thus her lack of ability to communicate. Repeatedly advised to use the call cord when needed, the patient seemed to understand by nodding her head in the affirmative. But her ongoing failure to actually do so, left staff to draw the conclusion that she was either stubborn, or that her cognitive functions were so impaired that she forgot.

But the woman was neither stubborn nor forgetful. The truth was, whenever she pulled the cord, she got no response—for what turned out to be a simple, basic-science reason that went uninvestigated for way too long. Consequently, she would give up pulling the cord when she needed to use the rest room, and attempted to get up and make the few steps on her own.

The upshot: several minor falls, followed by one mighty tumble that caused multiple fractures in her leg, in a failed attempt to get to the bathroom.

Nor was the facility negligent and uncaring. In fact, it was one of those rare facilities that put patients' needs first. It does not drug difficult patients, strap them down or ignore them. Somebody comes into each room every couple of hours just to chat, or to change out music and reading material. Most workers in the facility are Christians who see their job as a devout duty. They hug their bedridden charges, and find no request too trivial.

The cord problem occurred because no one could figure out a simple science dilemma.

The nurse "call" mechanism looked like a simple light switch with a small hole drilled through the little lever. A long, red string was attached by threading it through the hole. At the end of the string was a prominent red teddy bear that was secured to the patient's bed in such a way that it could be seen, and pulled. This action was supposed to lower the lever, just like turning off a light switch—an action which then activated another light in the nursing station. Every room had this setup. Whenever the "light switch" was pulled down, assistance was required in a specific patient's room.

The problem in this case was that the lever was directly in back, and just a little to the right of the headboard of the patient's bed. Thus, the cord needed to be pulled vertically to trip the lever (downward, like any light switch). But the placement of the bed with respect to this room's "switch" meant that the patient would be applying horizontal (sideways) force to the call cord, which of course would not trip the lever.

Unless the patient could physically turn around and look at the wall behind to see the problem, and then apply the necessary amount of downward pull on the string to trip the "light switch," the alert system at the nurse's desk wasn't going to work. A weak and elderly patient who isn't aware that a light isn't flashing down the hall is unlikely to make the connection with what looks like a light switch in back of her.

The solution was a basic "lever" problem. All that was required was either to move the bed, or place a simple eye hook—the kind used to fasten tie-backs on curtains and draperies—directly below the "light switch," and to run the thin, red cord through this eye hook *as well as* the hole in the switch. That way, whenever the string was pulled from any angle, the eye hook would convert the pull into a downward angle with respect to the "switch," and the nurse's station alert would then flash red. Not only that, but much less physical strength would be required by the patient to pull the string.

Here's the basic, 5th-grade science version of the same puzzle: The cord's horizontal force was translated into a vertical force by the use of a pulley. That's all any of the staff really needed to know to figure out why the patient wasn't alerting them. But nobody did; and, even when pointed out, *nobody could figure out a solution.* The patient's 64-year-old son-in-law had to demonstrate how to solve the problem.

In the 1950s and even the 60s, this lesson was usually taught as part of a basic science unit called "Levers and Pulleys." But most elementary schools today are too busy promoting goofy theories about "carbon footprints," and invoking Armageddon climate-change scenarios, to bother with basic science.

Yet, the fundamentals needed to master more advanced courses, like physics, later on, are being denied to pupils. They can take all the remedial courses they like, but still will probably never know where it was that their basic understanding of scientific principles got derailed.

Hopefully, they won't need to know when they are old and sick and can't get to the bathroom.

Case Study II: Real-World Results of "Junk Science".- According to a source who, for reasons that will become obvious, wishes not to be named, this incident occurred in a briefing for new congressional staffers at one of the NASA centers. The topic was the need for new and improved weather satellites. Representatives of the National Oceanic and Atmospheric Administration (NOAA) made the presentation.

In the midst of the lecture, a youngish staffer leaned toward his colleague and was overheard to say: "I don't see what we need all these satellites for when I can just download the weather any time I want to my cell phone." *And his colleague nodded in agreement!*

Here were *two* U.S. college graduates who apparently had never considered where, exactly, their vaunted weather downloads originated. They'd probably learned all about recycling and man-made global-warming "destroying the planet." Imagine how these staffers will advise their boss in Congress on energy and "sustainable development" issues.

Computerized, Politicized and Psychologized

The capability to computerized data collection, and cross-match that data with other information and curricular programs was a pipe dream, until a team comprised of former colleagues from Utah's World Institute for Computer-Assisted Technology (WICAT)—George Hall, Richard M. Jaeger, C. Philip Kearny and David E. Wiley—figured out how to do it. They wrote a ground-breaking paper[156] for the Education Department's old Office of Educational Research and Information in 1985. The paper (and the idea) was championed by Emerson J. Elliott,[157] who eventually headed up the vaunted National Center for Education Statistics, that critical component agency of the DoEd mentioned earlier (see "*A 'Test' or 'Not a Test': That is the Question*").

This cross-comparison capability virtually transformed the thrust of schooling in America—from excellence and hard knowledge, to functionality and family intervention. It also fulfilled the oft-quoted prophesy of Dustin Heuston, head of the Utah-based WICAT, who was famously quoted as having exclaimed during a panel discussion in the 1970s[158]:

Won't it be wonderful when no one can get between [the] child and that [computerized] curriculum?

The Curriculum-Control Game

The routes to federalizing schools are data collection, assessment and curriculum. We have discussed the first two. But how to control what is taught, specifically? Control of curriculum is unique in its complexity—but, then, if it weren't, the DoEd could never have pulled it off.

How the Left, in collusion with government agencies, sub-agencies (offices and bureaus) and influential foundations, took

---

[156] http://www.eric.ed.gov/PDFS/ED272576.pdf
[157] http://www.dataqualitycampaign.org/files/publications-the_time_has_come_finally.pdf
[158] http://www.crossroad.to/text/articles/cwhbcv3-98.html

advantage of the data-cross-matching breakthrough to transform society and ensure that parents were kept out of the loop represents a master stroke of subterfuge and government-aggrandizement that today serves as a model for other agencies hoping to enlarge their sphere.

First, be aware that with every incoming administration, component bureaus and offices that make up the "bureaucracy" typically get "reorganized" (and often renamed as well). The pretense of housecleaning entails reshuffling employees and tasks, but rarely eliminates any function. Rather, more are added. The point of this exercise is to confuse the media, watchdog organizations and average taxpayers so that by the time they catch on, there is yet another election and "restructuring"—complete with a "transition team" to implement the pseudo-changes—until sometimes even new appointees can't grasp it.

That's how the game was played out of the DoEd's now-renamed Office of Educational Research and Improvement (OERI)[159], utilizing its pivotal centerpiece: the National Diffusion Network (NDN)[160]. The NDN was a computerized repository of "*validated*" (government-approved) curricular programs costing taxpayers between $8 million and $14 million a year over a 20-year period[161].

Like so many other education projects, the NDN was created in 1965 under the Elementary and Secondary Education Act (ESEA)[162] — that marvelous piece of expandable, "enabling" legislation referred to earlier, devised under the Johnson Administration, when the DoEd was called the Office of Education and fell under the auspices of the Department of Health, Education, and Welfare[163]. This was prior to President Jimmy Carter's creation of the cabinet-level Department of Education (DoEd) in 1976.

---

[159]http://web.archive.org/web/20010413170851/http://www.ed.gov/offices/OERI/orgchart.html

[160] http://en.wikipedia.org/wiki/National_Diffusion_Network

[161] http://www2.ed.gov/pubs/FedStrat/newoeri.html

[162]http://en.wikipedia.org/wiki/Elementary_and_Secondary_Education_Act

[163]http://en.wikipedia.org/wiki/United_States_Department_of_Health,_Education,_and_Welfare

Once the NDN came online, regional, state and local educators were expected to select from the NDN's smorgasbord of curricular programs—not for every course, but at least for some of them. All programs had supposedly been vetted by *appointed* (not elected) members of a Joint Dissemination Review Panel, which would reward the curriculum with "*official recognition*" and include it in the network. Having been "*validated*" as successful, these curricular offerings were deemed in accordance with "What Works" and NGA's "Best Practices," alluded to earlier on.   This was how education officials made use of Section 209, the loophole in the ESEA law, discussed earlier, to get around Section 103b[164], which prohibits the federal government from involving itself in state or local curriculum choices. So, they produced a computerized catalogue of "recognized" (officially sanctioned) instructional *materials* through the NDN and called these "curricular *frameworks*."

What followed was even bolder. The federal government helped implement the programs in the states, often down to individual school districts, via a system of Developer Demonstration Projects (DDs), and "technical assistance." What happened is that a school district selecting one of the programs out of the NDN might ask for technical assistance.

With such an "invite" in hand, a team composed of State Facilitators (SFs) and Curriculum Coordinators (CCs) would descend upon the school district, with the federal government absorbing a percentage of the cost of these staff. OERI bureau heads hoped the public at large would remain unaware of the federal salaries just long enough to bring a system of 10 regional "Labs and Centers" up to speed so they could take over the job—thereby deflecting public attention, once again, from the direct involvement of the federal government.

Conveniently, the Labs and Centers were also a product of the landmark 1965 ESEA. Using Title III of that legislation—ostensibly aimed at culling "innovative ideas" (again under the umbrellas of "What Works" and "Best Practices")—what would actually be

---

[164] http://www.eric.ed.gov/PDFS/ED180121.pdf

promulgated was the content of curriculum, not "innovation." These curricular programs were often highly controversial. Diane Ravitch, former assistant secretary of OERI in the early 1990s, has since written[165] that most of the federal dollars went disproportionately for administration and *dissemination* rather than into fresh research—the intent of Title III.

By 1995, the cat was out of the proverbial bag, and the NDN was shuttered—officially, that is—under then-Speaker of the House Newt Gingrich's "Contract With America"[166]. However, by that time, dissemination of "validated" (federally recognized) curricular programs was virtually assured, *because the DoEd's network of regional Labs and Centers were now ready to provide the alternative route to dispersal*—and were these virtually impervious to shutdown. The Labs and Centers still exist today.

In typical fashion, OERI was "reorganized" in 2002 as the Institute of Education Sciences (IES)[167] under the Education Sciences Reform Act[168]. As usual, it re-assigned old staff and employed more. Under the Obama administration, IES was subdivided into four major research and statistics centers, but it remains, essentially, an expanded version of OERI—which brings us full circle, back to where we started. Enter Obama's Race to the Top (RTTT), Common Core of Standards (CCS), and Early Learning Challenge ECL).

As for the role of the National Governors Association[169] in all this, suffice it to say that the biggest teachers union is not the only power-player in town[170]. *State governors are the go-to persons for federal agency heads anxious to implement a piece of legislation nationwide.* That is why so many presidential contenders are former governors. It gives them huge credibility with their Party. A politician challenges NGA wisdom at his or her own risk, and only

[165] http://educationnext.org/files/ednext20041_34.pdf
[166] http://en.wikipedia.org/wiki/Contract_with_America
[167] http://ies.ed.gov/
[168] http://www2.ed.gov/policy/rschstat/leg/PL107-279.pdf
[169] http://www.nga.org/cms/render/live/about
[170] http://morgancountytax.org/index2.php?option=com_content&do_pdf=1&id=160

the strongest personalities—like Governor Chris Christie (R-NJ)—can do so and get away with it.[171]

So, when former Florida Governor Jeb Bush penned a piece[172] in *Politico* on August 4, 2011, calling for the reauthorization of the ESEA law, actually *giving the law credit* for decades of improved "student achievement across the nation" in the face of data from every direction saying otherwise[173], remember that, at the time, Jeb Bush was a possible presidential contender—and, as a governor, obligated to the NGA. If he expected support from his Party, he would have to ingratiate himself in some fashion with party hacks beholden to the Education Establishment.

Moreover, when fully enacted, RTTT, CCS, and ELC will be the culmination of a process that began in the wake of the Second World War, with the goal of producing an education system that molds public opinion and reverses "American exceptionalism" as a uniquely free nation.

Barack Obama's $4.35 billion Race to the Top is, in actuality, a Race to the *Trough*, the "public trough," with the amount sure to be doubled or tripled in successive administrations.

George Washington Didn't Sleep Here

Did you know that paintings and other depictions of George Washington have been quietly disappearing from school walls and texts? We all knew the Founders were under fire, from various liberal quarters—but our first President and Revolutionary War hero?

Turns out, the American Civil Liberties Union (ACLU) and the National Education Association (NEA) are behind it—no surprise there!—but since parents aren't particularly welcome in schoolhouses these days, it has gone more or less unnoticed.

Paintings and other depictions of George Washington were staples of every schoolhouse since 1932, when a more sensible

---

[171] Note to Readers: Upload Gov. Chris Christie's kenote speech to the Republican Nation Convention, Aug. 28, 2012, and you will see what is meant by "stong personality.

[172] http://www.politico.com/news/stories/0811/60651.html#ixzz1UJ1S34NF

[173] http://www.all4ed.org/files/IntlComp_FactSheet.pdf

Congress passed a mandate to commemorate the 200th anniversary of his birth. Since 1998, William Sanders[174] has been battling both groups over the issue. Over a period of 40 years, he says, paintings and pictures of our first President and Revolutionary War hero have been quietly removed from school walls and excised from history texts. Forty years neatly dovetails with the Left's effort to federalize schooling and rewrite history.

This mirrors the strategy employed following totalitarian coups—Maoist China and the Leninist-Stalinist takeover of neighboring countries being just two examples. Posters, statues and paintings of former national icons would be razed, their writings expunged and replaced.

By reducing the presence of George Washington's likeness, as well as the mention of other Founders, contempt is bestowed on the values and ideals they championed. As youngsters pass along from grade school into college and the workforce, the effect snowballs.

Dismantling evidence of George Washington is sometimes thought to be just another whack at "old, white, racist, Puritan Anglos"—no longer deemed by the Left as representative of America. But eradicating the familiar face of our nation's first president has more to do with mainstreaming progressivism than mainstreaming "diversity."

"Progressivism" by Any Other Name

The disastrous saga of progressivism began with John Dewey's education ideas, which featured socialization of the child as the primary goal of education. He is heralded in institutions of teacher training as "the father of modern education."

"Socialization" in the context he championed is not synonymous with good manners, fair play or even camaraderie. It is one part flexibility, one part acquiescence, and one part affability—creating the "collective spirit" of Marxist-Leninist idealism, as opposed to the

---

[174] http://www.georgewashingtonportrait.net/

model of individual initiative and opportunity that underlies the U.S. Constitution.

Although Dewey, a socialist-turned-Marxist, didn't coin the term "progressive education"[175], he inspired the movement. His core philosophy dictated that children should be socialized—much like puppies: thrown willy-nilly into a yard with lots of activity, critters and commotion. He considered this approach to schooling more advantageous to society than academics.

In 1896, Dewey wrote that the centrality of reading and writing was "one of education's great mistakes." He looked upon the schools as an opportunity to promote a worldview in which private property, free markets, competition and profits are passé. What we got in return was an America in which integrity, morality and self-discipline are passé—a situation remediable only with a ubiquitous government and vigorous enforcement of petty rules.

The late, iconic constitutional scholar, political theorist and author, Cleon Skousen[176] explains what came of this strategy: "a planned pattern of anarchy in education," where the new term "*self-realization* [self-absorption] became the focus of school." This vision rejects the older, universally accepted ideal of education as a "common body of knowledge," coined by Skousen's equally iconic colleague, Henry Steele Commager.

Dewey's latter-day disciples—among them, A. S. Neill (of Great Britain), Theodore Sizer, William Spady, Ralph Tyler, Francis C. Keppel, John Goodlad, William Glasser and Benjamin Bloom—all toiled behind the scenes in the 50s, 60s and 70s to enact Dewey's ideas about education and childrearing.

What Dewey Believed.- At its core, Dewey's progressivism was aimed at replacing the individual as the focus of good governance— including all its accompanying ideals, such as self-determination, personal responsibility and risk-and-reward—with a *dependent collective*. In that vein, progressive education gained traction at the

---

[175] http://www.bgsu.edu/departments/acs/1890s/dewey/educ.html
[176] http://en.wikipedia.org/wiki/Cleon_Skousen

prominent Teachers College (Columbia University), the primary entity churning out teachers in the 1930s and 40s[177], when most Americans were preoccupied with World War II.

Consequently, it went more or less unnoticed when influential educators started picking up the banner of socialist rhetoric. Most American mothers of the late 1950s and early 60s didn't connect the increasingly strident radicalism of the teachers union, much less John Dewey, with articles that appeared in childrearing magazines, penned by a new breed of "experts": child psychologists. Once parents realized that their Boomer offspring had nowhere near the grasp of basic subjects that they had had at the same age, and that their progeny were turning against family, God and country, progressivism was all but institutionalized.

By the mid-1960s, bad parenting advice, coupled to progressive education, was molding public opinion in a new generation of voters. Sam Weaver expressed the outcome well in a 2004 article[178]:

> Whenever you hear modern liberals proclaiming "American values," or "our values," you *must* understand that [they] are embracing the collectivist, secular, "progressive *'values'"* of John Dewey and his followers. After all, that is what they were taught American values have always been! When activist judges rule against the will of the American people, and discover new "rights" and "values" in the U.S. Constitution; those new "rights" and "values" represent—as far as *they* know—the secular, socialistic "values" which they have learned from the Ivy League schools [where] they received their law degrees....

So, one can't simply blame so-called liberals. "Today, people who call themselves conservatives...accept much of the Progressive view.... [It] has become the predominant view...." wrote Thomas West and William Schambra in a 2007 report[179] for the Heritage Foundation.

---

[177] http://www.crossroad.to/Books/BraveNewSchools/Chronology.htm
[178] http://www.renewamerica.com/columns/weaver/040308
[179] http://www.heritage.org/research/reports/2007/07/the-progressive-movement-and-the-transformation-of-american-politics

And this is the whole point: It is why education is the ultimate game-changer in American politics and governance.

All former Presidents since George H. W. Bush are Boomer-generation kids. Most political candidates today are unwitting beneficiaries of the "new thinking" that permeated society with the Boomer era—and all cut their teeth on progressivism, no matter where they were educated or how much money they have. They have spent more waking hours under the influence of their schools (and by extension the NEA and UNESCO) than under the tutelage of their families and forebears.

If a mere portrait of George Washington can be expunged from schools without an outcry, what are the chances of today's candidates being able to "connect" with Gen-X-ers and Millennials on the necessity of constitutional ideals, or the Founders' vision for our country? How does even a knowledgeable and patriotic CCCTP candidate communicate with a populace having virtually no "common body of knowledge"?

Mainstreaming Progressivism.- Although John Dewey defied most of the cultural, moral and economic norms of his era, his message somehow mainstreamed its way into K-12 schools nationwide. This was due in part to events that were taking place half a world away—with the Leninist-Stalinist Soviet Union at its pinnacle. Probably the best insight we have into the effect of these events on Dewey's thinking is his comment that "[t]he Russian educational situation is enough to convert one to the idea that only in a society based upon the coöperative principle can the ideals of educational reformers be adequately carried into operation"[180].

Dewey characterized himself as a "democratic socialist." Over the years, his writings increasingly underscored an aversion to the free-market system; an abhorrence of religion, especially Christianity; a distaste for educational basics like reading and writing; and finally,

---

[180] http://ariwatch.com/VS/JD/ImpressionsOfSovietRussia.htm

in 1928, outspoken admiration for Soviet schooling—especially its creation of a "collectivistic mentality"[181].

Dewey essentially agreed with the "father of experimental psychology," the German philosopher, professor and psychologist Wilhelm Wundt, that psychology was a rational alternative to "supernatural religion." Toward that end, he was among the signers of the original *Humanist Manifesto*[182] in 1933 (there is now a *Humanist Manifesto II* and *III*). Unless people actually read the Manifesto, most mentally translate the term "humanist" as either "humane," the "humanities," or maybe as a style of Renaissance art of the 14th and 15th centuries. So, when parents heard it in the context of education, no red flags went up.

"Functional Literacy" v. "Learning How to Live".- Throughout Dewey's voluminous writings—two themes recur: that (1) education and learning are interactive processes, which had some basis, and that (2) the school itself is a *social* institution through which social reform *can and should* take place. The latter paved the way for political opportunists.

Dewey averred that educational institutions should not just be a place to gain knowledge, but rather, be a place "where one *learns how to live*." Most Americans thought that was the family's prerogative.

Dewey coined the term "functional psychology" to describe this supposed key to living in a complex society[183]. The U.S. Department of Education quietly adapted that term as "functional literacy," replacing the old "excellence model," in a 1981 paper, "Measuring the Quality of Education."

The shift from knowledge-based schooling to a psycho-social model was the juncture at which everything started to go wrong in education. The heretofore inconspicuous contingent of American Communists seized upon psycho-social reform, ignoring other insights that Dewey proffered—many not unreasonable, such as

---

[181] Ibid, at Chapter 5.
[182] http://www.scribd.com/doc/24618012/1933-Humanist-Manifesto-I-John-Dewey-Et-Al
[183] http://en.wikipedia.org/wiki/John_Dewey

striking a balance between delivering knowledge and taking into account the interests and experiences of the student. Citing Dewey, Communist infiltrators turned the nation's schools into a political football steeped in the behavioral sciences instead of intellectual challenges.

A naïve Dewey and his colleagues envisioned a benevolent (as opposed to a coercive) welfare state, with schools serving as concealed-in-plain-sight "agents of change." The expectation was that these "enlightened change agents" would gently impose, through successive waves of graduating youth, a new social order on America within a couple of generations. These "change agents" would sweep away the ideals of the America's Founders under the cover of modernism and progress—thus the term "progressivism."

Today, even the trusty dictionary assigns positive synonyms to "progressivism," while "traditionalism," "individualism" and "conservatism" are depicted as backward.

Adult Guidance and Ingenuity Deemed Overrated.- Since most Americans at that time were focused on the carnage of World War II, an emerging "mental health" cabal began speaking out, advocating a society indifferent to nationality, sovereignty and bourgeois "morality." Among this cadre of behavioral psychologists are the same scoundrels we have met in previous chapters[184]—Drs. Brock Chisholm, J. R. Rees, and Even Cameron. Among such company, Dewey found a safe haven for his theories[185], but was alarmed by what he considered the excesses of "child-centered" pedagogues who claimed to be his followers. Dewey countered that *too much* reliance on the child could be detrimental to the learning process.

Dewey was admittedly ahead of his time in emphasizing "hands-on learning"[186], as opposed to teachers *always* standing at the front of the room doling out information to passive pupils. He insisted that "it is impossible to procure knowledge without the use of objects which

---

[184] See Chapter 4, "The Roots of Perception Management"; Chapter 5, "The Justice of Pretension"; and Chapter 6, "*Brown v. Board of Education* Fails to Foil Segregation."

[185] http://en.wikipedia.org/wiki/The_New_School_for_Social_Research

[186] http://en.wikipedia.org/wiki/Hands-on_learning

impress the mind." That is why many credit him with the Project Based Learning (PBL)[187], which places students in the active role, a concept not totally without merit.

But in the hands of left-leaning opportunists, PBL wound up emphasizing learning as a strictly *collective* process, with individual initiative suddenly becoming undesirable. When Dewey suggested that the teacher's role should be that of "facilitator" and "guide," the American Left had found its sales pitch. Ben D. Wood and Ralph W. Tyler, representing the new breed of behaviorist education-"reformers" in the Chisholm-Rees-Cameron mold, would promote it as "child-centered," "individualized" education in the 1960s.

These were PM slogans pure and simple; nevertheless, the claptrap about personalization and child-friendly fare were incorporated into every university teacher-preparation program nationwide, as well as into a new style of quasi-achievement testing known as "assessment." The Educational Testing Service, then headed by Tyler, in Princeton, New Jersey, was at the forefront of the assessment movement. By the mid-1970s, most educators wouldn't remember the rigorous learning environment of yesteryear.

Teachers' Union Swings Into Action

The primary enablers of left-wing opportunism, including the new breed of "child experts," was the National Education Association (NEA). Beginning in 1935, the NEA launched a campaign to see just how far they could go with socialist rhetoric before the public balked. At the NEA's annual meeting, incoming NEA Secretary Willard Givens said: "A dying laissez-faire must be completely destroyed; and all of us, including the 'owners,' must be subjected to a large degree of social control.... An equitable distribution of income will be sought." This was pure Marxist-Leninism.

The NEA had a friend in Louis Alber, head of National Recovery Act New York, who announced in 1933: "The rugged individualism

---

[187] http://en.wikipedia.org/wiki/Project_Based_Learning

of Americanism must go, because it is contrary to the purpose of the New Deal ... which is remaking America."

These kinds of pronouncements fueled a determination by leftist leaders to ensure that parental rights and religious ideals were swallowed up, the prerogatives of local communities usurped, and a "controlled collective" imposed. Americans had no clue how this rhetoric was expediting a pivotal shift and policy reversal under their noses. How many Americans, after all, would pick up a copy of *Psychiatry Magazine* in 1946 and read Dr. Chisholm's shocking speech to the World Federation of Mental Health?

> We have swallowed all manner of poisonous certainties fed us by our parents, our Sunday and day school teachers... The results are frustration, inferiority, neurosis and inability to... make the world fit to live in. ... The re-interpretation and eventually eradication of the concept of right and wrong which has been the basis of child training...these are the belated objectives of practically all effective psychotherapy....

By 1968, NEA president Elizabeth Koontz was alerting the American Association of Colleges for Teacher Education that the teachers union had "a multi-faceted program already directed toward the urban school problem, embracing every phase, from the Head Start Program (Title I of the Elementary and Secondary Education Act) to *sensitivity training for adults*—[aimed at] both teachers and parents."

Then, a bolder move: In the early 1970s, NEA president George Fischer told the union's annual assembly:

> ...a good deal of work has been done to begin to bring about uniform certification controlled by the unified profession in each state.... With these new laws, we will finally realize our 113-year old dream of controlling who enters, who stays and who leaves the profession.... we can also control the teacher training institutions.

Two years later, the NEA was at it again, when its president, Catharine Barrett, took an even more forceful tack, declaring: "We are the biggest potential political striking force in this country, and we are determined to control the direction of education." A year later, she called for *"de-emphasizing academic basics in favor of teachers becoming philosophical 'change agents'."*

By 1982, the education behemoth had grown intolerant of all but ultra-left ideas and individuals. Federal policy increasingly reflected the NEA's annual Legislative Agenda. Over the years, the NEA agenda items covered everything from national defense to social security to sexual orientation, but remarkably little about actual teaching[188].

The size of the NEA's political war chest doubled[189], even as its mission became only fleetingly focused on academics or finding and keeping competent teachers. Enormous amounts of its union dues made their way to state and local affiliates to ensure NEA-friendly school boards, via its various state Uniserve[190] offices, while the NEA's tax-exempt national headquarters in Washington, DC, continued to wield mounting influence on radical-left initiatives that eventually would crush the very pupils on whose behalf the organization pretended to function.

It didn't take long before the *NEA Journal* was endorsing the centerpiece of a morally corrupt ethical system: "values clarification"—a catch-phrase coined by leftist educators[191] as a stand-in for "affective-interactive educational psychology." The groundwork was laid by psychologist Lawrence Kohlberg in his controversial 1963 "Stages of Moral Development"[192], aimed at supplanting "conventional morality." With that, "progressive education" merged with humanistic psychology[193] and the "humanistic education movement." This marked the first open crusade to discourage adults from transmitting "good" values and

---

[188] http://www.heartland.org/custom/semod_policybot/pdf/3761.pdf
[189] http://www.eiaonline.com/archives/20110222.htm
[190] http://www.sussexcounty-ea.org/njea__uniserve_regional_office__stanhope.htm
[191] http://www.edpsycinteractive.org/topics/affsys/values.html
[192] http://psychology.about.com/od/developmentalpsychology/a/kohlberg.htm
[193] http://www.ahpweb.org/aboutahp/whatis.html

"empowering" small children to "develop their own valuing process" instead.

The 70s-era watershed book that made depravity, decadence and self-indulgence part and parcel of the school environment was *Values Clarification--A Handbook of Practical Strategies for Teachers and Students*[194]. It was aimed at speeding society's transformation to ethical relativism—which, of course, is antithetical to the Founders' vision for the country. Among the classroom exercises was Strategy #3: "values voting": the group "votes" a behavioral norm into existence, without any particular consideration as to its "rightness" or "wrongness," decency, propriety or morality. In other words, the child is encouraged to make up his "value system" as he goes along, rather than to judge it against any sort of benchmark or principle.

Today, we find the results of this lesson in the morning news: "flash mobs," theater killings, random attacks on innocents for no particular reason.

From there, progressivism was absorbed into the Marxist-socialist mold. The Soviet book, *The Scientific and Technological Revolution and the Revolution in Education*, was translated and imported to the U.S. It helped lay the foundation for a philosophy called Outcome-based Education, promulgated in America by William Spady. A 1988 *NEA Journal* published "The New Social Studies," urging that American education, especially the university departments of teacher education, be reorganized "using materials from the behavioral sciences," planting the tenets of social psychology firmly into elementary and secondary schools.

Ernest Boyer, president of Carnegie Foundation of the Advancement of Teaching (CFAT) pronounced that schools should no longer be treated as "academic centers," but as "social service centers," providing day-long health-care (now called *school-based health clinics*), day-care for preschoolers (now termed *early childhood education*), and other social services, such as healthy meals. John Goodlad, another influential voice among the new breed

---

[194] Text based on the work of Louis Raths, Vera Harmon, Sidney Simon, Howard Kirschenbaum, and Leland Howe

of "reformers," seconded these notions[195] in his 1984 tome, *A Place Called School*. Like his relativist colleagues, he believed that "[e]ducation is a never-ending process of developing characteristic ways of thinking and behaving...."

And on it went—precious little about education transmitting a common body of knowledge or culture.

The Public Becomes Alerted—Too Late.- It wasn't until parents began noticing an uptick in non-education-related data collectedn through quasi-educational surveys and assessments, together with blatant activities aimed at social engineering and promoting world government, that they started paying attention. Parent groups started cropping up and networking around the country, all of them comparing notes and "digging" for information about the forces behind new focus of schooling. They turned up more than they bargained for; among the culprits they found:

- the Education Commission of the States[196]
- the Rockefeller Foundation[197]
- the Robert Wood Johnson Foundation[198]
- the Jane Fonda Center[199]
- the American Psychological Association[200]
- the American Humanist Association[201]
- Sexuality Information & Education Council of the U.S.[202]
- Global Education Associates[203]
- Greenpeace[204]

[195] http://www2.selu.edu/Academics/Faculty/nadams/educ692/Goodlad.html
[196] http://www.ecs.org/ecsmain.asp?page=/html/issuesK12.asp
[197] http://www.rockefellerfoundation.org/who-we-are/our-history/
[198] http://www.rwjf.org/files/research/022208bunchanthology.pdf
[199] http://janefonda.com/tag/robert-wood-johnson-foundation/
[200] http://www.apadiv15.org/apa/
[201] http://www.americanhumanist.org/HNN/details/2011-04-aha-publishes-humanist-curriculum-manuals-for-childr
[202] http://www.siecus.org/index.cfm?fuseaction=Feature.showFeature&featureID=1730
[203] http://www.g-e-a.org/peace-ed/index.html
[204] http://www.stopclimatechaos.org/11/jun/action-keep-climate-change-school-curriculum-0

It was too late. By the year 2000, most government agencies had been infiltrated and virtually taken over by the Left, education being the most thoroughly compromised. Progressive education had gone "mainstream."

Preventative Psychology Makes Its Debut

For those wondering at the purpose of all this focus on children's attitudes, the expensive assessment of behaviors, and longitudinal (follow-on) surveys of student beliefs, they need look no further than Chris Mooney's new book, *The Republican Brain*. It is built around "facts" supposedly established recently by MRI scans and "gene sequencer" studies—that conservatives are closed-minded and resistant to change, and hence are anti-science and anti-fact, while "liberals consistently score higher on a personality measure called 'openness to experience,' one of the 'Big Five' personality traits, which are easily assessed through standard questionnaires."

Read that again—the last part, in particular: "...personality traits, which are easily assessed through standard questionnaires." That is why schools have converted so much of its academic testing to attitudinal assessment! What they are assessing is the child's "belief system" in an effort to launch a new field, ***preventative psychiatry***!

Before we get too far along in examining Mooney's thesis, let's harken back to chapter 5 ("The Justice of Harassment"), in which we covered the 2005 taxpayer-funded "study" out of the National Institute of Mental Health (NIMH) and the National Science Foundation, in which researchers representing three major universities worked to attribute notions about morality and individualism to "dogmatism," "uncertainty avoidance," and "mental rigidity." Then there was the work of the University of Manitoba's associate professor of psychology, Robert Altemeyer, who developed a Right Wing Authoritarian (RWA) Scale, to identify those harboring the same "mental illnesses." And let us not forget about scientists at the University of London's purported "findings" that conservatives have an enlarged "fear" area in their brains, with smaller areas associated with courage and optimism—also covered in chapter 5.

Mr. Mooney follows in the footsteps of these, and other, pronouncements, all arriving at the same general conclusions. In his April 15, 2012, column that appeared in several news forums, including such widely disparate venues as *Washington Post* and the *Bangor Daily News*, he averred[205]: "This means liberals tend to be the kind of people who want to try new things, including new music, books, restaurants and vacation spots—and new ideas."

As if to lend legitimacy to Mooney's thesis, psychologist Robert McCrae purportedly conducted voluminous studies on personality; he is quoted by Mooney as stating: "Open people everywhere tend to have more liberal values." Conservatives, of course, are characterized by Mooney as

> …less exploratory, less in need of change—and more 'conscientious,' a trait that indicates they appreciate order and structure in their lives. This gels nicely with the standard definition of conservatism as resistance to change.

Arie Kruglanski is another university psychologist who purportedly has pioneered research on liberal-conservative belief systems, and "worked to develop a scale for measuring the need for closure." He insists that there is a strong relationship between liberalism and openness, that "[t]he finding is very robust."

Who paid for this sort of "research"—or professional smear campaign? In large part, you did.

Mooney cites many other examples to support this claim, including the debate over global warming, writing that "tea party followers not only strongly deny the science but also tend to say that they 'do not need any more information' about the issue." This, despite the fact that there all kinds of information have been uncovered by highly credible scientists representing various political perspectives (see next chapter). They found that global-warming

---

[205]http://bangordailynews.com/2012/04/15/opinion/liberals-and-conservatives-vote-differently-because-they-think-differently/

science is statistically faulty and based on the wrong data. These are hardly the kind of people who do "not want any more information"!

Mooney's only weak attempt at appearing unbiased—with a book titled *The Republican Brain*, no less—is to say: "I'm certainly not saying that liberals have a monopoly on truth. Of course not. They aren't always right; but when they're wrong, they are wrong differently."

Differently in the sense of "more sanely"?

Anyone who is not troubled at the sudden confluence of these "studies" attempting to equate conservative, constitutional, Christian, traditional and patriotic values with mental illness is forgetting what horrors history has replayed concerning political "dissidents" and political prisons (or forced drugging) under the cover of mental instability—in particular the phrase "a danger to himself and others."

Moreover, the school has been secured as the primary vehicle to root out the "mentally unfit" conservative, traditionalist, constitutionalist and patriot.

Track Record of Failure Means Starting Over

Lawmakers know that schools have become the ultimate "hostile environments": hostile to learning, to Western culture, to individuality, to parents, to good manners, and to the much-ballyhooed self-esteem of pupils. Even Congress knows the Education Department is a failed agency, and that the only real justification for its continued existence is its data-collection systems (17 at last count), its babysitting-oversight function, and its questionable value as a tool of propaganda.

Even by the government's own measures, schools have failed. Juvenile crime has been linked to faulty "progressive" teaching methods, beginning with reading and spelling[206], as per a commissioned study by Michael S. Brunner for the U.S. Department of Justice's Office of Juvenile Justice and Delinquency Prevention in 1993. Police department and correctional statistics confirm Brunner's

---

[206] http://www.halcyon.org/reading.html

thesis, yet our government ignores its own experts whenever they contradict leftist dogma—mostly to acquire more tax dollars, directly or indirectly.

Pupils who spend day after day in a "captive" (a.k.a. compulsory) environment in which they can't learn become frustrated. Sustained frustration over a long enough timeframe produces one of two things: apathy (usually accompanied by withdrawal) or aggression (often featuring sudden, explosive violence). This is virtually the only issue on which educational researchers, theologians and psychologists agree.

Severely frustrated students will, therefore, misbehave—whether it means going to sleep at their desk, truancy, drug-abuse, or blowing up their school[207]. Ongoing misconduct typically lands a pupil in Special Education, where teachers have virtually no techniques at their disposal to correct, or even determine, a specific learning problem. Even if they did, the makeup of such classrooms today defies any means of maximizing the learning environment. Consequently, Special Education teachers are taught to use group-think and peer pressure as methods of control, which contributes to "flight-or-fight" reactions.

Students in these environments typically are referred for "counseling"—with child psychologists—who place them on a regimen of increasingly powerful psychiatric drugs that can ruin their lives, not to mention create an increasing cycle of dependency and criminality, at huge cost to society. Every year more children become "eligible" for Special Education "services," with a higher tax bite to accommodate it. Because the word "eligible" is one of those terms that carry a positive connotation, it fails to convey any disadvantages.

Worse, today's chaotic school day features non-stop distractions, noise and interruptions—none conducive to concentration, especially for younger children. Pupils who flit from one activity to another, often never learn to sustain an attention span. Then we "blame the victim," by medicalizing his or her condition as attention-deficit

---

[207] http://www.washingtontimes.com/news/2011/aug/17/teen-arrested-in-florida-bomb-plot/

disorder and attention-deficit-hyperactivity disorder. The "disorder" is not in the child; it is in the classroom.

Most children are by nature high-energy, easily distracted creatures. It is the *rare* child who sits alone and entertains himself (or herself) with some project for hours on end. Concentration is a *learned art*—and the school does not nurture it.

Moreover, government-subsidized education has, since the 1960s, fostered intellectual bankruptcy and lack of self-control. Schools steeped in progressivism and humanistic psychology convey the notion that there are no standards, academic or otherwise, that cannot be bent or broken.

Special programs for failure and bad conduct function as "negative rewards." Here is what our education tax dollars have subsidized:

- Brutal popularity contests that lead to school violence
- School days spent primping and jockeying for position
- Intractable peer pressure that trumps teacher authority
- Lack of respect for school and for learning
- Inability to hire and keep good teachers[208]
- Declining parental interest in,[209] and support for, schools and teachers
- Ongoing confrontations between parents, teachers and administrator
- Openings for radical opportunists (e.g., to insert their agenda)

The Education Department once declared it wanted "outcome-based" education. Here are the outcomes they got for their trouble (which is probably why the "outcome-based" catch-phrase fell out of favor):

---

[208] http://www.gpb.org/news/2010/12/14/poll-most-want-bad-teachers-fired
[209] http://www.adi.org/journal/ss03/Gonzalez-DeHass%20&%20Willems.pdf

- Delinquency
- Cynicism
- Unemployability
- Alienation
- Resentment
- Cultural decline
- Fatherless children
- Entitlement surges

All these lead inexorably to a future national security breakdown and economic crisis that requires an increasing large infusion of funds.

Government Strategies to Fight Education Reform

American education needs an "extreme makeover." Mostly, it needs to be privatized and not run by the federal government. If state and local governments are involved at all, inevitably they will seek federal tax dollars as well, and wind up with the same old carrot-and-stick situation we have now. The National Education Association must be defunded, with no "perks" whatsoever from government, federal, state or local. It is a traitorous organization that has caused incalculable damage to children, families and even the teachers they pretend to defend. Arguably, the organization would lose most of its membership overnight if it did not offer certain benefit programs and so-called collective bargaining rights. The NEA has turned professionals with masters and doctorate degrees into the equivalent of blue-collar workers.

There are many alternative approaches to the schooling of our nation's children, and these have been written up by many well-known educators and theorists, including this author.[210]

Big Government, of course, will battle these approaches tooth and nail—mainly due to the many vested interests in the status quo.

---

[210] http://www.thenewamerican.com/culture/education/item/341-an-extreme-makeover-for-us-education-%E2%80%94-can-we?-should-we?

A favorite ploy government uses to discourage schools seeking to incorporate the model above is to play **the accreditation game**: simply deny certain schools and venues accreditation. Government attempts to obstruct homeschoolers in much the same way.

But, ask yourself, exactly how much good has accreditation actually *done*?

The other tack the State will use is **the "compelling state interest" game**. That's how government took over curriculum, one "compelling state interest" at a time.

Citizens must start giving government its marching orders, reminding elected leaders and bureaucrats alike that *they* work for taxpayers; average citizens do not exist simply to accommodate the government! Certainly we hear comments to this effect from candidates for public office—until they get elected. That's why it will take more than reshuffling presidents and recycling politicians to turn things around. Citizens can no longer afford to play musical chairs at election time.

Reclaiming K-12 education is the first order of business for the nation's citizens—if nothing else, to prove we mean business! *The flip side is that if we don't change education, **nothing** else—no other crisis, not a single issue currently on the table—**can** be fixed.*

~

CHAPTER 8
THE GREEN GAME

Global warming, like Marxism, is a political theory of actions, demanding compliance with its rules....The global warming activists' target is the U.S. If America is driven to accept crippling restraints on its economy it will rapidly become unable to shoulder its burdens as the world's sole superpower and ultimate defender of human freedoms. We shall all suffer, however, as progress falters and then ceases and living standards decline. *-- Paul Johnson, British historian, author; in an article for* Forbes, *print magazine, Oct. 6, 2008*

"It's hard to be green," sang Jim Henson's most beloved Muppet, Kermit the Frog.

Barack Obama must be feeling Kermit's pain these days, as increasing numbers of respected scientists decided they'd had quite enough of the administration's twisted, politically correct versions of their hard-won research—data "rehabilitated" for the sole purpose of satisfying the environmental, or "green," agenda game.

Unlike Al Gore (who has no background in science), legitimate scientists are slowly coming to the realization that leftist elements, inside and outside of government, are giving all scientists a bad reputation, not to mention compromising the integrity of the "scientific method" itself. This places all scientists' careers on the chopping block unless they speak out now, collectively, ahead of the crash, when the masses finally grasp the fact that their lives have been turned upside down on the basis of phony data.

This chapter covers five overarching topics—**Agenda 21**, **Sustainable Development**, **Smart Growth** (also known under the names Urban Sprawl, Open Spaces and Livable Communities), **Green Energy** (or Clean Energy) and everybody's favorite, **Climate Change** (Global Warming). These, in turn, have important subcategories that affect large swaths of the population, but not equally for every category in all parts of the country. Consequently, some of them are not familiar to some Americans or equated with the environmental movement. Among these sub-issues are biodiversity, population control, water rights, "watersheds," land-use zoning, wetlands, pollution "monitoring" and regulation, conservation, drilling (oil), and "fracking" (coal).

Other issues can be more capricious: prohibitions against certain foods (e.g., "processed" and "sugary"), synthetic fuels, wind energy bunkum, and planned deterioration of critical infrastructures, such as power lines, power plants and grids, pipelines, water treatment plants, dams, etc. The point is, all are linked to the Environmental Movement, having become a joint venture between the United States and all its "member" nations, including, in particular, the United States.

All of the issues above encroach upon your property rights—not just your right to own property, but every use of that property once you have purchased it—down to and what kinds of light bulbs you use, and how you ranchers keep their cattle fed. The EPA is so powerful today that it can, without warning, declare your house and land a wetland preserve and force you out. It can starve a rancher's cattle by turning the water rights over to an Indian tribe miles away. It can suddenly take away a grazing permit—and doesn't need a reason. The federal government can trick you into "donating" your land, allowing a non-governmental organization (such as the Nature Conservatory) to rake in millions, even billions, off the deception.

Environmental Movement Morphs into Agenda 21

The environmental movement started out, ostensibly, as an anti-pollution campaign during the Nixon administration. It morphed into a United Nations construct called Agenda 21, the centerpiece of which is "sustainable development." Perception managers decided that had a nicer ring to it.

Unfortunately, too many politicians believe "sustainable development" is more trendy than treacherous—and turn it into a political bargaining chip.

Agenda 21, according to the U.N.'s own documents, is a "global plan of action" built around the U.N. Earth Charter, which includes all of the above issues, their subtopics and offshoots in some form, meaning that if you fight any of them, you will fight not only the U.S. government, but the United Nations, too.

Each of these issues is worthy of an entire book in itself. Obviously, lonely so much space can be allotted here, so this chapter will necessarily scratch the surface—with copious notes and links so that the reader can verify the content and seek additional information on facets of particular concern.

Agenda 21: America's Sovereignty at Risk

Most candidates for public office won't say the term "Agenda 21" out loud. They will claim, however, to be onboard with Sustainable Development, Smart Growth, Green Energy, or Climate Change—all part and parcel of Agenda 21. The number 21 refers to the 21st century.

The slogan "sustainable development" connotes, of course, *sustainability*. But, leftist leaders know most Americans and Brits also equate the term with "stability," as it sounds rather alike. Alas, it isn't true.

The term "sustainable development" first appeared in a 1987 report entitled "Our Common Future," produced by the United Nations World Commission on Environment and Development. It is impossible to overstate the importance of this document.

Michael Shaw, president of the Freedom Advocates[211] (an organizational network that advances constitutional principles), explains how this key work was used by the U.N. "as the virtual springboard for a 'wrenching transformation' (Al Gore's words) of human society." Shaw gives further evidence as to the sheer weight

---

[211] http://www.freedomadvocates.org/

Agenda 21 now has on U.S. policymaking (except, of course, for a selected elitists, like Al Gore, who "invented the Internet" and "re-invented government"), who are free to defy all its provisions):

> The term "sustainable development" is used in nearly every federal, state, and local development plan; on nearly every federal, state, and local government website; and in nearly every public statement on new development policies. [There is] even...a President's Council on Sustainable Development, created by an Executive Order of Bill Clinton, [its] stated purpose to impose the policies of Agenda 21 into United States law.
>
> The label "Agenda 21" was first presented as official U.N. policy in 1992 at the Earth Summit. In the report from that conference we read (emphasis added):
>
> Agenda 21 proposes an array of actions which are intended to be implemented by *every* person on Earth.... [I]t calls for specific changes in the activities if *all* people.... Effective execution of Agenda 21 will *require* a profound reorientation of *all* humans, unlike anything the world has ever experienced....[212]

So, the connection between the United Nations and Agenda 21 is undeniable and can easily be traced to the 1987 U.N. report, "Our Common Future." Heads of several environmental groups here at home were complicit in helping to pen Agenda 21, including John Sawhill of the Nature Conservancy, Jay Hair of the National Wildlife Federation and Michele Perrault, international Vice President of the Sierra Club.

Tom DeWeese, president of the American Policy Center[213], explains how Agenda 21 made its entrée onto the American stage:

> More than 178 nations adopted Agenda 21 as official policy during a signing ceremony at the 1987 Earth Summit. President George H.W. Bush signed the document for the U.S. In signing, each nation pledged to adopt the goals of Agenda 21. In 1995, President Bill Clinton ... signed Executive Order #12858 to create the President's

---

[212] Michael Shaw quoting and paraphrasing from *Agenda 21: The Earth Summit Strategy to Save Our Planet* (Earthpress, 1992).

[213] http://americanpolicy.org/

Council on Sustainable Development in order to "harmonize" U.S. environmental policy with U.N. directives, as outlined in Agenda 21. The Executive Order directed all agencies of the Federal Government to work with state and local community governments in a joint effort to "reinvent" government [former Vice President Al Gore's "baby"] using the guidelines outlined in Agenda 21.

A 300-page publication by the U.N. soon followed and can still be obtained, both in paperback and in HTML on the Internet: *Earth Summit AGENDA 21: The United Nations Programme of Action From Rio*. It is highly recommended that the reader order or download this document and keep it handy for meetings and focus groups. There have been several more conferences since that time, of course (in 2012, for example, in Rio de Janeiro), and predictably, the Agenda 21 mission has morphed. But the Rio document minces no words about its intent and is important for the terms it doesn't bother to "sanitize."

According to Cathie Adams of Sovereignty International, Inc.[214] in 2009, Barack Obama sent his Secretary of State, Hillary Clinton, to the U.N. Framework Convention on Climate Change Conference in Copenhagen, Denmark, to commit a whopping $30 billion to a new Fast Start fund for 2012, with a follow-up commitment to raise $100 billion annually from industrialized, developed nations to support a Green Fund by the year 2020.

The next year, at another conference in Cancun, Mexico, the U.N. began urging member nations to jump on the Green Fund bandwagon, apparently hoping to use it as a vehicle for its long-held global taxing scheme. A reading of its conference publication, revealingly entitled *Outreach, a Multi-Stakeholder Magazine on Environment and Sustainable Development*, made it clear that discussions revolved around what entity would govern the global tax system; through what channels the funds would flow; how "climate finance" would be monitored, reported and verified; and who would decide the recipients and purposes of each influx of funds.

---

[214] http://sovereignty.net/

Most readers probably recall the much-ballyhooed "carbon tax" idea—a concept favored by Al Gore and leftist influential billionaire George Soros. Other concepts on the table included international fees on shipping and aviation. The largesse, of course, would go either to Third World countries, to pay staff, or back into perception management for the causes themselves.

Thus, the U.N. has no reservations about admitting its Agenda 21 plan has social and economic consequences for industrialized, sovereign nations.

Technology Transfers and International Benefactors

At the top of Agenda 21's list for wealth redistribution is **technology transfer** to Third World countries. As detailed in chapter 7, U.S. **education** increasingly works in cooperation with UNESCO, which is why the largest teachers union, the National Education Association heavily promotes the tenets of "sustainable development" to teachers.

Agenda 21 also curries favor with **international institutions,** with ultra-wealthy benefactors (e.g., the Bill and Melinda Gates Foundation, George Soros[215] and his many leftist grant recipients[216] and other household-name groups like the Nature Conservancy, the National Wildlife Federation and the Sierra Club. This helps create U.S. and worldwide legitimacy. These tentacles facilitate the use of "financial wealth transfer mechanisms"—the International Monetary Fund, the World Bank, etc.)—most of which involve some share of U.S. taxpayer dollars as well as private philanthropies.

Third-Party Bureaucracies and Front Groups.- Agenda 21 usually doesn't advertise its vast network of U.N. front groups, such as

---

[215] László Pinté, Professor of Environmental Sciences, Central European University, is labeled a sustainability expert that worked with the United Nations. He focused on sustainable development in order to deal with environment problems such as climate change and biodiversity conservation and works hard with other CEU departments to promote, in particular, George Soros' vision, according to a June 2012 report of the Media Research Center. Find entire report at http://www.mrc.org/special-reports/special-report-george-soros-godfather-left.

[216] http://sorosfiles.com/soros/2011/10/open-society-institute-top-150-grantees.html

"International Council for Local Environmental Initiatives" (or ICLEI), which has infiltrated over 500 American cities, raking in federal and local tax dollars as it goes, to bring its socialist schemes to the American rank and file. For example, according to research located by the American Policy Center, ICLEI officials recently passed regulations in Oakland, California, forcing many homeowners to replace their windows, roofs and appliances, costing an average of $35,000 per household.

Unsurprisingly, the Environmental Protection Agency (EPA) actively supports the ICLEI agenda—via American tax dollars, of course—through Barack Obama's "Sustainable Development Challenge Grant Program." Thus, the Agenda 21 and the EPA are in strong alliance.

The U.S. House of Representatives, of course, which controls all the spending bills, could "simply vote to cut off all U.S. taxpayer funding of the United Nations' ICLEI agenda," writes Tom DeWeese, president of the American Policy Center. But if average Americans don't even know about ICLEI or its activities, that allows our representatives to simply play dumb, and pass the buck on American sovereignty issues.

Thus does the U.N. keep on compromising our citizens' rights—for example, through ICLEI's Intergovernmental Panel on Climate Change (IPCC). Many American who know about the panel, per se, and can even identify it as a U.N. agency, but they still don't get the ICLEI connection. This yet another instance what our Founders called an "entangling alliance." In the case of ICLEI, it adds a third layer (shield) of bureaucracy that makes it more difficult for average Americans to dis-engage from phony global-warming "science" and reject the mandates it imposes.

The American Planning Association (APA) is a different kind of third-party—a front group. Its purpose is to take the policy positions contained in Agenda 21 and get them accepted at the local level.

These heads of organizations like this usually recruit twenty-somethings graduating from liberal colleges and universities—young people who already have been "vetted" for their liberal-leftist viewpoints. Readers of the previous chapter already know how easy it is to ascertain, and collect this kind of information so that nobody is interviewed for a position who has not already passed muster. The only question for interviewers is, can the recruit perform well in local communities to change attitudes and secure consensus where there may be pockets of deep resistance.

Some of the larger front groups (such as APA, or the National Education Association's National Training Lab, or NTL) provide actual "boot camps" to teach operatives how to counter their opposition. NTL "graduates" go into the classroom and impose their various radical ideas on children; outfits like the APA head out to local forums posing as "facilitators"—which people take to mean "moderator of a discussion—then smoothly and deliberately pit one faction against another to make the favored side appear "sensible" and any opposing views out-of-touch. This particular approach is part of a strategy known as the Delphi Technique, but there are other manipulation tactics[217] as well.

Ron Ewart, president of the National Association or Rural Landowners[218] explains how representatives of front groups like APA "will say that what they are doing is all about inclusion and working at the local level, but what they don't say is they are implementing top-down international social and environmental policies (Agenda 21) and getting you to believe that you actually have a say in what they are doing at the local level. Activist front groups like the APA are surreptitious in their methods, and their functionaries are usually trained "change agents." They twist words and use phrases that dupe local citizens who generally have no idea they are dealing with professional manipulators tied to the U.N. and Agenda 21. They are typically clueless as to why some group they've never seen would be sent to ensure support for radical environmental "solutions," or "social justice" models—all "proposed" in the name of local communities.

---

[217] For a compendium of most professional manipulation strategies and how to counter them, see: http://www.amazon.com/Counter-Group-Manipulation-Tactics-Consensus-Building/dp/145051913X .

[218] http://www.narlo.org

What they do is preserve the pretense of public participation. Free and open discussion or debate is not in the interests of the U.N. or their front groups, yet in countries like the United States, an illusion of lay, or community, participation in policy-related decision-making must fulfill the requirements of state and local agencies. Once local communities are perceived to be onboard with an agenda item, then regulators can move in to impose it.

Countless citizens have engaged in focus groups and sat on committees only to find they agreed to something they never intended to approve. Only hours or days later do they realize they were hoodwinked. The ruse is successful because most groups tend to share a particular knowledge base and display a certain set of identifiable characteristics, which the facilitator researches well ahead of time. By the time the meeting takes place, smaller factions (and even individual ideologues) within the larger group have already been identified by the activist/"facilitator."

In getting local citizens onboard with an initiative or proposal (or at least acquiescent), activists take this "vote" to local and state representatives as "what the people want." At that point, the die is cast, and locals have no say at all. If anybody complains, they are reminded that it's what the community wanted.

Later, explains Tom DeWeese, the aforementioned president of the American Policy Center, "when local residents question their county commissioners, city councilmen, mayors, state legislators, and governors about the origins of their policies, it has become routine for these [so-called] representatives of the people to get a puzzled look on their faces and a wrinkle in their brows, as they say, 'I've never heard of Agenda 21. That's just a conspiracy theory.'"

Labels like American Planning Association are so innocuous-sounding that they don't raise any alarm bells in the community. Even if local citizens do a cursory check on the group, they will find only the usual public relations put out by the group itself: for example, that APA's mission is to "help create communities of lasting value."

Most citizens never see the group's actual training guide. If they did, they would find a memo entitled "Glossary for the Public" that lists words and terms which the APA leadership advises their members not to use anymore when they "engage" community focus groups, because Americans are catching on to them; for example: *affordable*, *consensus*, *density*, *public visioning*, *public-private partnership*, *eminent domain*, *police powers*, *green infrastructure*, *urban growth boundaries*, *regional planning*, *Smart Growth*, *stakeholders, regional, zoning* and even *sustainability* itself. Instead of *district* or *central*—now recognized by many locals as indicators of a "top down" or "Big Brother" process—APA advises switching to the more common words "downtown" or "business area" to appear as neutral as possible.

Some readers may wonder why terms like "regional" and "zoning" would be on this list: The explanations are further on.

So here, says DeWeese, "is…an organization that is supposed to be one of the most respected planning groups in the nation, operating in nearly every city, teach[ing] its people to lie at all costs in order to maintain their power and influence in our communities." [219]

In fact, activists like APA often do pose as "city planners," when they have no connection whatever to the city or town in question. Their real aim is to ram Agenda 21 policies down the throats of unsuspecting communities.

Thus has the U.S. government, in collusion with an international body, the United Nations, utilized a third-party approach to manipulate rank-and-file Americans into acquiescing on policy objectives based on highly questionable data.

What To Say to Storm-Troopers.- One method DeWeese suggests for challenging suspected activist front groups: "Ask them to name a single thing you can do on your private property without their permission. Ask them what guarantees for protection of private property rights they have included in their comprehensive plans."

Mr. DeWeese has found that disingenuous promoters of Agenda 21, when faced with obstinate criticism, will often deflect allegations with arguments like the following[220]:

---

[219] http://americanpolicy.org/2012/05/12/agenda-21-conspiracy-theory-or-threat/
[220] http://americanpolicy.org/2012/05/12/agenda-21-conspiracy-theory-or-threat/

- "Local planning is a local idea."
- "Agenda 21 is a non-binding resolution, not a treaty, so it carries no legal authority from which any nation is bound to act. There's nothing to worry about."
- "There are no 'Blue-Helmeted' U.N. troops [or 'black helicopters']" at City Hall" (i.e., an attempt at ridicule).
- "Planners are simply honest professionals trying to do their job, and that all these protests are wasting their valuable time."
- "The main concern of Agenda 21 is that man is fouling the environment and using up resources for future generations and we just need a sensible plan to preserve and protect the earth. What is so bad about that?"
- "I've read Agenda 21 and I can find no threatening language that says it is a global plot. What are you so afraid of?"
- And the old standby: "Agenda 21, what's that?"

After offering up these deflections, organizers may challenge locals to respond to their so-called "facts"—something that is particularly hard to do on the spot using quotes from U.N. documents. This is one reason that it is incumbent upon citizens to dig deeply into presenting groups before agreeing to participate in the meeting, task force or focus group. It is a reason to download or order a copy of key U.N. documents, such as the aforementioned *Earth Summit AGENDA 21: The United Nations Programme of Action From Rio*. Study it; underline and tab short passages you can quote; take it with you to the meeting if there is any suspicion that you will be dealing with U.N activists.

Mimicking the Tone (Not Substance) of U.S. Constitution

A major problem of trying to fend off Agenda 21—or, for that matter, any U.N. Declaration, Resolution or Proclamation—is that most people living today have not been taught anything about the makeup, background or core beliefs of that body, aside from the fact that it was created after World War II, ostensibly to promote and ensure world peace.

Most folks learned in school about the "model U.N.," as though that supersedes our Framers' model of a Legislative Branch—i.e., Congress. But, one of the down-sides of leftist incursions into our education system following the Second World War has been the careful avoidance by teachers of casting any world body in a negative light—be it the U.N., the World Federation on Mental Health, or something else. The Second World War, followed all too soon by the Korean War, served to shock Americans out of any complacency about the effect of world affairs upon the United States. That mind-set (and the Nuremburg Trials) made it easier to "sell" the idea of a transnational world entity, complete with its own policing agency that dispenses "global justice" above and beyond any rights enumerated in America's founding documents.

Consequently, when people read documents emanating from the U.N.—if, in fact, they *do* read them, *in their entirety* and with critical attention to detail—they appear, at first, to mimic the tone, of the U.S. Constitution and Bill of Rights. Each U.N. Declaration, Resolution or Proclamation is made to appear familiar on the surface, yet they are quite different on specifics, especially in matters relating to "individual" freedoms.

Universal Declaration on Human Rights (UDHR).- The UDHR is a primary example of a U.N. document penned to mimic our own Declaration of Independence. Thomas Jefferson's document espouses as a "moral truth" that "all Men are…endowed by their creator with certain unalienable Rights" including the "pursuit of Happiness." In 1776 this was considered a revolutionary idea—unheard of in the annals of government. But the U.N. steps beyond this in its UDHR by promoting the idea that government should somehow *guarantee* happiness, not just proclaim that people can pursue it.

Other substantive differences abound, despite the tone of the document:

- The right to bear arms -- UDHR has no right to bear arms.

329

- No double jeopardy under the law -- UDHR does not prohibit double jeopardy.
- Church-state separation -- UDHR promotes earth-worship "spirituality"
- Limited government -- UDHR has no limits on government.
- Guarantee that property cannot be taken by government without just compensation[221] -- UDHR has no such guarantee.

The UDHR reflects the United Nations' concept of justice, as noted in chapter 4 ("Justice in the Rear-View Mirror"), by replacing our action-based model of "equality before the law" with an *equity*-based model that hinges on parity and equality of social *outcomes*. This vision doesn't provide much "wiggle room" for *individual* freedom because the effect of equalizing social outcomes is to make as many people as possible "eligible" for some kind of government handout.

Agenda 21 Rejects American Ideals.- The U.N. aggressively stigmatizes the rugged individualism of frontiersmen like Davey Crockett and Andrew Jackson, the self-sufficiency, resourcefulness and self-reliance articulated in Benjamin Franklin's celebrated autobiography (as well as his *Poor Richard's Almanack*), and the self-determination deemed essential by Thomas Jefferson in the *Declaration of Independence*. The five values above contradict the Stalinesque view of "collective spirit" (which is purely political) and departs does not equate to Ben Franklin's reflections on "community spirit," which means "civic-mindedness" and presumes assimilation of immigrants.

In the U.N. worldview, attitudes like individualism, self-reliance, resourcefulness, self-sufficiency and self-determination, are considered markers of mental illness dangerous, if not social pathology. We have seen the results of this in the sudden emergence of "studies" in the 2000s aimed at discrediting these values as mental

---

[221] The U.S. slid closer to the U.N. position with the Supreme Court decision *Kelo v. New London* in 2005 and the EPA has repeatedly violated this individual property rights, as we shall see further on in at least two high-profile cases.

illnesses peculiar to political "conservatives" in an apparent effort to launch a new field directed toward preventive psychiatry: the 2005 NSF-NIMH "study," Chris Mooney, Robert McCrae, Arie Kruglanski, Robert Altemeyer, etc.

This outlook has completely penetrated U.S. government agencies. A humorous, but factually correct, article[222] by the inimitable Wesley Pruden (July 6, 2012), exemplifies the "new thinking." Pruden describes how "outreach workers" (another term for "operatives" and "change agents") at the U.S. Department of Agriculture's Supplemental Nutrition Assistance Program (a.k.a. the catchy acronym SNAP), have been working to root out cultural beliefs that oppose food stamps and other welfare benefits.

It seems that the "descendants of…[Scotch]-Irish settlers who pushed the frontier" and now inhabit the mountainous regions of some seven states still view it as an affront to their (and this nation's Founders') ethic of self-reliance to take public assistance, even if they are technically "eligible." The natives call it "mountain Pride." To that end, SNAP's organizers prepared a "tool kit" for their outreach staff to "counter myths…among those who…have beliefs that discourage them from enrolling."

Apparently, the SNAP workers were at least partially successful in their efforts to create the desired welfare mentality; they raised enrollments by 10 percent in just one year among this population using their "tool kit," which readers have probably surmised is another version of the manipulation and perception management strategies alluded to earlier.

The Earth Charter

The Earth Charter[223] is the backbone of the Agenda 21 science, ethics, and educational programs. The concept originated in 1987 along with the report "Our Common Future," alluded to earlier in this chapter, and was intended as a transitional guideline to sustainable development. In 1994, according to several sources, Maurice Strong

---

[222] http://www.washingtontimes.com/news/2012/jul/6/pruden-putting-us-all-on-the-dole/
223 (http://www.earthcharter.org/)

(founder of the Earth Council) and Mikhail Gorbachev (former president of the former Soviet Union and founder of Green Cross International), combined their efforts to get the Earth Charter on track as a "civil society" initiative. The Earth Charter, of course, reflects the U.N. policy. Briefly, the primary elements include:

- Earth worship (pantheism).
- Socialized medicine.
- World federalism.
- Income redistribution among nations and within nations.
- Information about contraception, all manner of sexual "gymnastics" and "reproductive health" rights for children, without regard to age-appropriateness.
- World-wide "education for sustainability" which means planned communities and citizens told where they must live.
- Debt "forgiveness" and different environmental standards for third-world nations.
- Elimination of any right to bear arms.
- Environmental extremist positions, including global warming and bans on all pesticides, including those that prevent malaria in third world countries.
- Setting aside "biosphere reserves" where no human presence is allowed, which means the government may come in and take land for its own higher purposes.

Policy Initiatives Under Sustainable Development

Wikipedia, like most texts that provide generic information on political topics, define Agenda 21 as "a program run by the United Nations related to sustainable development." A thorough reading of U.N.'s own texts reveals it is far from voluntary. As usual, there are carrots and sticks. Big sticks!

A long list of bills that have been introduced in Congress between 1987 and 2011 related specifically to "sustainable development" agenda items[224]. DeWeese details how foundations and government grants drive the process. The American Planning Association is just one of many operative groups that work to get local communities onboard. Others include the American Planning Council; the Renaissance Planning Group; the International City-County Management Group, aided by U.S. Mayors Conference; National League of Cities; National Association of County Administrators and (again!) the National Governors Association.

The sheer number of United Nations Association (UNA)-USA chapters throughout the U.S. is frightening in its sovereignty implications. (A state-by-state list[225] can be found appended to the National Association of Rural Landowners website.) The number, and kinds, of bills[226] enacted to institutionalize Agenda 21 is even more sobering (see highlighted sections at the site above), such as the World Environment Policy Act of 1989, sponsored by then-Senator Al Gore, global-warming alarmist-in-chief.

Fast-forward to 2011, with the State Department's Foreign Operations and Related Programs Appropriations Act, sponsored by the career politician, Sen. Patrick J. Leahy (D-VT); the Resolution the Official Designation of World Habitat Day, built around the theme of "Cities and Climate Change," compliments of Sen. John Kerry (D-MA); and others most people probably never heard of.

Sustainable development can be broken into four subcategories that account for most of the bills that either have already passed, or are still making their way through Congress, largely unknown and unchallenged by the public: the economy, natural resources, institutional changes and social changes. Here are a few of the slogans we hear often, but largely fail to place in the context of Agenda 21 or Sustainable Development:

- living wage
- comprehensive planning

---

[224] http://www.unausa.org/Page.aspx?pid=623
[225] http://www.unausa.org/Page.aspx?pid=623
[226] http://www.narlo.org/una21report.pdf

- affordable housing
- land-use patterns
- environmental equity

All these have origins in sustainable development jargon. A table on page 5[227] of the UNA-US document reveals the incredible level of detail and interconnectivity among the four categories—and Congress has signed on. The real losers, of course, are taxpayers, who have to fund this mess even as the U.S. experiences an economic downturn not seen since the Great Depression.

Rural landowners, in particular, are being hit with a disproportionate share of Agenda 21 policy restrictions, but as our style of government changes, so do all Americans' way of life, together with any hope for an upwardly mobile, peaceful future.

Biodiversity and Population Control

"Biodiversity is one of those terms that don't ring many bells with average taxpayers, except maybe inb the context of science fiction. But schoolchildren since the 1990s have been learning about *biodiversity* in their classrooms. The term translates to massive reduction of human populations, even though the original population scare, 1968 best-seller, *The Population Bomb*, by Stanford University Professor Paul R. Ehrlich and his wife, Anne Ehrlich has been discredited, even as the population stood at over 7 billion in August 2012, and the U.S. population at about 314 million.

When post-World War II Americans first saw pictures of starving children in Africa and other Third World populations in *National Geographic*, they heard proposals centered on population concerns. But they believed that the various suggestions were aimed at the typically large, and starving, families of 1940s-era China and sub-Saharan Africa. Even then, they didn't imagine "reductions" to mean forced abortions and sterilizations, one-child policies and infanticide.

---

227 http://www.narlo.org/una21report.pdf

Imagine their surprise to discover that such "reductions" were aimed at *them*—Americans.

Some proponents of Sustainable Development call for as much as an 85-percent reduction in human populations in order to "save the planet." David Brower of the Sierra Club said, *"Childbearing should be a punishable crime against society, unless the parents hold a government license."* The U.N.'s Biodiversity Assessment states: *"A reasonable estimate for an industrialized world society at the present North American material standard of living would be 1 billion."* So, that means some 6 billion lives fewer.

Many Americans more or less shrugged at these statements, if they heard them at all. They didn't pay attention to the further statement by Maurice Strong, head of the Earth Summit conference, who said: *"Isn't the only hope for the planet that the industrial nations collapse? Isn't it our responsibility to bring that about?*

Smart Growth: Dormitory-Style Living

Hidden among the various official documents of "sustainable development" (if you know where to look) is an agenda within an agenda: to make the price of single-family dwellings so expensive that all but a wealthy and "politically reliable" elite can afford it.

The concept of single-family residential neighborhoods, with automobiles and other big-ticket items, is considered wasteful, harmful to the environment, and not amenable to monitoring and surveillance by Sustainable Development advocates. Other factors are conservation, and increased the capability to impose energy "rationing."

Obviously, this belief is closely related to the hand-wringing over population. It also explains, in part, the reluctance to stem the deterioration of the nation's infrastructure, such as roads and power lines. If people want reliable power, water and transportation, maybe they will motivated to leave their neighborhoods for newer digs in "planned communities" and/or high-density urban metropolises.

The idea is for the population to forego their lawns, houses and garages for high-density living arrangements, where schools, public transportation and medical care are within walkable distance, public transportation, or at the very list, mini-cars.

This effort is known in Agenda 21 circles as "regional visioning projects" and "mega-regional zoning." That is why the terms "regional" and "zoning" are included in the APA Glossary's list of *verboten* terms when attempting to manipulate local community consensus for sustainable development objectives; some people have caught on to the buzz-terms.

An excellent book, *Eco-Tyranny*, by Brian Sussman, was recently published and is highly recommended here. He points to an internal document draft labeled "Not for Release" by the Department of the Interior, which places its Bureau of Land Management in a lead role in moving Americans toward large-city metrocomplexes that have easily accessed, mass-transportation stations to commute to work, grocery shopping, health services, and so on.

While such a concept obviously has its attractions for some people who like condominium-style arrangements, the American Dream (unlike in Europe) is built around the private land tract. The "mega-region" concept, on the other hand, is more on the order of a college dormitory with, maybe, a private kitchen and bath—what the British call "a flat."

If one is diligent, one can find documents showing the number of cities have signed on to "regionalization," or its more popular namesake, Smart Growth. Urban planners sloganized the phrase, "Smart Growth," to gain popular support for the creation of "livable communities." The National Governors Association put the concept under its "Best Practices" umbrella, the relevant document being "Regional Visioning Public Participation"[228].

Dr. Michael Coffman, president of Environmental Perspectives, Inc. [229], provides a reliable overview Smart Growth." He points out that government control over land-use has been part and parcel of socialist agendas everywhere. "But," cautions Coffman, "it creates the nightmares it is supposed to eliminate and subtly deprives urban

---

[228] http://www.sustainablepittsburgh.org/pdf/Regional_Visioning_Jan_05.pdf
[229] http://www.epi-us.com

residents of one of their property rights in the name of achieving economic equality and protecting the environment."

"Habitat" Concept Not So "Smart"

The idea for taking this concept to industrialized nations worldwide took shape in the early 1970s. Some of its anti-property rights features failed to gain support as proposed, so in 1976, at the Conference on Human Settlements (a.k.a. Habitat I), held in Vancouver, Canada, a working group came up with a slightly different angle. The Preamble of Agenda Item 10 of the 1976 Conference Report states:

> The provision of decent dwellings and healthy conditions for the people can only be achieved if land is used in the interests of society as a whole. Public control of land use is therefore indispensable...."

What Metroplex "Density" Really Entails.- The above statement jump-started a scheme built around "density," which, if rigorously followed, would eventually, according to a Heritage Foundation study, have most Americans living in areas that are 2.4 times denser than Manhattan in New York, or twice as dense as central Paris in France, or ten times the density of San Francisco, California.[230]

And that, according to Dr. Coffman, "is *after* the Sierra Club revised downward its definition of 'urban efficiency' to 100 housing units per acre, when critics complained that its original measurement of 500 housing units per acre would more than double the most squalid wards of Bombay, India!"

By comparison, the density of an average American suburb is between 1 and 3 units per acre. Dr. Coffman puts the scheme in context:

> Smart Growth advocates seek to preserve land in a natural...state by encouraging individuals to live in denser communities that take up smaller tracts of land per housing unit. Such communities encourage

---

[230] Ibid.

residents to rely more on walking or public transit than on cars for mobility, and they more closely mix retail and other commercial facilities with residential units to foster easy access to jobs and shopping.

...In order to plan and control growth in their enlightened way, government bureaucrats and planning advocates must control property rights. Private property rights and Smart Growth are therefore mutually exclusive.

Such policies do not permit Americans the freedom to live where they choose. They must live inside urban growth boundaries. Developers must provide open space around new development. Americans may not live in greenbelt areas around urban centers. They may not live in designated "viewsheds" of scenic highways, or in the buffer zone of a Heritage River or a designated stream.

Those advocating Smart Growth can become so obsessive they become irrational. For instance, on June 18, 2001, the Sierra Club [originally] defined "efficient urban density" as a city containing 500 housing units to the acre. Put another way, 500 families would have to live on an acre of land which is 209 x 209 feet! This would require a 14-story apartment building, if 36 very small 1,000 square-foot units (with hallways) occupied each floor! Increasing the apartment size to 1500 square feet would require a 21-story building!

Lest one imagine that legislators in America wouldn't take the idea very seriously (inasmuch as most of them in private land tracts, too) some 19 states already have growth-management laws or task forces. Even though Smart Growth has been grossly misrepresented in the media as a positive development, it is "Sustainable Development," writ large. Dozens of cities and counties have adopted urban growth boundaries to contain development and prevent the spread of urbanization to outlying and rural areas.

The Cost of Smart Growth to Taxpayers.- *Land-use zoning*, as it is termed, has had a devastating impact on the cost of land. Dr. Coffman points to a March 2002 study published by the Harvard Institute of Economic Research which showed early on how zoning artificially drove up the price of land. Everyone knows that the cost of a home ownership in California and New York is out-of-sight to the point where people no longer care to move there. Many businesses opted to open new offices elsewhere. In cities like San Francisco, Los Angeles, Anaheim, San Diego and New York City, "the difference in cost between an extra quarter-acre within the same lot, and a separate, buildable quarter-acre lot, is in the hundreds of thousands of dollars," says Dr. Coffman—a figure easily verifiable at any realty firm.

The Harvard study asserts that "only a small percentage of the value of the lot comes from an intrinsically high land price; the rest is due to restrictions on construction."

The Department of Housing and Urban Development (HUD) partially funded a 2002 report that is still the "bible" of the initiative here in America: "Growing Smart Legislative Guidebook: Model Statutes for Planning and the Management of Change."

The American Planning Association (APA), the aforementioned community-activist front group, is still using this guidebook. It hails the publication as "[t]he culmination of a seven-year research project. Growing Smart contains the next generation of model planning and zoning enabling legislation for the United States."

Readers of this chapter can purchase the updated, third edition on CD-ROM directly from the APA website[231]. It is advertised there as having "more than 500 pages of new information." At this writing, the site's right-hand sidebar features an ad for an online master's degree in Urban and Regional Planning, *with specialties in "Sustainability"* from the University of Florida. So, this plan is hiding in plain sight.

Major Political Parties Sign On to "Sustainability".-
It probably comes as something of a dilemma that the same man who, as governor of Massachusetts (2003-2007), balanced the budget every year of his administration without increasing taxes or increasing the state's debt, and turned a $3 billion budget deficit into a $500 million surplus, adding some 80,000 new jobs, would turn around and sign on to President Obama's "Partnership for Sustainable Communities." Unbelievably, he put the weight of both federal government and his Party firmly behind Smart Growth and "regional visioning."

---

[231] http://www.planning.org/growingsmart/

Mitt Romney pushed for Smart Growth policies in Massachusetts. In 2002, Romney actively fought sprawl and promoted density. In fact, he ran on a Smart Growth platform. He said: "Sprawl is the most important quality-of-life issue facing Massachusetts."

As reported in several news outlets, including a sustainable-development-friendly online publication, *Grist*[232], "Romney created a powerful new Office for Commonwealth Development, and appointed an aggressive environmental activist to run it—Douglas Foy." For 25 years, Foy had headed the Conservation Law Foundation, a litigious regional environmentalist group.

"The state's business community was appalled," wrote Lisa Hymas of *Grist*, which serves to substantiate Romney's tacit endorsement of the land-use facet of Agenda 21.

So, was Romney merely currying favor with internationalists? Did conservatives, Republican or Tea Party, ever address with Romney, especially during his 2012 presidential bid?

One answer is that some officials are consumed with other issues and not alarmed by the strength the U.N. influence over U.S. policymaking. They look at things like Smart Growth and global warming as "niche concerns"—important to a certain bloc of potentially helpful interest groups, but not a throw-away issue in the larger scheme of things. If Mitt Romney had "ticked off" every entity from the Wildlife Federation and the Sierra Club to front groups like the American Planning Association, his presidential candidacy would have been dead-in-the-water from the get-go, much like U.S. Rep. Ron Paul, who refuses to play these games. Agree with his positions or not, the reason why Ron Paul has been marginalized by his party and the media is solely his refusal to play agenda games. Consequently, he doesn't get to play in the "orchestra."

Romney was politically smart in pursuing Smart Growth in Massachusetts through *incentives* rather than through *regulation*, thereby deflecting attention from the link to sustainable development. Unlike Ron Paul, Romney was a governor, not just a U.S.

---

[232] http://grist.org/election-2012/romney-once-an-anti-sprawl-crusader-created-model-for-obama-smart-growth-program/

Representative, and he knew he had to play ball with the National governor's Association to some extent. It is hard to say whether Romney understands the full ramifications of the U.N.'s Sustainable Development scheme or not.

In any case, Romney's Agenda-21-friendly policy resulted in the Office for Commonwealth Development channeling hundreds of millions of dollars in state funds to cities and towns. The subsequent change in zoning rules allowed for more high-density housing and other Smart-Growth policies.

Global Warming on the Hot Seat

In 2007, the U.S. Supreme Court gave a virtual thumbs-up to the U.N.'s Intergovernmental Panel on Climate Change report that claimed human activity was warming the Earth and that environmental catastrophe was imminent. In *Massachusetts v. EPA*, the High Court ruled that the EPA was authorized to regulate carbon dioxide as a "pollutant," despite the well-known fact that the gas *is a naturally occurring chemical compound.* CO_2 is produced by every living, breathing human being and animal on the planet.

Then, three independent studies suddenly emerged showing that scientists were fairly sure that around 2020, sunspot activity would be lessening significantly. All the conditions for it were lining up. In layman's language, an active sun, devoid of sunspots, can produce cooling because solar flares are diminished. Technically, this condition is a "solar minimum." The last time it happened, scientists said, we had a "little Ice Age"[233].

Over a dozen scientists concurred that episodic sunspot activity lasting anywhere from 70 to 150 years is responsible for wild swings in weather on Earth, as well as on other planets within our solar system. This 70- to 150-year cycle has embedded within it several shorter-term, 11-year *solar cycles* ("mini-cycles," for lack of a better term), "that we all should have learned about in high school," said Dr. Michael Coffman.

---

[233] www.globalpost.com/dispatch/news/busines...spots-global-warming

Of course, given the school environment of the past 30 years, students probably *didn't* learn it. (They may even believe that the flatulence from cows contribute to global warming! Yes, that was really a theory; but it was supplanted at the July 6, 2012 Fourth International Conference on Climate Change, when "experts" insisted that "climate change" was stressing the cows!)

Still other studies started revealing that the correlation between increased levels of atmospheric carbon dioxide and rising temperatures didn't pan out. So, doomsayers who once thought that they had global warming "in the bag," had to abruptly switch the label to "Climate Change."

At that point, many scientific groups that didn't have any political axe to grind, and which had long harbored inconvenient misgivings about global-warming data, seized upon the term "human-caused." Okay, they said, maybe the climate is cycling back and forth; but even if it is, do climate variances have anything to do with human beings?

It turned out there were more non-concurring scientists on the issue of global warming than most people thought. When multiple scandals suddenly came to light in 2009, showing that various entities had either "doctored" their pro-global-warming data or had sent e-mails to one another alleging they had been pressured into skewing their conclusions to satisfy a political agenda, the entire house of cards began tumbling down: first Climategate, then Glaciergate, followed by Rainforestgate, Pachaurigate, and NASAgate. Even the ultra-liberal Supreme Court Justice Ruth Bader Ginsburg was moved to back off the Court's 2007 decision. She hedged her bets in *American Electric Power v. Connecticut* on June 20, 2011, by stating for the record that "[t]he Court...endorses no particular view of the complicated issues related to carbon dioxide emissions and climate change."

Steve Milloy[234]—an expert with two masters degrees, a doctorate and two highly acclaimed books on the subject (*Green Hell* and *Junk Science Judo*)—cheered both the Supreme Court's decision in that

---

[234] http://www.junkscience.com

case and Justice Ginsburg's comment. He declared that environmental activist-extremists would no longer be able to "claim that the Supreme Court has validated the science of climate alarmism and [order] the EPA to regulate greenhouse gases."

Even the U.N.'s Intergovernmental Panel seemed to back off its human-activity-based stance in a Special Report released March 28, 2012, stating: "There is medium evidence and high agreement that long-term trends in normalized [property] losses have not been attributed to natural or anthropogenic [human-influenced] climate change."

The final nail in the coffin seemed to come the same day, when 50 scientists and astronauts penned a letter to NASA Administrator Charles Bolden, Jr., to:

...respectfully request that NASA and the Goddard Institute for Space Studies (GISS) refrain from including unproven remarks in public releases and websites. We believe the claims by NASA and GISS, that man-made carbon dioxide is having a catastrophic impact on global climate change, are not substantiated, especially when considering thousands of years of empirical data.

With hundreds of well-known climate scientists and tens of thousands of other scientists publicly declaring their disbelief in the catastrophic forecasts, coming particularly from the GISS leadership, it is clear that the science is NOT settled.

The unbridled advocacy of CO_2 being the major cause of climate change is unbecoming of NASA's history of making an objective assessment of all available scientific data prior to making decisions or public statements.

As former NASA employees, we feel that NASA's advocacy of an extreme position, prior to a thorough study of the possible overwhelming impact of natural climate drivers is inappropriate. We request that NASA refrain from including unproven and unsupported remarks in its future releases and websites on this subject. At risk is damage to the exemplary reputation of NASA, NASA's current or former scientists and employees, and even the reputation of science itself.

All 50 signed the letter, and further recommended known professionals within the close-knit scientific community that Bolden might contact to expand upon the signatories' position. They wondered if the EPA would change its website to reflect this re-assessment.

It didn't.

Disappointingly, just three months later, the U.S. Court of Appeals in Washington, D.C., ruled[235] that the EPA was "unambiguously correct" in applying the Clean Air Act to combat carbon dioxide!

The Appeals Court had essentially harkened back to the Supreme Court's 2007 ruling, which deferred to political correctness in supporting the EPA's intransigent position on global warming, despite evidence to the contrary.

So, who is having difficulty "processing reality" now? Who is expressing the "dogmatism," "mental rigidity," "fear," and "decreased cognitive function," so artfully characterized as faulty hard-wiring by Chris Mooney's book, *The Republican Brain*? Whose turn is it to be smeared as "mentally unbalanced"?

Different Studies, Different Data

Global-warming theory is based on the argument that mankind's overuse of fossil fuels has resulted in a combustion effect, in which carbon dioxide is released in excess, trapping the sun's energy in the atmosphere, and resulting in a so-called "greenhouse effect." Anyone who has ever been inside a greenhouse knows that it just keeps getting warmer inside—which is fine for some plants, but not so great for humans. Using this model, rising temperatures worldwide eventually would cripple the planet's ecosystem.

Unfortunately for global-warming activists, their computer model failed to take in a complete range of data. A June 15, 2011, *Los Angeles Times* article explains how sunspots "are caused by pockets

---

[235] http://www.washingtontimes.com/news/2012/jul/5/court-decrees-global-warming/

of intense magnetic activity that disrupt the normal circulation of heated gases on the sun's surface, leading to areas of cooling[236]."

In recent decades, researchers have been using sunspots to track the sun's magnetic highs and lows[237]: "When there are very few sunspots, solar flares, and coronal mass ejections, the earth cools. In the case of the 'little Ice Age'," says Dr. Michael Coffman, "the 3-degree Celsius cooling period caused the Thames River and the Holland canals to freeze over every year."

Moreover, global cooling is much more dangerous to humanity than global warming, he says—a point absent from most discussions on the subject.

But, neither global warming nor global cooling has anything to do with human activity. Taken together, the studies showing the temperatures vis-à-vis carbon dioxide are seriously out of whack, calling into question not only the whole dogma of global warming per se, but even the capability of human beings to produce any effect at all upon climate.

Thus did man-made climate change begin to look increasingly foolish—with ulterior motives galore. Global-warming alarmists seemed to be selling hysteria.

An Intransigent, Irrational EPA

Fast-forward again to the last week of June 2012. Because everyone was awaiting the decision on ObamaCare with bated breath, few followed the case against the EPA brought by the Coalition for Responsible Regulation,[238] which is composed of industry organizations and several states. The group had sued the EPA, arguing that the 2009 imposition of ever-more-stringent air-quality regulations had relied on highly questionable scientific evidence and, in the process, damaged economic growth.

---

[236] http://www.gazettenet.com/2011/06/16/researchers-foresee-weaker-sunspot-cycle

[237] http://news.nationalgeographic.com/news/2011/06/110614-sun-hibernation-solar-cycle-sunspots-space-science/

[238] http://www.washingtontimes.com/topics/coalition-for-responsible-regulation/

In attempting to quell growing resistance to global-warming dogma in the wake of the series of Climategate scandals, the EPA had again insisted that greenhouse gases posed a danger to human health. The EPA wanted to buy time for Barack Obama and the rest of his administrative agencies to craft legislation (some version of "Cap and Trade," or possibly a carbon tax) that would both satisfy Agenda 21 goals and make it difficult or impossible for individuals and groups to challenge regulations or taxes on activities related to global warming.

The June 26, 2012, Appeals Court ruling: "This is how science works. EPA is not required to re-prove the existence of the atom every time it approaches a scientific question."

Really?

U.S. Rep. Ralph Hall (R-TX and former Democrat) is chairman of the House Committee on Science, Space and Technology. In 2012, he was interviewed by Brett M. Decker, editorial page editor of the *Washington Times*, in which he characterized the EPA as an "out-of-control agency" with an "unscientific attitude." He castigated the EPA for its lack of transparency, its "anti-fossil-fuel policies," its contradictory energy rhetoric, its utilization of "secret data," and its conflicts of interest in procuring "supposedly independent advisory panels [comprised of] members who are EPA grant recipients." With all that, if Rep. Hall can't cause an investigation and shutdown of the EPA, nobody can—save a national uprising.

Eventually, the U.S. Supreme Court will have no choice but to make a determination on this issue. But, as we have seen with ObamaCare, the socialist-left has managed to prevail, regardless of whether individual Justices choose to be tagged as left-of-center or right-of-center. Issues of constitutionality are being bypassed.

An Embarrassing "Apology

Because people tend not to connect the dots between news stories that are written more than two weeks apart, most Americans didn't realize that this intransigence on the part of the EPA could affect the campaign of Republican nominee, Mitt Romney, who ill-advisedly released his memoir, *No Apology: The Case for American Greatness*, in 2010 to boost his then-fledgling presidential bid. In it, he stated:

> I believe that climate change is occurring—the reduction in the size of global ice caps is hard to ignore. I also believe that human activity is a contributing factor. Scientists are nearly unanimous in laying the blame for rising temperatures on greenhouse gas emissions.

Alas, Mr. Romney may end up wishing he could apologize for the comment, as it brought kudos from Al Gore.

Case Studies in Property Rights Abuses

Smart Growth may still be a work-in-progress, but a now completely unbridled (if not "unhinged") EPA is pressuring state regulators to locate landowners and homeowners they can intimidate into abandoning their property rights in the face of some obscure regulation that requires huge court costs to fight. The following case studies are powerful, each more outrageous than the one before it, and unprecedented in the nation's history.

If this is what Americans can now expect from government agencies adopting SS tactics in a random effort to score "points" with Agenda 21's international bigwigs, the country has more to worry about than falling off the financial "cliff."

Before we begin, let's review exactly how the game is played: ***Start small, using several "trial balloons" to gauge the level of resistance; then once a gambit works, cite it as a "precedent."*** Got it?

In this first one, *Sackett v. EPA*, the EPA overplayed its hand. It didn't figure on the notoriety that took the case all the way to the U.S. Supreme Court, and lost (thankfully) on March 21, 2012.

Case Study I: EPA Gets Doused in Wetlands Scandal.-

The high-profile case of Michael and Chantell Sackett of Bonner County, Idaho, began when the EPA delivered a "compliance order" to the Sacketts. It demanded that they renovate their entire site so as to meet the standards of EPA's so-called Restoration Work Plan, or pay a fine of as much as $75,000 per day! Of course, no normal couple could possibly afford that!

The EPA effectively seized Mike and Chantell Sackett's Idaho land and ordered them to stop building a house on the half-acre lot, *even though it was already zoned for residential use and situated between other houses in a suburban neighborhood, complete with a sewer hookup*. The reason? The EPA decided, *after* their purchase, that the lot was a federally designated wetland and in violation of the Clean Water Act[239]!

Then the Sacketts were told that the EPA's special-permit application would cost some $200,000—*more than the value of the property*. Their rebuffed efforts to challenge "compliance" requirements in court put the total cost into the stratosphere.The EPA even went so far as to deny the Sacketts a hearing.

The always outrageous 9th Circuit Court of Appeals (pejoratively referred to as the "Circus Court" for its goofy determinations over the years), happened to cover the Sackett's part of the country, and it rejected their plea for a review. The Sackett's rightfully filed on the basis of their Fifth Amendment rights, relating to denial of life, liberty or property without due process.

In the four-year legal tug-of-war, The Sackett's attorney, Damien Schiff, said, "Charging property owners a sky-high admissions fee [merely] to get into court isn't just wrong, it's flat-out unconstitutional."

Fortunately, the High Court agreed—this time.

Case Study II: A Foiled Attempt to Incite Hysteria.- This case started when the Florida Department of Environmental Protection (FDEP) a draft proposal on May 24, 2012, to impose ridiculously strict mercury limitations on Florida's rivers, lakes, streams and coastal waters. The proposed new rules would not only have raised electricity costs enormously for Florida's citizens, but would have harmed human health.

---

239 (http://www.washingtontimes.com/news/2011/ jun/28/couples-case-against-epa-to-be-heard/)

What the FDEP didn't count on was renowned scientist, Dr. Willie Wei-Hock Soon.

Willie Soon is a geoscientist and astrophysicist at the Solar and Stellar Physics Division at the Harvard-Smithsonian Center for Astrophysics—hard to ignore that! In addition to his other scientific research, Dr. Soon had, coincidentally, spent a decade studying the effect of mercury (and its toxic form, methylmercury) on the environment and human health. Thus, he was exactly the right person, in the right place, at the right time to challenge the FDEP. His investigative piece on this, the FDEP's seditious attempt to limit in water rights and compromise the fishing industry, appeared in the *Washington Times*, *Science and Public Policy*, *Canada Free Press* and the *Wall Street Journal Online* (the latter with columnist Paul Driessen). These articles exemplify the lengths to which environmental extremists will go for the purpose of satisfying a price-gouging, leftist agenda.

Without getting into too many scientific technicalities, the FDEP's first mistake, according to Dr. Soon, was to claim that that "mercury pollution is a new, man-made phenomenon." It's not.

The agency's second error was its failure to take into account "studies that found no significant increase in mercury levels for tuna caught between 1971 and 1998, demonstrating that mercury in fish is not related to human emissions," which was the connection the FDEP was hoping to make here.

A third mistake was ignoring "a 17-year-long...study that found no harm from mercury in children whose mothers [had eaten] five to 12 servings of fish per week—far more than most Floridians consume." In fact, Dr. Soon (and any medical doctor worth his salt) knew that it had long since been established that prenatal consumption of ocean fish is *beneficial* to a developing fetus. So, scaring pregnant women into *avoiding* fish would harm their health—especially given that the fish Florida women would be eating were already well below the *federal* EPA's own "safe" limits for mercury.

Fourth, the FDEP based their proposal on the false assumption "that mercury levels in water are directly related to mercury levels in fish tissue." Wrong again.

Moreover, mercury pollution had not increased in either Florida's waters or its fish. Even if one could eliminate mercury from every natural and man-made source, wrote Dr. Soon, it "would bring trifling environmental and health benefits—[but would raise] electricity rates for the state's families, retirees, schools, hospitals and businesses...."

Well, of course, raising utility rates—the real motive behind launching such a ridiculous proposal in the first place!

Case Study III: Troubled Waters.- Any debate over water rights may come as news to East Coast residents, and indeed to most folks east of the Mississippi River. But states like Montana, Colorado, Nevada, Arizona and Oregon, to mention just a few, are under the government boot—with the rest of America too taken up with other concerns to notice their plight. Montana, for example, was sending out this SOS in 2012:

**HUMANS SIMPLY CANNOT CARRY ON
NORMAL LIFE WITHOUT WATER.
ITS OWNERSHIP, CONTROL AND
MANAGEMENT IS NOW IN TRANSITION**.

If one goes to websites such as SmartPlanet, the arguments from the "sustainable development" faction become a bit clearer—if disquieting. In an October 28, 2010, piece, online journalist Andrew Nusca gets a discussion going among several heads of organizations that reveals some interesting rationales:

Some believe that water should not be a question of ownership at all, with its distribution and management being through government regulation. Among this faction, there are those who think there should be a price on water. But others disagree—especially when it comes to water that has been "treated," to make it drinkable.

Then there are strict environmentalists like ITT[240] senior vice president Gretchen McClain, who claims say there is a larger, "global

---

[240] ITT is a diversified manufacturing firm specializing in global energy infrastructure markets.

issue"—and that "water usage needs to be reduced." Inevitably, that brings up some degree of rationing.

Pacific Institute (PI)[241] president Peter Gleick pointed to California's state constitution, where water use is based on its being "reasonable and beneficial"; meaning that, as SmartPlanet journalist Mr. Nusca understood it, if you don't have a good reason, you can't use it.

In Nusca's SmartPlanet discussion forum, Gleick said: "So take a farmer growing four acres. If they can grow it in three, that last acre is not reasonable. [The issue of] rights is unresolved, and it's wrapped up in this public-private question."

So, Gleick is on the environmental-extremist side of the policy question, implying that government gets to decide how much water is "reasonable" for a framer. This is completely in line with Agenda 21 thinking.

But then a surprise statement: former Arizona governor and World Wildlife Fund trustee Bruce Babbitt declared that "global water crisis" was merely "Leninist history." He said the "relentless talk" of a crisis was, in effect, scaremongering.

"There is no lack of water on this globe," he said. "There is not a water supply crisis. Water is a renewable resource. There are some distributional issues, yes. But we're not going to make any progress buying into this notion [of water crisis]."

To Babbitt, if there was a global aspect, the real issue there was sanitation and accessibility in the Third World.

Unfortunately, that has little to do with water rights Montana and Colorado—yet somehow the EPA has managed to draw them into the global policy debate.

This is where the water gets, um, cloudy—the issue, that is:

"Montanans Water Permits Get Redirected to Indian Tribes" announced one headline. Clarice Ryan, columnist and a director of

---

[241] Pacific Institute's website describes the organization as being heavily into "environmental protection," "social equity" and "social and political change." Readers already recognize "social equity" as part of the U.N. concept of "Justice." So, it should come as no surprise that PI worked with the U.N. Global Compact to release the publication "Water as a Casualty of Conflict" and advocates central planning, management and operation of water systems.

<u>Montanans For Multiple Use</u> has taken this, and other, topics to clueless audiences nationwide.

In Montana, among other states, she says, the *uses* of water are not only under debate, but the *quantity to be made available* as well. Ryan alleges that State regulators, in collusion with federal, and (all of a sudden) Indian Tribes, have produced rulings that will have profound, long-term impacts on the state and local economy, as well as on citizen activities and livelihoods in western region of Montana. If so, the impact on ownership rights, irrigation and distribution is criminal.

Ryan reported on July 9, 2012, that a Water Compact was being negotiated between the federal government and the State of Montana, including indigenous Indian tribes. It contained a huge "gotcha." It seems that not just *part*, but *all* irrigation rights were stipulated as being "held in trust" by the federal government *on behalf of* the Indian Tribe in question, making the Tribe—not the bulk of western Montana citizens—the senior rights holder.

This meant that out of nowhere an Indian Tribe—more or less an anachronism as far as the rest of the nation is concerned, which is why most media outlets didn't pick up on the story—was about to receive the authority to approve or deny permits for everybody's ground wells! The Tribe would also reserve the right to meter the wells, thus directly affecting land values in a large swath where a majority of Montanans live and work their ranches. In the end, all residents of Montana would be affected, because the State, in collusion with the federal government, was pledging water rights to *off-reservation* water, which affects at least eight major waterways and their tributaries.

So, in July 2012 an emergency meeting was called for well owners, irrigators and other citizens, in advance of the Flathead (County) Joint Board of Control meeting. What these citizens decided may well seal residents' fate, adversely affecting farming, ranching and tourism statewide.

Tourism?

For those unacquainted with that part of the country, places like Hungry Horse is built around a beautiful body of water, Glacier Park, and is a favorite vacation destination.

Why should the rest of the country care about this? Because inevitably, this will affect not only your travel plans, but your food prices, and maybe even where the foods you eat come from. Government may prefer that all your fruits and vegetables come from Mexico, or some other country, under the cover of boosting a struggling nations' economy instead of our own.

Of course, this is the same government that howls about local citizens supplementing their diet (especially their children's diet) with lots of locally grown fruits and vegetables. The trick is *locating* "locally grown" products. Read the labels on the little plastic cartons of fruit sold in your grocery store chains: They say "Product of Mexico," or Canada, Argentina, Bolivia and only occasionally, the "USA"—which may mean clear across the country from wherever you live. Floridians may grow enough fruit to feed the East Coast—but chains will buy from Watsonville, California. ***That's global planning in action.*** And the same logic applies to water rights.

Montana is hardly alone. "Government Shuts off Water Pumps in South Platte River Basin, Colorado" is another case most of the country missed.

Here, a Colorado judge had effectively shut down the wells (i.e., pumping) in 2006, claiming that "depletions were harming lower-end users." He was referring to allegedly unprecedented (called "non-historic") drying and flooding along the South Platte River Basin.

But, there was nothing exceptional about such oscillations—until two Colorado governors decided to pull a fast one. Having the river go dry past the town of Greeley is normal (i.e., "historic"), not unprecedented (or, "non-historic").

But Governor Bill Owens signed the South Platte Recovery Act in 2006, which *gave away* approximately 40,000 acre feet water that *crossed the border* all the way to North Platte, Nebraska, *ostensibly to accommodate the Endangered Species Act.*

Turned out, this effort was initiated by Owens' predecessor, three-term governor Gov. Roy Romer (1987-1999). Thus, both governors were complicit in committing a state asset (i.e., water) and making a financial commitment without a vote of its Colorado citizenry.

In committing this water to the South Platte River Implementation Recovery Program, a tri-state Colorado-Nebraska-Wyoming agreement emerged. So, instead of a state matter, it was now a multiple-state arrangement, which brought Colorado ranchers' and farmers' water rights under the auspices of—guess what?—the Commerce Clause. That, of course, constitutes an entrée for the federal government.

As we have seen with ObamaCare (chapter 2), the Commerce Clause was used to take a state issue to the federal level—an action that dovetails with the goals of Agenda 21: namely, to federalize as many state and local issues as possible.

Readers will recall the role and influence of the National Governors Association (chapter 7): that *State governors are the go-to persons for federal agency heads anxious to implement specific legislation nationwide.* So, in this case, we have not one, but two, Colorado governors who set up this agreement, with just enough years elapsing between the original initiative by Gov. Romer and the actual signed agreement by Gov. Owens to deflect attention from individual rights—unless one happened to live north and west of Denver!

On July 2, 2012, Land and Water USA, (a.k.a LAW USA[242]) challenged the Agreement. The action by the Governor Owens, critics claimed, essentially violated the Colorado Constitution. State's rights are slowly being obliterated by the federal government, because they stand in the way of federal objectives.

The federal government does not own water. The States own water. The only way the federal government can obtain water is by purchasing from what are called "Decree Owners." These ownership rights date back to the 1860s. Everyone in that part of the country understand that it is in everyone's interests—Senior Owners and (latecomers, by date) Junior Holders—to take up the slack whenever a

---

[242]   http://www.LandAndWaterUSA.com

water property goes dry—an arrangement that it has worked well for 140 years.

Now, with the two Governors tri-state shenanigans, water took the river from historic *intra*state into non-historic *inter*state status— not only inviting clueless federal oversight under the Commerce Clause, but altering water-level trends in ways they never were before. All to satisfy some obscure passage in the Endangered Species Act.

Heretofore unheard-of technical problems were encountered— having mostly to do with growing seasons, and ensuring that lower-end users do not suffer harm—all initiated by government meddling. Solving them, of course, would be left to federal bureaucracies that are totally out of their element and cannot relate even to the key terms used by old, experienced hands.

So, LAW USA petitioned the Governor to withdraw from the South Platte River Implementation Recovery and re-start the pumping of the wells. Once well pumping is re-activated, any "non-historic flooding and drying" along Colorado's South Platte River Basin would be resolved, and life would get back to normal for everyone.

Unfortunately, as we shall see in the following case—worst-case scenarios, by any measure—once federal agencies get involved, they stay, refuse to learn anything and wreak havoc.

Case Study IV: It "Couldn't Happen in America"

There is no improvement this author could make to the following case, written up as a book by the victim, Wayne Hage, *Storm Over Rangelands*[243], and reported by Dr. Michael Coffman in *Range Magazine* (complete story at[244]). For corruption of justice and outright viciousness of U.S. government agencies, this case has no match.

Wayne and Jean Hage purchased Pine Creek Ranch (northern Nye County, central Nevada), in 1978. Confrontations began in 1979, when a self-important U.S. Forest Service took it upon itself to fence off a major spring from the Hages' cattle and pipe their water into the

---

[243] http://www.amazon.com/Storm-over-Rangelands-Private-Federal/dp/0939571153
[244] http://www.rescuingamericabook.com/opeds/federal_landlord3.pdf

federal ranger station without permission. Over some 105 days, the couple received 70 visits and 40 certified letters from the Forest Service citing various violations, most of which either did not exist at all or were created by the Forest Service out of thin air. One involved maintenance of the drift fences on Table Mountain.

After two days riding the fence [by horse], one of the Hages' hands found the Forest Service flag marking a single missing staple. They also charged the Hages with trespass citations, where they cattle were in forbidden locations. They dropped these charges once they realized the Hages had eyewitnesses watching Forest Service employees *move our cattle into these areas* within hours notifying the couple of the alleged offense.

From there it got worse—much worse.

The short version is that the federal government spent 18 years harassing Wayne and Jean Hage via operatives at the Bureau of Land Management and the U.S. Forest Service over trifling or nonexistent regulations, egged on by several major environmental organizations. Among other outrages, the government sent 30 staff armed with semi-automatic rifles and bullet-proof vests to attack (literally) their ranch; physically killed their a cow, thanks to sheer incompetence, by running it to death; put the Hages out of business due various permit delays, suspensions and cancellations; inundated the Hages with court costs.

"Even when the government had driven the Hages were out of business in 1991, the federal Gestapo did not let up," wrote Dr. Coffman in his article for *Ranger Magazine*.

In a tremendous victory for American landowners, and a staggering defeat for the environmentalists' agenda, a court found in *Hage v. United States*[245] [that] "the property rights owned by Hage were pre-existing ... by the Act of 1866.... The Hages owned the water rights and all their improvements."

Finally, on Aug. 2, 2010, 18 years[246] after it was started, Claims Court Judge Loren Smith awarded[247] the Hage estate $14,240,853.92

[245] http://caselaw.lp.findlaw.com/data2/circs/fedclaim/2008/911470lp.pdf
[246] http://americanstewards.us/about-us/historical-victories/hage-v-united-states/briefs-and-opinions/final-decision-aug-2-2010

and ruled the federal agencies must pay all legal fees. (By then, the Hages were dead.)

This was the first time a federal agency had been taken to the United States Court of Federal Claims on the grazing and water right issue, says their daughter, Margaret Hage-Byfield.

Predictably, with every win for the Hages, a new round of harassment would begin, resulting in criminal charges against BLM and the Forest Service.

The case is too long to go into further in this book, but it is not too long for a magazine article. The reader is strongly urged to read the story in its entirety (and its various twists and turns, see footnotes) to fully comprehend just one fact: *the level of retribution that rains down from environmentally aligned government entities, even whenever they lose.* Unbelievably, the case is still being pursued by the feds, says daughter Margaret Hage-Byfield.

You won't find anything closer to the old German Gestapo than this. The enviro-extremists, led by the EPA at the behest of Agenda 21 and its toady organizations here in America, don't take kindly to losing—and our nation's leaders are either too distracted, or just plain out of their league, like U.S. Rep. Ralph Hall (R-TX), chairman of the House Committee on Science, Space and Technology (whom we met through a Washington times interview earlier in the chapter), to forcefully put a stop to it.

This case is so crucial that ever since the publication in 1989 of the late Wayne Hage's book, *Storm over Rangeland*, judges and lawyers have used arguments in the book in court cases. The federal agencies were not pleased with the book.

Conservation Easements

Water rights aren't the only thing baffling to East-Coasters. Most also have no idea what a Conservation Easement is, the concept affecting them personally. Merging the definition in Wikipedia with other sources, a "conservation easement" (a.k.a. *conservation*

---

[247] http://americanstewards.us/news-publications/archives/liberty-matters/2010/lmaug4/hage-v-us-moves-to-the-next-round

covenant or *conservation restriction*) is a legal liability on property which, in this case, includes a transfer of usage rights. It entails a legally enforceable land preservation agreement between a landowner and a government agency (i.e., a municipality, county, state, federal) <u>or</u> a qualified **land protection organization** (that is, a second party), ostensibly for the purpose of conservation.

The decision to place a conservation "easement" (i.e., "land trust") on a property is supposed to be voluntary. The land, including any structures on it, is donated. But the restrictions of the easement, once set in place are legally binding.

Again, Montana columnist and speaker Clarice Ryan explains, for the uninitiated, the incredibly fraudulent nature of this scheme, which is linked to "sustainable development." The following September 16, 2009, column for Canada Free Press[248], below, is excerpted with punctuation changes added for clarity:

> Unsuspecting landowners, especially in rural areas, are led to believe they are helping…environmental efforts, while obtaining in return personal financial benefits and security. In some cases, there is a public recognition program via a Certificate of Appreciation or notice in the media "for a person's noble, unselfish 'contribution'."

Unknowingly, writes Ryan, the landowner-donor essentially becomes a victim "of legalized fraud."

Meanwhile, non-governmental organizations—for example, the aforementioned Nature Conservancy, with its close ties to "sustainable development" and Agenda 21—can "become wealthy in the billions," says Ryan, while "the land [that] innocent victims have committed in perpetuity is doomed to *federal* ownership."

Ryan's explanation here serves as a warning to anyone being approached about a "conservation easement contract." A landowner's signature, states Ryan, will, in essence:

> …be releasing to a "land trust," the controlled "use" of the land and development rights, while you retain title to the "land" and remain

---

[248] http://www.canadafreepress.com/index.php/article/14768

responsible for all costs of ownership—FOREVER. It will be virtually impossible for you, your heirs or a purchaser, regardless of circumstance, to over-ride this contract agreement.

Differences of opinion with the "land trust" concerning interpretation of contract terms may eventually lead you to seek court settlement. Unfortunately you, the owner of the land, are committed to bearing all court costs if you lose, which in all likelihood you will. Furthermore, they can take you to court if they decide you are not adequately meeting contract obligations. You will bear all legal costs, including their high-priced attorneys. And if your current friendly land trust shows too much leniency, another more demanding third party agency can step in, take over and rule with a firmer hand, [typically] in the interests of "the environment."

For various reasons…, you or your heirs may attempt to sell all or part of the property. [But] the contract prevents dividing or selling off portions….

By law, the conservation easement can only be extinguished when the entity holding the easement (the land trust) becomes the full owner of the property, both the land [itself] and its controlled use. The friendly land trust will probably be happy to purchase your land at the greatly reduced value. However, once purchased, and with the easement restriction removed, this non-profit, non-taxpaying land trust is legally free to resell at [the] high market value of [any] adjoining property. Or [the "land trust"] can develop subdivisions; perform timber harvests, [run] lumber mills, mining [operations] …— at a profit.

All of this, of course, is in direct conflict with your original noble intent when you donated the conservation easement. Sadly the idealistic, worthy causes you had envisioned through the land trust—environmental protection, preserve for wildlife, a bulwark against urban sprawl—will no longer exist, except as they may be initiated and enforced *by environmental agencies at your expense.*

The War Against Energy Independence

Brian Sussman, author of *Climategate* and most recently, *Eco-Tyranny*, is by no means alone in pointing out that there is no reason whatsoever why the U.S. should be dependent upon the Middle East (specifically, the Organization of Petroleum Exporting Countries, or OPEC) for its energy needs. We have more than enough resources to do the job. It's amazing, in fact, that Americans have allowed its educators and legislators to hijack the enormous technological capability of our fossil fuel industry on the basis of preposterous climate change scenarios and wildly exaggerated pollution scares. Our "progressive" liberals are anti-progress, anti-technology, anti-growth and anti-science.

Thus, do existing oil wells stand abandoned and natural gas deposits go unexploited. The U.S. has one of the largest oil reserves in the world, but we hardly hear a peep about it.

American Policy Center president, Tom DeWeese, cites statistics showing that even before the June 29 reinstituted moratorium announcement, some "*67 percent of our oil reserves and 40 percent of our natural gas reserves are locked away on federal lands in America's western states.* Yet, so conditioned have Americans become from years of government propaganda, they have become irrational."

For every oil spill and mine explosion, America has hundreds of VIPs (Very Intelligent People) in fields like robotics, engineering and geology to avert these tragedies if it weren't for the politically correct carrot of "green energy" alternatives that provide, at best, only about 1 percent of our energy needs.

Eradicating the Fossil Fuel Industry

In 2008, we got a president who campaigned on an "all-of-the-above" energy platform. Then he colluded with Interior Secretary, Kenneth L. Salazar, to restrict as much as possible any access to offshore oil and gas resources. Throughout Mr. Obama's presidency, he has rebuffed even some among his own Party, who supported efforts to open America's enormous offshore resources for energy development. On June 29, 2012, sneaking it in the day following the Supreme Court's onerous ObamaCare decision, the Administration announced that it would re-institute the 30-year moratorium on offshore energy exploration. That meant cutting off access to a whopping 98 percent of U.S. energy potential on the region known as the Outer Continental Shelf (OCS).

One accident (the 2010 Deepwater Horizon oil spill) in the Gulf, caused by failure of government to oversee its own safety regulations, resulted in a complete ban on pursuing America's vast off-shore supply. British Petroleum, which by then had merged with Amoco and acquired both ARCO and Burma Castrol, had had safety issues in the past. But, as punishment for this large spill off our coast, it was coerced into publicly acknowledging phony climate change and establish target dates for reducing emissions of greenhouse gases—as if that had anything to do with the accident.

We have seen this game before: diversion. Mr. Obama knew BP's money and time would have been better spent correcting the actual cause of the Horizon explosion, but that wasn't his agenda.

The Institute for Energy Research's Senior Vice President Dan Kish released a statement responding to the continued moratorium:

"President Obama's offshore charade continues today with the formal announcement of the 2012-2017 leasing plan for the outer continental shelf. With this plan, the administration reinstitutes the 27-year moratorium that was lifted in 2008, and turns its back on potentially enormous energy resources that could provide jobs and energy security for America....

"The president has cancelled lease sales, delayed others, and imposed a unilateral executive embargo on the oil resources that our most promising public lands could provide. With 98 percent of the U.S. offshore [areas] currently unleased for energy exploration, Secretary Salazar has finalized this plan to continue the administration's war against affordable energy. In the end, Americans will pay more for the energy they need.

Even during the Carter administration, when the initial oil crisis created angry gas lines throughout America, Congress was prevailed upon to create a series of five-year plans that allowed for a regularly scheduled release for the sale of gas and oil to meet consumers' expectations. But the EPA and its Agenda 21 allies were not as powerful as they are today, and the U.N. had not yet advanced its disingenuous global-warming hysteria. In fact, that was when experts were first predicting the Earth's cooling![249]

Declaring moratoriums is not going to make an innovative breakthrough happen any sooner, nor will such any such breakthrough, when it does come, necessarily be "ready for prime time" when needed.

Meanwhile, nearly every month there is one or more new instances fighting fossil fuel development at the state level, complimenting those at the federal level. For example, in Maryland in 2012, the Sierra Club fought the exploitation of booming natural gas supplies at Cove Point, Maryland. Ben Wolfgang reported in the *Washington Times* on the effort to halt construction of a combination natural-gas-liquefaction and export facility by Dominion, an "industry giant."

The reason? To change "the footprint" of Cove Point.

"Fracking" Technology

About the same time, in Ohio, geologists claimed that hydraulic fracturing, or "fracking," is causing tiny earthquakes—a claim that has not been substantiated via properly replicated studies. Other environmentalist extremists allege contamination of ground water, risks to air quality, the migration of gases and chemicals to surface areas, and health hazards from all of the above—again unproven in replication studies.

Most people are unfamiliar with the term "fracking"—unless they were fans of the hit science fiction series *Battlestar Galactica*, in which case they think it is a futuristic curse word. The process of fracking extracts natural gas from shale rock layers deep within the earth. This releases petroleum, natural gas (including shale gas, tight gas and coal seam gas)—vast amounts that were formerly inaccessible.

---

[249] http://denisdutton.com/newsweek_coolingworld.pdf

Fracking creates fractures from a wellbore drilled into reservoir rock formations. This is the closest we have gotten to a "breakthrough technology," even though it was essentially a 1947 invention. In any case, "fracking" is on the chopping block, with some U.N. member nations either suspending or banning it altogether, as is the regulatory onslaught against coal in general. The industry is slowly being killed by the EPA, even though its latest overreach was stopped by the U.S. Court of Appeals in August 22, 2012, when the agency tried to regulate coal-fired power emissions across state lines.[250]

Some problems do exist with fracking, however. These relate to local citizens in and around the areas where engineers must move materials and work. For example, around Appalachian, New York, many farmers that once pushed for development and selling rights later complained that the practice was hurting their farms. Some farms close to the action actually did suffer some damage from fracking, which apparently wasn't explained beforehand as a possibility.

Other side issues include: Constant lines of very heavy equipment traveling long distances over mere two-lane highways and roads already heavily traveled. Much of the movement occurs at night and is very noisy for areas with homes close to the road. Some roads, not built to withstand the pummeling, have too many potholes and cracks. In a few instances, drilling vehicles have broken down and dumped liquid chemicals or waste-water into roadside creeks.

These are legitimate issues that *should* be addressed and are probably resolvable.

But experts can't resolve valid issues like these if Energy Secretary Steven Chu is going to dump millions of "stimulus" dollars and bad loans to "green energy" schemes. Columnist Victor Davis Hanson points to a revealing comment that Chu made prior to his post as Energy Secretary—that he would like to see U.S. gas prices reach European levels!

---

[250]

http://www.tulsaworld.com/business/article.aspx?subjectid=46&articleid=20120826_46_E4_CUTLIN260954

Well, of course: That would reflect the administration's goal of egalitarianism, wouldn't it?

Obama's "Crackdown" on Oil Investors

Meanwhile, on April 17, 2012, the Obama administration called for "a crackdown on oil speculators," with a proposal to deter so-called market manipulation. The administration asked Congress to fund yet another war on oil investment with $52 million in taxpayer dollars—funds that could have gone into producing more oil!

Susan Crabtree, a reporter for the *Washington Times*[251] cited Joe Pounder, a Republican National Committee spokesman, who responded to the announcement: "Barack Obama must believe the American people can be fooled into thinking he actually has an energy policy."

But the truth is, between propagandizing and disinformation, Americans have been fooled into believing that America—and the world, for that matter—are out of fossil fuel resources. They believe that skyrocketing prices for oil and gas—regardless of end-use by consumers—are a natural consequence of a global "energy crisis" and "global warming." They are conditioned to suspect technologies that would increase production and reduce prices, as being a threat to their health, directly or indirectly.

"Today our education system is promoting all things 'renewable'," says John Droz, North Carolina physicist. "So-called science teachers have kids going door-to-door in their neighborhoods getting people to sign petitions for renewable energy, more recycling laws, bans on nuclear power, and 'going green'. As for the basics of science and the scientific method, well, those are on the back burner."

What about "Renewable" Energy?

Some ask: "What's the matter with renewable energy?"

---

[251] http://www.washingtontimes.com/news/2012/ apr/17/obama-wants-52m-crack-down-oil-speculation/

What's the matter is, that the over-emphasis on "renewability" is regressive, not innovative, and never a permanent fix. "This 'Band-Aid' thinking," says Dr. Droz, "has unfortunately become embedded into our thinking…. America's defenses are not just under attack, they have been breached—in the least expected way." Droz explains further:

> So-called "renewable" energy is completely devoid of a scientific basis. We have been so successfully indoctrinated that we now believe that widespread adaptation of a fifteenth century technology (such as wind energy) is actually necessary and progressive! Even wind-energy's promoters acknowledge its limitations (cost, reliability, transmission, etc.), but their answer is always the same: spend more money on it, even if it's outdated.
>
> Every billion dollars the U.S. spends on wind energy development not only increases our debt, but causes more money to be borrowed from China, of all places. Our money and effort goes down a rat hole, because it is not a comprehensive answer to a problem that cries out for real action, and the effect is putting the brakes on innovation.

Windy Propositions

Texas icon T. Boone Pickens was among the first big-name advocates of wind energy—a move that was lauded by the alternative energy and "green" cartel, here and at the United Nations. He had to revise his thinking in the wake of reality.

According to Wikipedia, and confirmed in numerous news outlets, in June 2007 Pickens announced the intention to build the world's largest wind farm by installing large wind turbines in parts of four Texas Panhandle counties. The project was supposed to produce up to four gigawatts of electricity. Pickens' "Mesa Power LP" would undertake the construction. If completed, he said, the farm would generate more than five times the 735 megawatts produced at the largest such farm near Abilene, Texas.

On August 16, 2007, Pickens' Mesa Power announced that it had filed documents with the state of Texas to add four gigawatts of electricity to the state grid. The filing with the Electric Reliability

Council of Texas (ERCOT) projected that the project would be completed in 2011 and would include up to 2,700 turbines on up to 200,000 acres.

"We are now meeting with Panhandle landowners and negotiating wind lease and easement agreements," said Pickens. "We are excited at how quickly the pieces are falling into place." He called the new venture the Pickens Plan.

By July 17, 2009, the *Wall Street Journal* was reporting that Pickens had postponed plans to build his Texas wind farm. He said the project was stopped partly because existing transmission line capacity wasn't available. Consequently, Pickens couldn't obtain financing. But, the *New York Times* reported the same day that Pickens was still committed to purchasing 667 turbines and developing wind projects.

On December 15, 2010, Nathanael Baker wrote[252] that Pickens had scrapped plans for wind farms and would instead focus exclusively on natural gas. MSNBC reported that "Pickens said low natural gas prices have made utility companies view wind power as too expensive."

Now that natural gas exploitation is being crushed by the environmental movement, too, Mr. Pickens is probably not a happy man—and certainly not "excited" about how "the pieces are falling into place."

That point aside, Pickens should have picked better experts to advise him before he started hyping his expectations from wind technology.

According to a long list of experts, wind turbines require fossil fuels. Paul Driessen, author of *Eco-Imperialism: Green Power, Black Death* (2010), and senior policy advisor to the Committee for a Constructive Tomorrow, wrote a critical piece that appeared June 7, 2012, in the *Washington Times*[253]. It was picked up in other publications as well. He noted that "hydrocarbon-fired backup generators must run constantly, to avoid brownouts, blackouts and

---

[252] http://en.wikipedia.org/wiki/T._Boone_Pickens

[253] http://www.washingtontimes.com/news/2012/jun/6/wind-down-wind-subsidies/

grid destabilization owing to constant surges and fall-offs in electricity to the grid." Driessen explains further:

> Turbines average only 30 percent of their "rated capacity," and less than 5 percent on the hottest and coldest days, when electricity is needed most. ... Despite tens of billions in subsidies, wind turbines still generate less than 3 percent of U.S. electricity. Thankfully, conventional sources keep our country running—and America still has centuries of hydrocarbon resources, if only our government would make them available.

In the article, he cites a laundry list of down-sides associated with power from wind turbines, even if you assume nonstop backup generators. On the health front, says Driessen, "[a]udible and inaudible turbine noise causes fatigue, headaches, dizziness, irritability, sleep problems and vibro-acoustic effects on people's hearts and lungs."

According to both Droz and Driessen, some wind turbines, apparently, are even drawing electricity *from existing power grids*, to keep blades turning when the wind is not blowing so as to reduce the strain on turbine gears, as well as to prevent icing during periods of winter calm, wrote Driessen in another article for the Canada Free Press.

But the most important fact is that even at peak performance, in locations like the Texas Panhandle, where presumably weather conditions are more favorable to wind power, wind turbines don't generate enough energy to meet our needs or pay for themselves.

As for the irresponsible endorsement of wind power by U.N. climate change and environmental hawks, they would be very dead hawks anywhere near a wind farm. Nearly a *half a million* flying critters on the U.N.'s "endangered" and "protected" lists are killed annually by U.S. wind turbines.

Thankfully, opposition is growing to continued funding of this ill-conceived idea, which got a jump-start not only from Mr. Pickens in Texas, but from aggressive recruiting of well-connected party leaders and political operatives by the American Wind Energy

Association—under the cover of disappearing fossil fuels and global warming alarmism.

Unsurprisingly, many schools nevertheless have availed themselves of the organization's teachers' guide[254].

Thus, the U.N. and its fellow travelers still stand by discredited wind technology that Driessen labels, quite aptly, a "racket."

Our Love-Hate Relationship with Environmentalism

DeWeese gives this hilarious, but priceless, characterization of the American psyche:

> The real political parties in America are the NIMBYs (Not In My Back Yard) and the BANANAs (Build Absolutely Nothing Anywhere Near Anything).... They want to build their homes in rural areas with beautiful vistas, yet complain when someone else wants to do the same thing. They argue that a neighbor's new home has blocked their "viewshed," never considering that their home used to be someone else's viewshed, or open space.
>
> Americans support programs to lock away land to keep wilderness pristine, free of human development, power lines and cell towers. Yet they want to use their cell phones and computers wherever they go. They want three car garages to house the family van, the daughter's little bug and the husband's sports car; but don't blight the landscape with filling stations, refineries or power plants.
>
> [In short,] there's no place in our pretty, clean, politically correct, well-ordered world for industry to make the things we need, yet when all of our toys don't work, Americans are outraged....

~

---

[254] http://www.ocgi.okstate.edu/owpi/EducOutreach/ Documents/AWEATeachersGuide.pdf

Chapter 9
THE FAMILY VALUES GAME

...the general public wanders around in [art] museums trying to make sense of a pile of coat hangers (or worse), without daring to call it nonsense.

Our social air is polluted far more from the rotting refuse of human values than it is from car emissions. -- *Alexandra York, president of* **American Renaissance for the 21st Century (ART***), from her book,* **From the Fountainhead to the Future***, 2000*

"Family values," like "Western Culture" has become a catch-phrase among conservatives and liberals alike. The difference is that liberals (especially the large, far-left faction) want to break up the family, while social conservatives and traditionalists want to "save" it—or, rather, what remains of it.

Values are what give a family cohesiveness, of course, but what does that mean? Values go beyond "morals." Families require shared experiences outside of food, shelter and an occasional trip to the beach for entertainment. If that's all a family's got, it soon will devolve into a collection of people who happen to live under the same roof.

"Family," "social issues" and "culture," of course, are inextricably linked. The Left knows this—as did Marx, Lenin, Stalin and all their latter-day, respective "progressive" disciples (see chapter 7). This is why the newer generations of socialist leaders simultaneously go after all three, with special focus on education and justice systems.

This chapter covers threats to the *family*, *Western culture*, and *religious/philosophical ideals*, with special attention give to *role models and entertainment*. Obviously, the government, the schools and media have a profound effect upon all these.

The Left's recent gambits to redefine families and marriage, and to expand "gender identities," are only the latest in a long string of attacks on the nuclear family unit. The purpose, as always, is to shift loyalties away from relatives and place more power in the hands of the State. To accomplish that, emotional bonds to loved ones must be loosened, the authority of parents undermined, and family cohesion weakened.

We have come a long way from the days when the daily ritual of every school child included pledging allegiance to the flag, reciting the Lord's Prayer and/or reading a biblical verse of the day. Such was par for the course as late as the mid-1960s, even at average public schools in liberal enclaves like Washington, D.C. In those days, sexual activity was still equated with love and romance; and all homosexuals wanted was simply to be left alone.

Today, every person, from the senior citizen to the youngest school child (now beginning at age 3 or less) is under intense pressure to abandon "bourgeois" concepts about what is considered "fine culture," "talent," "music," and "morality."

Schools, the media, clothing designers, child "protection" agencies and even some churches—all these have long been inoculating Americans with a "value-neutral" message: the message of "politically reliability," or political correctness, if you prefer. But, it wasn't until fairly recently that the tactics associated with these efforts turned downright vicious.

Merchants of Violence, Degeneracy, Score Big Wins

In 2005, then-Governor Arnold Schwarzenegger of California signed a law introduced that year by California Senator Leland Yee, prohibiting sales (AB 1179) of violent video games to minors without parental consent. Given Schwarzenegger's Hollywood background—usually playing the violent protagonist or antagonist in "Terminator-"style in films—he knew the power of visual entertainment. He was in the right place at the right time. He realized that interactive video games had gone a step beyond the action films in which he starred. He agreed with Lee that the entertainment industry had upped the ante to the point where it was delivering criminality, not just harmless amusement.

An angry video-gaming industry insisted the law would criminalize the sale or rental of interactive entertainment labeled to minors as "Mature" or "Adults Only," and therefore was an unconstitutional infringement of the First and Fourteenth Amendments. Everyone knew, of course, that these ratings usually serve as enticements to children, and that sales staff rarely ask or care about the buyer's age.

Gov. Schwarzenegger, like Sen. Yee, paid attention to the studies showing a connection between violent video games and aggressive behavior in children. They hoped, at minimum, to enforce the video game industry's voluntary ratings review system, established by the Entertainment Software Rating Board.

Although laws similar to Sen. Yee's had been passed in other States, they were always challenged by industry groups, like the Entertainment Software Association (EMA), and defeated in lower courts. So, it wasn't surprising when a lower court also overturned Sen. Yee's law and rebuked Schwarzenegger, ruling that video games were protected speech under the First Amendment, as were other forms of media.

Undeterred, Schwarzenegger took the case to the U.S. Supreme Court in 2009. He was succeeded by a new governor, Jerry Brown, as the case was pending, so it was renamed *Brown v. EMA*.

The landmark case was decided on June 27, 2011. The Supreme Court, in a 7-2 decision, upheld the lower court's decision, again invalidating Sen. Yee's attempt to rein in the violent interactive "entertainment" industry. Some viewed the ruling as a victory for the video game (and entire entertainment) industry, with the same protections as movies, books, and television. But, both concurring and dissenting opinions from the Justices suggested that the issue deserved to be revisited in future case law, considering the disparities between community standards regarding violence, as compared with, say, pornography—not to mention the ever-morphing technology that could now be applied to both.

Either way the decision went, of course, would be of no help to parents battling the ongoing surge of Aurora, Colorado[255]; Tucson, Arizona[256]; and Virginia Tech[257]-style random, mass killings, or the sex-torture abductions of children (described in chapter 5). Politicians have largely distracted the public by focusing their rhetoric on ever-more stringent *rating systems*, which is worthless as a strategy. Every entity from the Federal Trade Commission, the Entertainment Software Rating Board, to household-name federal legislators like Hillary Clinton, Joseph Lieberman, and Evan Bayh, has played this game. Ratings systems are a ruse. As pointed out earlier, marketing experts will tell you "Mature" labels actually boost the sales, and ensure that products are passed along to children..

Pros and Cons of Violent Play-Acting

Of more interest than the passage or failure of the bill is the long list of Amicus ("Friend of the Court") Briefs went into both sides of the Lee/Schwarzenegger violent video game case[258]. We have already discussed Lee's and Schwarzenegger's views. Representative of the EMA side of the case is a recent article by self-described video-game creator, Daniel Greenberg, who chairs the anti-censorship and social issues committee of the International Game Developers Association. He took on the pro side of violent video-games in a column for the *Washington Post*[259]:

"I express myself through the creation of video games, including violent ones…," he wrote. He challenged government bureaucrats to figure out how they were going to assess the "artistic value" of a video game for "a 17-year-old."

---

[255] http://denver.cbslocal.com/2012/07/20/aurora-colorado-mall-shooting-town-center-century-16/
[256] http://en.wikipedia.org/wiki/2011_Tucson_shooting
[257] http://en.wikipedia.org/wiki/Seung-Hui_Cho
[258] http://www.scotusblog.com/case-files/cases/eanf/
[259] http://www.washingtonpost.com/wp-dyn/content/article/2010/10/29/AR2010102905315.html

The term "artistic value," applied to violent video gaming may seem a bit of a stretch, but the remark reflects the industry's marketing and advertising savvy. Notice he did not choose ages such as 10 or 12 or 14, much less 7 or 8. Yet, his gory products will no doubt be passed around among those age groups.

Daniel Greenberg's arguments and justifications concerning the *benefits*—yes, ***benefits***—to children of violent video-gaming are breath-taking:

- ...children can "build original worlds";
- ...they can "cooperate with or compete against friends, acquaintances or strangers";
- ...they can "tell their own stories."
- [Violent videos] "give players meaningful consequences for the choices that they make";
- ... allow for "a truly meaningful moral choice [such as whether] to save [a player's "virtual"] family from death or save thousands of ["virtual"] innocent people—but not both" (as per a game entitled *Fable 2*).
- ..."make-believe violence" can "relieve stress," "release anger," and "help children cope with difficult feelings such as powerlessness and fear of real violence."
- [Violent games] can "actually reduce violent tendencies and...be used as a therapy tool for teens and young adults."

Greenberg points an accusatory finger at former Governor Schwarzenegger. As star of the box office hit, *The Terminator*, wrote Greenberg, "even Schwarzenegger should understand the thrill of a good fake explosion."

What the Research, Testimonies Say.- Unsurprisingly, Daniel Greenberg didn't cite a single study or testimony from the avalanche of contradicting research: for example, the finding that during adolescence there is a general increase in aggression[260]; or that such

---

[260] Lindemann, Harakka, & Keltikangas-Jaervinen, *Journal of Youth and Adolescence,* vol. 26, 339-351, 1997

aggression, combined with the exposure to violent media, tends to "reinforce and increase aggressive cognitions, affects and arousal"; or that the interactive nature of super-realistic games "have a negative effect on the internal state, leading to increased aggression"[261]. Perhaps Greenberg didn't read about the ramifications of this exposure, which are greater during early adolescence than in mid- to-late adolescence, due to the increased amount of physiological arousal during this time period[262].

Then there was the research study, published in the journal *Pediatrics*, and subsequently reported in one of the same publications in which Greenberg's articles have appeared. It brought together three longitudinal studies, one from the U.S. and two from Japan, examining the content of violent video games, how often they are played and citing links to aggressive behavior later in a school year.

The study concluded that children and teens who played violent video games demonstrated increased physical aggression even months afterward. It was a finding particularly significant in Japan, which experiences a generally lessened crime-aggression than in America and is a hugely popular consumer of video games. Yet when it comes to *violent* video games, the outcomes in both countries were the same[263].

Daniel Greenberg and his EMA colleagues clearly take the view that if parents do not have to give approval for minors to play bingo, then children don't need their parents' consent to play video games depicting decapitation, torture or rape.

Ever since 1999's horrific shootings at Columbine High School touched off a wave of copycat rampages nationwide, some young perpetrators have told authorities outright that they got their ideas from a violent video game. There are far too many instances to list, but here are just two: "Teen boys admit to murder of Victoria

---

[261] http://www.personalityresearch.org/papers/kooijmans.html

[262] L. P. Spear, "The adolescent brain and age-related behavioral manifestations," *Neuroscience and Biobehavioral Reviews, vol. 24,* 417-463, 2000.

[263] http://www.washingtonpost.com/wp-dyn/content/article/2008/11/02/AR2008110202392.html

girl,"[264] and "Teens moved from online violence to real-life murder"[265].

When Games Are More Violent Than Challenging.-   James Carmichael, writing for *Slate* (now a publication of the *Washington Post*) on July 15, 2012, discussed[266] the effect his favorite violent video games had on him as a child—something his mother apparently put a stop to "after watching her otherwise cheerful son seethe and curse at *Prince of Persia* [in 1990]." What kept him playing in those days, he said, was the challenge he experienced at the more difficult, advanced levels—the kind "that made you want to bash your controller and head through the television." The more demanding ones like *Battletoads* and *Mega Man*, he wrote, took hours.

Then he found *Max Payne 3*. It was the sort "that makes your loved ones fear for your health and sanity." Mr. Carmichael says the player acts out the part of "a gun-toting lunatic whose shattered life has developed into a series of bloody firefights he doesn't fully understand. ...You survive by murdering gunmen before they can murder you. [But you] don't automatically heal, and it takes just a few shots to ice you. ...After a few hours, you feel the way Max is supposed to feel: hounded, confused, adrenalized."

A Step Too Far.-   Moreover, these "toys" go way beyond early fare like *Dungeons and Dragons* in 1974 (which many parents rightly criticized back then as being the opening salvo in a flurry of prurient entertainment), and even later varieties like the blatantly crime-glorifying *Grand Theft Auto* (1997).

Then along came *Soldier of Fortune* in 2000, to accommodate the personal computer. It was among the first of the super-realistic

---

[264] http://www.cbc.ca/canada/british-columbia/story/2010/10/27/bc-proctor-murder-guilty-pleas.html
[265] http://www.ottawacitizen.com/news/Killers+were+avid+gamers+self+described+nihilistic+atheist/3737201/story.html
[266] http://www.slate.com/articles/technology/gaming/2012/07/max_payne_3_how_a_monstrously_hard_video_game_made_me_a_better_person_.html

interactive violent games, providing each character with 26 "kill zones"—that is, areas on which a "person" can be hit by a bullet.[267]

This game also was among the first to utilize a first-person perspective, making it seem as though the player was actually seeing *through the eyes of* the in-game character. This means the new models were functioning as simulators, such as those used to train military personnel. Among the latest of the enhanced survival-horror genre is *Silent Hill: Downpour*. Most parents haven't got a clue as to how high the malevolence factor has been raised.

Mr. Carmichael says in his article that he stopped playing after *Max Payne 3*—which, remember, in 1990 was still approached from a third-person perspective. He claims the incredible difficulty of the game made him "a better person."

What isn't really clear from his article is whether he was disappointed in subsequent games due to the quality of the narratives, their lack of "challenge," and the (up to that time) built-in capability to "master" extreme difficulty levels—or whether the emotional toll the games took finally got to him. Toward the end of his article he remained insistent that it was all fun: "Bonkers fun." As if his gaming was a substitute for a boxer's punching bag.

Mr. Carmichael's view is noteworthy because, to *him*, the real-life lessons he took away from the games embodied the values of "challenge" and "hard work." Only in passing, does the reader catch a glimpse now and then that maybe he became uneasy about "the hours" he spent playing them—immersed in moral turpitude. Without the boost of a challenge to spur him further, maybe there was just no reason to play.

The Parent's Dilemma

Even if parents don't read specific studies showing harm, or hear admissions from child-players themselves, it is obvious to most adults (like Mr. Carmichael's mother?) that children—particularly more sensitive kids—who get hold of today's deceptively marketed

---

[267] http://www.personalityresearch.org/papers/kooijmans .html

violent video games are at once repulsed and transfixed by the graphic displays they encounter. In the hands of youngsters who then encounter problems at home, in school, or who are egged on by not-so-stable pals, these games can result in real-time tragedy.

Moreover, modern video games are a far cry from the cartoonish caricatures of yesteryear's novelties like *Pac-Man*, *Space Invaders*, and *Shootout* (two cowboys dueling) that were played on Atari setups by the whole family. The new models feature spinal cords being ripped out; rapists stalking and/or sexually mutilating terrified, often nude, girls and women; abductions similar to the real-life ones described in chapter 5; and graphic torture scenarios of every description.

Even two stay-at-home parents with extended family (such as grandparents) at beck and call are no match for today's plethora of "virtual" simulation technologies; much less the enticements of resourceful advertisers and game creators, such as Daniel Greenberg, who seem to take special delight in contributing to the delinquency of minors. The best grown-ups can do is to restrict their children's access to money; and inculcate moral and ethical principles, early and often.

A typical approach for many parents is to keep their kids so busy with structured activities that they have no opportunity to deviate from a pre-selected set of options. *In other words, a parent's best defense is to strip all the joy (and certainly the freedom) out of childhood*, until they have turned kids into detached, isolated beings leading demanding, hectic lives.

Constitutional Ramifications of Brown v. EMA

Obviously, interactive video games did not exist in 1787, or 1887, or even 1987 in the terms we think of today. But the wording of the various state challenges to violent, interactive videos brings up serious Tenth Amendment questions: Does a State of the Union have a right to satisfy the childrearing principles of its own population in areas not specifically addressed in the U.S. Constitution? The Tenth Amendment says it does.

Where, pray tell, is a family supposed to move in order to escape the easy accessibility of violent video games? That, right there, is the crux of the matter, and the reason why the case *Brown v. EMA* is important: A parent—the family—no longer has the support of government or its major institutions, and there is no place to run to that is outside the purview of the radical, "anything goes" agenda.

That alone makes this issue worth "revisiting."

Celebrity "Packaging"

American Idol. America's Top Model. The Apprentice. The Bachelor. Survivor. The Biggest Loser. Ah, now *there's* a double entendre—assuming anyone under 40 knows what that means!

What it means, at least in this context, is that we have met the losers, and they are us!

Record Companies Go Out of Business

It wasn't surprising to learn that household-name recording retailers like Tower Records, Sam Goody, the Wiz and Virgin Megastores started going out of business beginning about 2006. This occurred despite their shift from old-fashioned record albums, to audiotapes, to CDs, to DVDs and finally, the MP3 and iPod. The most obvious reasons, of course, are online retailing and file-sharing, which includes the capability to access just one song, without necessarily, purchasing an entire "album" (or "collection"); and satellite/cable TV channels that play nonstop selections in the genre of one's choice, often without any need for a separate subscription.

A third reason is more muted in the public dialogue. Music creativity is being strangled. So, there's little new in the "popular" genre that actually listeners.

The Artificially Subsidized "Market"

Weekly Standard writer Philip Terzian opined in an article concerning the Public Broadcasting Corporation that. the kind of radio and television he likes—classic jazz and classical music, as well as documentaries on history, literature, and science—were nearly nonexistent on the air, *except on PBS and NPR*, but then he averred that "the market has demonstrated that no private broadcaster would [ever] fill the vacuum.[268]"

Really? What "market" is he talking about?

Terzian is far from alone in his basic complaint—as proved by all those channels (TV and SiriusXM radio) that *do* play the kinds of music he likes. So, it is not clear that the "market" per se has "demonstrated" anything.

However, if Mr. Terzian is correct in his view that the typical fare presented on commercial radio and television is "predominantly...or relentlessly lowbrow" whereas "the kind of elitist fare" he likes is found only on PBS and NPR, then it might be because the "market" for lowbrow entertainment has been ***artificially subsidized***.

Ya think?

Beginning in the 1960s, disc jockeys were lambasted for taking kickbacks from managers and other interested parties to play certain songs and music, to feature the works of particular entertainers, and, finally, to offer only "reliable" genres to the public. (Politically reliable, perhaps?) Stations were often bought and sold with that in mind.

By the 1990s, many people were sick of the nonstop howling and screeching of so-called popular entertainers; the lack of old favorites; and the noisy, crass commercials. They didn't want to set their alarms and wake up to such cacophony.

So, radios started being sold that had an accompanying audiotape feature so one could awake to a favorite tape, commercial-free. As digital came along, Sirius and XM satellite providers added the capability to access one's favorite genre 24/7, even in their car. No more station fade-out problems on the road or local jabber when traveling through an unfamiliar part of the country.

---

[268] http://www.npr.org/2011/03/10/134433836/weekly-standard-npr-and-pbs-need-welfare-reform

The problem was that one didn't get any weather, traffic updates or news that way. Thus, local radio stations stayed in business by default.

Mr. Terzian insisted, that PBS and NPR, however, should go private, if for no other reason than to "end the perpetual tension…between taxpayer funds and public accountability [and] exempt them from political pressure and interference" so they could air whatever they wanted. He assumed that "marginal markets would succumb [without government subsidies]," and was unhappy that this was so. But he never stopped to think, apparently, that the trash assaulting his ears might not represent "the market" so much as a planned effort to lower the standards of the culture.

Not everyone, of course, can be one-man or one-woman Annie B. Casey Foundation or a Pew Charitable Trust. But conservatives of all stripes—CCCTPs—are missing an opportunity, again! Instead of dumping so much largesse into Party offices and campaign committees, they could work to raise the level of the culture by serving as benefactors for up-and-coming individuals of real talent. It is not as though there is a dearth of such people, or that media wouldn't air them—providing something was in it for them. If you look closely at the audiences that populate shows like "American Idol" and "Britain's Got Talent," you will notice that the occasional standout, who cannot only carry a tune but blow the competition, such as it is, out of the water (whether they win or not, as most of these shows have their element of politically correct quotas—you will notice that regardless of age, they clearly recognize a singer with "perfect pitch" when they hear it. Recent examples include Scotland's Susan Boyle and Australian tenor Mark Vincent

There are many more like them: Josh Grobin, the female cast of "Celtic Woman," Sarah Brightman, Andrea Boccelli, Jackie Evancho, Michael Bublé, Billy Gilman, the male group "Rolling Thunder." And these are just the relative newcomers. There are hundreds of others—seasoned performers, not just "acts"—from the 1960s who are still raking in audiences: among them, Michael Feinstein, Patti LuPone, David Foster, Tommy Tune, Barbra Streisand (politics notwithstanding) who are still at the top of their game. Others, of course, have passed away or are retired, but that has not kept people from downloading their works on their iPods and MP3s. It has not stopped PBS from successfully forming reunions from old groups.

Conservatives need not complain about bias at CPB and their PBS and NPR components if they are not working to create something better, immune to politics. Conservative ought to be seeking out talent like a football agent scouts for players.

"Presence" Versus "Performances"

Youngsters today are typically taken in by "acts" over "performances." Unschooled in the finer points of culture, they are easy prey for hyped-up rubbish.

This has had an adverse effect on society and founding American values. Families do not, for the most part, attend concerts or listen to musicians and other artists as a family. Again, we see the pattern of shifting loyalties emerging under still another venue.

Adults beyond a certain age cannot (and don't wish to) acclimate themselves to lyrics and sounds that, frankly, make them nervous and agitated. Their youngsters often demonstrate signs of becoming nervous and agitated, too, but being young, they adapt out of a perceived need to "fit in" and be "popular."

Over the past three decades (beginning with the 1970s reject, *The Gong Show*), audiences have seen dozens of mega-hyped "artists"—most of them phony, scripted, talent-challenged, and rude to paying spectators, who are either too unschooled (or maybe too addled) to notice. In an era when even a burger or beer joint carries several large-screen TVs, even a commercial seems to have a hallucinogenic effect on the patrons. Perhaps this is to be expected. How does one ignore ubiquitous large-screen TV monitors?

The outpouring of tears following the drug-induced death of pop icon Michael Jackson brings another dimension to the debate over cultural decline.

Clearly, Michael Jackson was appreciated by countless young people, and no doubt he possessed some degree of talent, had it been channeled, refined and nurtured. However, "talent" today is confused with "presence." Like Britney Spears, what Michael Jackson actually demonstrated was "stage presence." His voice and even his range of dance steps were mediocre—nothing approaching the skill levels of Ben Vereen, the late Bob Fosse or Sammy Davis, Jr.

Spears' voice is similarly challenged, even off-key, requiring an echo chamber and special effects (and a lot of "jiggling") to detract from the fact that her singing borders on downright awful. She has plenty of company—Christina Aguilera comes to mind: another pretty face with minimal talent and an overabundance of promotion.

Understanding any words from most of these pop artists requires closed-captioning. But the lyrics are pretty depressing and uninspiring anyway, so young listeners are more or less conditioned to watching singers sway, bounce round and make grotesque faces into the camera.

"Talent" Versus "Exhibitionism"

A truly superior voice (or proficiency with a musical instrument, for that matter) is distinguished first by its uniqueness. If a musical score no one has heard before is played over the airwaves, the listening audience ought to be able to recognize the composer instantaneously. Stephen Sondheim comes to mind. *That* is uniqueness. This is true of singers as well. Even when the artist in question lacks "perfect pitch" — Maurice Chevalier, Ray Charles and Louis Armstrong were decidedly lacking in the "pitch" department—yet they continue to be instantly recognizable. *All* three could make any song a winner, hands down.

The uniqueness factor holds even if a musical piece is not quite orchestral quality. Take, for example, the late Jack Benny's signature violin spoof ("The Kreutzer Etude"), or today's female prodigy, Máiréad Nesbitt, the Welsh fiddler/dancer/violinist of "Riverdance" and "Celtic Woman" fame, who somehow manages to play her chosen instrument almost flawlessly and perform difficult dance steps at the same time.

Timeless favorites like Bing Crosby, Frank Sinatra, Frankie Avalon, Johnny Mathis, Roy Orbison, Barbra Streisand, Michael Feinstein and even the late Jerry Lee Lewis and Elvis Presley are additional examples of unique *style*, more than quality of voice per se. Each is so memorable that once a person has heard any of them, they recognize the voice whether or not they actually see the person—or even particularly like the singer.

Extraordinary talent, on the other hand, (as opposed to "style") is distinguished by perfect pitch (or "perfect ear" in the case of musical composition). Even toddlers often pick up on it—and there's no explanation, really, as to why. To appeal to mass audiences, however, this perfection usually must be accompanied by an ability to express a piece and "touch" an audience. This aptitude can be honed, but it is usually innate and virtually unteachable to those who don't come by it naturally.

If you watch their performances you will notice something that maybe doesn't "click" right away: None makes much use of hand gestures, or superfluous facial expressions, which is a departure from the norm.

Why? Quite simply, they don't need to. They're that good.

In dance, neither Michael Jackson's "moonwalk" nor Britney Spears' gyrations (based initially on her early gymnastics training) approach the precision and complexity of virtuoso dance artists like the three named earlier, or Michael Flatley, Gwen Verdon, Ginger Rogers, Fred Astaire, Lisa Minnelli, Ann Miller, and the newly inspirational J. R. Martinez (a wounded Iraq War veteran).

Michael Jackson, like Britney Spears, is more properly classified as an exhibitionist—much like the "KISS" group (circa 1972, New York City, recently having revived its act under the moniker "Monster"—which is at least apt). To sell tickets, individuals and groups like these rely on outrageous costuming, crotch-grabbing, mock strip-teases and other shock-jock effects. "Madonna" was of the same mold until someone got hold of her and provided some lessons, at which point she moved on to legitimate theater and did a passable job. Too bad they didn't give her lessons in humility and propriety.

Over the past three decades, what has been marketed to the masses has been primarily "exhibitions," not *performances* in the true sense of the word. Jumpstarted via modern technology—psychedelics, pyrotechnics, etc.—professional handlers and managers discovered they could rake in a fortune by deflecting attention from the fact that their "stars" had little actual talent. The old "mob psychology" factor could be made to drive younger audiences into a frenzy, even when there was nothing of substance there.

Old newsreels show fans of Frank Sinatra, Elvis Presley and the Beatles swooning and screaming with delight—but they *did* listen to the songs. The addle-brained appearance of today's youthful audiences is reminiscent of Woodstock-inspired recreational drugs, which augmented spectators' "entertainment experience."

Thus, the emergence of the term "celebrity packaging": a pejorative, of sorts, coined to describe talentless performers who are almost entirely dependent upon the skills of marketing-managers. These are magnates who gear their human "product" to the "lowest common denominator"—which is to say, to the great untaught masses—and hope the hype, tabloid and otherwise, will sells false goods.

The mainstream media has "bought": nobodies like 50 Cent, Jay-Z, Eminem, Christine Aguilera, stardom based an ability to degrade and offend; or MSNBC host known simply as "Touré," noted recently in a story for *Washington Post* story[269]: "gruesome first-person accounts of selling [drugs], addiction, gangs, guns, the police and prison...."

Touré was describing the genre known as hip-hop, which has served to stereotype blacks in a shockingly negative way. Even the usually ever-so politically correct *Washington Post* published Touré's, allowing him to add: "Hip-hop could have grown into a challenge to the war on drugs but instead accepted [drugs] as a fact of life and told bluesy, or braggadocious, stories about its part in it."

---

[269] http://www.washingtonpost.com/opinions/how-hip-hop-lost-the-war-on-drugs/2012/07/13/gJQAlcsJiW_story.html

Touré's article carefully avoided mentioning that the genre contained little or no actual music, that hip-hop, like "rap," is more like a rhythmic chant—the auditory equivalent of graffiti.

One side-effect of this was to stimulate a rash of compositions incorporating such tiny fragments of musicality that most pieces one hears in malls, and over the radio in the morning, contain as few as six notes. In other words, the selection is nearly flat, or monotone. This has become par for the course throughout post-90s "popular" music.

How popular? It's hard to tell. The tunes aren't "catchy," so nobody hums them; the lyrics aren't decent, memorable or even, in many cases, comprehensible, so sing-alongs are pretty much a "no-go." Yet, obviously hear this stuff coming and going. Is it any wonder they download it to their iPods and MP3 Players? Adults over age 35 can't relate to them—again another good way to separate generational loyalties and create alienation.

Censuring Western—and American—Culture

Most schools today do not teach *any* culture, much less Western culture or uniquely American art and literature. Elementary and secondary school students do not, and have not for a long time, partaken of daily (or even weekly) lessons in music, painting, dance and sculpture. Most know nothing about the "greats" in these areas; thus, there is little common body of cultural knowledge beyond "packaged pulp."

Art: Beyond "Band" and "Finger-Painting"

In looking over vintage yearbooks from the late 1930s-1950s recently, a lot more than something called "band" leaped off the pages. Apparently, entire student bodies (both elementary and high school) in Maryland, Virginia and Indiana, to name a few, would gather in a large room or auditorium on a regular basis to sing staples from Americana as well as British, Scottish and even Stephen Foster mainstays of blacks—in their way, folk songs as well, which defined an era every bit as much as "Old Suzanna" (from Alabama with a banjo on her knee").

More than this, pupils learned to recognize the difference between a Monet and a Renoir painting; there were small violin ensembles and piano recitals that put on display the talents of "the best of best" for a particular year. In some states, students graduated also with a bit of architectural knowledge. They learned the difference between Tudor, Victorian and Georgian-style structure; between ancient Greek and Roman styles. They were taught to recognize Baroque, Renaissance, and Neoclassical designs.

Alexandra York, president of American Renaissance for the Twenty-first Century, headquartered in New York City, is an internationally recognized author and lecturer on the arts. She is also outspoken on the need to revive Western culture, especially art, in the nation's schools, and to make fine arts, in general, an important part of family activities. "Art, in its most uplifting form, can communicate life-affirming ideas to any audience, inspiring them … toward laudable goals."

"It can also do the opposite," York cautions. Totalitarian societies—including "left-wing advocates in America [who] have *always* understood the persuasive power of art and used it to promulgate their agendas and ... intimidate their opponents…."

A Case for New Philanthropy.- In her poignant anthology, *From the Fountainhead to the Future*, Alexandra York recaps a delightful story from a 1997 speech she gave at Hillsdale College, entitled "The Fourth 'R' in Education." She describes "a barefoot woman walking along the beach…picking up star fish that had been washed ashore by the tide, and one by one, throwing them back into the sea…. Intrigued, [a man who was watching this] scrambled down from the bank of a cliff and [asked her what she was doing]."

"I'm saving star fish," she answered, gently tossing another into the water.

The man let his eyes drift over the … shoreline in wonder. "But," he stammered, "there are *thousands* of starfish stranded on this beach. You can't save them all."

"I know," smiled the woman. …"But I'm saving *this* one. And *this* one. And *this* one."

No one individual can hope to influence, or mentor, every child, but they can mentor one, or maybe a handful.

The Prodigies Among Us.- One never knows where genius is going to crop up. Take Jay Greenberg, the 12-year-old who composes entire symphonies in his head. CBS' *60 Minutes* presented him to its audience in 2009.

Jay's works are not just *any* symphonies: "We are talking about a prodigy [on a] level of the greatest prodigies in history…," says Sam Zyman, a composer. "I am talking about the likes of Mozart, and Mendelssohn, and Saint-Sans."

But how many youngsters—or adults, for that matter—can identify either the composers or the pieces from any of those cited above by Zyman?

Zyman teaches music theory to Jay at the Juilliard School in New York City, where he's been teaching for 18 years. He never expected what he found in "Bluejay":

"This is an absolute fact," he told *60 Minutes* correspondent Scott Pelley in an interview. "This is objective. This is not a subjective opinion. Jay could be sitting here, and he could be composing right now. He could finish a piano sonata before our eyes in probably 25 minutes. And it would be a great piece."

For those who didn't catch the *60 Minutes* segment, Rebecca Leung wrote about it in an online journal article: "Jay wrote a piece, "The Storm," in just a few hours. It was commissioned by the New Haven Symphony in Connecticut. When the last note sailed into the night, Jay navigated an unfamiliar stage, and then took a bow."

Jay Greenberg (nicknamed "Bluejay") is studying at New York's renowned Juilliard School. Some say he is the greatest talent to come along in 200 years. The 14-minute video[270] from *60 Minutes* is still making the rounds on the Internet.

---

[270] "*BlueJay*: The Mind of a Child Prodigy," 60 Minutes, http://www.twylah.com/glosjazz/tweets/38326781824073728

This young boy isn't alone. Such standouts are all over the place. There's Benjamin Grosvenor, a classical musician who won BBC's Young Musician of the Year award in 2010 at age 11. And Shuan Hern Lee, the 6-year-old classical pianist. The list goes on, Yet, America's schoolchildren sit in a sea of squalid lyrics and five-note melodies.

How many unknown Mozarts might be among "gang-banger" subculture; how many Michelangelos, Rodins, Denyce Graveses, Carusos—and even comedians, like Bill Cosby, who, by the way, doesn't have to rely on off-color material?

Just air quality entertainment. Nothing else. "If you build it, they will come."

The Religion Game

It's not exactly *Kristallnacht* for Christianity—yet. But it's getting eerily close to something similar.

For those who don't quite recall, *Kristallnacht* refers a "pogrom" (series of coordinated attacks) against Jews throughout Nazi Germany and parts of Austria on November 9 and 10, 1938. Also called "Night of Broken Glass," or *Reichskristallnacht*, the perpetrators were both civilian and paramilitary. German authorities looked on, but declined to intervene—something we have seen here in America vis-à-vis law enforcement and other violent attacks (see chapter 5).

While "special groups" are protected, at least ostensibly, a law enforcement community that focuses its efforts primarily on parking tickets, children's lemonade stands and seat-belt violators, but declines to investigate burglaries and prevent abductions, is a hair's-breadth away from ignoring attacks on out-of-favor congregations and their properties.

There was a pretext for the 1938 *Kristallnacht* attacks, of course—there is always a pretext for violence, and for lack of police response. There is a pretext for the hostility to Christianity, too: its traditional stances on casual sex, promiscuity, child discipline and other matters—all of which meet with the approval of a certain leftist cadre of psychologists and psychiatrists. The reader will recall that these "experts" went public with their ideas in 1947 at the World Federation of Mental Health (see chapters 5 and 6), shortly following the Second World War. They were decidedly anti-Christian, American's largest religious contingent up to that time, and probably today as well.

Some activists, mainly in the self-awareness movement, recanted later, such as Drs. Abraham Maslow and William Coulson (who actually tried to warn people), but it was already too late. The groundwork had been prepared for a de-Christianized America.

Why should non-Christians care?

Non-Christian, and even the non-religious across-the-board, needs to care about this issue because too many of the values and ideals we take for granted, attitudes that undergird the Declaration of Independence, the U.S. Constitution and other documents, including state constitutions, are direct or indirect outgrowths of Christianity. One of our nation's founders, Patrick Henry, put it plainer than anyone: "It can not be emphasized too strongly or too often that this great nation was founded, not by religionists, but by Christians, not on religions, but on the gospel of Jesus Christ!"

Needless to say, this line is not one specifically taught to schoolchildren.

Nevertheless, once America's courts and national leaders start marginalizing Christianity wholesale, on the basis of whatever a few factions don't like, our entire system of individual liberties and protections will be dismantled, one at a time. This is something predicted by John Adams (see chapter 1).

The process has already begun, and is presently accelerating at a fast clip. Whereas Ronald Reagan and the two Bush presidencies always closed their addresses to the nation with "God bless America," we have seen, since 2008, a sitting president who refrains from uttering those words. The three little words, in themselves, may be viewed by cynics as hackneyed and trite; but the 20-year affiliation with of a U.S. President with a "Reverend" Jeremiah

Wright, who made use of a decidedly different three words, "God damn America," is a wake-up call. Mr. Obama made several thousand dollars' worth of contributions over the years to Wright's Trinity United Church.

This is hardly the time for such "lapses" in judgment—in an age of Middle Eastern religious fanaticism. Yet, videotapes recently have surfaced of Mr. Obama openly condemning[271] the Bible, before he became President. As President, he has taken pains on many occasions to validate[272] radicalized Islam, the centerpiece of which is now a threat to our national security.

Case Study I: The Candy Cane Case.- The "Candy Cane Case," or *Morgan v. Swanson (and Plano Independent School District)*, began in 2003. It involved the politically correct censorship of six- and seven year-olds engaging in open Christmas merriment. The outcome in this case hinged on whether elementary schoolchildren have First Amendment rights under the U.S. Constitution—again, an attempted twisting of our constitutional freedoms to advance hostility to Christianity.

In May 2011, the case was heard by all 17 judges on the Fifth Circuit Court of Appeals, sitting *en banc*, a rare occurrence that is usually reserved for cases having national impact.

According to the Liberty Institute, the case involved several students who were discriminated against because their "speech," as it were, was religious in nature. One youngster, Jonathan Morgan, was rebuked for handing out candy cane pens and a bookmark bearing a typical religious Christmas message at his class's "winter party". A little girl was threatened for handing out tickets to a religious play on (horrors!) school property. An entire class of children was prohibited from writing "Merry Christmas" on holiday cards to American troops serving overseas.

Government officials argued that elementary students are too young to have First Amendment rights. Their legal counterpart on behalf of the students was the famous Kenneth W. Starr—best-

---

[271] http://youtu.be/Hi-V_ilJu0w
[272] http://www.youtube.com/watch?v=tCAffMSWSzY& feature=related

known, perhaps, for his investigation of figures associated with the Monica Lewinsky-Paula Jones scandals during the Clinton administration. He is also former U.S. Solicitor General from 1989-93.

Currently, Starr serves as president of Baylor University. But in the "Candy Cane" case he was among two former U.S. Solicitors General who assisted the Liberty Institute on May 23, 2011, in presenting oral arguments before the Fifth Circuit Court of Appeals. Starr stated in his argument: "This is 'cold on the docks' unconstitutional."

In a Liberty Institute video about the case, Judge Starr explained:

> For over a half century, the Supreme Court and other courts have held that schoolchildren have constitutional rights, especially the rights of freedom of speech, freedom of conscience, and that's what's at stake here. And so a ruling to the effect that schoolchildren don't have those rights would really represent, in my view, a very significant departure from settled law, and more than that, it…would give enormous power to schools and school districts in ways that are really incompatible with the spirit of liberty that informs a constitutional republic.

Now get this: The Fifth Circuit Court of Appeals found the school principals *were within their rights in stopping the candy canes*, <u>but</u> also found *restrictions on student speech unconstitutional*. In other words, they hedged their bets and tried to have it both ways.

Why?

More like: Why not?" The judges knew that the principals were already exempt under "qualified immunity," *which protects government officials*."

Where have we seen this before? In chapter 5, "The Justice Game"—in particular, the case of Jaycee Lee Dugard.

So, the Appeals court handed government schools a win, sort of. So, the "Candy Cane" case was appealed to the U.S. Supreme

Court. Continuing the ongoing rotten month for any kind of justice from the High Court, on June 11, 2012, the Justices *denied* Liberty Institute's petition to hear oral arguments in the case, putting the religious freedoms of our nation's 50 million public school students at risk.

Case Study II: Valedictorian Reprimanded for Recognizing Jesus in Speech.- In 2006, Erica Corder, a high school valedictorian at Lewis-Palmer High School in Colorado, was reprimanded, harassed and intimidated by school officials for alluding to Jesus in a 30-second "speech", and told her diploma could be withheld unless she apologized publicly (sounds like the Romans asking Christians to recognize Caesar or face flogging). School officials called her references to Christianity "immature." Most readers probably already know that there's a history behind the characterization of anything "Christian" as "unenlightened" and "immature," implying anti-intellectualism on the part of the believer.

In 2008, her attorneys filed a lawsuit—which was thrown out in federal court. She appealed to the 10th U.S. Circuit Court of Appeals, which also sided against Ms. Corder, citing a standing policy of religious-neutrality. Although she did not submit her speech ahead of time, which might have changed the outcome, it is probably fair to say that if a student had advocated for homosexuality or said something positive about a local mosque, officials would have been hesitant to reprimand them.

The U.S. Supreme Court refused to revive Erica Corder's lawsuit[273].

Case Study III: The Left Casts Lots for Churches They Break.- On Mar 2, 2012, seven breakaway Anglican churches in Virginia lost their final appeal to keep their personal property, including Bibles, office supplies and cash donations. By the vote of an overwhelming majority of parishioners—in the 90-percent range—the churches broke away from the Episcopal Diocese in Virginia in 2006-2007,

---

[273] http://www.huffingtonpost.com/2009/11/30/erica-corder-has-case-aga_n_374030.html

and, by extension, from the Episcopal Church in the United States of America, or (ECUSA). Grievances were long-standing, as the larger ECUSA had been promoting theological politics since the 1970s. Issues surrounding actual ordination of openly homosexual bishops were only the last straw. They knew it wouldn't stop there.

The Falls Church (now the Falls Church Anglican) was located in the city of Falls Church, Virginia, its namesake, and was one of the largest to break ties with the diocese and the national ECUSA in the wake of the consecration of a homosexual (and divorced) priest, Gene Robinson, as Bishop in New Hampshire in 2003. In December 2006, its congregation voted 1,221 to 127 to affiliate instead with the Convocation of Anglicans in North America, or CANA. Thus, the word "Anglican" was affixed to the church's name. The huge congregation was characterized as "dissidents" by the smaller, but more powerful, liberal-left faction. (This scenario begins to sound familiar, doesn't it?)

The breakaway church—located near the Nation's Capital—had been thriving in a locale known for its cynicism toward religion in general and for its left-leaning politics. Obviously, the area's liberal reputation was a bit exaggerated, inasmuch as so many had selected a traditional church.

George Washington is said to have worshipped there; its cemetery was dotted with gravestones dating back to the early 1700s. The church was on the cusp of another expansion project, having purchased several adjacent, run-down properties for development as a school and activities center.

The vote and official break touched off a years-long legal battle, despite initial assurances by Virginia's then-Bishop, Peter Lee, that if some congregations chose to leave the larger body, their disaffiliation would be respected and "an amicable settlement" reached. But, once the votes were counted, and nine parishes actually defected, he reneged and threatened litigation.

Maybe Bishop Lee wrote his threatening letter under pressure—it really didn't sound like him; or maybe he was trying to curry favor with the ECUSA's Presiding Bishop, Katherine Jefferts-Schori (a long-time supporter of ordaining partnered homosexuals). Maybe he was worried about legal action against him personally by ECUSA.

In any case, the ensuing furor over whether the overseeing diocese owned the buildings and contents, or whether the congregations did, led to mega-lawsuits. Some structures on the property had been separately funded by parishioners with monies specifically targeted to expansion projects and other materials, not for general purposes. Very large churches of 2,000 members or more, like the Falls Church Anglican, took the hardest hits—but, then, they had more to lose.

The Falls Church Anglican had their last, standing-room only services on May 13, 2012, before turning the church over to a considerably smaller, sexual-identity-obsessed congregation—a "legitimacy," "politically reliable," congregation.

The Falls Church Anglican filed a writ of appeal with the Virginia Supreme Court on June 1, 2012, but court costs in the intervening years had pretty much depleted their resources (over $22 million). That outcome, of course, is a familiar strategy that liberal-leftists use, and it is not limited to churches.

With the likes of presiding Bishop Katharine Jefferts-Schori sitting in the National Cathedral in Washington, D.C. (she once said she'd rather have the disputed properties become Baptist churches, or even saloons, than continue as sanctuaries for fellow Anglicans), winning the appeal will be, well, miraculous.

Meanwhile, the smaller, liberal group will find it difficult to maintain the large historic church and its expanded properties. Most people following the case expect the "ministry" to devolve into a social club, perhaps selling off the property later.

Mollie Ziegler Hemingway, writing for *The Wall Street Journal* on October 7, 2011, reported that average Sunday attendance (having several services per Sunday) for the now-removed congregation was at least 2,000. The liberal congregation which has taken over the property, on the other hand, reported a firm membership of 178, with an average Sunday attendance of 74—an attendance of less than 4 percent of what its Anglican counterpart typically saw.

Hemingway added in a later online piece, by way of comparison:

> When the Church of the Good Shepherd in Binghamton, [New York], left the Episcopal Church over disagreements about what the Bible says about sexuality, the congregation offered to pay for the building in which it worshiped. In return the Episcopal Church sued to seize the building, then sold it for a fraction of the price to someone who turned it into a mosque.

The writer says that while she was researching the above information for the *Wall Street Journal* article, she "heard other stories about what happens to the buildings that are taken by the Episcopal Church [ECUSA] and its dioceses.... Many are sold or shuttered, unable to keep up with basic maintenance expenses. One was [apparently] leased to a dog kennel."

Maybe it's in better, er, paws. Who knows?

Whether one views the issues surrounding homosexuality as "religious," depraved, or just a huge health risk, it is Christianity that is being blamed for the resistance. That serious Christians also oppose casual sex, another important cause of the Left, seems to seal the link between orthodox Christianity and animosity toward homosexuality. Therefore, the implications for Christianity as anything more than a social club aren't encouraging.

The case above represents only one out of some 1,000 confrontations in the U.S. and Canada over various liberal-left positions. When you add all the other Christian denominations, including Episcopalians, which have splintered over political radicalism, the numbers are staggering.

Case Study IV: "Useful Idiots" Help Sustain Anti-Christian Fervor.- By 2011, anti-Christian forces had become so good at their game that, on May 25 of that year, one the best-known of the radical front-groups, Americans United for Separation of Church and State, managed to locate a couple of "useful idiots," Christa and Danny Schultz, and financed their lawsuit to remove invocations and benedictions from a student commencement exercise in Texas—on the school district's historic 50th anniversary, no less. This action denied the vast majority of parents and students *their* right to a traditional, and Christian, graduating ceremony. The parents in question had two children, only one of whom was graduating at the Medina Valley Independent School District, according to the *San Antonio Express*.

Moreover, a couple having only one child graduating in a school district of over a thousand was allowed to intimidate all the rest into providing a forum for radical extremism[274].

Coming Soon: Arrests for Being "Too Christian"?

Almost weekly, another instance of "Christianity Under Fire" makes news. Everyone, from the youngest child to the senior citizen, is under threat of being deemed "too religious" and placed in violation. Sometimes that means measuring, in inches, what kind of Christmas decoration one can place on a private lawn without "encroaching" upon County property in the street. Other times, it means limits on the number of folks who attend a weekly Bible study group at your house using the excuse of zoning laws.

Taken together, all this portends a frightening picture for 20 years down the road, and certainly was never advocated by the Framers.

The $5 "Pole" Tax: Society's Cure for Sexual Abuse

The Texas Supreme Court has its priorities straight.

In August 2011, the Court determined that something derisively referred to as a "pole" tax—a $5 entrance fee per customer at strip clubs—is constitutional.

This decision came after some two years of wrangling and *outrage* on the part of some 8 million strip-club regulars. (Yes, you

---

[274] http://www.foxnews.com/us/2011/05/28/lawsuit-filed-texas-school-district-stop-prayer-graduation/?test=latestnews

read that right: 8 million.) The case began in 2007, when state legislators passed the Sexually Oriented Business Fee Act.

Legislators intoned that their intentions were, um, pure, inasmuch as the small fee collected would raise some $44 million for—now hear this!—***sexual-assault prevention***[275]! *USA Today* was the first to eagerly seize on the story, followed quickly by *The Wall Street Journal*, *The Washington Times*, and ABC News.

This wasn't the first time the state had tried to cash in on the sex trade. In 2004, a similar small strip club fee sought to donate the proceeds to—***schools***!

Customers apparently resented the implication that strip clubs spur men to commit sex crimes. Strange, then, that prostitutes (which include street walkers, escorts, and call girls, as well as brothel and massage parlor workers) are "disproportionally" subjected to sexual violence and murder[276].

Teenagers might want to consider the statistics when deciding whether to work their way through college by stripping[277]. According to a study involving 130 sex workers in San Francisco, 82 percent had been physically assaulted, 83 percent had been threatened with a weapon and 68 percent raped, all while plying their trade[278]—huge numbers by any measure.

Moreover, in the Texas case, money was basically being collected by government to subsidize the same depravity that kills and debilitates women. Great agenda!

Whatever Happened to Mommy?

The *Washington Post* called it "a sign of the times" when 3-year-old Zoe Rosso was suspended from her elementary pre-school for a month in 2011 because she didn't quite make it to the bathroom in time to avoid an "accident."[279]

---

[275] www.nytimes.com/2011/08/27/us/27texas.html
[276] http://en.wikipedia.org/wiki/Violence_against_prostitutes
[277] http://abcnews.go.com/Business/story?id=4045606&page=1
[278] http://www.prostitutionresearch.com/prostitution_research/000021.html
[279] http://www.pressherald.com/news/nationworld/
three-year-old-suspended-for-preschool-potty-accident_2011-01-31.html#

Betsy Rosso, the child's mother, paid $835 a month to send her child to Claremont Elementary, a Montessori preschool that is part of the Arlington County, Virginia, public school system. She continued to pay that astronomical fee during the child's suspension, in addition to virtually shutting down her business and rushing about trying to find suitable child-care substitutes.

To put the financial outlay alone in perspective, in 1960 the tuition for an entire *year* at a top private school in the Washington, DC Metro area (of which Arlington County is a part) was about $600.

Lost in the debate over small bladders, fairness, school policies and the inevitable teasing by peers once the child returns to preschool—readers can "google" some 13 pages of listings on the story—is that government has essentially replaced Mommy as caretaker and nurturer.

Back when birth control first became a viable alternative for women seeking a life that included more than homemaking and childrearing, theologians, family experts and moralists all worried that the warm-and-fuzzy memories of past generations of children would vanish, and that persons unrelated to the child, would be less sensitive to youngsters in their care because they would lack any real personal and intimate connection with them. This, so the thinking went, would have a deleterious effect on society as a whole as time went on.

It seems that day has arrived. All the government's prattle about "individual differences" dissolves into thin air if every event—down to bathroom breaks—must be codified in policies, programs and rules. The process, having trickled down to the 3-year-old level, does something else, too: It trains the toddler to expect a lifetime of senseless regimentation at the hands of a mindless government bureaucracy.

Just 40 years ago, common wisdom had it that children went to school at age 4, 5 or 6, depending on when *Mommy* determined the child was ready. Today, progressive "experts" have determined that parents stand in the way of child development, and that toddlers should be "socialized" as quickly as possible.

And what of little Zoe, who didn't make it to the bathroom in time...again!! Well, you see, Zoe is a product of government's one-size-fits-all "individualized learning" model—including her bladder. Government says, essentially: *Who cares about Mommy, now stuck with $835-a-month for day care? She **chose** to have that kid, didn't she?*

Such thinking will take a new twist, however, as we move farther into the socialist agenda of government "health" care. At that point, "choice" will be about government's willingness to pay, not a mother's choice to conceive.

Little Zoe's beleaguered mother, of course, doesn't 'get' it. Unaccustomed to a life where mommies wipe runny noses, change yucky diapers, select their children's little friends, push them on swings at the playground, place them on the potty at specific times of day, and sing the 'a,b,c' song till they're blue in the face, she probably considers $835 a bargain in comparison to giving up her business.

As for Zoe, she'll probably make it through this troublesome ordeal. But will she have the warm-and-fuzzy feeling once associated with childhood?

Doubtful.

~

EPILOGUE:
THE "IT" YEAR OF 2012

First, the "It" girl—a concept that means more than mere "perfection." The "It" factor captures that certain "something" one can't quite define, but that redirects the attention from anything else whenever "It" appears.

Professional entertainers and those celebrity-centric people who follow this sort of thing attribute the term to Elinor Glyn, who wrote the magazine article that inspired the *It* film in 1927 starring Clara Bow—although the honors for this particular perception of "It" actually go to Rudyard Kipling.

But no matter. In frenzied succession, there followed a series of "Its": female celebrities, "It" hairdos, "It" fashions, "It" songs, foods, and even exercise regimens. All seemed to define their era, the prevailing mentality, or even an entire generation.

By extension, the "It" phenomenon took on another meaning, as in "This is 'it'!" Whenever "It" appeared, everyone was to understand that "It" was irreplaceable; that "It" would never be—and *could* never be—superseded. So, "It" also took on yet another connotation: "The End," or "The Defining Moment."

In American politics, the "It" moments came with the close of World War II ("happy days" were here again), with the Communist takeover Saigon (the first "war" America ever "lost")—and in 2012, the first time the Republic had ever been thought of as "threatened." The "It" years—the years everything changed, up close and visible.

Since the 1970s, traditionalists and patriots have seen "It" coming, and dreaded that there would come a time when American ideals would not just be ridiculed in the media, but dismantled by the courts. They worried that elections would eventually be manipulated to such a degree that American values and ethics could no longer be sustained. In the year 2012, the crossroads became clear.

But for this author, it happened in a most unexpected way.

The following is a true story:

I was sitting with a neighbor in a café over lunch. It was the week before Christmas, 2011. Though this neighbor had never been a particularly close friend (given our wildly divergent political views), we had lived in the same community for so many years, and even helped each other on out so many occasions, that we were, one could say, on very good terms as long-time acquaintances, if not exactly confidantes.

Many of my other neighbors jokingly called this woman the "resident Commie" behind her back, mostly because she proudly and openly admitted to being a Marxist in the hippie-dippy days of our 1960s youth. She had participated in protests and demonstrations, somehow managing to squeeze them in amongst her college studies and various doctoral degrees.

But on this particular day, she was protesting something altogether different. She confided, to my astonishment, that she was leaving the Washington area—this place where everything is vital and "happening": the museums, the Kennedy Center, the Fireworks over the Capital on the Fourth of July, the plentiful ethnic restaurants, and Capitol Hill. She was headed for fairer fields in the Great Southwest, of all places—home to the same Confederacy and "rednecks" she had often denigrated.

"But why?" I asked, perplexed. "I mean, you just revamped your entire house two years ago!"

Because, she said, "I don't like the turn the lifestyle has taken here." What's more, she saw "no change in sight, regardless of who's elected."

My neighbor was blissfully unaware, apparently, that the District of Columbia and its surrounding bedroom communities exemplified the very lifestyle for which she had once demonstrated, marched and chanted slogans during our coming-of-age years—the only era, we both once thought, that really mattered.

Regardless of our politics (we didn't even know each other then), we imagined ourselves on the cusp. We were first-wave Baby Boomers, born immediately after the War. The "times, they were a-changin'," and lucky us, we were part of "It"! We were the "It Generation," the Ones Who'd Change the World.

The disappointed, graying visage looking at me from across the table came as something of a shock. Instead of being a smug representative of our "It" generation—her side had "won," after all—there was only "Me."

Despite her multiple Ph.D.'s in cutting-edge disciplines such as women's studies, political "science" and environmentalism, in my neighbor's mind, the "Its" had accomplished next to nothing, leaving the "Me Generation" in charge.

Like most young people our age, I was never part of the "It" crowd, having stupidly declared a major in a financially responsible (if not particularly emotionally satisfying) career. I'd looked around for (and gratefully found) Mr. Right, rewarded my parents with respectable, if not exactly stellar, grades, and "ate my peas" (to use a quip from President Obama).

So, I was mightily disturbed to hear that now, nearing retirement age, anybody at all was actually in charge, much less this "Me Generation."

"It" was all very confusing... When did "It" turn into "Me"?

Was it merely "all so simple then," as per the song from the tear-jerker film, *The Way We Were*, starring Barbra Streisand and Robert Redford?

Well, from the way my neighbor was now shaking her gray locks, things certainly hadn't turned out as expected.

"Too many rules...," she complained. "And surveillance cameras—can you believe it, @#$% surveillance EVERYWHERE?" In cathartic-like fashion, she elaborated:

... Can't even take your dog for a romp in the woods without some @#$% lazy pig snooping around making sure you have a baggie clipped to your belt! And no trash cans! All these taxes, and not a single @#$% garbage bin to dump your baggie full of droppings! Do they really think people want to walk for an hour in the great, *green* outdoors with a bag full of p_ _p in their hands? And speaking of TAXES! For what? The lights go out every time we have a little *rain*! In the Capital of the Nation, for God's sakes! I mean, this isn't 1950! Aren't we due a few upgrades for all this money we're shelling out? And my prescriptions...."

By now my neighbor's voice had reached enough pitch to draw attention:

"Do you believe," she continued, "that just two weeks after being hospitalized for a hysterectomy, my pharmacy gets grief from the frigging government over a two-bit bottle of pain medication! I mean, you'd think I was asking for *crack*, when all I wanted was a refill that my doctor had already approved!"

I smiled. In commiseration...among other things....

As my neighbor carried on with her laundry list of grievances, my mind wandered: For some reason, I fancied how she might have looked as a 10-year-old, riding a bike and thrilling to the feel of the wind blowing through her hair. I imagined her frolicking into the school building in the morning, flagging down a friend in the hallway—no gauntlet of metal detectors and pat-downs standing in her way. No concerns that some monster would jump out of nowhere and start shooting.

I imagined her laughter and delight as she and her siblings lighted "sparklers" on the Fourth of July. She might have caught me smiling, but it was not at her rant. Rather, it was at the image of her enjoying buying a gooey ice-cream sandwich from a machine at the local theater on a Saturday afternoon, with no notion of some entity called the "food police." Or as a teenager, with a bunch of other kids at Tops Drive-in, ordering a burger—and the best, thickest milkshake in town.

I pictured her...or maybe I was picturing *us*—or maybe the little girl in my mind's eye was...*me*...?

The 1960s Boomers. The "Me Generation."

Whatever became of those of us who were hopelessly...well, "nerdy" in today's lingo? Never "brave" enough, or "popular" enough, or self-serving enough to qualify for the "It" crowd. All *those* "Me's" who didn't have the leisure (much less the parental support) to demonstrate against anything! We didn't know it then, but *We* were still in the majority—on our way to independence, self-sufficiency and self-reliance. Unfortunately, press accounts of the 60s pretended otherwise, so we had no idea. "Changes ... they were a-comin'," the pundits said. And the world would belong to the counterculture radicals. It would be the "It" kids—like my now-grown neighbor—the "radicals" and the "counterculture" fighting against the Establishment—who would rule America.

Yet, somehow "We, the People" had found each other and reconnected, in cities all around the country via the Internet. We may not have been actual classmates, but we had similar stories, and deep down each of us knew an "It" day is a-comin'.

And now, apparently, so did my left-leaning neighbor.

So, she had decided to run, to run away—down to "Dixie," of all places.

I wondered if she realized that the great liberal activist folk singer we all loved, Joan Baez—even with her astonishing voice and range—today would never make it past the stage door with her signature piece, "The Night They Drove Old Dixie Down." The word "Dixie," in any context, is so politically incorrect that it cannot be uttered in public. Like the old Christmas standby, "I Saw Mommy Kissing Santa Claus," Baez's "Dixie" song is a relic of the past, when terms like "husband," "wife" and "fiancé" were not referred to as "partners" in TV ads.

What a difference a few years makes! I mused.

My neighbor, unfortunately, will not escape the rules she helped precipitate—and now despises—in the Great Southwest. So, who, will stand as the "resisters" now? Which side will throw in the towel—or maybe throw down the gauntlet? "It" was kind of hard to say.

The world's billionaires and the "mainstream" media work long and hard to narrow America's choice of candidates, be it national, state or local races—and no matter who, technically, sits atop the heap with the most endorsements from average Americans. Yet, both the media and the political parties tell us, over and over, that "every vote counts." Most people think it doesn't.

Unless.

What if "We, the People" did the unexpected? What if a candidate played the game and tricked the pollsters? Polls, after all, are mostly extrapolations from a sampling of a few hundred individuals. The media pays attention to them? Should we?

With a start, my attention returned to my grumbling neighbor. Just how "radical" was she? Would someone like her—a member of the "It" 60s-counterculture—be a help or a hindrance now?

Maybe my neighbor's frame of mind was merely signaling a "fight or flight" response—like before the Nazis invaded Poland in the 1930s, or before the tanks rolled into Hungary in the 50s, or ahead of the Rwandan genocide in the 1990s... Maybe she'd go to the polls at election time and vote the way she always had—Left.

In any case, my neighbor's angst made me think: Maybe this was really "It"!

~

ACKNOWLEDGMENTS

Dr. Jane M. Orient, executive director of the Association of American Physicians and Surgeons; and Chip Mellor, president and general counsel of the Institute for Justice, brought much-needed lucidity to certain elements of Barack Obama's health care reform package.

Judiciary Committee Chairman Lamar Smith showed a side of national security that pretty much neutralizes the whole Patriot Act. Andrew "Andy" Ramirez, founder and president of the Law Enforcement Officers Advocates Council (LEOAC), was a tremendous help in understanding issues surrounding our border with Mexico, and added to the sorry role the "Fast and Furious" scandal has played in national security.

Michael Coffman, president of Environmental Perspectives, Inc., and Michael Shaw, Freedom Advocates, are simply the "best of the best" when it comes to explaining property rights and complex environmental issues.

Columnists Joseph Curl and Donald Lambro helped take the bureaucrat-ese out of complex budget issues, and Dr. Milton Wolf (Barack Obama's cousin) penned some exquisite pieces on how government encroachment occurs.

A word of thanks also goes to Paul Driessen and John Droz for their insights on wind energy.

Finally, last but certainly not least, it is my privilege to acknowledge my proofreader, Joan Battey, my long-suffering publisher, Jon Batson, and publicist and cover artist, Eileen Batson.

~

About the author...

Beverly Eakman is the author of six other books which began with education issues (she taught for 8 years). She left teaching to become a technical writer with the space program. As editor-in-chief of NASA's newspaper in the 1970s, she penned the technical piece, "David the Bubble Boy," which was turned into a motion picture.

Mrs. Eakman left technical writing when she was tapped for a position as a speechwriter. She spent some 13 years in top posts as writer for the Director of Voice of America, for the late Chairman of the Bicentennial Commission of the U.S. Constitution, and for various officials at the U.S. Dept. of Justice.

Mrs. Eakman was the first to expose federal and state complicity in collecting psychological information on children and their parents under the cover of academic testing and placing it in non-secure, cross-matchable databanks—an activity eventually acknowledged as "data-mining" after 9/11. By 1998, she was on the lecture circuit explaining the particulars of "predictive psychology" and tracking technology. Mrs. Eakman's subsequent research took her into the realm of political strategy. She has become an expert on countering professional agitation techniques and "perception management."

Based in Washington, D.C., Mrs. Eakman is a veteran of some 750 radio and television talk shows. She has served as Executive Director of the National Education Consortium, a think-tank specializing in education law. She has been called to testify on education panels against child drugging for misbehavior, including preparing the legal case that resulted in a surprise win for the plaintive. It was written up in *Chronicles Magazine* in a piece entitled "Uncle Sam's Classroom."
Website: BeverlyE.com
To schedule media interviews
E-Mail: bkeakman@gmail.com

Also by B. K. Eakman

A Common Sense Platform for the 21st Century
Midnight Whistler Publishers

How To Counter Group Manipulation Tactics
The Techniques of Unethical Consensus-Building Unmasked
(Seminar Workbook)
Midnight Whistler Publishers

WALKING TARGETS:
How Our **Psychologized Classrooms are Producing a Nation of Sitting Ducks**
Midnight Whistler Publishers

Cloning of the American Mind: Eradicating Morality Through Education,
Huntington House Publishers
(limited copies available through Midnight Whistler)

Educating for the New World Order
Huntington House Publishers
(limited copies available through Midnight Whistler)

Microchipped: How the Education Establishment Took Us Beyond Big Brother
Halcyon House Publishers

These books can be ordered through Amazon, at Barnes & Noble online bookstores, and by special order at most specialty and independent bookstores.

For bulk orders or special requests, contact the publisher:

http://www.midnightwhistler.com
info@midnightwhistler.com

About the author…

Beverly Eakman is the author of six other books which began with education issues (she taught for 8 years). She left teaching to become a technical writer with the space program. As editor-in-chief of NASA's newspaper in the 1970s, she penned the technical piece, "David the Bubble Boy," which was turned into a motion picture.

Mrs. Eakman left technical writing when she was tapped for a position as a speechwriter. She spent some 13 years in top posts as writer for the Director of Voice of America, for the late Chairman of the Bicentennial Commission of the U.S. Constitution, and for various officials at the U.S. Dept. of Justice.

Mrs. Eakman was the first to expose federal and state complicity in collecting psychological information on children and their parents under the cover of academic testing and placing it in non-secure, cross-matchable databanks—an activity eventually acknowledged as "data-mining" after 9/11. By 1998, she was on the lecture circuit explaining the particulars of "predictive psychology" and tracking technology. Mrs. Eakman's subsequent research took her into the realm of political strategy. She has become an expert on countering professional agitation techniques and "perception management."

Based in Washington, D.C., Mrs. Eakman is a veteran of some 750 radio and television talk shows. She has served as Executive Director of the National Education Consortium, a think-tank specializing in education law. She has been called to testify on education panels against child drugging for misbehavior, including preparing the legal case that resulted in a surprise win for the plaintive. It was written up in *Chronicles Magazine* in a piece entitled "Uncle Sam's Classroom."
Website: BeverlyE.com
To schedule media interviews
E-Mail: bkeakman@gmail.com

Also by B. K. Eakman

**A Common Sense Platform
for the 21st Century**
Midnight Whistler Publishers

**How To Counter Group
Manipulation Tactics**
The Techniques of Unethical Consensus-Building Unmasked
(Seminar Workbook)
Midnight Whistler Publishers

WALKING TARGETS:
How Our **Psychologized Classrooms are Producing a
Nation of Sitting Ducks**
Midnight Whistler Publishers

**Cloning of the American Mind:
Eradicating Morality Through Education,**
Huntington House Publishers
(limited copies available through Midnight Whistler)

Educating for the New World Order
Huntington House Publishers
(limited copies available through Midnight Whistler)

**Microchipped:
How the Education Establishment
Took Us Beyond Big Brother**
Halcyon House Publishers

These books can be ordered through Amazon, at Barnes & Noble online bookstores, and by special order at most specialty and independent bookstores.

For bulk orders or special requests, contact the publisher:

http://www.midnightwhistler.com
info@midnightwhistler.com

7794567R00242

Made in the USA
San Bernardino, CA
17 January 2014